FIFTH EDITION

Nutrition Diet Therapy

Self-Instructional Approaches

Peggy S. Stanfield, MS, RD/LD, CNS

Dietetic Resources
Twin Falls, Idaho

Y. H. Hui, PhD

West Sacramento, California

JONES AND BARTLETT PUBLISHERS

Sudbury, Massachusetts

BOSTON   TORONTO   LONDON   SINGAPORE

World Headquarters
Jones and Bartlett Publishers
40 Tall Pine Drive
Sudbury, MA 01776
978-443-5000
info@jbpub.com
www.jbpub.com

Jones and Bartlett Publishers Canada
6339 Ormindale Way
Mississauga, Ontario L5V 1J2
Canada

Jones and Bartlett Publishers
International
Barb House, Barb Mews
London W6 7PA
United Kingdom

Jones and Bartlett's books and products are available through most bookstores and online booksellers. To contact Jones and Bartlett Publishers directly, call 800-832-0034, fax 978-443-8000, or visit our website, www.jbpub.com.

Substantial discounts on bulk quantities of Jones and Bartlett's publications are available to corporations, professional associations, and other qualified organizations. For details and specific discount information, contact the special sales department at Jones and Bartlett via the above contact information or send an email to specialsales@jbpub.com.

The authors, editor, and publisher have made every effort to provide accurate information. However, they are not responsible for errors, omissions, or for any outcomes related to the use of the contents of this book and take no responsibility for the use of the products and procedures described. Treatments and side effects described in this book may not be applicable to all people; likewise, some people may require a dose or experience a side effect that is not described herein. Drugs and medical devices are discussed that may have limited availability controlled by the Food and Drug Administration (FDA) for use only in a research study or clinical trial. Research, clinical practice, and government regulations often change the accepted standard in this field. When consideration is being given to use of any drug in the clinical setting, the health care provider or reader is responsible for determining FDA status of the drug, reading the package insert, and reviewing prescribing information for the most up-to-date recommendations on dose, precautions, and contraindications, and determining the appropriate usage for the product. This is especially important in the case of drugs that are new or seldom used.

Production Credits
Publisher: Kevin Sullivan
Acquisitions Editor: Amy Sibley
Acquisitions Editor: Emily Ekle
Associate Editor: Patricia Donnelly
Editorial Assistant: Rachel Shuster
Senior Production Editor: Tracey Chapman
Marketing Manager: Rebecca Wasley
V.P., Manufacturing and Inventory Control: Therese Connell
Composition: Auburn Associates, Inc.
Cover Design: Timothy Dziewit
Cover Image: © inacio pires/ShutterStock, Inc.
Printing and Binding: Malloy, Inc.
Cover Printing: Malloy, Inc.

Library of Congress Cataloging-in-Publication Data
Stanfield, Peggy.
  Nutrition and diet therapy : self-instructional approaches / Peggy Stanfield, Y.H. Hui.—5th ed.
      p. ; cm.
  Includes bibliographical references and index.
  ISBN-13: 978-0-7637-6137-0 (pbk.)
  ISBN-10: 0-7637-6137-0 (pbk.)
  1. Diet therapy—Programmed instruction. 2. Dietetics—Programmed instruction. I. Hui, Y. H. (Yiu H.) II. Title.
  [DNLM: 1. Nutritional Physiological Phenomena—Programmed Instruction. 2. Diet Therapy—Programmed Instruction. QU 18.2 S785n 2009]
  RM218.S73 2009
  615.8'54—dc22
                                                                                        2008051158

6048
Printed in the United States of America
13 12 11 10 09   10 9 8 7 6 5 4 3 2 1

This fifth edition of Nutrition and Diet Therapy *is dedicated with appreciation to our dear friend and first editor, James Keating, who many years ago started our writing careers. His unfailing support and encouragement enhances our endeavors and his friendship gives us great pleasure.*

Much love to you, Jim.

Peggy and Y. H.

Contents

PART III Nutrition and Diet Therapy for Adults   215

PART IV   Diet Therapy and Childhood Diseases   351

About the Authors

Peggy Stanfield is a Registered Dietitian and Professor Emeritus from the College of Southern Idaho, Twin Falls. She is a Certified Nutrition Specialist, a professional member of the Institute of Food Technology (IFT), and has recently completed a second term as president of Text and Academic Authors (TAA), an organization devoted to advancing quality education materials for students and advocating for authors' rights. Following her retirement from CSI, she taught at the University of Hawaii, Manoa, Honolulu.

While at CSI, she helped develop and implement the nutrition component of the nursing curriculum, taught nutrition theory, and supervised nursing students during their clinical experience in teaching diet therapy to selected patients. She transferred from the Nursing Department into the Allied Health division, and while continuing to teach nursing students also taught students with majors in other health professions.

During the years that she taught at CSI, she wrote *Nutrition and Diet Therapy with Self-Instructional Modules, Introduction to the Health Professions, Mastering Medical Terminology,* and *Essentials of Medical Terminology* (Jones and Bartlett Publishers). These books continue to be revised, and most are in their third and fourth editions.

She is one of the editors in *Food Borne Diseases, vol. 1* (Marcel Dekker, New York, 2000) and has also contributed chapters on food safety, food regulations, and good manufacturing practices in books written or edited by her coauthor, Dr. Y. H. Hui. She remains active in all aspects of nutrition education.

Y. H. Hui received his doctoral degree in nutrition biochemistry from the University of California at Berkeley in 1970.

Dr. Hui taught nutrition and food science at Humboldt State University from 1971 to 1987. Since 1987, he has devoted himself to writing full time, also serving as a publishing consultant. From 1992–1995 he was Editor-in-Chief for the United States Association for Food and Drug Officials.

Dr. Hui has authored or edited more than 30 books in nutrition, food science, health sciences, medicine, and law. In 2000, he published his first book as a publisher; currently, he acts as both an author and publisher. His current areas of interest are: health science, nutrition, food science, food technology, food engineering, and food laws.

Preface

Many thanks to students and instructors for their continued support of our book, *Nutrition and Diet Therapy: Self-Instructional Modules.* Your insight and information have been very helpful to us in preparing this fifth edition. This book has been in print for over 20 years, and it is gratifying to know that it has benefited thousands of students entering the health professions over these years.

Sweeping changes have occurred in the field of nutrition since this book first went to print, and they continue to occur with great rapidity as increasing knowledge of the subject and its effects on our health and longevity are scientifically established. There is no doubt that every new edition will contain even more changes.

Upon suggestions from instructors and reviewers, we have made three changes on the overall format of the book:

1. The title of the book has changed slightly to: *Nutrition and Diet Therapy: Self-Instructional Approaches.*
2. Each module in the book has been changed to a chapter.
3. The suggestion in previous editions at the beginning of each chapter on credits has been eliminated.

The technical contents of the following chapters received major changes:

1. Chapter 1, Introduction to Nutrition, has been completely rewritten to reflect current thinking on Dietary Reference Intakes, MyPyramid, Dietary Guidelines, Food Exchanges, and Food Labeling
2. Chapter 4, Carbohydrates and Fats: Implications for Health
3. Chapter 11, Dietary Supplements
4. Chapter 13, Food Ecology
5. Chapter 14, Overview of Therapeutic Nutrition

New references have been provided for all chapters in the book.

Small or minor—but significant—changes have been made to all other chapters. Appendix F provides the 2007 Food Exchange Lists from the American Dietetic Association and the American Diabetes Association.

We hope that the revised contents will expand your knowledge and make the basics of nutrition and diet therapy a little easier to understand. Please continue to give us feedback; your constructive suggestions enable us to improve each succeeding edition.

Peggy Stanfield
Y. H. Hui

Acknowledgments

We all know how hard it is to prepare the manuscript for a technical book. Actually, the production of a book poses equal difficulty, though the challenges are of a different type. Many people are involved in the production of a book, and we have been fortunate to have had a number of committed people who gave their support and lent their expertise to the finished product. You are the best judge of the quality of their work.

We also thank the students who helped research and compile new information that appears in this edition. We are especially appreciative of the invaluable assistance of Dr. Wai-Kit Nip (Professor Emeritus, University of Hawaii) for his participation in preparing this manuscript.

And last, may we again extend thanks to the students and their instructors for continued use of *Nutrition and Diet Therapy* and valuable feedback through the last four editions. We have tried in this fifth edition to again provide you with the kinds of learning activities and new information that you have asked for, and hope that our mutual relationship continues for another 20 years!!

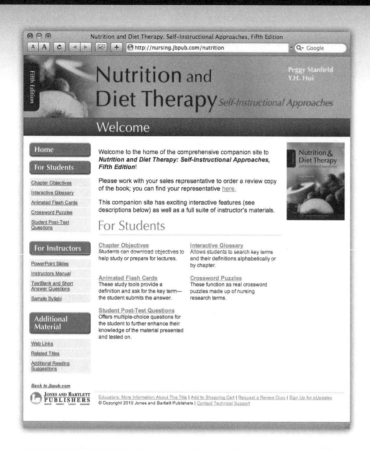

A companion Web site where students and instructors will find complete, current material to support the text!

For Students

Chapter Objectives
Students can download objectives to help study or prepare for lectures.

Interactive Glossary
Allows students to search key terms and definitions alphabetically or by chapter.

Animated Flash Cards
These study tools provide a definition and ask for the key term; the student types in the answer.

Crossword Puzzles
These function as real crossword puzzles made up of nursing research terms.

Student Posttest Questions
Multiple-choice questions for students that further enhance their knowledge of the material.

Additional Material

Web Links
Applicable evidence-based nursing Web resources for easy clicking and linking!

Related Titles
Additional Jones and Bartlett titles in related areas that might be of interest to the student and the instructor.

Additional Reading Suggestions
A list of chapters from other Jones and Bartlett titles in related areas—great for further study or research projects. Instructors can ask their Jones and Bartlett sales rep to package these, or other, chapters with this textbook for required reading on a particular topic.

For Instructors

PowerPoint Slides
Download our slides and use them in your course!

Instructor's Manual
A comprehensive tool for instructors that includes classroom discussion questions, classroom activities, and lecture ideas.

TestBank
A TestBank for instructors to pull questions from and assist in preparing tests for their students. Includes critical-thinking short-answer questions as well.

Sample Syllabi
A handful of sample syllabi for instructors to get new ideas for presenting the information in their classes.

Nutrition Basics and Applications

CHAPTER 1

Introduction to Nutrition

Time for completion
Activities: 1½ hours
Optional examination: ½ hour

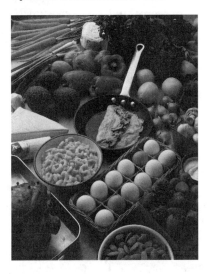

OBJECTIVES

Upon completion of this chapter, the student should be able to do the following:

1. Define major concepts and terms used in nutritional science.
2. Identify guidelines and rationale used for planning and evaluating food intake.
3. Describe some major concerns about the American diet.
4. Use appropriate sources and services to obtain reliable nutrition information.

GLOSSARY

#5 **Adequate diet:** one that provides all the essential nutrients and calories needed to maintain good health and acceptable body weight.

Adequate Intake (AI): an estimate of average requirements when evidence is not available to establish an RDA.

#1 **Calorie (Cal):** unit of energy, often used for the term *kilocalorie* (*see also* kilocalorie). Common usage indicating the release of energy from food.

Culture: the beliefs, arts, and customs that make up a way of life for a group of people.

3

Daily Reference Values (DRVs): a set of values that covers nutrients, such as fat and fiber, that do not appear in the RDA tables. Expressed as % Daily Value (%DV).

Diet: (a) the foods that a person eats most frequently; (b) food considered in terms of its qualities and effects on health; (c) a particular selection of food, usually prescribed to cure a disease or to gain or lose weight.

Dietary Guidelines for Americans: dietary recommendations to promote health and to prevent or delay the onset of chronic diseases.

Dietary Reference Intakes (DRIs): a set of dietary reference values including but not limited Adequate Intake (AI), Estimated Average Requirement (EAR), Recommended Dietary Allowance (RDA), and Tolerable Upper Intake Level (UL) used for planning and assessing diets of individuals and groups.

Energy: capacity to do work; also refers to calories, that is, the "fuel" provided by certain nutrients (carbohydrates, fats, proteins).

Estimated Average Requirement (EAR): intake that meets the estimated nutrient needs of one half of the individuals in a specific group. Used as a basis for developing the RDA.

Food: any substance taken into the body that will help to meet the body's needs for energy, maintenance, and growth.

Good nutritional status: the intake of a balanced diet containing all the essential nutrients to meet the body's requirements for energy, maintenance, and growth.

Gram (g): a unit of weight in the metric system. 1 g = .036 oz. There are 28.385 grams to an ounce. This conversion is usually rounded to 30 g for ease in calculation, or rounded down to 28 g.

Health: the state of complete physical, mental, and social well-being; not merely the absence of disease and infirmity.

Kilocalorie (kcalorie, kcal): technically correct term for unit of energy in nutrition, equal to the amount of heat required to raise the temperature of 1 kg of water 1°C.

Malnutrition: state of impaired health due to undernutrition, overnutrition, an imbalance of nutrients, or the body's inability to utilize the nutrients ingested.

Microgram: a unit of weight in the metric system equal to 1/1,000,000 of a gram.

Milligram: a unit of weight in the metric system equal to 1/1,000 of a gram.

Monitor: to watch over or observe something for a period of time.

National Cholesterol Education Program (NCEP): program designed to educate the public and healthcare providers about the risks of an elevated cholesterol level and methods to lower it.

Nutrient: a chemical substance obtained from food and needed by the body for growth, maintenance, or repair of tissues. Many nutrients are considered essential. The body cannot make them; they must be obtained from food.

Nutrition: the sum of the processes by which food is selected and becomes part of the body.

Nutritional status: state of the body resulting from the intake and use of nutrients.

Optimum nutrition: the state of receiving and utilizing essential nutrients to maintain health and well-being at the highest possible level. It provides a reserve for the body.

Overnutrition: an excessive intake of one or more nutrients, frequently referring to nutrients providing energy (kcalories).

Poor nutritional status: an inadequate intake (or utilization) of nutrients to meet the body's requirements for energy, maintenance, and growth.

Recommended Dietary Allowances (RDAs): levels of nutrients recommended by the Food and Nutrition Board of the National Academy of Sciences for daily consumption by healthy individuals, scaled according to sex and age.

Tolerable Upper Intake Level (UL): maximum intake by an individual that is unlikely to pose risks of adverse health effects in a healthy individual in a specified group. There is no established standard for individuals to consume nutrients at levels above the RDA or AI.

Undernutrition: a deficiency of one or more nutrients, including nutrients providing energy (calories).

BACKGROUND INFORMATION

The subject of nutrition is both exciting and confusing to the beginning student. Nutrition has become a major topic of conversation at places of work, at social gatherings, and in the media. We are living at a time when the focus is on prevention of disease and responsibility for one's own health. The newest trends in health care emphasize the importance of nutrition education.

Throughout history, food and its effects on the body have been studied and written about, but most of the information gathered was based on trial and error. Many superstitions regarding the magical powers and healing capabilities of food also evolved.

The study of nutrition as a science is relatively new, developing only after chemistry and physiology became established disciplines. Its growth begins with the end of World War II. Nutrition science is now a highly regarded discipline. The progressive advances in the science and technology of this discipline offer us hope in controlling our destiny by preventing or delaying the onset of a number of chronic diseases related to nutrition, food, and lifestyle.

Every specialized field has its own language. A beginning student in nutrition needs to comprehend the language used in this discipline and to understand some basic concepts upon which the science is based. The activities in this chapter should assist you in gaining the knowledge and vocabulary necessary to understand the science of nutrition.

ACTIVITY 1:

Dietary Allowances, Eating Guides, and Food Guidance System

The appropriate diet at any stage of life is one that supplies sufficient energy and all the essential nutrients in adequate amounts for health. For more than 50 years, professionals from the government and academics have made recommendations on such basic needs.

For more than two decades there has been increasing concern about the eating patterns of American people. National health policy makers have linked several specific dietary factors to chronic diseases among the population. This connection between diet and disease has, in turn, led to publication of guidelines to promote healthier eating habits. Most of these publications have been issued by relevant units within the following national agencies:

1. U.S. National Academy of Sciences (NAS)
2. U.S. Department of Agriculture
3. U.S. Department of Health and Human Services
4. U.S. National Institute of Health
5. U.S. Surgeon General

According to these agencies, the major chronic diseases in the United States are coronary heart disease, strokes, hypertension, atherosclerosis, some cancers, obesity, and diabetes. Several high-risk factors for these diseases are linked to the American diet. A discussion of these health factors and a proper diet presented in such national publications as *Healthy People 2000*, *American Dietary Guidelines*, and *MyPyramid* will be presented in this chapter. We will first look into the concept of dietary standards in the United States.

DIETARY STANDARDS

There are two basic questions regarding dietary standards: What are the nutrients in food? How much of each nutrient do we need everyday to be healthy? Collectively, this information is the core of the U.S. Dietary Standards. Each country has its own dietary standard, and no two countries have the same standards, for a variety of reasons.

For more than half a century the U.S. National Academy of Sciences (NAS) has been the major scientific arm of the federal government to provide answers to these questions. The NAS in turn depends on one of its institutes, the Institute of Medicine (IOM), to review scientific literature to arrive at the appropriate conclusions. IOM has developed many boards of experts to perform such scientific investigations. One such board is the Food and Nutrition Board (FNB) which is the actual scientific body that develops most of the U.S. dietary standards.

At present the FNB is using the concept of dietary reference standards to define the terms describing the amount of nutrients we consume, such as *recommen-* *dation, requirement, dietary allowances, adequate intake, upper limits, tolerance, estimation, average requirements,* and so on. In general, there are four sets of reference data, collectively called Dietary Reference Intakes or DRIs: Estimated Average Requirement (EAR), Recommended Dietary Allowance (RDA), Adequate Intake (AI), and Tolerable Upper Intake Level (UL). They are defined as follows:

- Estimated Average Requirement (EAR): The intake that meets the estimated nutrient needs of half of the individuals in a specific group. This figure is to be used as the basis for developing the RDA and is to be used by nutrition policy makers in evaluating the adequacy of nutrient intakes of the group and for planning how much the group should consume.

- Recommended Dietary Allowance (RDA): The intake that meets the nutrient needs of almost all of the healthy individuals in a specific age and gender group. The RDA should be used in guiding individuals to achieve adequate nutrient intake aimed at decreasing the risk of chronic disease. It is based on estimating an average requirement plus an increase to account for the variation within a particular group.

- Adequate Intake (AI): When sufficient scientific evidence is not available to estimate an average requirement, Adequate Intakes (AIs) have been set. Individuals should use the AI as a goal for intake where no RDAs exist. The AI is derived through experimental or observational data that show a mean intake that appears to sustain a desired indicator of health, such as calcium retention in bone for most members of a population group. For example, AIs have been set for infants through 1 year of age using the average observed nutrient intake of populations of breastfed infants as the standard. The committee set AIs for calcium, vitamin D, and fluoride.

- Tolerable Upper Intake Level (UL): The maximum intake by an individual that is unlikely to pose risks of adverse health effects in almost all healthy individuals in a specified group. This figure is not intended to be a recommended level of intake, and there is no established benefit for individuals to consume nutrients at levels above the RDA or AI. For most nutrients, this figure refers to total intakes from food, fortified food, and nutrient supplements.

There are nine tables of DRIs that are of interest to this book. They are all issued and distributed by the National Academy Press, the publishing arm of NAS. The data are prepared by the FNB of the NAS. The tables are described below:

Presented inside the front cover of this book:

1. Table F-1: Dietary Reference Intakes (DRIs): Recommended Intakes for Individuals, Vitamins.
2. Table F-2: Dietary Reference Intakes (DRIs): Recommended Intakes for Individuals, Elements.

Accessible at the National Academies of Science Web site (www.nas.edu):

1. Dietary Reference Intakes (DRIs): Tolerable Upper Intake Levels (UL), Vitamins
2. Dietary Reference Intakes (DRIs): Tolerable Upper Intake Levels (UL), Elements
3. Dietary Reference Intakes (DRIs): Estimated Energy Requirements (EER) for Men and Women
4. Dietary Reference Intakes (DRIs): Acceptable Macronutrient Distribution Ranges
5. Dietary Reference Intakes (DRIs): Recommended Intakes for Individuals, Macronutrients
6. Dietary Reference Intakes (DRIs): Additional Macronutrient Recommendations
7. Dietary Reference Intakes (DRIs): Estimated Average Requirements for Groups

Because nutritional requirements differ with age, sex, body size, and physiological state, all data are presented for males and females in different age and weight groups. Nutrition-related health problems such as premature birth, metabolic disorders, infections, chronic diseases, and the use of medications require special dietary and therapeutic measures. The amount of nutrients in each table is determined through scientific research and varies from nutrient to nutrient.

To be valuable from a practical standpoint, the technical information supplied by the dietary standards must be interpreted in terms of a selection of foods to be eaten daily. The RDAs and other standards should be met by consuming a wide variety of acceptable, tasty, and affordable foods and not solely through supplementation or the use of fortified foods. Various basic diet patterns may be devised to serve as guides in food selection.

There are many applications of the DRIs, some of which will be discussed in various chapters in this book.

DIETARY GUIDELINES

The *Dietary Guidelines for Americans* (*Dietary Guidelines*), first published in 1980, provides science-based advice to promote health and to reduce risk for chronic diseases through diet and physical activity. The recommendations contained within the *Dietary Guidelines* are targeted to the general public over 2 years of age who are living in the United States. Because of its focus on health promotion and risk reduction, the *Dietary Guidelines* form the basis of federal food, nutrition education, and information programs.

By law (Public Law 101445, Title III, 7 U.S.C. 5301 et seq.), the *Dietary Guidelines* is reviewed, updated if necessary, and published every 5 years. The content of the *Dietary Guidelines* is a joint effort of the U.S. Department of Health and Human Services (HHS) and the U.S. Department of Agriculture (USDA). Visit www.healthierus.gov/dietaryguidelines. The information in this section has been modified from this document, 2005 edition.

Major causes of morbidity and mortality in the United States are related to poor diet and a sedentary lifestyle. Some specific diseases linked to poor diet and physical inactivity include cardiovascular disease, type 2 diabetes, hypertension, osteoporosis, and certain cancers. Furthermore, poor diet and physical inactivity, resulting in an energy imbalance (more calories consumed than expended), are the most important factors contributing to the increase in overweight and obesity in this country. Combined with physical activity, following a diet that does not provide excess calories according to the recommendations in this document should enhance the health of most individuals.

The intent of the *Dietary Guidelines* is to summarize and synthesize knowledge regarding individual nutrients and food components into recommendations for a pattern of eating that can be adopted by the public. In this publication, key recommendations are grouped under nine interrelated focus areas. It is important to remember that these are integrated messages that should be implemented as a whole. Taken together, they encourage most Americans to eat fewer calories, be more active, and make wiser food choices.

A basic premise of the *Dietary Guidelines* is that nutrient needs should be met primarily through consuming foods. Foods provide an array of nutrients and other compounds that may have beneficial effects on health. In certain cases, fortified foods and dietary supplements may be useful sources of one or more nutrients that otherwise might be consumed in less than recommended amounts. However, dietary supplements, while recommended in some cases, cannot replace a healthful diet.

Key recommendations of the *Dietary Guidelines* are presented below.

Adequate Nutrients Within Calorie Needs

Key recommendations for the general public:

- Consume a variety of nutrient-dense foods and beverages within and among the basic food groups while choosing foods that limit the intake of saturated and trans fats, cholesterol, added sugars, salt, and alcohol.
- Meet recommended intakes within energy needs by adopting a balanced eating pattern, such as the USDA Food Guide or the DASH Eating Plan.

Key recommendations for specific population groups:

- People over age 50—Consume vitamin B_{12} in its crystalline form (i.e., fortified foods or supplements).
- Women of childbearing age who may become pregnant—Eat foods high in heme-iron and/or consume iron-rich plant foods or iron-fortified foods with an enhancer of iron absorption, such as foods rich in vitamin C.

- Women of childbearing age who may become pregnant and those in the first trimester of pregnancy—Consume adequate synthetic folic acid daily (from fortified foods or supplements) in addition to food forms of folate from a varied diet.
- Older adults, people with dark skin, and people exposed to insufficient ultraviolet band radiation (i.e., sunlight)—Consume extra vitamin D from vitamin D-fortified foods and/or supplements.

Weight Management

Key recommendations for the general public:

- To maintain body weight in a healthy range, balance calories from foods and beverages with calories expended.
- To prevent gradual weight gain over time, make small decreases in food and beverage calories and increase physical activity.

Key recommendations for specific population groups:

- Those who need to lose weight—Aim for a slow, steady weight loss by decreasing calorie intake while maintaining an adequate nutrient intake and increasing physical activity.
- Overweight children—Reduce the rate of body weight gain while allowing growth and development. Consult a healthcare provider before placing a child on a weight-reduction diet.
- Pregnant women—Ensure appropriate weight gain as specified by a healthcare provider.
- Breastfeeding women—Moderate weight reduction is safe and does not compromise weight gain of the nursing infant.
- Overweight adults and overweight children with chronic diseases and/or on medication—Consult a healthcare provider about weight loss strategies prior to starting a weight-reduction program to ensure appropriate management of other health conditions.

Physical Activity

Key recommendations for the general public:

- Engage in regular physical activity, and reduce sedentary activities to promote health, psychological well-being, and a healthy body weight.
- To reduce the risk of chronic disease in adulthood, engage in at least 30 minutes of moderate-intensity physical activity, above usual activity, at work or home on most days of the week.
- For most people, greater health benefits can be obtained by engaging in physical activity of more vigorous intensity or longer duration.
- To help manage body weight and prevent gradual, unhealthy body weight gain in adulthood, engage in approximately 60 minutes of moderate- to vigorous-intensity activity on most days of the week while not exceeding caloric intake requirements.
- To sustain weight loss in adulthood, participate in at least 60 to 90 minutes of daily moderate-intensity physical activity while not exceeding caloric intake requirements. Some people may need to consult with a healthcare provider before participating in this level of activity.
- Achieve physical fitness by including cardiovascular conditioning, stretching exercises for flexibility, and resistance exercises or calisthenics for muscle strength and endurance.

Key recommendations for specific population groups:

- Children and adolescents—Engage in at least 60 minutes of physical activity on most, preferably all, days of the week.
- Pregnant women—In the absence of medical or obstetric complications, incorporate 30 minutes or more of moderate-intensity physical activity on most, if not all, days of the week. Avoid activities with a high risk of falling or abdominal trauma.
- Breastfeeding women—Be aware that neither acute nor regular exercise adversely affects the mother's ability to successfully breastfeed.
- Older adults—Participate in regular physical activity to reduce functional declines associated with aging and to achieve the other benefits of physical activity identified for all adults.

Food Groups to Encourage

Key recommendations for the general public:

- Consume a sufficient amount of fruits and vegetables while staying within energy needs. Two c of fruit and 2-½ c of vegetables per day are recommended for a reference 2000-calorie intake, with higher or lower amounts depending on the calorie level.
- Choose a variety of fruits and vegetables each day. In particular, select from all five vegetable subgroups (dark green, orange, legumes, starchy vegetables, and other vegetables) several times a week.
- Consume 3 or more ounce-equivalents of whole-grain products per day, with the rest of the recommended grains coming from enriched or whole-grain products. In general, at least half the grains should come from whole grains.
- Consume 3 c per day of fat-free or low-fat milk or equivalent milk products.

Key recommendations for specific population groups:

- Children and adolescents—Consume whole-grain products often; at least half the grains should be whole grains. Children 2 to 8 years should consume 2 c per day of fat-free or low-fat milk or equivalent milk products. Children 9 years of age and older should consume 3 c per day of fat-free or low-fat milk or equivalent milk products.

Fats

Key recommendations for the general public:

- Consume less than 10% of calories from saturated fatty acids and less than 300 mg/day of cholesterol, and keep consumption of trans-fatty acids as low as possible.
- Keep total fat intake between 20% to 35% of calories, with most fats coming from sources of polyunsaturated and monounsaturated fatty acids, such as fish, nuts, and vegetable oils.
- When selecting and preparing meat, poultry, dry beans, and milk or milk products, make choices that are lean, low fat, or fat free.
- Limit intake of fats and oils high in saturated and/or trans-fatty acids, and choose products low in such fats and oils.

Key recommendations for specific population groups:

- Children and adolescents—Keep total fat intake between 30% to 35% of calories for children 2 to 3 years of age and between 25% to 35% of calories for children and adolescents 4 to 18 years of age, with most fats coming from sources of polyunsaturated and monounsaturated fatty acids, such as fish, nuts, and vegetable oils.

Carbohydrates

Key recommendations for the general public:

- Choose fiber-rich fruits, vegetables, and whole grains often.
- Choose and prepare foods and beverages with little added sugars or caloric sweeteners, such as amounts suggested by the USDA Food Guide and the DASH Eating Plan.
- Reduce the incidence of dental caries by practicing good oral hygiene and consuming sugar- and starch-containing foods and beverages less frequently.

Sodium and Potassium

Key Recommendations for the general public:

- Consume less than 2300 mg (approximately 1 tsp of salt) of sodium per day.
- Choose and prepare foods with little salt. At the same time, consume potassium-rich foods, such as fruits and vegetables.

Key recommendations for specific population groups:

- Individuals with hypertension, blacks, and middle-aged and older adults—Aim to consume no more than 1500 mg of sodium per day, and meet the potassium recommendation (4700 mg/day) with food.

Alcoholic Beverages

Key recommendations for the general public:

- Those who choose to drink alcoholic beverages should do so sensibly and in moderation—defined as the consumption of up to one drink per day for women and up to two drinks per day for men.
- Alcoholic beverages should not be consumed by some individuals, including those who cannot restrict their alcohol intake, women of childbearing age who may become pregnant, pregnant and lactating women, children and adolescents, individuals taking medications that can interact with alcohol, and those with specific medical conditions.
- Alcoholic beverages should be avoided by individuals engaging in activities that require attention, skill, or coordination, such as driving or operating machinery.

Food Safety

Key recommendations for the general public (*also see* Chapter 13):
To avoid microbial food-borne illness:

- Clean hands, food contact surfaces, and fruits and vegetables. Meat and poultry should not be washed or rinsed.
- Separate raw, cooked, and ready-to-eat foods while shopping, preparing, or storing foods.
- Cook foods to a safe temperature to kill micro-organisms.
- Chill (refrigerate) perishable food promptly, and defrost foods properly.
- Avoid raw (unpasteurized) milk or any products made from unpasteurized milk, raw or partially cooked eggs or foods containing raw eggs, raw or undercooked meat and poultry, unpasteurized juices, and raw sprouts.

Key recommendations for specific population groups:

- Infants and young children, pregnant women, older adults, and those who are immunocompromised—Do not eat or drink raw (unpasteurized) milk or any products made from unpasteurized milk, raw or partially cooked eggs or foods containing raw eggs, raw or undercooked meat and poultry, raw or undercooked fish or shellfish, unpasteurized juices, and raw sprouts.
- Pregnant women, older adults, and those who are immunocompromised: Only eat certain deli meats and frankfurters that have been reheated to steaming hot.

FOOD GUIDANCE SYSTEM

The USDA has released the MyPyramid Food Guidance System (www.mypyramid.gov). Along with the new MyPyramid symbol, the system provides many options to help Americans make healthy food choices and to be active every day. Figures 1-1 and 1-2 provide visual presentations of the general goals and food groups or system of MyPyramid. Consult these two figures as you follow the discussion in this section.

The general messages in the MyPyramid symbol are: physical activity, variety, proportionality, moderation, gradual improvement, and personalization. The specific messages are about healthy eating and physical activity, which apply to everyone. MyPyramid helps consumers find the kinds and amounts of foods they should eat each day. The Food Guidance System is the core of MyPyramid.

The 2005 *Dietary Guidelines for Americans* are the basis for federal nutrition policy. The Food Guidance System provides food-based guidance to help implement the recommendations of the *Dietary Guidelines*. The system was based on both the *Dietary Guidelines* and the Dietary Reference Intakes from the National Academy of Sciences, while taking into account current consumption patterns of Americans. The system translates the *Dietary Guidelines* into a total diet that meets nutrient needs from food sources and aims to moderate or limit dietary components often consumed in excess. An important complementary tool to the system is the nutrition data displayed on the labels of food products.

The Food Guidance System provides Web-based interactive and print materials for all citizens: consumers, news media, and professionals. They include the following:

- Food intake patterns identify what and how much food an individual should eat for health. The amounts to eat are based on a person's age, sex, and activity level. These patterns have been published in the 2005 *Dietary Guidelines*.

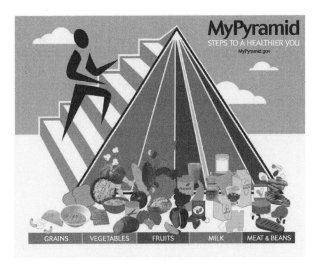

FIGURE 1-2   MyPyramid: The Food Groups
Source: Courtesy of the USDA.

- An education framework explains what changes most Americans need to make in their eating and activity choices, how they can make these changes, and why these changes are important for health.
- A glossary defines key terms used in the Food Guidance System documents.

The education framework provides specific recommendations for making food choices that will improve the quality of an average American diet. These recommendations are interrelated and should be used together. Taken together, they would result in the following changes from a typical diet:

- Increased intake of vitamins, minerals, dietary fiber, and other essential nutrients, especially of those that are often low in typical diets
- Lowered intake of saturated fats, trans fats, and cholesterol, and increased intake of fruits, vegetables, and whole grains to decrease risk for some chronic diseases
- Calorie intake balanced with energy needs to prevent weight gain and/or promote a healthy weight

The recommendations in the framework fall under four overarching themes:

- Variety—Eat foods from all food groups and subgroups.
- Proportionality—Eat more of some foods (fruits, vegetables, whole grains, fat-free or low-fat milk products), and less of others (foods high in saturated or trans fats, added sugars, cholesterol salt, and alcohol).
- Moderation—Choose forms of foods that limit intake of saturated or trans fats, added sugars, cholesterol, salt, and alcohol.
- Activity—Be physically active every day.

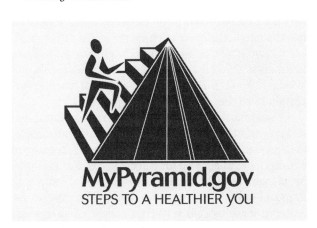

FIGURE 1-1   MyPyramid: Steps to a Healthier You
Source: Courtesy of the USDA.

The framework's recommendations are presented as key concepts for educators. The key concepts are organized by topic area: calories; physical activity; grains; vegetables; fruits; milk, yogurt, and cheese; meat, poultry, fish, dry beans, eggs, and nuts; fats and oils; sugars and sweets; salt; alcohol; and food safety. Under each topic area, information is presented on the following:

- What actions should be taken for a healthy diet
- How these actions can be implemented
- Why this action is important for health (the key benefits)

Food Groups

The core of MyPramid is the Food Guidance System as indicated in Figure 1-2. A brief discussion of the food groups follows.

Calories and Physical Activity

One must balance calorie intake from foods and beverages with calories expended and engage in regular physical activity and reduce sedentary activities.

Grains

The grains group includes all foods made from wheat, rice, oats, cornmeal, barley, such as bread, pasta, oatmeal, breakfast cereals, tortillas, and grits. In general, 1 slice of bread, 1 c of ready-to-eat cereal, or ½ c of cooked rice, pasta, or cooked cereal can be considered as 1 ounce-equivalent from the grains group. At least half of all grains consumed should be whole grains.

Consume 3 or more ounce-equivalents of whole-grain products per day. Since the recommended 3 ounce-equivalents may be difficult for young children to achieve, they should gradually increase the amount of whole grains in their diets. An ounce-equivalent of grains is about 1 slice of bread, 1 c of ready-to-eat cereal flakes, or ½ c of cooked pasta or rice, or cooked cereal.

Vegetables

The vegetable group includes all fresh, frozen, canned, and dried vegetables and vegetable juices. In general, 1 c of raw or cooked vegetables or vegetable juice, or 2 c of raw leafy greens can be considered as 1 c from the vegetable group.

Eat the recommended amounts of vegetables, and choose a variety of vegetables each day. For example, those needing 2000 calories per day need about 2-½ c of vegetables per day. See food intake patterns in the next section for other calorie levels.

Fruits

The fruit group includes all fresh, frozen, canned, and dried fruits and fruit juices. In general, 1 c of fruit or 100% fruit juice, or ½ c of dried fruit, can be considered as 1 c from the fruit group.

Eat recommended amounts of fruit, and choose a variety of fruits each day. For example, people who need 2000 calories per day need 2 c of fruit per day. See food intake patterns in the next section for other calorie levels.

Milk, Yogurt, and Cheese

The milk group includes all fluid milk products and foods made from milk that retain their calcium content, such as yogurt and cheese. Foods made from milk that have little to no calcium, such as cream cheese, cream, and butter, are not part of the group. Most milk group choices should be fat free or low fat. In general, 1 c of milk or yogurt, 1-½ ounces of natural cheese, or 2 ounces of processed cheese can be considered as 1 c from the milk group.

Consume 3 c of fat-free or low-fat (1%) milk, or an equivalent amount of yogurt or cheese, per day. Children 2 to 8 years old should consume 2 c of fat-free or low-fat milk, or an equivalent amount of yogurt or cheese, per day. Consume other calcium-rich foods if milk and milk products are not consumed.

Meat, Poultry, Fish, Dry Beans, Eggs, and Nuts

For the meat and beans group in general, 1 ounce of lean meat, poultry, or fish; 1 egg; 1 tbsp peanut butter; ¼ c cooked dry beans; or ½ ounce of nuts or seeds can be considered as 1 ounce-equivalent from the meat and beans group.

One should make choices that are low fat or lean when selecting meats and poultry. Choose a variety of different types of foods from this group each week. Include fish, dry beans, peas, nuts, and seeds, as well as meats, poultry, and eggs. Consider dry beans and peas as an alternative to meat or poultry as well as a vegetable choice. Keep the overall amounts of foods eaten from this group within the amount needed each day. For example, people who need 2000 calories per day need 5-½ ounce-equivalents per day. See food intake patterns in the next section for other calorie levels.

Fats and Oils

Oils include fats from many different plants and from fish that are liquid at room temperature, such as canola, corn, olive, soybean, and sunflower oil. Some foods are naturally high in oils, such as nuts, olives, some fish, and avocados. Foods that are mainly oil include mayonnaise, certain salad dressings, and soft margarine.

Choose most fats from sources of monounsaturated and polyunsaturated fatty acids, such as fish, nuts, seeds, and vegetable oils. Keep the amount of oils consumed within the total allowed for caloric needs. For example, people who need 2000 calories per day can consume 27 grams of oils (about 7 tsp). See food intake patterns for amounts for other calorie levels. Choose fat-free, low-fat, or lean meat, poultry, dry beans, milk, and milk products. Choose grain products and prepared foods that are low in saturated and trans fat.

Limit the amount of solid fats consumed to the amount within the discretionary calorie allowance, after taking into account other discretionary calories that have been consumed. For example, people who need 2000 calories per day have a total discretionary calorie allowance of 267 calories.

Sugars and Sweets

Choose and prepare foods and beverages with little added sugars or caloric sweeteners. Keep the amount of sugars and sweets consumed within the discretionary calorie allowance, after taking into account other discretionary calories that have been consumed. For example, people who need 2000 calories per day[1] have a total discretionary calorie allowance of 267 calories. See food intake patterns in the next section for amounts for other calorie levels. Practice good oral hygiene and consume sugar- and starch-containing foods and beverages less frequently.

Salt

Choose and prepare foods with little salt. Keep sodium intake less than 2300 mg per day. At the same time, consume potassium-rich foods, such as fruits and vegetables.

Alcohol

If one chooses to drink alcohol, consume it in moderation. Some people, or people in certain situations, should not drink. Keep consumption of alcoholic beverages within daily discretionary calorie allowance. For example, people who need 2000 calories per day[1] have a total discretionary calorie allowance of 267 calories.

Food Intake Patterns

The suggested amounts of food to consume from the basic food groups, subgroups, and oils to meet recommended nutrient intakes at 12 different calorie levels are provided in Table 1-1. Nutrient and energy contributions from each group are calculated according to the nutrient-dense forms of foods in each group (e.g., lean meats and fat-free milk). The table also shows the discretionary calorie allowance that can be accommodated within each calorie level, in addition to the suggested amounts of nutrient-dense forms of foods in each group. Table 1-2 shows the vegetable subgroup amounts per week. Table 1-3 shows the calorie levels for males and females by age and activity level. Calorie levels are set across a wide range to accommodate the needs of different individuals. Table 1-3 can be used to help assign individuals to the food intake pattern at a particular calorie level.

Discretionary calorie allowance is the remaining amount of calories in a food intake pattern after accounting for the calories needed for all food groups—using forms of foods that are fat free or low fat and with no added sugars.

Table 1-4 shows some weekly sample menus for a daily 2000 calorie intake diet. Table 1-5 describes the nutrient contribution from these weekly menus.

The original MyPyramid contains many more details about the Food Guidance System. The best sources are your instructors and the Web site MyPyramid.gov.

At this Web site, consumers can enter their age, gender, and activity level, and they are given their own plan at an appropriate calorie level. The food plan includes

TABLE 1-1 Daily Amount of Food from Each Group

Calorie Level	1000	1200	1400	1600	1800	2000
Fruits	1 cup	1 cup	1.5 cups	1.5 cups	1.5 cups	2 cups
Vegetables	1 cup	1.5 cups	1.5 cups	2 cups	2.5 cups	2.5 cups
Grains	3 oz–eq	4 oz–eq	5 oz–eq	5 oz–eq	6 oz–eq	6 oz–eq
Meat and Beans	2 oz–eq	3 oz–eq	4 oz–eq	5 oz–eq	5 oz–eq	5.5 oz–eq
Milk	2 cups	2 cups	2 cups	3 cups	3 cups	3 cups
Oils	3 tsp	4 tsp	4 tsp	5 tsp	5 tsp	6 tsp
Discretionary calorie allowance	165	171	171	132	195	267
Calorie Level	**2200**	**2400**	**2600**	**2800**	**3000**	**3200**
Fruits	2 cups	2 cups	2 cups	2.5 cups	2.5 cups	2.5 cups
Vegetables	3 cups	3 cups	3.5 cups	3.5 cups	4 cups	4 cups
Grains	7 oz–eq	8 oz–eq	9 oz–eq	10 oz–eq	10 oz–eq	10 oz–eq
Meat and Beans	6 oz–eq	6.5 oz–eq	6.5 oz–eq	7 oz–eq	7 oz–eq	7 oz–eq
Milk	3 cups	3 cups	3 cups	3 cups	3 cups	3 cups
Oils	6 tsp	7 tsp	8 tsp	8 tsp	10 tsp	11 tsp
Discretionary calorie allowance	290	362	410	426	512	648

Source: Courtesy of the USDA.

TABLE 1-2   Vegetable Subgroup Amounts per Week

Calorie Level	1000	1200	1400	1600	1800	2000
Dark green veg.	1 c/wk	1.5 c/wk	1.5 c/wk	2 c/wk	3 c/wk	3 c/wk
Orange veg.	.5 c/wk	1 c/wk	1 c/wk	1.5 c/wk	2 c/wk	2 c/wk
Legumes	.5 c/wk	1 c/wk	1 c/wk	2.5 c/wk	3 c/wk	3 c/wk
Starchy veg.	1.5 c/wk	2.5 c/wk	2.5 c/wk	2.5 c/wk	3 c/wk	3 c/wk
Other veg.	3.5 c/wk	4.5 c/wk	4.5 c/wk	5.5 c/wk	6.5 c/wk	6.5 c/wk
Calorie Level	**2200**	**2400**	**2600**	**2800**	**3000**	**3200**
Dark green veg.	3 c/wk	3 c/wk	3 c/wk	3 c/wk	3 c/wk	3 c/wk
Orange veg.	2 c/wk	2 c/wk	2.5 c/wk	2.5 c/wk	2.5 c/wk	2.5 c/wk
Legumes	3 c/wk	3 c/wk	3.5 c/wk	3.5 c/wk	3.5 c/wk	3.5 c/wk
Starchy veg.	6 c/wk	6 c/wk	7 c/wk	7 c/wk	9 c/wk	9 c/wk
Other veg.	7 c/wk	7 c/wk	8.5 c/wk	8.5 c/wk	10 c/wk	10 c/wk

Source: Courtesy of the USDA.

TABLE 1-3   The Calorie Levels for Males and Females by Age and Activity Level

	Males				Females		
Activity level Age	Sedentary*	Mod. active*	Active*	Activity level Age	Sedentary*	Mod. active*	Active*
2	1000	1000	1000	2	1000	1000	1000
3	1000	1400	1400	3	1000	1200	1400
4	1200	1400	1600	4	1200	1400	1400
5	1200	1400	1600	5	1200	1400	1600
6	1400	1600	1800	6	1200	1400	1600
7	1400	1600	1800	7	1200	1600	1800
8	1400	1600	2000	8	1400	1600	1800
9	1600	1800	2000	9	1400	1600	1800
10	1600	1800	2200	10	1400	1800	2000
11	1800	2000	2200	11	1600	1800	2000
12	1800	2200	2400	12	1600	2000	2200
13	2000	2200	2600	13	1600	2000	2200
14	2000	2400	2800	14	1800	2000	2400
15	2200	2600	3000	15	1800	2000	2400
16	2400	2800	3200	16	1800	2000	2400
17	2400	2800	3200	17	1800	2000	2400
18	2400	2800	3200	18	1800	2000	2400
19–20	2600	2800	3000	19–20	2000	2200	2400
21–25	2400	2800	3000	21–25	2000	2200	2400
26–30	2400	2600	3000	26–30	1800	2000	2400
31–35	2400	2600	3000	31–35	1800	2000	2200
36–40	2400	2600	2800	36–40	1800	2000	2200
41–45	2200	2600	2800	41–45	1800	2000	2200
46–50	2200	2400	2800	46–50	1800	2000	2200
51–55	2200	2400	2800	51–55	1600	1800	2200
56–60	2200	2400	2600	56–60	1600	1800	2200
61–65	2000	2400	2600	61–65	1600	1800	2000
66–70	2000	2200	2600	66–70	1600	1800	2000
71–75	2000	2200	2600	71–75	1600	1800	2000
76 and up	2000	2000	2400	76 and up	1600	1800	2000

*Calorie levels are based on the Estimated Energy Requirements (EER) and activity levels from the Institute of Medicine's *Report on Dietary Reference Intakes—Macro Nutrients,* 2002.

Sedentary = less than 30 minutes a day of moderate physical activity in addition to daily activities.

Mod. active = at least 30 minutes up to 60 minutes a day of moderate physical activity in addition to daily activities.

Active = 60 or more minutes a day of moderate physical activity in addition to daily activities.

Source: Courtesy of the USDA.

TABLE 1-4   Sample Weekly Sample Menus for a Daily 2000 Calorie Intake Diet

Day 1	Day 2	Day 3	Day 4	Day 5	Day 6	Day 7
BREAKFAST	BREAKFAST	BREAKFAST	BREAKFAST	BREAKFAST	BREAKFAST	BREAKFAST
Breakfast burrito 1 flour tortilla (7" diameter) 1 scrambled egg (in 1 tsp soft margarine) ⅓ cup black beans* 2 tbsp salsa 1 cup orange juice 1 cup fat-free milk	Hot cereal ½ cup cooked oatmeal 2 tbsp raisins 1 tsp soft margarine ½ cup fat-free milk 1 cup orange juice	Cold cereal 1 cup bran flakes 1 cup fat-free milk 1 small banana 1 slice whole wheat toast 1 tsp soft margarine 1 cup prune juice	1 whole wheat English muffin 2 tsp soft margarine 1 tbsp jam or preserves 1 medium grapefruit 1 hard-cooked egg 1 unsweetened beverage	Cold cereal 1 cup shredded wheat cereal 1 tbsp raisins 1 cup fat-free milk 1 small banana 1 slice whole wheat toast 1 tsp soft margarine 1 tsp jelly	French toast 2 slices whole wheat French toast 2 tsp soft margarine 2 tbsp maple syrup ½ medium grape-fruit 1 cup fat-free milk	Pancakes 3 buckwheat pancakes 2 tsp soft margarine 3 tbsp maple syrup ½ cup strawberries ¾ cup honey-dew melon ½ cup fat-free milk
LUNCH	LUNCH	LUNCH	LUNCH	LUNCH	LUNCH	LUNCH
Roast beef sandwich 1 whole grain sandwich bun 3 ounces lean roast beef 2 slices tomato ¼ cup shredded romaine lettuce ⅛ cup sauteed mushrooms (in 1 tsp oil) 1 ½ ounce part-skim mozzarella cheese 1 tsp yellow mustard ¾ cup baked potato wedges* 1 tbsp ketchup 1 unsweetened beverage	Taco salad 2 ounces tortilla chips 2 ounces ground turkey, sauteed in 2 tsp sun-flower oil ½ cup black beans* ½ cup iceberg lettuce 2 slices tomato 1 ounce low-fat cheddar cheese 2 tbsp salsa ½ cup avocado 1 tsp lime juice 1 unsweetened beverage	Tuna fish sandwich 2 slices rye bread 3 ounces tuna (packed in water, drained) 2 tsp mayonnaise 1 tbsp diced celery ¼ cup shredded romaine lettuce 2 slices tomato 1 medium pear 1 cup fat-free milk	White bean-vegetable soup 1 ¼ cup chunky vegetable soup ½ cup white beans* 2 ounce breadstick 8 baby carrots 1 cup fat-free milk	Smoked turkey sandwich 2 ounces whole wheat pita bread ¼ cup romaine lettuce 2 slices tomato 3 ounces sliced smoked turkey breast* 1 tbsp mayo-type salad dressing 1 tsp yellow mustard ½ cup apple slices 1 cup tomato juice*	Vegetarian chili on baked potato 1 cup kidney beans* ½ cup tomato sauce w/ tomato tidbits* 3 tbsp chopped onions 1 ounce lowfat cheddar cheese 1 tsp vegetable oil 1 medium baked potato ½ cup cantaloupe ¾ cup lemonade	Manhattan clam chowder 3 ounces canned clams (drained) ¾ cup mixed vegetables 1 cup canned tomatoes* 10 whole wheat crackers* 1 medium orange 1 cup fat-free milk
DINNER	DINNER	DINNER	DINNER	DINNER	DINNER	DINNER
Stuffed broiled salmon 5 ounce salmon filet 1 ounce bread stuffing mix 1 tbsp chopped onions 1 tbsp diced celery 2 tsp canola oil ½ cup saffron (white) rice 1 ounce slivered almonds ½ cup steamed broccoli 1 tsp soft margarine 1 cup fat-free milk	Spinach lasagna 1 cup lasagna noodles, cooked (2 oz dry) ⅔ cup cooked spinach ½ cup ricotta cheese ½ cup tomato sauce tomato bits* 1 ounce part-skim mozzarella cheese 1 ounce whole wheat dinner roll 1 cup fat-free milk	Roasted chicken breast 3 ounces boneless skinless chicken breast* 1 large baked sweet potato ½ cup peas and onions 1 tsp soft margarine 1 ounce whole wheat dinner roll 1 tsp soft margarine 1 cup leafy greens salad 3 tsp sunflower oil and vinegar dressing	Rigatoni with meat sauce 1 cup rigatoni pasta (2 ounces dry) ½ cup tomato sauce tomato bits* 2 ounces extra lean cooked ground beef (sauteed in 2 tsp vegetable oil) 3 tbsp grated Parmesan cheese Spinach salad 1 cup baby spinach leaves ½ cup tangerine slices	Grilled top loin steak 5 ounces grilled top loin steak ¾ cup mashed po-tatoes 2 tsp soft margarine ½ cup steamed carrots 1 tbsp honey 2 ounces whole wheat dinner roll 1 tsp soft margarine 1 cup fat-free milk	Hawaiian pizza 2 slices cheese pizza 1 ounce canadian bacon ¼ cup pineapple 2 tbsp mushrooms 2 tbsp chopped onions Green salad 1 cup leafy greens 3 tsp sunflower oil and vinegar dressing 1 cup fat-free milk	Vegetable stir-fry 4 ounces tofu (firm) ¼ cup green and red bell peppers ½ cup bok choy 2 tbsp vegetable oil 1 cup brown rice 1 cup lemon-flavored iced tea

(continues)

TABLE 1-4   (continued)

Day 1	Day 2	Day 3	Day 4	Day 5	Day 6	Day 7
			½ ounce chopped walnuts 3 tsp sunflower oil and vinegar dressing 1 cup fat-free milk			
SNACKS	SNACKS	SNACKS	SNACKS	SNACKS	SNACKS	SNACKS
1 cup cantaloupe	½ ounce dry-roasted almonds* ¼ cup pineapple 2 tbsp raisins	¼ cup dried apricots 1 cup low-fat fruited yogurt	1 cup low-fat fruited yogurt	1 cup low-fat fruited yogurt	5 whole wheat crackers* ⅛ cup hummus ½ cup fruit cocktail (in water or juice)	1 ounce sunflower seeds* 1 large banana 1 cup low-fat fruited yogurt

*Starred items are foods that are labeled as no-salt-added, low-sodium, or low-salt versions of the foods. They can also be prepared from scratch with little or no added salt. All other foods are regular commercial products that contain variable levels of sodium. Average sodium level of the 7 day menu assumes no-salt-added in cooking or at the table.
Source: Courtesy of the USDA.

TABLE 1-5   Nutrient Contribution from Weekly Menus in Table 1-4

Food Group	Daily Average Over One Week	Nutrient	Daily Average Over One Week
Grains	Total Grains (oz–eq) 6.0	Calories	1994
Vegetables*	Whole Grains 3.4	Protein, g	98
Fruits	Refined Grains 2.6	Protein, % kcal	20
Milk	Total Veg* (cups) 2.6	Carbohydrate, g	264
Meat & Beans	Fruits (cups) 2.1	Carbohydrate, % kcal	53
Oils	Milk (cups) 3.1	Total fat, g	67
	Meat/Beans (oz–eq) 5.6	Total fat, % kcal	30
	Oils (tsp/grams) 7.2 tsp/32.4 g	Saturated fat, g	16
		Saturated fat, % kcal	7.0
		Monounsaturated fat, g	23
		Polyunsaturated fat, g	23
		Linoleic Acid, g	21
		Alpha-linolenic Acid, g	1.1
		Cholesterol, mg	207
		Total dietary fiber, g	31
		Potassium, mg	4715
		Sodium, mg*	1948
		Calcium, mg	1389
		Magnesium, mg	432
		Copper, mg	1.9
		Iron, mg	21
		Phosphorus, mg	1830
		Zinc, mg	14
		Thiamin, mg	1.9
		Riboflavin, mg	2.5
		Niacin Equivalents, mg	24
		Vitamin B_6, mg	2.9
		Vitamin B_{12}, mcg	18.4
		Vitamin C, mg	190
		Vitamin E, mg (AT)	18.9
		Vitamin A, mcg (RAE)	1430
		Dietary Folate Equivalents, mcg	558
*Vegetable subgroups			(weekly totals)
Dk-Green Veg (cups)			3.3
Orange Veg (cups)			2.3
Beans/Peas (cups)			3.0
Starchy Veg (cups)			3.4
Other Veg (cups)			6.6

Source: Courtesy of USDA.

specific daily amounts from each food group and a limit for discretionary calories (fats, added sugars, alcohol). Their food plan is one of the 12 calorie levels of the food intake patterns from the *Dietary Guidelines*. Visitors to the Web site can print out a personalized miniposter of their plan and a worksheet to help them track their progress and choose goals for tomorrow and the future.

FOOD EXCHANGE LISTS

The Food Exchange Lists are the basis of a meal planning system designed by the American Dietetic Association and the American Diabetes Association. They are based upon principles of good nutrition for everyone. There are 11 lists, of which the last one is alcohol. For some lists, each contributes an *approximate* level of nutrients for each food: calories, carbohydrates, proteins, and fats. For others, the contribution of nutrients varies within or between lists. Every time you replace one food item with another item in the same or different list, you know approximately the change in levels of nutrients you will be consuming.

Choices from each group balance the meal. Health practitioners use the exchange system because it is an easy tool to work with and teaches food selection in a practical way. It also meets the guidelines for limiting saturated fat and cholesterol intake.

The associations revise and update the exchange system regularly to reflect current nutrition research and the national dietary guidelines for health promotion and reduction of chronic disease risk factors as new information becomes available.

The 2007 edition of the Food Exchange Lists continues the basic principles of 2003 edition, arranging the food groups into 11 broad categories or listed based on their nutrient content. Subcategories that appear within these categories provide additional information to assist clients in choosing more healthful foods, as well as more choices. They reflect today's consumers' changing dietary habits and lifestyles. The 11 lists in this document are described below, with alcohol as the last category:

Starch list
  Bread
  Cereals and grains
  Crackers and snacks
  Starchy vegetables
  Beans, peas, and lentils
Sweets, desserts, and other carbohydrates list
  Beverages, sodas, and energy/sports drinks; brownies, cake, cookies, gelatin, pie, and pudding
  Candy, spreads, sweets, sweeteners, syrups, and toppings
  Condiments and sauces
  Doughnuts, muffins, pastries, and sweet breads
  Frozen bars, frozen desserts, frozen yogurt, and ice cream
  Granola bars, meal replacement bars/shakes, and trail mix
Fruit list
  Fruits
  Fruit juices
Vegetables (nonstarchy) list
Meat and meat substitutes list
  Lean meat
  Medium-fat meat
  High-fat meat
  Plant-based proteins (for beans, peas, and lentils, see starch list)
Milk list
  Fat-free and low-fat milk
  Reduced fat
  Whole milk
  Dairy-like foods
Fat list
  Monounsaturated fats list
  Polyunsaturated fats list
  Saturated fats list
Fast-foods list
  Breakfast sandwiches
  Main dishes/entrees
  Oriental
  Pizzas
  Sandwiches
  Salads
  Sides/appetizers
  Desserts
Combination foods list
  Entrées
  Frozen entrées/meals
  Salads (deli-style)
  Soups
Free foods list
  Low-carbohydrate foods
  Modified-fat foods with carbohydrate
  Condiments
  Free snacks
  Drinks/mixes
Alcohol list

Chapter 18 and Appendix F provide more details on these lists concerning food, nutrient data, and applications.

RESPONSIBILITIES OF HEALTH PERSONNEL

1. Assume responsibility for one's own health through changes in eating habits and lifestyle patterns.
2. Select, prepare, and consume an adequate diet.
3. Promote good eating habits for all age groups.

4. Use appropriate guidelines when teaching clients regarding food selection.
5. Facilitate healthy lifestyles by encouraging clients to expand their knowledge of nutrition.
6. Use approved food guides when assessing, planning, and evaluating a client's intake.

PROGRESS CHECK ON ACTIVITY 1

SHORT ANSWER

Define the following terms:

1. Calorie _____

2. Health _____

3. Nutrient _____

4. Optimum nutrition _____

5. Appropriate diet _____

FILL-IN

6. Dietary recommendations to promote health and prevent or delay the onset of diseases are known as _____.

7. The recommended dietary allowances (RDAs) are

_____.

8. Tolerable Upper Intake Levels (ULs) are

_____.

9. Dietary Reference Intakes (DRIs) are

_____.

10. An adequate intake is defined as what?

_____

DEFINE THESE ACRONYMS

11. FNB _____

12. ADA _____

13. EAR _____

14. USDA _____

15. AHA _____

16. NCEP _____

17. UL _____

MULTIPLE CHOICE

Circle the letter of the correct answer.

18. Energy is:

a. the capacity to do work.
b. food that provides calories.
c. chemical substances in the body.
d. heat required to raise body temperature.
e. a and b
f. a, b, c, and d

19. There are _____ grams in one ounce.

a. 2.285
b. 28.385
c. 1000
d. 36

20. Malnutrition is defined as:

a. impaired health due to undernutrition.
b. imbalance of nutrients.
c. excessive nutrients.
d. the inability of the body to use ingested nutrients.
e. all of the above.

21. Nutritional requirements vary from nutrient to nutrient because of which of these factors?

a. age
b. gender
c. physiological state
d. size
e. a, b, and d
f. a, b, c, and d

GENERAL QUESTIONS

22. What is MyPyramid? _____

23. How does MyPyramid help the consumers?

_____

24. Define the milk, yogurt, and cheese group according to MyPyramid.

_____

25. The Food Guidance System is based on two important food guides. They are:

_____.

26. Name the seven chronic diseases in the United States that are linked to risk factors associated with diet.

_____

27. List four nutrition health problems that require special dietary measures. _____

28. Explain the difference(s) between the *Dietary Guidelines for Americans* and MyPyramid Food Guidance System. _____

29. List the 11 primary lists in the 2007 Food Exchange Lists. _____

30. Name three approved food guides you would use when assessing, planning, or evaluating a client's diet: (a) _____ (b) _____

    (c) _____

SELF-STUDY

Use Table 1-3 to determine your approximate daily caloric need. Write down everything you ate or drank in the last 24 hours for meals and snacks. Then do the following:

1. Did you have the number of servings from the five major food groups that are right for you according to MyPramid.gov?
2. At approximately which of the three calorie levels was your 24-hour intake? Was the number of servings you ate greater, less, or about right for your age, gender, and activity?
3. Using the *Dietary Guidelines*, look at your diet to see if you should make any substitutions regarding your salt, sugar, or fiber content (clue: visit the Web site given for the *Dietary Guidelines*).
4. Write a short summary of things you could do to improve your present diet if improvement is needed.

Self-Study: Your individual answers will provide information for your personal health status.

ACTIVITY 2:
Legislation and Health Promotion

At present, there are national policies and recommendation on nutrition labeling, dietary supplements, and educational programs on cholesterol and our health. In the last decade, a new concept of bioactive food ingredients (nutraceuticals) and functional foods has developed and will be discussed with other national policies in this activity.

FOOD LABELING

In general, food and nutrition labeling is now mandatory for many foods excluding meat and poultry, with special considerations for seafood and other fresh foods.

The information in this section has been modified from the document issued by the U.S. Food and Drug Administration, *How to Understand and Use the Nutrition Facts Label*. This document was published in June 2000 and updated twice, July 2003 and November 2004. See www.cfsan.fda.gov/label.html for the latest updates and other legal announcements related to food labeling.

People look at food labels for different reasons. But whatever the reason, many consumers would like to know how to use this information more effectively and easily.

The food label is headed with the title, "Nutrition Facts." It describes the nutrients, among other data, including the following:

Total calories
Calories from fat
Calories from saturated fat
Total fat
Saturated fat
Polyunsaturated fat
Monounsaturated fat
Cholesterol
Sodium
Potassium
Total carbohydrate
Dietary fiber
Soluble fiber
Insoluble fiber
Sugars
Sugar alcohol (for example, the sugar substitutes xylitol, mannitol, and sorbitol)
Other carbohydrate (the difference between total carbohydrate and the sum of dietary fiber, sugars, and sugar alcohol if declared)
Protein
Vitamin A
Vitamin C
Calcium
Iron
Other essential vitamins and minerals

Listing of most of the above nutrients is mandatory. Some are voluntary listings, and others require special consideration. Let us look at a sample label of macaroni and cheese. Refer to Figure 1-3.

The information in the main or top section (see Step 1 through Step 4 and Step 6 on the sample nutrition label that follows), can vary with each food product; it contains product-specific information (serving size, calories, and nutrient information). The bottom part (see Step 5 on the sample label that follows) contains a footnote with Daily Values (DVs) for 2000 and 2500 calorie diets. This footnote provides recommended dietary information for important nutrients, including fats, sodium, and fiber. The footnote is found only on larger packages and does not change from product to product.

The Contents of a Food Label

Only selected information is included. Refer to Figure 1-3.

Step 1.   Start here.
        The first place to start when you look at the Nutrition Facts label is the serving size and the

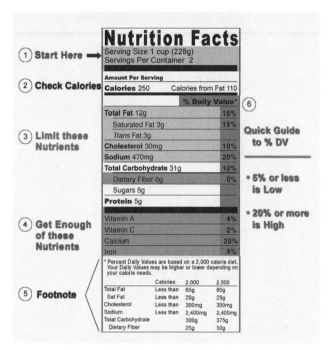

FIGURE 1-3   Sample Label of Macaroni and Cheese
Source: Courtesy of the FDA.

number of servings in the package. Serving sizes are standardized to make it easier to compare similar foods; they are provided in familiar units, such as cups or pieces, followed by the metric amount (the number of grams).

The size of the serving on the food package influences the number of calories and all the nutrient amounts listed on the top part of the label. *Pay attention to the serving size, especially how many servings there are in the food package. Then ask yourself, "How many servings am I consuming"? (e.g., ½ serving, 1 serving, or more).* In the sample label, one serving of macaroni and cheese equals 1 c. If you ate the whole package, you would eat *2* c. That doubles the calories and other nutrient numbers, including the %DVs as shown in the sample label. Table 1-6 compares the nutritional contributions for a single or double serving.

Step 2. Check calories.

Calories provide a measure of how much energy you get from a serving of this food. Many Americans consume more calories than they need without meeting recommended intakes for a number of nutrients. The calorie section of the label can help you manage your weight (i.e., gain, lose, or maintain). *Remember: The number of servings you consume determines the number of calories you actually eat (your portion amount).*

In the example, there are 250 calories in one serving of this macaroni and cheese. How many calories from fat are there in *one* serving? Answer: 110 calories, which means almost half the calories in a single serving come from fat. What if you ate the whole package content? Then, you would consume two servings, or 500 calories, and 220 would come from fat.

Box 1-1, General Guide to Calories, provides a general reference for calories when you look at a Nutrition Facts label. This guide is based on a 2000-calorie diet.

Eating too many calories per day is linked to overweight and obesity.

Look at the top of the nutrient section in the sample label (Figure 1-3). It shows you some key nutrients that affect your health and separates them into two main groups.

Step 3. Limit these nutrients.

The nutrients listed first are the ones Americans generally eat in adequate amounts, or even too much. Eating too much fat, saturated fat, trans fat, cholesterol, or sodium may increase your risk of certain chronic diseases, such as heart disease, some cancers, or high blood pressure.

Important: Health experts recommend that you keep your intake of saturated fat, trans fats, and cholesterol as low as possible as part of a nutritionally balanced diet.

Step 4. Get enough of these nutrients.

Most Americans don't get enough dietary fiber, vitamin A, vitamin C, calcium, and iron in their

TABLE 1-6   Single vs. Double Serving

	Single Serving	Double %DV	Serving	%DV
		Example		
Serving Size	1 cup	2 cups (228 g)	(456 g)	
Calories	250	500		
Calories from Fat	110	220		
Total Fat	12 g	18	24 g	36
Trans Fat	1.5 g		3 g	
Saturated Fat	3 g	15	6 g	30
Cholesterol	30 mg	10	60 mg	20
Sodium	470 mg	20	940 mg	40
Total Carbohydrate	31 g	10	62 g	20
Dietary Fiber	0 g	0	0 g	0
Sugars	5 g		10 g	
Protein	5 g		10 g	
Vitamin A		4		8
Vitamin C		2		4
Calcium		20		40
Iron		4		8

Source: Courtesy of the FDA.

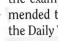

BOX 1-1 General Guide to Calories

40 calories is low

100 calories is moderate

400 calories or more is high

Source: Courtesy of the FDA.

diets. Eating enough of these nutrients can improve your health and help reduce the risk of some diseases and conditions. For example, getting enough calcium may reduce the risk of osteoporosis, a condition that results in brittle bones as one ages. Eating a diet high in dietary fiber promotes healthy bowel function. Additionally, a diet rich in fruits, vegetables, and grain products that contain dietary fiber, particularly soluble fiber, and low in saturated fat and cholesterol, may reduce the risk of heart disease.

Remember: You can use the Nutrition Facts label not only to help limit those nutrients you want to cut back on but also to increase those nutrients you need to consume in greater amounts.

Step 5. Footnote.

Note the asterisk (*) used after the heading "% Daily Value" on the Nutrition Facts label. It refers to the footnote in the lower part of the nutrition label, which tells you "Percent Daily Values are based on a 2,000 calorie diet." This statement must be on all food labels. But the remaining information in the full footnote may not be on the package if the size of the label is too small. When the full footnote does appear, it will always be the same. It doesn't change from product to product, because it shows recommended dietary advice for all Americans—it is not about a specific food product.

Look at the amounts or the Daily Values (DV) for each nutrient listed. These are based on public health experts' advice. DVs are recommended levels of intakes. DVs in the footnote are based on a 2000 or 2500 calorie diet. Note how the DVs for some nutrients change, while others (for cholesterol and sodium) remain the same for both calorie amounts.

Look at Table 1-7 for another way to see how the DVs relate to the %DVs and dietary guidance. For each nutrient listed there is a DV, a %DV, and dietary advice or a goal. If you follow this dietary advice, you will stay within public health experts' recommended upper or lower limits for the nutrients listed, based on a 2000 calorie daily diet.

The nutrients that have upper daily limits are listed first on the footnote of larger labels and on

the example. Upper limits means it is recommended that you stay below—eat less than—the Daily Value nutrient amounts listed per day. For example, the DV for saturated fat is 20 g. This amount is 100%DV for this nutrient. What is the goal or dietary advice? To eat less than 20 g or 100%DV for the day.

Now look at the entry where dietary fiber is listed. The DV for dietary fiber is 25 g, which is 100%DV. This means it is recommended that you eat at least this amount of dietary fiber per day.

The DV for the entry Total Carbohydrate is 300 g or 100%DV. This amount is recommended for a balanced daily diet that is based on 2000 calories, but can vary, depending on your daily intake of fat and protein.

Now let's look at the %DVs.

Step 6. The percent daily value (%DV).

The % Daily Values (%DVs) are based on the Daily Value recommendations for key nutrients but only for a 2000 calorie daily diet—not 2500 calories. You, like most people, may not know how many calories you consume in a day. But you can still use the %DV as a frame of reference whether or not you consume more or less than 2000 calories.

The %DV helps you determine if a serving of food is high or low in a nutrient. Note: A few nutrients, like trans fat, do not have a %DV—they will be discussed later.

You don't need to know how to calculate percentages to use the %DV? The label (the %DV) does the math for you. It helps you interpret the numbers (grams and milligrams) by putting them all on the same scale for the day (0–100%DV). The %DV column doesn't add up vertically to 100%. Instead each nutrient is based on 100% of the daily requirements for that nutrient (for a 2000 calorie diet). This way you can tell high from low and know which nutrients contribute a lot, or a little, to your *daily* recommended allowance (upper or lower).

TABLE 1-7 Examples of DVs vs. %DVs, Based on a 2000 Calorie Diet

Nutrient	DV	%DV	Goal
Total Fat	65 g	= 100%DV	Less than
Sat Fat	20 g	= 100%DV	Less than
Cholesterol	300 mg	= 100%DV	Less than
Sodium	2400 mg	= 100%DV	Less than
Total Carbohydrate	300 g	= 100%DV	At least
Dietary Fiber	25 g	= 100%DV	At least

Refer to Step 6 in Figure 1-3, as shown below:
Quick Guide to %DV:

- 5% or less is low
- 20% or more is high

This guide tells you that 5%DV or less is low for all nutrients, those you want to limit (e.g., fat, saturated fat, cholesterol, and sodium), or for those that you want to consume in greater amounts (fiber, calcium, etc.). As the Quick Guide shows, 20%DV or more is high for all nutrients.

Example: Look at the amount of total fat in one serving listed on the sample nutrition label. Is 18%DV contributing a lot or a little to your fat limit of 100%DV? Check the Quick Guide to %DV, and you'll see that 18%DV, which is below 20%DV, is not yet high, but what if you ate the whole package (two servings)? You would double that amount, eating 36% of your daily allowance for total fat. Coming from just one food, that amount leaves you with 64% of your fat allowance (100% − 36% = 64%) for *all* of the other foods you eat that day, snacks and drinks included. See Figure 1-4.

The %DV can be used for:

Comparisons: The %DV also makes it easy for you to make comparisons. You can compare one product or brand to a similar product. Just make sure the serving sizes are similar, especially the weight (e.g., gram, milligram, ounces) of each product. It's easy to see which foods are higher or lower in nutrients because the serving sizes are generally consistent for similar types of foods, except in a few cases such as cereals.

Nutrient Content Claims: Use the %DV to help you quickly distinguish one claim from another, such as "reduced fat" vs. "light" or "nonfat." Just compare the %DVs for total fat in each food product to see which one is higher or lower in that nutrient—there is no need to memorize definitions. This works when comparing all nutrient content claims, such as less, light, low, free, more, or high.

Dietary Trade-Offs: You can use the %DV to help you make dietary trade-offs with other foods throughout the day. You don't have to give up a favorite food to eat a healthy diet. When a food you like is high in fat, balance it with foods that are low in fat at other times of the day. Also, pay attention to how much you eat so that the total amount of fat for the day stays below 100%DV.

Health Claims

You may have noticed that some labels have health claims and some do not. At present, the FDA permits six groups of qualified health claims subject to enforcement discretion. They include the following.

1. Qualified Claims About Cancer Risk
   a. Tomatoes and/or tomato sauce and prostate, ovarian, gastric, and pancreatic cancers
   b. Calcium and colon/rectal cancer and calcium and recurrent colon/rectal polyps
   c. Green tea and cancer
   d. Selenium and cancer
   e. Antioxidant vitamins and cancer
2. Qualified claims about cardiovascular disease risk
   a. Nuts and heart disease
   b. Walnuts and heart disease
   c. Omega-3 fatty acids and coronary heart disease

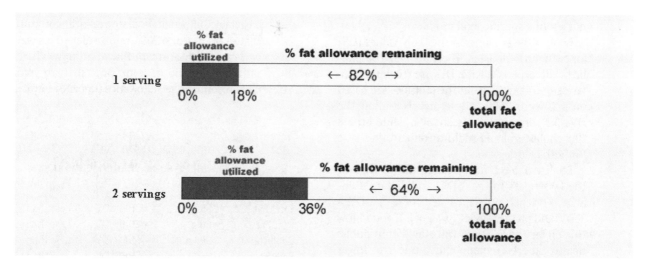

FIGURE 1-4   Fat Allowance and %DV: Low vs. High Consumption
Source: Courtesy of the FDA.

   d. B vitamins and vascular disease
   e. Monounsaturated fatty acids from olive oil and coronary heart disease
   f. Unsaturated fatty acids from canola oil and coronary heart disease
   g. Corn oil and heart disease
3. Qualified claims about cognitive function
   a. Phosphatidylserine and cognitive dysfunction and dementia
4. Qualified claims about diabetes
   a. Chromium picolinate and diabetes
5. Qualified claims about hypertension
   a. Calcium and hypertension, pregnancy-induced hypertension, and preeclampsia
6. Qualified claims about neural tube birth defects
   a. 0.8 mg folic acid and neural tube birth defects

Space limitation does not permit a detailed discussion of different aspects of food and nutrition labeling. You may obtain more details in two ways:

1. The instructors will provide more information where applicable.
2. Visit the Web site www.cfsan.fda.gov/label.html for reference.

DIETARY SUPPLEMENT LAW

The Dietary Supplement Health and Education Act (DSHEA) was signed into law in October 1994. While it is a compromise between the supplement industry and the FDA position, it still preserves the standards set by the FDA in the Nutrition and Labeling Act of 1990. It provides consistency between food regulations and regulation of dietary supplements. Chapter 11, "Dietary Supplements," provides a detailed discussion of this law.

NATIONAL CHOLESTEROL EDUCATION PROGRAM (NCEP)

The NCEP is one of three principal programs administered by the Office of Prevention, Education, and Control of the National Heart, Lung, and Blood Institute (NHLBI) of the National Institutes of Health (NIH). The program came about after years of trials and scientific evidence that linked blood-cholesterol levels to coronary heart disease. The trials showed that levels could be lowered safely by both diet and drugs. Hence, the National Cholesterol Education Program, today known as the NCEP, came into being. This became known as Adult Treatment Panel 1 (ATP 1). In 1989 the first guidelines were issued for the adult population. In 1991 the NCEP drafted an additional report that included children and adolescents.

Three ATP reports have been issued. ATP 1 outlined a major strategy for primary prevention of coronary heart disease (CHD) in persons with high levels of low density lipoprotein (LDL) ($>$ 160 mg/dl) or borderline LDL of 130–159 mg/dl. ATP 2 affirmed this approach and added a new feature: the intensive management of LDL cholesterol in persons with CHD. It set a new goal of $<$ 100 mg/dl of LDL.

The third ATP report (May 2001) updates the existing recommendations for clinical management of high blood cholesterol as warranted by advances in the science of cholesterol management. ATP 3 maintains the core of ATP 1 and 2, but its major new feature is a focus on primary prevention in persons with multiple risk factors. It calls for more intensive LDL lowering therapy in certain groups of people and recommends support for implementation. This approach includes a complete lipoprotein profile, high density lipoprotein (HDL) cholesterol and triglycerides, as the preferred initial test. It encourages the use of plants containing soluble fiber as a therapeutic dietary option to enhance lowering LDL cholesterol and presents strategies for promoting adherence. It recommends treatment beyond LDL lowering in people with high triglycerides.

Chapter 16, "Diet Therapy for Cardiovascular Disorders," discusses the diet therapy associated with ATP guidelines in detail.

FUNCTIONAL FOODS AND NUTRACEUTICALS

In the last 15–25 years, two new concepts, functional foods and nutraceuticals, have been slowly developing with important ramifications to our health. To understand their origins and meanings, we must be familiar with "bioactive ingredients" found in traditional foods and other edible or nonedible items. What are bioactive active ingredients? Examples include some of most popular items in the news media, printed or electronic:

1. Omega-6 polyunsaturated fatty acids (PUFA) come from liquid vegetable oils, including soybean oil, corn oil, and safflower oil. Fish that naturally contain the same ingredient, including salmon, trout, and herring, are higher in EPA and DHA than are lean fish (e.g., cod, haddock, catfish). According to scientists, limited evidence suggests an association between consumption of fatty acids in fish and reduced risks of mortality from cardiovascular disease for the general population. Such acids form a group of bioactive ingredients.
2. Folic acid is a water-soluble vitamin found in green vegetables. Its benefit for pregnant women is getting increasing attention from the government, academic, and industrial scientists, not to mention the general public. There are other claims about their positive effects on clinical disorders such as birth defects. This vitamin is a bioactive ingredient.
3. Green tea contains three chemicals: epicatechin (EC), epicatechin gallate (ECG), eigallocatechin

gallate (EGCG). The claims are that they can neutralize free radicals (responsible for aging) and may reduce risk of cancer. Some consider them as bioactive ingredients.

4. The botanical ginkgo contains chemicals known as flavone glycosides. The claims are that they can improve memory and blood flow to the brain and may help cure Alzheimer's disease. Thus, these chemicals are considered by some to be bioactive ingredients from a nonfood substance.

The printed and electronic media have listed hundreds of these bioactive ingredients found in foods (plant and animal), spices, herbs, and so on. Industries engaged in food products, dietary supplements, and over-the-counter (OTC) drugs have expressed tremendous interests in these bioactive ingredients because of their potential ramifications in manufacturing products that have appeal to the consumers because of health implications.

Most popular bioactive ingredients are already sold in traditional foods, dietary supplements, and OTC drugs. We will exclude prescription drugs. All three categories are strictly controlled by the FDA. The industry must comply with all requirements governing labeling. At present, there are many items in food labeling regulated under federal and state agencies. Most of them are not familiar to consumers. The three most important items in food labeling regulated by the FDA and directly related to the consumers are the following:

1. Name of the food, supplement, and drug
2. Health claims
3. Ingredients added

This brings us back to the two concepts mentioned earlier: functional foods and nutraceuticals. Scientifically, they have been used to mean the following, among many other definitions:

1. Functional foods refer to "legal" conventional foods (natural or manufactured) that contain bioactive ingredients. One example is adding PUFA to a traditional TV dinner of roast beefs. Another example is adding EC, ECG, or EGCG to any instant tea.
2. Nutraceuticals refer to adding a bioactive ingredient, especially one with nutritional value, to a dietary or an OTC drug, such as adding ginkgo or ginseng extracts. Such a product is claimed as a nutraceutical.

Assuming the new product complies with all requirements of the FDA, the logical question is: Can the product be marketed as a functional food or nutraceutical? The FDA is now undergoing the legal process to settle this issue. At the time of printing this book, the FDA is soliciting comments from the public. The FDA hopes that a dialogue among government, academia, industry, and the general public will facilitate the process to reach a final legal decision.

RESPONSIBILITIES OF HEALTH PERSONNEL

1. Become an informed consumer. Use the new regulations to promote better health for yourself and family.
2. Become an informed educator. Teach others to make healthy choices for a healthier lifestyle.

PROGRESS CHECK ON ACTIVITY 2

FOOD AND NUTRITION LABEL:

1. One serving of macaroni and cheese equals

   _____.

2. The number of calories you actually eat is determined by _____.

3. Americans should limit the intake of these nutrients if they wish to reduce the risk of certain chromic diseases: _____, _____, _____, _____, or _____.

4. Most Americans do not get enough of the following nutrients: _____, _____, _____, _____, and _____.

5. The meaning of upper limits is

   _____.

6. The %DV helps you to determine

   _____.

Functional foods and nutraceuticals:

7. One meaning for functional foods is

   _____.

8. One meaning for nutraceuticals is

   _____.

What is the potential health benefit offered by each of the following bioactive ingredient:

9. Omega-6 PUFA: _____.

10. Folic acid: _____.

11. Green tea: _____.

12. Ginkgo: _____

Cholesterol education:

13. What was the major thrust of ATP 1?

    _____

14. What was the new added feature in ATP 2?

    _____

15. In addition to retaining the core of ATP 1 and ATP 2, ATP 3 focused on yet another new feature. Name the new feature in ATP 3 and the three approaches used to implement it.

    _____

16. Define these acronyms:
    a. NIH_____
    b. CHD_____
    c. LDL_____
    d. HDL_____
    e. FDA_____
    f. NCEP_____
    g. ATP_____

REFERENCES

Bendich, A. & Deckelbaum, R. J. (Eds.). (2005). *Preventive Nutrition: The Comprehensive Guide for Health Professionals* (3rd ed.). Totowa, NJ: Humana Press.

Caballero, B., Allen, L., & Prentice, A. (Eds.). (2005). *Encyclopedia of Human Nutrition* (2nd ed.). Boston: Elsevier/Academic Press.

Eastwood, M. (2003). *Principles of Human Nutrition* (2nd ed.). Malden, MA: Blackwell Science.

Food and Agriculture Organization. (2001). Human energy requirements: Report of a Joint FAO/WHO/UNU expert consultation. Rome: Food and Agriculture Organization of the United Nations.

Haas, E. M. & Levin, B. (2006). *Staying Healthy with Nutrition: The Complete Guide to Diet and Nutrition Medicine* (21st ed.). Berkeley, CA: Celestial Arts.

Hargove, J. L. (2006). History of the calorie in nutrition. *Journal of Nutrition, 136*: 2957–2961.

Hark, L. & Morrison, G. (Eds.). (2003). *Medical Nutrition and Disease* (3rd ed.). Malden, MA: Blackwell.

Healthy People. www.healthypeople.gov.

Klein, S. (2007). Waist circumference and cardiometabolic risk: A consensus statement from shaping america's health: Association for Weight Management and Obesity Prevention: NAASO, The Obesity Society: The American Society for Nutrition and The American Diabetes Association. *American Journal for Nutrition, 85*: 1197–1202.

Knukowski, R. A. (2006). Consumers may not use or understand calorie labeling in restaurants. *Journal of American Dietetic Association, 106*: 917–920.

Lane, H. W. (2002). Water and energy dietary requirements and endocrinology of human space flight. *Nutrition, 18*: 820–828.

Mahan, L. K. & Escott-Stump, S. (Eds.). (2008). *Krause's Food and Nutrition Therapy* (12th ed.). Philadelphia: Elsevier Sauders.

Mann, J. & Truswell, S., (Eds.). (2007). *Essentials of Human Nutrition* (3rd ed.). New York: Oxford University Press.

Moore, M. C. (2005). *Pocket Guide to Nutritional Assessment and Care* (5th ed.). St. Louis, MO: Elvesier Mosby.

MyPyramid food guide. www.mypryamid.gov.

Ormachigui, A. (2002). Prepregnancy and pregnancy nutrition and its impact on women health. *Nutrition Reviews, 60* (5, pt. 2): s64–s67.

Otten, J. J., Pitzi, J., Hellwig, & L. D. Meyers, (Eds.). (2006). *Dietary Reference Intakes: The Essential Guide to Nutrient Requirements*. Washington, DC: National Academy Press.

Park, M. I. (2005). Gastric motor and sensory functions in obesity. *Obesity Research, 13*: 491–500.

Payne-James, J. & Wicks, C. (2003). *Key Facts in Clinical Nutrition* (2nd ed.). London: Greenwich Medical Media.

Sardesai, V. M. (2003). *Introduction to Clinical Nutrition* (2nd ed.). New York: Marcel Dekker.

Shils, M. E. & Shike, M. (Eds.). (2006). *Modern Nutrition in Health and Disease* (10th ed.). Philadelphia: Lippincott, Williams & Wilkins.

Stewart-Knox, B. (2005). Dietary strategies and update of reduced fat foods. *Journal of Human Nutrition and Dietetics, 18*: 121–128.

Stover, P. J. (2006). Influence of human genetic variation on nutritional requirements. *American Journal of Clinical Nutrition, 83*: 436s–442s.

Temple, N. J., Wilson, T., & Jacobs, D. R. (2006). *Nutrition Health: Strategies for Disease Prevention* (2nd ed.). Totowa, NJ: Humana Press.

Thomas, B. & Bishop, J. (Eds.). (2007). *Manual of Dietetic Practice* (4th ed.). Ames, IA: Blackwell.

United States Department of Health and Human Services and United States Department of Agriculture. (2005). *Dietary Guidelines for Americans* (6th ed.). Washington, DC: Government Publishing Office.

U.S. National Cholesterol Education Program (NCEP), National Heart, Lung, and Blood Institute (NHLBI). (2001). Third report of the expert panel on detection, evaluation, and treatment of high blood cholesterol in adults (Adult Treatment Panel III). www.NIH.gov.

Webster-Gandy, J., Madden, A., & Holdworth, M. (Eds.). (2006). *Oxford Handbook of Nutrition and Dietetics*. Oxford, England: Oxford University Press.

CHAPTER **2**

Food Habits

Time for completion

Activities: 1 hour

Optional examination: ½ hour

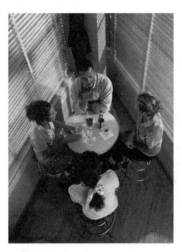

OBJECTIVES

Upon completion of this chapter, the student should be able to do the following:

1. Describe the cultural, social, and psychological factors that influence food behavior.
   a. Distinguish between biological necessity and cultural patterning.
   b. Identify the use of food in a culture.
   c. Explain the symbolism of food in a culture.
   d. Identify the social influences of food in a culture.
   e. Evaluate the psychological influence of food.
2. Determine the economic considerations that affect food intake.
3. Identify some common problems in the nutritional status of individuals in the United States.
4. Explain the ways that illness affects food acceptance.
5. Identify the dietary patterns of some ethnic, cultural, and religious groups in the United States.

GLOSSARY

Culture (or acculturation): traditions, values, or religions that make up a way of life.

Food behaviors: result of the social, physiological, psychological, environmental, and sociocultural impact on a person's food preferences.

Foodways: way(s) in which a distinct group selects, prepares, consumes, and uses food.

Heritage: that which is transmitted from preceding generations.

Physiological: physical development, state of health, mental attitudes.

Psychological: body image, perception of self, ways of coping.

Society (sociological): interactions between people, governments, and so forth.

Suboptimal: below desirable, as in below desirable intake.

BACKGROUND INFORMATION

Biologic necessity refers to the nutrient balance that the body requires in order to maintain life and health. Cultural patterning, on the other hand, establishes values, feelings, attitudes, and beliefs regarding food consumption. The required nutrient levels may or may not be met under influences of cultural patterning.

In recent years, because of improved research and interpretation of data regarding the nutritional status of individuals, scientists are sure that primary malnutrition exists in the United States. It is recognized that overnutrition, misinformation, ignorance, poor economic status, and poor eating habits are prevalent in this country. Malnutrition is difficult to manage in the United States because of the diverse cultures, subcultures, values, and experiences present in the country. Common nutritional problems are obesity; iron-deficiency anemia, especially among low-income women of childbearing age and among infants; and suboptimal intakes of calcium, ascorbic acid, and vitamin A. Also, special nutritional problems affect the poor, the elderly, and the adolescent.

ACTIVITY 1:

Factors Affecting Food Consumption

Eating behaviors develop from cultural, societal, and psychological patterns. These patterns, reflecting food habits that have been transmitted from preceding generations, are the heritage of any given ethnic group. They may be influenced by interactions with other groups, so that some intermingling of patterns is inevitable, but modifications are worked into the total structure over long periods of time and are acceptable only if they fit the existing customs.

Food patterns reflect a people's social organization, including their economy, religion, beliefs about the health properties of foods, and attitudes about family. Great emotional significance is attached to the consumption of certain foods.

FOOD AND SYMBOLS

Eating behaviors are derived from many sources. To become part of a group's eating pattern, a food must be available and acceptable within the cultural context. The ways in which a food is determined to be acceptable vary greatly among societies and among individuals, and both conscious and unconscious criteria are applied. One such criterion is food symbolism, which is the meaning attached to food. Those foods symbolically designated as positive are acceptable, whereas a negative evaluation causes rejection.

Most food symbolism is related to security. This security can be emotional, biological, or sociological, or any combination of the three. For instance, foods believed to have safety and health benefits offer biological security. An example is food faddism—the belief that eating certain foods will bring special health benefits.

Great numbers of food taboos and superstitions are associated with biological symbolism. Food taboos are based on beliefs that certain foods or food combinations are bad or unsafe. Superstitions arise from beliefs about magical powers of foods. For example, certain herbs are believed to ward off old age. It does not matter that there may be little or no scientific basis for these beliefs; it is what the individual thinks that influences his or her choice.

Nowhere is food symbolism more pronounced than in the context of emotional security. A deep emotional attachment to food begins from the moment an infant receives his or her first food from a significant other. Eating is associated with love, caring, attention, and satisfaction. One of the causes of obesity may be a response to this emotional association. Food may also be used for discipline, punishment, reward for moral virtue, and bribery; hence, the response elicited by such uses of certain foods may be frustration, anger, and rejection.

Food is often used as a weapon or a crutch. A child learns the hidden meanings of food very quickly and will use this tool for power and manipulation—for example, refusing to eat, throwing a tantrum, or developing sudden whims. For teenagers, strenuous dieting, refusal to eat healthy foods, and voracious overeating are weapons that gain them attention, enable them to manipulate or avoid situations, and often give them a feeling of control over their bodies. Used this way, food becomes an emotional outlet for boredom, frustration, anxiety, and other stresses. Using food as a crutch is also a contributing factor in obesity.

Food and religion are linked symbolically with emotional security. In all religions, certain foods are used in ceremonial rites as a means of demonstrating faith and commemorating events. Prohibition of certain foods is also common practice. Examples of religious food symbolism include Holy Communion in Christian churches, the Jewish dietary laws, and the exclusion of animal flesh by Hindus and Buddhists. Fasting is common to most religions. Often the reasons for food prohibitions are obscure.

Sociological symbolism can include the use of food as status symbols—that is, certain foods are considered desirable because of high cost, difficulty in obtaining or preparing them, and superior quality. Examples include prime rib, imported wines, truffles, caviar, fancy and complicated desserts, and other such food choices.

Also of sociological significance is the use of foods as a means of communication. Eating together denotes acceptance. Almost all social occasions involve some sort of food or drink. Examples include refreshments at meetings, weddings, and feasts. Dinner parties and dinner dates are socially significant events. Foods communicate roles in life often as clearly as actions do.

Of the various kinds of security-related food symbolism, sociological symbolism is the one most likely to change. Social meanings attached to food are not as deeply imbedded in the psyche as are emotional and biological meanings. Social symbols change as situations and experiences change.

Illness modifies food acceptance. Anxiety, loneliness, lack of activity, and the disease process all contribute to an alteration of usual eating patterns. Appetite may diminish, and hostility and apathy about food may occur. Children may regress to an earlier developmental stage, and adults may regress to less mature states.

Some examples should help the student to understand the forces at work in the development of eating behaviors.

EXAMPLES OF FOOD BEHAVIORS

Example A

Mary W., age 65, states that she takes 2 tbsp of lecithin, 1200 mg of organic vitamin E, plus a cup of rose hips tea each day to "keep her arteries cleared out" and "prevent arthritis."

1. What eating behavior is being manifested by Mary?
2. Is this a superstition or a taboo?

Example B

Jane is your roommate. The night before the final exam in anatomy and physiology, the two of you go to the store and purchase six doughnuts, four candy bars, a bag of popcorn, a pound of peanuts, and a carton of cola beverages because you do not plan to take time out for dinner.

3. What eating behavior are you manifesting?
4. Was the choice of foods based on scientific evidence of the need for extra energy while studying strenuously?

Example C

Jesus Martinez, age 35, is admitted to your floor in the hospital for lab tests tomorrow. His lunch tray contains broiled fish, asparagus, baked potato, Jell-O, and milk. It is an attractive tray. He does not touch the food. As he speaks no English and the nurse speaks no Spanish, there is a communication gap.

5. What may you assume is the cause of this rejection?

Example D

Ellen confides to you that her mother once made her sit at the breakfast table for three hours until she ate her bowl of oatmeal and that she will never touch another bite of oatmeal as long as she lives. "The thought of cold, sticky, nasty oatmeal makes me want to throw up," she says.

6. What factors are involved in Ellen's feelings about the oatmeal?

Example E

Mrs. Theo F. Jones III, wife of a prominent government official, is the guest of honor at a luncheon where hamburger casserole is the main entrée. She barely touches any of her food and leaves immediately afterward, even though she had planned to speak on a pet project.

7. Was Mrs. Jones ill, allergic to hamburger, or angry?
8. What type of food symbolism is manifested here?

Answers to Examples

1. Biological food symbolism. Food faddism—the belief that certain foods bring special health benefits—is very prevalent.
2. Superstition—a set of beliefs about the magical powers of food. There does not have to be a scientific basis for such beliefs.
3. Emotional food symbolism. Students' eating patterns change during exam time. They usually eat more, and the choices are usually high-calorie items. Such eating seems to help relieve strain.
4. There is no scientific evidence of need for extra calories while studying. One peanut would probably furnish enough energy for the entire study period.
5. There could be several causes, including anxiety, fear, unfamiliar surroundings, and strange people presenting the food, but the major cause is probably that these foods are not culturally acceptable.
6. Ellen is projecting an unpleasant memory associated with oatmeal. This frequently causes a food once eaten to become unacceptable. Psychotic patients often show great agitation by spitting on a food or dashing the tray to the floor when it brings back unpleasant memories. This is another example of emotional food symbolism.
7. Angry. Food is used as a status symbol, and hamburger is not included among status foods in our society. She felt rejected and humiliated by this menu because she felt it did not reflect her social standing.
8. Sociological food symbolism.

POVERTY, APPETITE, AND BIOLOGICAL FOOD NEEDS

Economics is a very strong factor in the determination of food consumption. The costs of producing, transporting, and distributing food determine how much and what types of food are available. Lack of money affects not only the prices that people can pay for food but also the kinds of storage facilities they can afford to have within the household. Poor people often must buy cheap foods in small quantities and purchase items that do not require special storage facilities such as freezers or refrigerators. The cost of transportation may prohibit going to a large market, where volume purchases permit cheaper prices. Poverty is sometimes classified as a subculture in our society, and different attitudes and adaptations about foods emerge from this class than those found in the middle or upper classes. Nurses should have an extensive knowledge of these differences.

Eating is generally prompted by hunger or appetite. Hunger is a physiological mechanism, controlled by the central nervous system. It is an unpleasant sensation. Appetite is a desire for food related to past experiences in response to stimuli such as smell, taste, and appearance. Appetite is not necessarily related to biological needs. People who are really hungry will eat many things not within their cultural frame of reference. They adapt physiologically and psychologically in order to survive. Appetite, on the other hand, can become uncontrolled behavior and can result in obesity. Obesity is a form of malnutrition, usually resulting in a deficiency of some essential nutrients in addition to excess fat in the body.

The biological food needs of a person throughout the life cycle have one requirement. The food consumed must provide essential chemical substances— nutrients—which the body can digest, absorb, and metabolize. To maintain life and health, the nutrients must reach the cells. Adequate nutrient intake depends on many factors, including age, sex, activity, size, and individual variations. The amounts of required nutrients may vary, but the types and kinds of nutrients established as being essential to life and health will remain the same throughout life. Research may add other, as yet unrecognized, essentials as scientific investigation progresses.

SUMMARY

Feelings, attitudes, conditioning, and economics continually affect one's food consumption throughout life. Except for health professionals, who are very aware of the vital role that nutrition plays in the maintenance of health and the recovery from illness, most people give other aspects of food a priority over its importance for health.

Culture is a way of life. It is useful in adapting a person to his or her environment. Beginning with an infant's earliest experiences, individuals acquire customs and attitudes which they begin to internalize. Along with food, the child receives information that helps form his or her feelings and values; these remain on a subconscious level and are therefore very difficult to change. Eating habits, then, develop as a complex pattern of feelings, values, and customary behavior.

Abstract knowledge is rarely sufficient in itself to motivate someone to make a change. All the scientific knowledge and reasoning that can be brought to a person's attention will have little effect unless these facts can be related intimately to the individual's culture and eating habits. The person will respond more favorably if new knowledge is presented within the framework of the individual's culture, along with social and psychological conditioning, and situational dimensions. It is essential to encourage whatever good elements are found in the person's present eating pattern and to motivate the individual to change those elements that require alteration.

PROGRESS CHECK ON ACTIVITY 1

SELF-STUDY

Analyze your eating patterns. Be as objective as possible. Answer the following questions about your behaviors.

1. What are the determining factors in the way you eat? _____

_____

_____

2. What are the determining factors in the amount you eat? _____

_____

_____

3. What determines your likes and dislikes? _____

_____

_____

TRUE/FALSE

Circle T for True and F for False.

4. T F Food habits result from human beings' instinctive behavior responses throughout life.
5. T F Social class structure in American society is largely determined by income, occupation, education, and residence.
6. T F Lifestyles change as society's values change.
7. T F From the time of birth, eating is a social act, building on social relationships.
8. T F High-status foods usually become so because they have higher nutritional food values.
9. T F Food fads are usually long lasting and seldom change.

10. T F Special food combinations are effective as reducing diets and have special therapeutic effects.
11. T F Citrus fruits make the body acidic and produce "acid stomach."
12. T F Lean meat does not contribute to sexual potency or virility.
13. T F Gelatin builds strong fingernails.

MULTIPLE CHOICE

Circle the letter of the correct answer.

14. Food fads are likely to develop in response to all of these except:

    a. the striving of aging persons to regain their youth.
    b. different physiological requirements in certain individuals.
    c. peer group pressure on teenagers for social acceptance.
    d. the struggle of obese persons to lose weight.

15. The healthy body requires:

    a. specific foods to control specific functions.
    b. certain food combinations to achieve specific physiological effects.
    c. "natural" foods to prevent disease.
    d. specific nutrients in a number of different foods to perform specific body functions.

16. Which of the following foods carries the most feminine symbolism?

    a. meat
    b. peaches
    c. cheese
    d. bread

17. Food habits in a given culture are largely based on all of these factors except:

    a. food availability and agricultural development.
    b. genetic group differences in food tastes that lead to development of likes and dislikes.
    c. food economics, market practices, and food distribution.
    d. lifestyles and value systems.

18. Which principle(s) should guide the health worker in helping patients with different cultural food habits meet their nutritional needs? (Circle all that apply.)

    a. Learn as much as possible about the person's cultural habits related to nutrition and health.
    b. Encourage traditional practices that are beneficial.
    c. Do not interfere with practices that are harmless.
    d. Try to overcome harmful practices by persuasion and demonstration.

19. Common nutritional problems among the many cultures in the United States include:

    a. obesity.
    b. iron-deficiency anemia.
    c. calcium deficiency.
    d. all of the above

20. Ascorbic acid (vitamin C) deficiency among the lower economic classes is not due to:

    a. dislike of citrus fruits.
    b. inability to digest foods containing vitamin C.
    c. ignorance of the daily need for vitamin C.
    d. lack of funds to purchase citrus fruits.
    e. any of the above.

21. Some diseases that are directly linked to eating patterns in the United States include (circle all that apply):

    a. heart disease.
    b. high blood pressure.
    c. cancer.
    d. diabetes.

ACTIVITY 2:

Some Effects of Culture, Religion, and Geography on Food Behaviors

BASIC CONSIDERATIONS

Large cultural groups are often subdivided into distinctive subcultures in the United States, and each has an effect on the group's eating patterns. While many differences exist among small cultural groups, we will not attempt here to identify each separately. Religious group affiliations within cultural groups also change the patterns of eating as do occupation, income, and social class. Foodways can be changed as family units diversify, either perpetuating or modifying cultural practices. The influence of advertising, the tendency to move long distances, intermarriage, the employment of women, and the disruption of families often lead to more diversity within a group.

When first viewing cultural food practices, it may appear that nutrient intake is substandard. Closer examination, however, often reveals that this is not the case, and that, in fact, the culture has adapted certain practices peculiar to that group that make up for nutrients appearing to be missing or limited in the diet.

REFERENCE TABLES ON FOOD PATTERNS

Table 2-1 describes the typical eating patterns of some prominent cultures in the United States and compares the foods used with the basic four food groups, with comments regarding certain adaptations. Regional differences are noted.

Table 2-2 describes some religious dietary practices.

TABLE 2-1   Comparison of Eating Patterns of Certain U.S. Cultural Groups with the Basic Four Food Groups

Culture Group	Foods Widely Used	Foods Seldom Used	Comments
1. European American a. Western Region	*Meat Group:* beef, pork, poultry, fish, shellfish, eggs *Fruit/Vegetable Group:* all *Bread/Cereal Group:* bulgar, dark breads, wheat *Milk Group:* all cheeses, milk		Western European diet similar to U.S. pattern Rich desserts popular (strudel, kuchen [cake], butterhorns, pies, etc.) Diet tends to be high in fat, sugar
b. Central Region	*Meat Group:* sausages, pork, beef *Fruit/Vegetable Group:* sauerkraut, potatoes, onions, carrots, beans *Bread/Cereal Group:* all dark breads, especially rye *Milk Group:* cheeses more popular than milk		Seasonings include many highly salted items, garlic salt, celery salt, etc. Diet high in sodium
c. Italians	*Meat Group:* spiced sausages, meat sauces with peppers, cheeses, onions, tomato, fish *Fruit/Vegetable Group:* root vegetables, tomatoes *Bread/Cereal Group:* all pasta, yeast breads *Milk Group:* cheese *Other:* olive oil, spices	Milk	Calcium-rich diet Cheeses popular Diet high in sodium
2. Mexican American	*Meat Group:* meat, poultry, eggs (if income permits), dried beans *Fruit/Vegetable Group:* chili peppers, corn, tomatoes, potatoes, onions *Bread/Cereal Group:* tortillas *Milk Group:* cheeses (if income permits)	Milk	Foods are usually fried in animal fats. Green peppers, as well as tomatoes, good source of vitamin C; garlic used heavily. Lime-soaked corn tortillas supply a good course of calcium. Coffee used by children and adults. Diet is high in fat and sodium, low in calcium and folacin.
3. Southern Black	*Meat Group:* dried beans/peas, fish, pork *Fruit/Vegetable Group:* corn, yams, greens *Bread/Cereal Group:* cornbread, biscuits, white bread *Milk Group:* buttermilk occasionally *Other:* heavy seasonings (smoked foods, barbecue sauce, pickled, salt pork cured in brine)	Milk	Long cooking time for vegetables destroys some nutrients. Protein intake may be low if income is low. Common food preparation is frying in lard. All parts of the hog are used. Blacks have high incidence of lactose intolerance. Calcium-rich greens are popular. Diet contains excessive starch, sodium, and fat.
4. Asian a. Cantonese (Southern Chinese)	*Meat Group:* beef, pork, poultry, seafood *Fruit/Vegetable Group:* mushrooms, bean sprouts, Chinese greens, bok choy *Bread/Cereal Group:* rice predominately *Milk Group:* limited quantity ice cream	Milk	All parts of the animal used, including blood. Vegetables are quickly cooked, conserving nutrients. Soy sauce used for seasoning; high salt content in the diet.
b. Northern Chinese	*Meat Group:* beef, poultry, seafood, pork, eggs, tofu *Fruit/Vegetable Group:* soybeans, Chinese greens, bamboo and alfalfa sprouts, bok choy *Bread/Cereal Group:* rice, noodles, bread, dumplings *Milk Group:*	Milk	Diet low in total fat. A high incidence of lactose intolerance is found among the Chinese people. Tea is a favorite beverage. Daily meals try to balance the *yin* (cold) and *yang* (hot) concepts. This is not related to the temperature of foods.

TABLE 2-1   (continued)

Culture Group	Foods Widely Used	Foods Seldom Used	Comments
c. Japanese Americans	*Meat Group:* salt and fresh-water fish, both steamed and eaten raw (sushi); beef, pork, eggs, poultry *Fruit/Vegetable Group:* all vegetables and fruits, soy bean products, sesame seeds *Bread/Cereal Group:* all complex carbohydrates, especially rice *Milk Group:*	Milk	The Issei retains the traditional food pattern: Nisei, Sansei, and especially Yansei likely to mix patterns or follow Western eating patterns. Traditional diet low in total fat, cholesterol, and animal protein (because only small amounts used mixed with other foods). Diet is low in sugar. Tea is a favorite beverage. Soy sauce and teriyaki sauce are used liberally. High incidence of lactose intolerance. The diet is high in sodium. Certain food combinations are thought harmful or healthful, i.e., *harmful:* cherries and milk; *helpful:* pickled plums and rice gruel.
5. Native American a. Reservation and Rural	*Meat Group:* wild game, waterfowl, fish, beef *Fruit/Vegetable Group:* nuts, roots, berries, squash, beans, corn and blue cornmeal *Bread/Cereal Group:* mostly from cornmeal, but wheat products are also used. *Milk Group:*	Milk	Some tribes do not eat fish. Corn and blue cornmeal are used in childbirth and healing practices.
b. City	Generally assimilated into the predominant culture: retains many traditional foods and food practices in home		Restrictions on normally acceptable foods are sometimes imposed by Shaman as a healing in pre- and postnatal periods. High incidence of lactose intolerance among Native American tribes.

TABLE 2-2   Some Religious Practices That Affect Dietary Habits in U.S.

Religion	Foods and Beverages Prohibited	Comments
Orthodox Jewish	All pork and pork products; all fish without scales or fins; improperly slaughtered meats; food containing blood; meats and poultry if combined with dairy products; all milk, cream and other dairy products with a meat meal or for 6 hrs. following	Kosher (Kashruth Laws) regulations are strict regarding slaughter and preparation of animal products and also regulate separation of milk and meat. Certain foods are designated pareve (neutral): fruits, uncooked vegetables, grains, tea, coffee. Two separate sets of dishes, utensils and cooking equipment maintained in kosher households. 24-hour fast on Yom Kippur.
Muslim	All pork and pork products; meat not slaughtered by a Muslim, Jew, or Christian; alcoholic beverages; stimulant beverages	Fast from dawn to dusk during the month of Ramadan (9th month of the Islamic calendar). Only kosher gelatin used: this eliminates marshmallow, gelatin desserts, and many candies. Only vegetable oils used in food preparation.
Seventh Day Adventist	Pork, pork products, shellfish, blood, all flesh foods (if strict), dairy products and eggs (if very strict), highly spiced foods, meat broths, stimulant and alcoholic beverages	Cereal-based beverages used. Children from strict vegetarian homes may be low in some nutrients.
Christian	Meats may be prohibited on certain religious occasions, alcohol and stimulant beverages prohibited by some denominations	Moderation in food and beverage intake is encouraged in amost denominations.

RESPONSIBILITIES OF HEALTH PERSONNEL

Healthcare personnel have often treated clients with the assumption that they all share the same background and value systems. The influence of religion and culture on a client's attitude toward food is often overlooked.

It is not possible to be familiar with the dietary practices of all religions and cultures, and there remains a shortage of published information for the health practitioner on the subject. However, health practitioners need to be aware of dietary variations of groups and the diets most likely to be adhered to in order to give the best treatment. For example, an individual's refusal to eat a particular food or adhere to a particular diet may be due to restrictions imposed by the individual's religion or culture.

Some of the health problems of ethnic groups living in the United States are due to religious and cultural customs, as well as genetic differences. Measures for alleviating some of these problems are discussed below.

1. Those people whose diets may be low in calcium because they are lactose-intolerant can frequently tolerate buttermilk, yogurt, and fermented cheeses.
2. If changes in family eating patterns must be made, include the whole family when possible. In many cultures, children share in the preparation of food.
3. The diets of Native Americans tend to be deficient in calories, calcium, riboflavin, vitamin C, and vitamin A. Native Americans living on reservations show increased incidence of malnutrition, tuberculosis, and diabetes. Children often have kwashiorkor, a severe form of malnutrition. Because of religious as well as social requirements, Native Americans seldom follow a modified diet. Adding hot spices such as chili peppers to the required foods sometimes helps in making foods more acceptable to them.
4. Yin and yang are somewhat complex concepts representing opposite conditions. In the Chinese culture, these conditions should balance each other. Pregnancy and birth are yin conditions for the Chinese. Therefore, the prescribed diet during this period balances out with yang foods. The yang foods given are rich in protein and calcium, which are beneficial. Pregnant women may refuse iron supplements for fear of hardening fetal bones.
5. The typical Chinese diet may be low in protein, calcium, and vitamin D. Many Asians are vegetarians, and when meat is used, it is used in limited quantity. Tofu (soybean curd) is a good source of protein and iron. If calcium salts are used to precipitate curd, tofu is also a good source of calcium. Some milk may be acceptable in custards.
6. Soy sauce is a favorite Asian condiment and should be included in limited amounts instead of eliminated in a sodium-restricted diet. Rice and tea should also be included whenever possible. Alternate seasonings to soy and teriyaki sauce should be encouraged.
7. Garlic, wine, and unsalted tomato puree can be suggested as ways of lowering the high-sodium content of the Italian diet. Elimination of cold cuts and sausages may also be necessary.
8. The Jewish diet will usually be high in saturated fats and cholesterol. Jewish people have a high incidence of diabetes mellitus, obesity, and lactose intolerance. If feeding an orthodox Jewish client in a medical facility, a complete line of kosher frozen foods may have to be purchased. Pareve used on a food label means that the product contains no dairy, meat, or poultry products.
9. The diet of Mexican Americans tends to be high in fats and sodium and low in calcium and folacin. The practice of using the refined wheat tortilla instead of the lime-soaked corn tortilla should be discouraged. If spicy foods are limited or omitted from the Mexican diet, the health practitioner should be aware that this practice will decrease vitamins A and C in the diet, as the red and green peppers used are good sources of these vitamins.
10. Adaptations of diet for Muslims should not be difficult if kosher foods are available. Foods considered as being healthy by Muslims include honey, dates, and sweets. These can be added to the modified diet unless contraindicated (as with diabetes, for example).
11. A hospitalized vegetarian should not have difficulty selecting from a hospital menu. Vegetarian diets, as practiced by religions such as the Seventh Day Adventist, tend to be low in saturated fats and cholesterol and high in fiber. Vegetarians are also taught how to combine plant proteins to obtain adequate essential amino acids. Between-meal feedings are discouraged by the Adventist faith and five- to six-hour meal intervals are practiced. This should be taken into consideration when hospital routine conflicts with their practice.

PROGRESS CHECK ON ACTIVITY 2

QUESTIONS

The following menu is an example of meeting a cultural variation when planning a nutritionally adequate diet for a Native American woman, age 25. Using it as a guide, plan a day's menu that meets the RDAs for any two cultural groups studied in this chapter. State the age, sex, and culture or religion of the group about which you are writing.

Breakfast	Lunch
1 c cornmeal mush	1 slice fried Indian bread
1 tbsp sugar	1 c pinto beans
1 tsp margarine	½ squash
*1 c milk, fresh, or ½ c evaporated	1 apple
	1-½ oz cheese
1 c orange juice	coffee, if desired
coffee, if desired	

	Dinner	Snacks (if desired)

Dinner

3 oz venison roast
½ c fried potatoes
greens of choice
blackberries
yogurt or buttermilk

Snacks (if desired)

any fruits
oatmeal/raisin cookies

*If tolerated

REFERENCES

Archer, S. L. (2004). Differences in food habits and cardiovascular disease risk factors among native Americans with and without diabetes: The inter-tribal heart project. *Public Health Nutrition, 7*: 1025–1032.

Ashley, B. (2004). *Food and Cultural Studies: Studies in Consumption and Markets.* New York: Routledge.

Berner, L. et al. (1999). Food choices for the 21st century. *Journal of Nutraceuticals, Functional Food and Medical Foods, 1*(4): 89.

Chern, W. S. & Rikertsen, K. (Eds.). (2003). *Health, Nutrition and Food Demand.* Cambridge, MA: CABI.

Contento, I. R. (2007). *Nutrition Education: Linking Research, Theory, and Practice.* Sudbury, MA: Jones and Barlett Publishers.

Counihan, C. & Van Esterik, P. (Eds.). (2007). *Food and Culture: A Reader.* (2nd ed.) New York: Routledge.

Drewnowski, A. (1997). Taste preference and food intake. *Annual Review of Nutrition 17*: 237.

Eastwood, M. (2003). *Principles of Human Nutrition.* (2nd ed.). Malden, MA: Blackwell Science.

Elmadfa, I. (Ed.) (2005). *Diet Diversification and Health Promotion.* Basel, NY: Karger.

Franz, M. J. (1997). *Exchange for All Occasions: Your Guide to Choosing Healthy Foods Anytime.* Minneapolis, MN: IDC.

Germov, J. & Williams, L. (Eds.). (2004). *A Sociology of Food & Nutrition: The Social Appetite.* New York: Oxford University Press.

Guillano, M. (2005). *French Women Don't Get Fat.* New York: Knopf.

Kittler, P. G. & Sucher, K. P. (2004). *Food and Culture* (4th ed.). Belmont, CA: Thomson/Wadsworth.

Lallukka, T. (2007). Multiple socio-economic circumstances and healthy food habits. *European Journal of Clinical Nutrition 61*: 701–710.

MacClancy, J., Henry, J. & Macbeth, H. (2007). *Consuming the Inedible: Neglected Dimensions of Food Choice.* New York: Berghahn Books.

MacFie, H., Thomson, D. M. H, & Thomson, J. H. (1994). *Measurement of Food Preference.* London: Blackie Academic.

Mann, J. & Truswell, S. (Eds.). (2007). *Essentials of Human Nutrition.* (3rd ed.). New York: Oxford University Press.

Mela, D. J. (Ed.). (2005). *Food, Diet and Obesity.* Boca Raton, FL: CRC Press.

MyPyramid food guide. www.mypryamid.gov.

Otten, J. J., Pitzi Hellwig, J., & Meyers, L. D. (Eds.). (2006). *Dietary Reference Intakes: The Essential Guide to Nutrient Requirements.* Washington, DC: National Academy Press.

Parasecoli, F. (2008). *Bite Me: Food in Popular Culture.* Oxford, London: Berg.

Pollan, M. (2006). *The Omnivore's Dilemma: A Natural History of Four Meals.* New York: Penguin Press.

Pollan, M. (2008). *In Defense of Food: An Eater's Manifesto.* New York: Penguin Press.

Shils, M. E. et al. (ed.). (1999). *Modern Nutrition in Health and Disease* (9th ed.). Baltimore: Lippincott, William & Wilkins.

Somer, E. (1999). *Food & Mood: The Complete Guide to Eating Well and Feeling Your Best.* New York: Henry Holt.

United States Department of Health and Human Services and United States Department of Agriculture. (2005). *Dietary Guidelines for Americans* (6th ed.). Washington, DC: Government Publishing Office. www.healthypeople.gov.

United States National Cholesterol Education Program (NCEP), National Heart, Lung, and Blood Institute (NHLBI), National Institutes of Health (NIH). (2001). Third report of the expert panel on detection, evaluation, and treatment of high blood cholesterol in adults (Adult Treatment Panel III). www.NIH.gov.

Webster-Gandy, J., Madden, A. & Holdworth, M. (Eds.). (2006). *Oxford Handbook of Nutrition and Dietetics.* Oxford, London: Oxford University Press.

CHAPTER 3

Proteins and Health

Time for completion
Activities: 1 hour
Optional examination: ½ hour

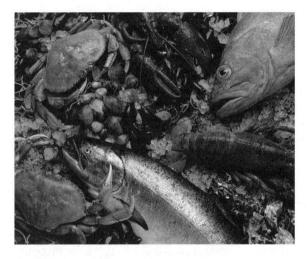

OBJECTIVES

Upon completion of this chapter the student should be able to do the following:

1. Identify the structure of proteins and their fuel value.
2. Define complete and incomplete protein and essential amino acids.
3. Discuss protein quality and the concept of limiting amino acids.
4. Describe the amino acid requirements of humans and their RDAs for protein.
5. Explain the method of measuring protein in the body.
6. Summarize the major functions and food sources of protein.
7. Analyze the all-or-none law in protein metabolism and the concept of protein sparing.
8. Recognize various vegetarian diet regimes and their relationship to adequate protein intake.
9. Compare the effects on health of inadequate or excessive protein intake.
10. Specify certain conditions where alteration in protein intake may be needed.

GLOSSARY

Amino acids: compounds containing nitrogen that are the building blocks of the protein molecule.

Antibody: a protein substance produced within the body that destroys or weakens harmful bacteria.

Biologic value of protein (BV): the ability of a protein to support the formation of body tissue.

Complementary proteins: two or more protein foods whose amino acid compositions complement each other so that one has what the other lacks.

Complete protein: a protein containing all the essential amino acids.

Essential amino acids: amino acids that cannot be synthesized by the body and must be provided by food.

Immobility: the condition of being inactive owing to disability, such as that experienced by the person confined to bed or a wheelchair.

Incomplete protein: a protein lacking one or more of the essential amino acids or containing some of the amino acids in only very small amounts.

Kwashiorkor: a severe protein deficiency disease that occurs in infancy or early childhood and in high-risk hospitalized patients.

Marasmus: a condition characterized by a loss of flesh and strength due to underfeeding; a lack of sufficient calories for a prolonged period of time.

Meat analogs: *See* TVP.

Nonessential amino acids: amino acids that can be synthesized by the body to meet its needs.

Synthesis: the process of building complex compounds from simple ones when they are furnished to the body.

Textured vegetable protein (TVP): protein that is drawn from plant protein, spun into fibers, and manufactured into products that imitate animal protein foods. Also called meat analogs.

Vegetarianism: the practice of eating no animal flesh.

BACKGROUND INFORMATION

Genetics involves the passing of characteristics from one generation to the next. These characteristics make a person unique. The entire genetic process creates one important substance: protein. Each protein molecule is made of many units, called amino acids. There are 20 to 25 different amino acids in nature. The word protein comes from the Greek word *protos*, which means *primary*.

All living substances, including plants and viruses, contain protein. Approximately 18% to 20% of the human body is protein. It is present in all body tissues and fluids except bile and urine. Protein is made up of about 16% nitrogen, in both body tissue and food. The quantity of protein in a given sample, therefore, is measured by the amount of nitrogen it contains. Nitrogen or protein balance of the body is an important factor in determining the body's health.

Protein is an important factor in the American diet. Individuals' use and abuse of protein due to misconceptions and inaccurate information about it have led to unusual and sometimes dangerous eating practices. Many athletes take powdered protein supplements in the hope of increasing their muscle size or strength. The liquid-protein crash diets many people have tried have caused some deaths. Some types of protein foods are completely avoided by some religious sects. The use of protein foods to denote masculinity (meats) and femininity (eggs, milk), and for status symbols (lobster instead of sardines) is significant in learning about people's lifestyles and cultural patterns.

The role that protein plays in the healthy diet is an important one, but should not be exaggerated. Without an adequate supply of this essential compound, all growth, repair, and maintenance of the body cells cease, and the body dies. On the other hand, excessive consumption of protein, or protein foods eaten to the exclusion of other types of food, is not healthy.

All proteins are not alike. The health practitioner needs a thorough knowledge of the functions, requirements, and sources of protein to counsel clients on how to meet their protein needs.

ACTIVITY 1:

Protein as a Nutrient

DEFINITIONS, ESSENTIALITY, AND REQUIREMENT

Proteins are composed of carbon, hydrogen, oxygen, and nitrogen; they provide the foundation for every cell in the body. Proteins are broken down to amino acids by the body.

Amino acids are classified as essential—that which cannot be produced by the body and must be obtained from food; and nonessential—that which can be produced by the body.

Proteins are also categorized as complete or incomplete. Whether a protein food can be used for the growth and repair of tissue depends upon its biological value. Proteins of high biological value are complete proteins and contain all essential amino acids in adequate amounts to promote growth. Those of low biological value are called incomplete proteins; they may not supply all the essential amino acids or may supply some of them in limited amounts.

The essential amino acid that provides the least adequate kind of protein in meeting human nutritional needs is termed the limiting amino acid. In a complete protein, the limiting amino acid poses no problem. In an incomplete protein, the limiting amino acid is responsible for the poor utilization of its fellow essential amino acids.

Individuals consuming this incomplete protein must be provided a source of the limiting amino acid. Animal proteins (except gelatin) are complete proteins; vegetable proteins (for example, dried beans and peas) are incomplete.

Protein of high biologic value can result from complementary mixtures of vegetable proteins, in which one vegetable protein supplies the amino acid that the other vegetable protein is lacking.

Foods containing a combination of the essential amino acids from plant sources need to be consumed over the course of a day. A pool of essential amino acids must be present in the blood to make complete proteins for protein synthesis. Therefore, the complete proteins should be mixed with the incomplete ones in order to achieve adequate growth and repair. Vegetarians must be especially careful to consume complementary proteins. The recommended daily protein intake for adults is 0.8 g per kg of body weight. Clinical factors such as surgery, burns, disease, medications (such as chemotherapy), and fevers will increase the protein need. The extent of increase should be predicated on the individual problem. Pregnancy and lactation require more protein; RDA requirements are set at 15 to 20 g above those for the nonpregnant adult female, but should be altered according to individual need. Requirements during infancy, childhood, and adolescence vary with the growth pattern. Daily protein intake should be in the form of complete good-quality protein and/or complementary protein foods.

PROTEIN SPARING

There are 20 to 25 amino acids, 20 of which are commonly found in food. When an amino acid is considered nonessential, it can be produced by the body using available oxygen, carbon, hydrogen, and nitrogen. Essential amino acids must be supplied by the diet. Eight essential amino acids are required by adults; nine are required by infants.

The distinction between essential and nonessential requires further amplification. Individuals cannot survive without a dietary supply of the proper amounts of the essential amino acids. However, our bodies need the nonessential amino acids to achieve optimal protein metabolism. Biochemically, we need the carbon skeleton and amino groups of the essential and nonessential amino acids, respectively.

It is of great importance, then, to have good sources of both essential and nonessential amino acids to provide sufficient nitrogen. The ratio of ingested amino acids, which is dependent on adequate food sources, must be present in proper proportion to permit efficient manufacture and repair of all the tissues in the body. In addition, there must be sufficient carbohydrate available to meet energy needs; otherwise, body protein will be broken down for energy use. This is the protein-sparing action of carbohydrate that is discussed in Chapter 4. Most edible plant products contain more carbohydrate than protein which is incomplete. However, animal or muscle foods contain only little carbohydrate and a large amount of protein which is complete. Thus, a diet containing both plant and animal products means we will consume an adequate amount of complete protein and carbohydrate. The animal protein will complete the inadequate amino acids pattern of plants, and plant sources will provide the needed carbohydrates. Clinical evidence indicates that the human body can deteriorate when fed only essential amino acids.

FUNCTIONS, STORAGE, SOURCES, AND UTILIZATION

Functions

The main function of protein is to provide the body with the amino acids necessary for growth and maintenance of body tissues. Cells, enzymes, hormones, antibodies, muscles, blood, and all tissues and fluid except bile and urine require protein.

Storage

Proteins in the form of amino acids are the building blocks of the body. Protein as such is not stored; therefore, a daily intake is required.

Sources

Animal sources of protein include milk and milk products, meat, fish, poultry, and eggs. Plant sources include breads and cereal products, legumes, nuts and seeds, and textured vegetable protein. Cereal grains are the primary source of protein for the majority of the world's population. The production of large animals for protein will become less practical as the world's population grows and space for humans must take precedence over space for raising large animals.

The health practitioner should be familiar with the complementary proteins in foods. Animal protein is relatively expensive. As the world's protein supply diminishes, an understanding of complementarity will become increasingly important. The proper mixing of ingested plant protein foods can provide nutritional value similar to that of animal protein.

Adequate amounts of high-quality protein are not difficult to obtain in diets that contain dairy products and eggs. However, achieving nutritional balance in a strict vegetarian diet requires considerable knowledge of the contributions of various foods to our dietary requirements. Activity 2 discusses the use of vegetarian diets.

Utilization

To be absorbed, proteins must be broken down to individual amino acids or small peptides (by-products of protein digestion composed of 2 to 10 amino acids).

The products of protein digestion are absorbed into the bloodstream as amino acids and are transported via the portal vein to the liver and then to all the body cells. Some amino acids stay in the liver to form liver tissue itself or to produce a wide variety of blood proteins. The remaining amino acids circulate in the bloodstream, from which they are rapidly removed and utilized by the tissues.

When amino acids are broken down, the nitrogen-containing part is split off from the carbon chain. Most of the nitrogen is converted to urea in the liver and excreted via the kidneys. Then the carbon-containing portion that remains is utilized for energy. Proteins provide 4 kcal per g, the same as carbohydrates.

AMINO ACID SUPPLEMENTS

Of all the supplements that have come to market since people have been attempting to find magic bullets to prevent aging, increase their libido, and improve their bodies, amino acid supplements have been at the top of the list. This phenomenon has been greatly enhanced by competitive athletes, both professional and amateur, and their coaches. Some 25 to 30 amino acid supplement advertisements can be found in any one body building or popular health magazine each month. Two major reasons are given by athletes for using amino acid supplements: (1) the belief that it gives them the "competitive" edge, and (2) the belief that amino acids build muscle and are a major energy source. Neither of these beliefs is correct. Exercise builds muscle, not protein, and carbohydrates are the body's major energy source. Excess protein (amino acids) is detrimental in that it places an undue burden on the kidneys to excrete the excess nitrogen, and on the metabolism of the body. Excess protein will also convert to fat.

Two other groups most vulnerable to the claims made by companies for their products are the elderly, who are attempting to avoid health problems and retain their youth, and persons with chronic diseases or terminal diseases such as AIDS.

Nutritional supplements have never been regulated by the FDA, and so have not been evaluated for safety or effectiveness. With the passage of the 1994 Supplement Bill (see Chapter 1), they will now come under that scrutiny. This may control future product development and sales, but the existing supplements are not covered, and there are at least 300 of these supplements already on the market. The burden of proof for health claims made for supplements will fall on the FDA, and these criteria are still to be determined. It will take a few more years before the public will know which ones are safe and effective. In the meantime, all health professionals should be aware of the attitudes and beliefs of many of their clients and should attempt to educate them about potential health risks.

PROGRESS CHECK ON ACTIVITY 1

SHORT ANSWERS

1. Keep a 24-hour food record.

   a. List all the complete proteins you consumed.

   _____

   _____

   _____

   b. List all the incomplete proteins you consumed.

   _____

   _____

   _____

   c. Identify which food(s) has the highest quality protein. _____

   _____

2. Why is it important to spread consumption of good-quality protein throughout the day?

   _____

   _____

3. Is protein deficiency common in the United States?

   _____

MULTIPLE CHOICE

Circle the letter of the correct answer.

4. Substances are classified as protein when they contain:

   a. carbon, oxygen, and nitrogen.
   b. carbon, oxygen, hydrogen, and sulfur.
   c. carbon, hydrogen, oxygen, and nitrogen.
   d. carbon, calcium, phosphorus, and iron.

5. Adults require _____ essential amino acids, and infants require _____ essential amino acids.

   a. 8, 7
   b. 8, 9
   c. 7, 8
   d. 6, 7

6. An amino acid is said to be essential if it:

   a. is needed by the body.
   b. cannot be synthesized by the body.
   c. contains vitamins and minerals.
   d. combines with nonessential amino acids.

7. On days when a person exercises strenuously, his or her protein intake should be:

a. increased greatly.
b. reduced sharply.
c. about the same as usual.
d. reduced by half.

8. For protein synthesis to occur:

a. all the essential amino acids must be present.
b. sufficient nitrogen to form nonessential amino acids is needed.
c. the diet must have adequate calories from carbohydrate and fat.
d. all of the above.

TRUE/FALSE

Circle T for True and F for False.

9. T F Foods of animal origin contain substantial quantities of high-quality protein.
10. T F Malnutrition affects physical and mental development.

ACTIVITY 2:

Meeting Protein Needs and Vegetarianism

REQUIREMENTS FOR PROTEIN AND AMINO ACIDS

Recommended protein intakes are based on the amount of nitrogen (quantity) and kind of amino acids (quality) consumed. The quantitative value of protein foods is made by comparing the amount of protein in a serving of food to the amount required by humans. Animal protein sources are highly concentrated, with the single exception of bacon, which is considered a fat in the Food Exchange Lists. Soybean products are quite concentrated in protein, although they contain a limiting amino acid, which reduces the quality of the product.

The protein content of some common foods is compared in Table 3-1.

The quality of a protein is dependent upon the essential amino acids it contains compared to the essential amino acid needs of the body. Quality is sometimes expressed as biological value (BV). This is a measure of the body's retention of the nitrogen contained in the ingested protein. Eggs, with a BV of 100, have the highest quality of any dietary proteins. Milk, at 93, follows a close second. Most meats, fish, and poultry have a BV of about 75. Any BV of 70 or above is considered sufficient for sustaining growth and maintenance of body tissue. Requirements for protein differ by age, sex, and physical state of the body. Factors influencing protein utilization can be modified by the digestibility of the protein and the overall composition of the diet, as well as the source of the protein and its amino acid balance.

The RDA for protein is set by nitrogen-balance studies. A healthy adult should be in nitrogen balance. When new tissue is being formed, the body retains more nitrogen than it excretes, creating a positive nitrogen balance. This is the case during periods of growth such as pregnancy and childhood. Negative nitrogen balance occurs when muscles are breaking down, such as with bedridden persons or when very low-calorie reducing diets are used. More nitrogen is excreted than is taken in.

To calculate the protein need of an adult, we need two items of information:

• Body weight, using the body mass index (*see* Chapter 7).
• The requirement of protein per kg body weight.

Accordingly for an adult 19–30 years of age, the (Dietary Reference Intakes/Estimated Average Requirement) DRI/EAR is:

• Man: 0.66 g/kg/day
• Nonpregnant woman: 0.66/kg/day
• Pregnant woman: 0.88/kg/day
• Lactating woman: 1.05/kg/day

For details on the protein requirements (DRI/RDA) for different age groups (males and females), consult the Web site www.nas.edu.

TABLE 3-1 Protein Content of Some Selected Foods Using the Exchange List Values*

Food	Serving Size	Protein (g)
Cheese, cheddar	1 oz	7
Cheese, cottage	¼ c	7
Cheese, parmesan, grated	2 tbsp	7
Milk	1 c	8
Egg	1	7
Asparagus, cooked	½ c	2
Leafy green vegetable, cooked	½ c	2
raw	1 c	2
Green peas, cooked	½ c	3
Potato, baked	1 small	3
Squash, winter, cooked	1 c	3
Beef, pork, lamb	1 oz	7
Poultry	1 oz	7
Bread	1 slice	3
Crackers, saltines	4	3
Wild game, any	1 oz	7
Fish, any	1 oz	7
Tuna, canned	¼ c	7
Peanut butter	1 tbsp	7
Tomato juice/vegetable juice	½ c	2
Broccoli, cooked	½ c	2

*This list does not differentiate the amount or type of fat in any of the products, the biological value, or amino acid balance. Modified from data in Appendix F.

The requirement for protein and each essential amino acid varies with age in absolute and relative quantities. Approximately 40% of an infant's protein must be from essential amino acids, but only 20% for an adult. A food that may be an adequate protein source for adults may be inadequate for the young child. Protein requirements increase in certain kinds of illnesses or malnutrition.

Protein consumption in the United States is quite high, ranging between 100 to 120 g per day. This exceeds the DRI/RDAs shown previously. Approximately two thirds of the protein consumed in the United States is from animal sources. Excess protein intake has raised questions about health risks. These risks will be discussed later in this activity.

For optimal use of protein, intake should be spread throughout the day rather than being consumed at one meal.

VEGETARIANISM: RATIONALE AND CLASSIFICATION

There are many reasons why individuals eliminate animal foods from their diets. The most common reasons are economic concerns, religious guidelines, health considerations, and concern for animal life.

When a vegetarian consumes no meat, fowl, or fish as food, the further restrictions on the remaining part of the diet can be classified as follows:

1. Fruitarians: individuals who eat only fruit.
2. Vegans: individuals who eat no animal flesh nor any food of animal origin. They are sometimes called strict vegetarians.
3. Lacto-vegetarians: individuals who eat plant proteins, and also use milk.
4. Ovo-vegetarians: individuals who eat plant proteins, as well as eggs.
5. Lacto-ovo-vegetarians: individuals who eat both milk and eggs along with plant proteins.

Semivegetarians restrict red meats only—that is, beef, pork, lamb, and game animals. Fish, poultry, dairy foods, eggs, and plants furnish proteins for their diet.

VEGETARIANISM: DIET EVALUATION

Generally, the more restrictive the vegetarian's diet is, the more likely it is to be deficient in one or more major nutrients. The simplest and easiest of the vegetarian diets to balance is the lacto-ovo-vegetarian, with its use of eggs and milk. This diet offers high-quality protein for both children and adults, but may be low in iron if nonmeat sources of this mineral are not included. Both milk and eggs are poor sources of iron. A high intake of legumes, seeds, nuts, and enriched grains will increase iron intake substantially. Vegetarian diets may contain so much bulk that the stomachs of children are full before they get enough calories. If this happens, protein may be inefficiently used for energy instead of building. The semiveg-etarian diet presents no nutritional problems, if the iron intake is sufficient.

Those people who follow either lacto- or ovo-vegetarian diets must plan more carefully. While the protein content of either diet is adequate, the ovo-vegetarian may be low in calcium and phosphorus intake because of avoidance of milk. Cases of rickets (vitamin D deficiency disease) have been reported in vegetarian children who have no milk intake.

The strict vegetarian (vegan) diet presents several problems. It tends to be low in calcium, vitamin D, vitamin B_{12}, riboflavin, and zinc. None of the vegetable sources furnishes adequate calcium. Calcium is poorly absorbed from vegetables because of the fiber content of the calcium-binding oxalic acid found in some greens. Also, a vegan may be lacking in vitamin D, since it is obtained from animal sources only. If the person does not receive adequate sunlight, which can help vitamin D synthesis under the skin, any existing calcium deficiency will be compounded by a dietary lack of vitamin D.

Problems with protein quality and quantity often occur among vegans. If vegetables and cereals are the only sources of protein, not only will they be of low quality but the digestibility factor is often low. Because of high fiber content, many nonmeat sources are not well digested. Beans are especially difficult for children. Although soybean protein is fairly similar to animal protein, its low digestibility and a lack of flavor prohibit its consumption as such. Soybeans are usually consumed in a highly processed and value-added form, for example, tofu or soy milk. Soy products are derived from soybeans; they are not soybeans. Also, soybeans contain a trypsin inhibitor that interferes with the function of trypsin, a major enzyme for digesting protein. Some vegetarian children tend to be smaller and show symptoms of undernutrition, but nutrient deficiencies vary with the number of dietary items restricted and the children's overall meal plans. Complementary protein mixes do not give an amino acid pattern fully usable by the body as animal protein does, but correct combinations can increase protein quality by up to 50%. Children should not be put on a vegan diet unless medical and nutritional expertise is available to monitor their health. When foods are chosen wisely, a vegetarian child can meet his or her nutritional needs.

Vegetarianism, when properly managed, can be a healthy way to eat. Children are especially at high risk of failure to thrive if they are not supplemented with fortified foods containing essential nutrients missing from their diets. Vegetarians may be at lower risk for gastrointestinal disorders (such as constipation, diverticulitis) and colon cancer because of the high fiber content of the diet. On the other hand, osteoporosis, which affects three out of five women over the age of 60, is a high risk factor among many vegetarians. The avoidance of animal products with their high saturated fat content may lower the risk of coronary heart disease. Because of less fat in the diet, vegetarians also tend to have a lower incidence of obesity.

VEGETARIANISM: DIET PLANNING

To assure adequate intake of nutrients, vegetarians must carefully follow certain guidelines:

1. Include 2 c legumes daily to meet calcium and iron requirements.
2. Include 1 c dark greens daily to meet iron requirements for women.
3. Include at least 1 tbsp fat daily for proper absorption of vitamins.

Tables 3-2 and 3-3 indicate the food groups for lacto-ovo- and strict vegetarians. Table 3-4 provides sample menus.

Figure 3-1 shows some complementary protein combinations. There are many vegetarian cookbooks available today. They have also become quite popular among non-vegetarians who wish to change their eating patterns by increasing fiber and lowering cholesterol and saturated fat. Evaluation of some of the recipes included is advised before choosing a cookbook, because not all of them meet the criteria of the dietary guidelines.

The health professional should be aware that some vegetarians believe that all medical problems can be prevented or cured by their diet and fail to seek help when they need it.

While some religious groups that are vegetarian or semivegetarian show a lower incidence of certain diseases that afflict the U.S. population (such as colon cancer, coronary heart disease), it must be remembered that these groups' general lifestyles also differ from others.

TABLE 3-2   Food Groups for Lacto-Ovo-Vegetarians

Food Groups	Major Products	Daily Servings
Meat equivalents	Legumes, peas and beans, nuts, textured vegetable proteins (soy meat analogs and other formulated plant protein products and spun soy isolates), eggs	2
Milk and dairy products	Milk, cheese, yogurt, many other milk products (8 oz = 1 serving)	2
Breads and cereals	All varieties	4–6
Fruits and vegetables	All varieties	Vegetables: 3 Fruits: 1–3

TABLE 3-3   Food Groups for Strict Vegetarians

Food Groups	Major Products	Daily Servings
Meat equivalents	Legumes, peas and beans, nuts, textured vegetable proteins (soy meat analogs and other formulated plant protein products and spun soy isolates)	*2
Milk equivalents	Soybean milk, preferably fortified with calcium, vitamins B_2 and B_{12} (if not fortified, supplements, especially vitamin B_{12}, may be necessary)* (8 oz = 1 serving)	*2
Breads and cereals	All varieties	4–6
Fruits and vegetables	All varieties	Vegetables: 4 Fruits: 1–4**

*Nut milks are nutritionally inadequate, especially for infants.
**Including a source of vitamin C.

TABLE 3-4   Sample Vegetarian Menus

Vegan	Lacto-Ovo-Vegetarian
Breakfast	
Orange juice	Orange juice
Oatmeal/honey	Cheese/mushroom omelet
Soy milk	Whole wheat toast
Toasted soy wheat bread	Tea
Tea	
Lunch	
Split pea soup	Split pea soup
Peanut butter sandwich on soy wheat bread	Peanut butter sandwich on wheat bread
Fruit salad with sunflower seeds	Fruit and cottage cheese
Almonds/raisins	Salad/mayonnaise
Tea	Milk
Dinner	
Vegetable soup	Vegetable soup
Green salad with nuts and seeds	Green salad with nuts and seeds
Soybean croquettes fried in oil	Whole wheat bread with margarine
Pears	Yogurt with oranges and strawberries
Soybean milk	Tea or milk

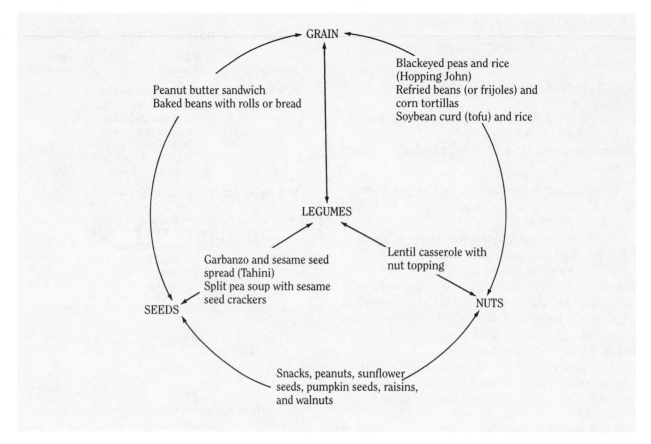

FIGURE 3-1   **Complementary Vegetable Proteins**
Examples of Common Foods Eaten Together That Supply Essential Amino Acids

They generally avoid tobacco and alcohol, suffer few stresses, and exercise regularly. These factors contribute to a lower risk for these diseases.

It is not possible to document that a vegetarian diet alone promotes better health, but this practice together with other lifestyle changes may lead to healthy habits.

EXCESSIVE AND DEFICIENT PROTEIN INTAKE

Normal tissue growth in infancy and childhood and during pregnancy and lactation requires more amino acids than those needed for tissue maintenance. As has been demonstrated in many laboratory studies, in the absence of adequate protein, growth is slowed down or even stopped.

The feeding of infants in strict vegetarian families is of particular concern to the health professional. If breastfeeding is not possible, a formula such as nutritionally fortified soybean milk should be provided. The soybean formula fortified with vitamin B_{12} should continue to be given by cup after the child is weaned. A wide variety of foods should be chosen, with emphasis on those that are high in iron and vitamins A, B complex, and C. In addition to soybean milk, mixtures of legumes and cereals are needed to supply sufficient protein.

Excesses

Questions raised about excessive protein intake of Americans include the following:

1. Excess nitrogen must be cleared by the kidneys. This may negatively affect kidneys that are malfunctioning, damaged, or underdeveloped.
2. High protein consumption has recently been cited as one factor in bone demineralization, especially if coupled with low calcium intake.
3. While inconclusive at this time, research indicates that high protein consumption may increase risks of colon cancer by changing the internal environment and altering the bacteria of the colon.
4. Large amounts of protein, especially of animal origin, also contain saturated fats. Most authorities are convinced that saturated fats contribute to a high incidence of heart disease.
5. Since excess protein from any source is converted to fat and stored as adipose tissue, it can contribute to obesity.

Deficiencies

Large losses of protein may occur during illness or surgical procedures. These situations require substantial increases in protein consumption. Lack of increased protein intake during illness will result in delayed wound healing, slow convalescing, low resistance to infections, and inability to return to optimum health.

Protein energy malnutrition (PEM) is the most serious and widespread deficiency disease in developing countries. The two major types are nutritional marasmus, due primarily to caloric deficiency, and kwashiorkor, due primarily to a deficiency of protein.

The clinical features of kwashiorkor and marasmus are illustrated in Figure 3-2. Although they are treated as two separate diseases, they are closely related. Diets low in calories will almost always be low in protein. Even if there is adequate protein, the body will use it for energy instead of for growth and development.

While primarily considered a child's disease, PEM also develops in adults. Adults with PEM exhibit weight loss, fatigue, and other symptoms of acute malnutrition. A low intake of protein and calories also results in the deficiency of three nutrients: vitamin A, iron (causing anemia), and iodine (causing endemic goiter). Vitamin A, being a fat-soluble vitamin, will be low in a protein-restricted diet. Vitamin A deficiency negatively affects growth, skin, and vision, sometimes causing blindness. Many women die in childbirth from low iron levels. If there is an infection from parasites such as hookworm, even less iron is available. PEM will produce stunted growth and mental retardation. A malnourished woman is likely to give birth to a premature, often retarded infant with less resistance to infection and illness. Poorly nourished persons have a shortened life expectancy, and common childhood diseases are often fatal to the malnourished child. Enzyme and hormone production is inadequate in these victims. Although they badly need extra nutrients, they are unable to digest and absorb them.

Some infants are born with an inability to metabolize phenylalanine, an essential amino acid. Mental retardation results if the disease is not treated. Phenylketonuria will be discussed in Part IV. The protein in specific foods is considered to be the cause of food allergies. In this case, careful addition of protein foods to an infant's diet must be practiced.

RESPONSIBILITIES OF HEALTH PERSONNEL

The health professional should do the following:

1. Recommend moderate amounts of animal protein. Excess protein is wasteful, since the excess is converted to energy, and excess energy is converted to fat. Protein food is an expensive form of energy.
2. Be aware that protein foods are not low in calories. They provide the same number of calories per gram as carbohydrates. Furthermore, protein foods from animal sources (such as meats, cheese) frequently contain excessive calories from fat.
3. Advise clients to eat good-quality protein at each meal to provide a consistent supply of essential amino acids. Protein cannot be stored in the body and is used constantly in its major functions.

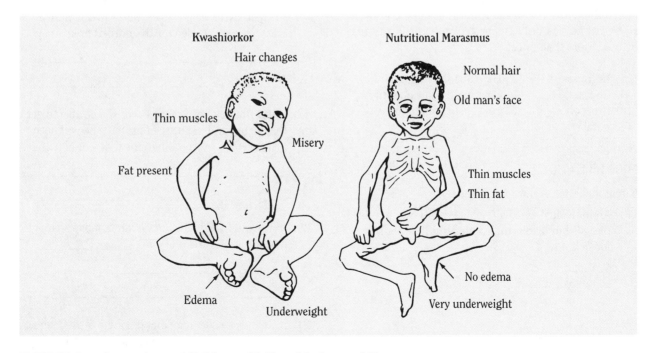

FIGURE 3-2   Comparison of Children with Kwashiorkor and Marasmus
Source: D. B. Jelliffe. Clinical Nutrition in Developing Countries, 1968. U.S. Department of Health, Education and Welfare, Public Health Service.

4. Plan some meals for clients around complementary vegetable protein foods for variety, economy, and increased fiber.
5. Be aware that meals containing legumes and grains are very nourishing and less expensive than meals containing meat.
6. Be aware of the importance of eating extra protein during illnesses, which cause excessive breakdown of body tissue.
7. Recognize that certain illnesses require alterations in amounts and types of protein ingested.
8. Ask clients questions regarding their use of supplements and advise them of any undesirable side effects.

PROGRESS CHECK ON ACTIVITY 2

MATCHING

Match the nutrient listed in Column A to the statement that best describes it in Column B. Terms may be used more than once.

Column A	Column B
1. Calcium	a. Strict vegetarian diets are at risk of being deficient in this nutrient.
2. Vitamin A	
3. Iron	
4. Vitamin B$_{12}$	b. Strict vegetarian diets are generally adequate in this nutrient.
5. Thiamin	
6. Riboflavin	
7. Vitamin D	

Match the food item on the left to the statement on the right that best describes its protein content. Terms may be used more than once.

8. Legumes	a. High quality, high quantity
9. Cheese	b. Low quality, low quantity
10. Broccoli	c. Low quality, high quantity
11. Potato	
12. Tuna	

MULTIPLE CHOICE

Circle the letter of the correct answer.

13. An individual who will not eat meat, fish, poultry, or eggs but drinks milk with his or her plant foods is a(n):

a. vegan.
b. ovo-vegetarian.
c. fruitarian.
d. lacto-vegetarian.

TRUE/FALSE

Circle T for True and F for False.

14. T F Excessive protein intake may place a strain on the kidneys.

Case Study

Mary and Leon are married college students, both 21 years of age. They are living on a limited income and became vegetarians 2 years ago when they became involved in the ecological movement on campus. Mary, who at 5'9" weighs 110 lb., has just discovered that she is pregnant with her first child. She requests advice about an appropriate diet. Using the above information and research data from other sources (other chapters in this book, instructor, relevant Web sites, and so on), answer the following:

15. List other data you will need to gather about her diet habits before you can assist her. _____

_____

_____

16. What is the basic nutritional increase she will need during her pregnancy? How much increase?

_____

_____

17. What is her general protein requirement according to her weight? _____

_____

_____

18. Is her weight appropriate for her height? Should she gain extra weight over the 24 to 30 lb. increase recommended for the normal pregnancy?

_____

_____

19. If she and Leon are vegans, will she be able to get the quality and quantity of protein she will need? List several food combinations that would help.

_____

_____

20. Why would adequate carbohydrate foods be important in her prenatal diet? _____

_____

_____

21. If she has an adequate diet during her pregnancy, will she be in positive or negative nitrogen balance? Explain your answer. _____

_____

_____

REFERENCES

Anderson, G. H. (2004). Dietary proteins in the regulation of food intake and body weight in humans. *Journal of Nutrition, 134*: 974s–979s.

Bauer, J. D. (2007). Nutritional status of patients who have fallen in an acute care setting. *Journal of Human Nutrition and Dietetics, 20*: 558–554.

Bilsborough, S. (2006). A review of issues of dietary protein intake in humans. *International Journal of Sport Nutrition and Exercise Metabolism, 16*: 129–152.

Caballero, B., Allen, L., & Prentice, A. (Eds.). (2005). *Encyclopedia of Human Nutrition* (2nd ed.). Boston: Elsevier/Academic Press.

Di Pasquale, M. (2008). *Amino Acids and Proteins for the Athlete: The Anabolic Edge* (2nd ed.) Boca Raton, FL: CRC Press.

Driskell, J. A. (2007). *Sports Nutrition: Fats and Proteins.* Boca Raton, FL: CRC Press.

Eastwood, M. (2003). *Principles of Human Nutrition* (2nd ed.). Malden, MA: Blackwell Science.

Houston, M. S., Holly, J. M. P., & Feldman, E. L. (2006). *IGF and Protein in Health and Disease.* Totowa, NJ: Humana Press.

Kerstetter, J. E. (2006). Meat and soy protein affect calcium homostasis in healthy women. *Journal of Nutrition, 136*: 1890–1895.

Li, P. (2007). Amino acids and immune function. *British Journal of Nutrition, 98*: 237–252.

Ling, J. R. (Ed.). (2007). *Dietary Protein Research Trends.* New York: Nova Science.

Mann, J. & Truswell, S. (Eds.). (2007). *Essentials of Human Nutrition* (3rd ed.). New York: Oxford University Press.

Martin, D. S. (2003). Dietary protein and hypertension: Where do we stand? *Nutrition, 19*: 385–389.

Miller, G. D., Janis, J. K., & McBean, L. D. (2007). *Handbook of Dairy Foods and Nutrition* (3rd ed.). Boca Raton, FL: CRC Press.

Otten, J. J., Hellwig, J. P., & Meyers, L. D. (Eds.). (2006). *Dietary Reference Intake: The Essential Guide to Nutrient Requirements.* Washington, DC: National Academics Press.

Randi, G. (2007). Lipid, protein and carbohydrate intake in relation to body mass index: an Italian study. *Public Health Nutrition, 10*: 306–310.

Roboud-Ravaux, M. (Ed.). (2002). *Protein Degradation in Health and Disease.* New York: Springer.

Rose, H. J. (2005). Fat intake of children with PKU on low phenylalanine diets. *Journal of Human Nutrition and Dietetics, 18*: 395–400.

Stipanuk, M. H. (Ed.). (2006). *Biochemical, Physiological and Molecular Aspects of Human Nutrition* (2nd ed.). St. Louis, MO: Elsevier Sauders.

Tores, N. (2007). The role of dietary protein in lipotoxicity. *Nutrition Reviews, 65*: s64–s68.

CHAPTER 4

Carbohydrates and Fats: Implications for Health

Time for completion
Activities: 1 hour
Optional examination: ½ hour

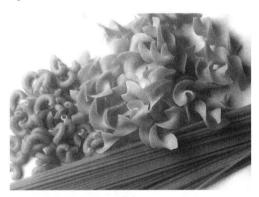

OBJECTIVES

Carbohydrates and Health

Upon completion of this chapter the student should be able to do the following:

1. Identify the types of carbohydrates, their fuel value, and storage methods.
2. Summarize the major functions and food sources of carbohydrates.
3. Discuss nutritive and nonnutritive sweeteners.
4. Evaluate blood glucose level as an indicator of certain body conditions.
5. Define fiber and list its functions and food sources.
6. Discuss health problems associated with excess sugar or low-fiber intake.
7. Describe the effects of carbohydrate consumption on athletic activity.

Fats and Health

Upon completion of this chapter the student should be able to do the following:

1. Classify fats and state their fuel value.
2. List the major functions and food sources of fats.
3. Discuss body utilization of essential fatty acids and cholesterol.
4. Explain the difference between saturated and unsaturated fatty acids and identify their food sources.
5. Evaluate storage of fat in the body and the relationship of fat to normal body weight.
6. Relate a body's health to excess total fat intake and excess saturated fat intake.

GLOSSARY

Carbohydrates

Cellulose: a fibrous form of carbohydrate that makes up the framework of a plant. A component of fiber.

Complex carbohydrates: a class of carbohydrates called polysaccharides; foods composed of starch and cellulose.

Cruciform: cross shaped; bearing a cross. The name *cruciferous* is given to certain vegetables, namely broccoli, cabbage, Brussels sprouts, and cauliflower. These plants have four-petaled flowers that resemble a cross, hence the botanical name *cruciferal*, and the term *cruciferous vegetables*.

Diabetes mellitus: a condition characterized by an elevated level of sugar in blood and urine, increased urination, and increased intake of both fluid and food, with an absolute or relative insulin deficiency. Complications include heart disease, high blood pressure, and kidney disease. Diabetes can cause blindness and is frequently associated with severe infections.

Diverticulitis: inflammation of the sacs that form at weakened points along the colon lumina, especially in older people.

Fiber: a group of compounds that make up the framework of plants. Fiber includes the carbohydrate substances (cellulose, hemicellulose, gums, and pectin) and a non-carbohydrate substance called lignin. These compounds are not digested by the human digestive tract.

Glycogen: the form in which carbohydrate is stored in humans and animals.

Insulin: a hormone secreted by the pancreas that is necessary for the proper metabolism of blood sugar.

Ketosis: an accumulation of ketone bodies from partly digested fats due to inadequate carbohydrate intake.

Lactose intolerance: a condition in which the body is deficient in lactase, the enzyme needed to digest lactose (the sugar in milk). Leads to abdominal bloating, gas, and watery diarrhea. Affects 70%–75% of blacks, almost all Asians, and 5%–10% of whites.

Naturally occurring sugars: sugars found in foods in their natural state; for example, sugar occurs naturally in grapes and other fruits.

Refined food: food that undergoes many commercial processes resulting in the loss of nutrients in the food.

Fats

Atherosclerosis: thickening of the inside wall of the arteries by fatty deposits, resulting in plaques that narrow the arteries and hinder blood flow. Can lead to heart disease.

Bile salts: the substance from the gallbladder that breaks fats into small particles for digestion.

Cholesterol: a fatlike compound occurring in bile, blood, brain and nerve tissue, liver, and other parts of the body. Cholesterol comes from animal foods and is used by the body for the synthesis of necessary tissues and fluids. Cholesterol is also found in plaques that line the inner wall of the artery in atherosclerosis.

Fatty acids: the basic unit of all fats. Essential fatty acids are those that cannot be produced by the body and must be obtained in the diet. A saturated fatty acid is one in which the fatty acids contain all the hydrogen they can hold. A monounsaturated fatty acid is one into which hydrogen can be added at one double bond. Polyunsaturated fatty acids have two or more double bonds into which hydrogen can be added.

Hydrogenation: the addition of hydrogen to a liquid fat, changing it to a solid or semisolid state. Generally, the harder the product, the higher the degree of saturation with hydrogen.

Lipoproteins: transport form of fat (attached to a protein) in the bloodstream.

Satiety value: a food's ability to produce a feeling of fullness.

BACKGROUND INFORMATION

Carbohydrates

Carbohydrates are the most abundant organic substances on Earth, comprising approximately 70% of plant structure. They are the main source of the body's energy.

In the United States, about 50% of dietary energy comes from carbohydrates. This level of intake is considered acceptable, but the type of carbohydrates consumed has caused concern among health professionals. Although both starches and sugars are carbohydrates, they differ in food sources and nutrient values. Starches are mainly found in certain fresh and processed products such as vegetables, breads, and cereals. They provide a large amount of calories and lesser amounts of protein, vitamins, minerals, and water. Sugars, on the other hand, furnish only calories and no nutrients. They are derived from sugar cane and sugar beets. The typical Western diet contains more carbohydrates from sugary foods than from starches. The government guidelines for healthy eating strongly recommend the reverse. Fiber, another plant component, is also an important carbohydrate. Although it neither furnishes energy nor is digestible, it is important for health. All plant foods contain fiber, and we obtain it mainly from cereal grains, especially unrefined ones.

Fats

Fats, chemically termed *lipids*, are also organic compounds. They are insoluble in water. Most fat in the diet is in the form known as triglycerides. Fats differ in chemical structure from carbohydrates, though both contain carbon, hydrogen, and oxygen. Based on their chemical bonding arrangements, fats can be saturated, monounsaturated, or unsaturated. Many different properties of fats are determined by the degree of saturation.

The typical Western diet derives approximately 38%–40% of its total daily calories from fats, mainly saturated fats. Ninety percent of fats in the American diet come from fats and oils, meat, poultry, fish, and dairy products. We are advised to eat about 30% of our total daily calories from fat, with no more than 10% in saturated forms.

Dietary fats are important because they serve as stored energy reserves and as carriers of essential fatty acids and fat-soluble vitamins. Fats must combine with bile from the gallbladder to be digested. Since they are not soluble in water, they must attach themselves to proteins before they can travel through the intestinal walls, lymph system, and bloodstream. From the bloodstream they are delivered to body tissues.

Cholesterol, which is a cross between fat and alcohol, is derived both from foods and body synthesis. Although much maligned because of its implication in heart disease, cholesterol is an important body component and is transported by low-density or high-density lipoproteins in body circulation. Lipoproteins are discussed in Chapter 16 in relation to cardiovascular disease, and will not be explored here.

TABLE 4-1   Classification of Carbohydrates

Carbohydrates	
Starches **Kinds and Sources**	**Sugars** **Kinds and Sources**
Polysaccharides	Monosaccharides

1. Starch—cereals
    grains
    vegetables
	1. Glucose—blood sugar

	2. Fructose—sugar found in fruit

2. Dextrin—digestion
    product
    infant formula
	3. Galactose—digestion
	    product

	Disaccharides

3. Cellulose*—stems, leaves
    coverings
    seeds
    skins, hulls
	1. Sucrose—table sugar

	2. Lactose—sugar found in milk
4. Pectin*—fruits	3. Maltose—germinating seed
5. Glycogen—muscle and liver	

*Nondigestible.

ACTIVITY 1:

Carbohydrates: Characteristics and Effects on Health

DEFINITIONS, CLASSIFICATION, AND REQUIREMENTS

Carbohydrates are composed of carbon, hydrogen, and oxygen. Sugars, starches, and fiber are the main forms in which carbohydrates occur in food. Starches and sugars are the major source of body energy. They are the cheapest and most easily used form of fuel for the body. Fibrous materials provide bulk and aid digestion. Although most carbohydrates occur in plant foods, a few are of animal origin. These include glycogen, which is stored in the liver and muscle as a small reserve supply, and lactose, a sugar found in milk.

Carbohydrates are classified as monosaccharides (simple sugars), disaccharides (double sugars), and polysaccharides (mainly starches). All carbohydrates must be reduced to simple sugars (monosaccharides) in the intestine before they can be absorbed into the bloodstream. Glucose, a simple sugar, is the form in which carbohydrates circulate in the bloodstream. Glucose is commonly referred to as blood sugar. Table 4-1 classifies carbohydrates according to their chemical structures.

The nutrients and calories contributed by different carbohydrates vary. For example, whole grains, enriched cereal products, fruits, and vegetables provide vitamins, minerals, fiber, and energy. Sugars, sweets, and unenriched refined cereals provide calories only.

Carbohydrates are also good sources of fiber, which is the nondigestible part of plant foods. It is nutritionally significant in gastrointestinal functioning. Fiber is classified as soluble or insoluble.

Insoluble fiber (cellulose and hemicellulose) is found in legumes, vegetables, whole grains, fruits, and seeds. Soluble fibers are the pectins, gums, mucilages, and algae and are found in vegetables, fruits, oats and oat bran, legumes, rye, and barley.

The NAS has established DRIs/RDA for carbohydrates for individuals at different stages of life. For example, for an adult aged 19–30 years:

- Males: RDA is 130 g/day
- Females, not pregnant: RDA is 130 g/day

The NAS has established DRIs/AI for total fiber for individuals at different stages of life. For example, for an adult aged 19–30 years:

- Males: AI is 38 g/day
- Females, not pregnant: AI is 25 g/day

FUNCTIONS
Energy Source

Carbohydrates are the most economical and efficient source of energy. They furnish 4 kcal/g of energy. The body requires a constant source of energy to support its vital functions.

Protein-Sparing Action

Carbohydrates prevent protein from being used as energy. Carbohydrate, protein, and fat can all be used to produce energy. However, the body utilizes carbohydrate first. When not enough carbohydrate is present, the body uses protein and fat for its energy needs. Thus, an adequate amount of carbohydrate can spare protein that can then be used for tissue building and repair rather than energy.

Metabolic Functions

Under normal conditions, the tissues of the central nervous system (especially the brain) can use only glucose as an energy source. Muscles can use either glucose or fats as fuel. Body fat is used by the muscles only during physical activity varying from walking up stairs to lifting weights.

Some carbohydrate is needed for the proper utilization of fat. In the absence of carbohydrate, fats are not completely burned, and ketosis results (see later discussion). Severe restriction of carbohydrate in reducing diets can cause ketosis, which can produce adverse effects.

Carbohydrates are important components of certain substances needed for regulating body processes. They also encourage the growth of beneficial bacteria involved in the production of certain vitamins and in the absorption of calcium and phosphorus.

Fiber and Health

Insoluble fiber has a laxative effect. It provides bulk, leading to regular elimination of solid wastes. By promoting normal function, insoluble fiber is useful in reducing pressure on the lumina of the colon, thus helping prevent diverticulitis. Insoluble fiber provides a feeling of fullness, thereby reducing the amount of food eaten. Most food sources of insoluble fiber such as legumes, vegetables, and fruits are not calorie dense. These factors are helpful when weight-reduction diets are needed. Insoluble fibers also exert a binding effect on bile salts and cholesterol, preventing their absorption. Excessive ingestion of fiber, however, is undesirable, as this fiber also binds with minerals such as calcium, zinc, and iron, which are essential for body function.

Soluble fibers are important factors in preventing diseases such as heart disease, colon cancer, and diabetes mellitus. They form soft gels by absorbing water, which slows carbohydrate absorption and binds cholesterol and bile acids. Slow absorption reduces fasting blood sugar and lowers insulin requirements. Binding of the bile acids and cholesterol permits cholesterol to be excreted instead of absorbed. Studies indicate that bile acids may contribute to colon cancer; therefore, this binding capacity is important. Major sources of soluble fiber include vegetables and fruits.

Combinations of both soluble and insoluble fibers produce the best effects; many of the recommended foods contain both types of fiber. The recommended daily intake of fiber, consumed from plant sources, varies though our DRI/AI requirements are defined as mentioned previously. Our actual consumption of fiber is unknown and influenced by such factors as gas formation. The fermentation of carbohydrate by intestinal bacteria produces volatile gases that are socially unacceptable and may occasionally cause bloating and pain, especially in those persons who decide to drastically increase their fiber intake. Clients are advised to do so gradually, to eat a variety of fiber-containing foods and avoid just one source, such as bran, for all their fiber intake.

The NCI dietary guidelines, directed especially toward the prevention of colon cancer, recommend high intakes of vegetables (especially cruciferous), fruits, and whole grains, which facilitate the removal of bile salts and cholesterol, along with a low-fat diet. The *Dietary Guidelines for Americans* and MyPyramid also highly encourage eating these foods and reducing fat in the diet.

Blood Glucose

The form of carbohydrate used by the body is a monosaccharide—glucose. All forms of carbohydrate except fiber eventually are broken down by the body to glucose. Glucose is the form of sugar found in the blood, and its control at normal blood levels is important to health. Without sufficient glucose, the body will use its protein to make glucose, since the brain requires glucose to function. This diverts protein from its important functions of building and repairing tissues. When carbohydrate is insufficient, the body metabolizes fat differently to produce ketosis, a condition in which unusual by-products of fat metabolization break down into ketones and accumulate in the blood. Ketosis during pregnancy can result in brain damage and irreversible mental retardation in the infant. Some experts suggest that ketosis is potentially dangerous for all adults.

Blood glucose levels vary. Normal levels range between 70 to 120 mg per 100 ml of blood. When blood sugar is less than 70 mg, hunger occurs. After eating, blood sugar levels normally rise. The beta cells in the pancreas respond to the increase by secreting insulin. Insulin causes the liver, muscle, and fat cells to increase their uptake of sugar, which in turn reduces the blood sugar levels to normal. The glucose entering the cells is then converted to glycogen or fat or is used for energy if the body needs it. Insulin also assists in regulating the metabolism of fat by the body.

Insulin is the only hormone that directly lowers blood sugar levels. If there is insufficient production of insulin by the pancreas, or if it is unavailable, the blood cannot be cleared of excess glucose. This condition is hyperglycemia, the term used to describe blood glucose levels above the normal range. It occurs in diabetes mellitus. This abnormal response to glucose can sometimes be controlled by diet therapy and weight control, but in certain types of diabetes, insulin may have to be administered to help lower blood glucose levels.

When blood glucose drops below the normal limits, the condition is called hypoglycemia. Symptoms of hypoglycemia vary, depending on blood sugar level. Early symptoms include weakness, dizziness, hunger, trembling, and mental confusion. If the levels drop very low, convulsions or unconsciousness may occur. Although it can occur, as a spontaneous reaction in some people, most often it happens when a diabetic uses excess insulin and/or has not eaten for a long period. A glucose-tolerance test will determine true hypoglycemia. People who are not diabetic but are sensitive to changes in blood sugar levels should follow a calculated diet much the same as a diabetic, avoiding sweets and eating regular, balanced meals.

SOURCES, STORAGE, SWEETENERS, AND INTAKE

The major food sources of carbohydrate are plants, which vary in the amounts of sugar and starches they provide. Milk and milk products containing lactose are the only significant animal sources of carbohydrates. Food sources of carbohydrate include cereal grains, fruits, vegetables, nuts, milk, and concentrated sweets. Table 4-2 compares the carbohydrate content of selected foods.

TABLE 4-2   Carbohydrate Content of Some Selected Foods

Food	Serving Size	Carbohydrate Content
Milk, skim	1 c	12 g
Milk, whole	1 c	12 g
Bread (white or whole wheat)	1 slice	15 g
Oatmeal	½ c (cooked)	15 g
Green peas (frozen or canned)	½ c	15 g
Puffed wheat	1½ c	15 g
Popcorn (popped)	3 c	15 g
Yam, sweet potato	⅓ c	15 g
Mushrooms, cooked	½ c	5 g
Asparagus	½ c	5 g
Green beans	½ c	5 g
Strawberries, raw/ whole/unsweetened	1¼ c	15 g
Pineapple juice (unsweetened)	½ c	15 g
Cantaloupe, cubed	⅓ melon	15 g
Angel food cake	½₂ cake	15 g
Ice cream, any flavor	½ c	15 g
Granola	¼ c	15 g
Cheese pizza, thin crust	¼ of 10″ pie	30 g
Chile, with beans	1 c	30 g
Frozen fruit yogurt	⅓ c	15 g

Nutritive sweeteners provide calories. Examples include sugar, honey, molasses, and syrup (corn, maple). The most common is table sugar, which comes from sugar beets or sugar cane. Table sugar is sucrose, two simple sugars chemically joined. Sugar can be white or brown. White sugar contains mainly sucrose. Brown sugar contains trace amounts of protein, minerals, vitamins, water, and pigment in addition to sucrose.

Synthetic sweeteners are nonnutritive and furnish no calories. They have been used for many years by diabetics and dieters. Since 1969 saccharin was the only legal nonnutritive sweetener until the recent availability of aspartame. Cyclamates were used until 1969, when they were banned because they were shown to cause bladder cancer in rats. Since the consumption of artificially sweetened beverages and foods has increased drastically in recent years, the Food and Drug Administration (FDA) is studying saccharin and aspartame carefully. Aspartame is made from the amino acids aspartic acid and phenylalanine. Although it is on the GRAS (generally recognized as safe) list, precautions are advised about the use of aspartame by pregnant women and young children. Other people may be sensitive to aspartame and should avoid using it. Products sweetened with aspartame carry a warning label for people who have phenylketonuria (PKU) to avoid the use of the product. PKU is an inherited disorder of defective protein metabolism. It is discussed in Chapter 29. The newest synthetic sweetener on the market is acesulfame K (potassium). Brand names are Sweet One and Sunette.

In general, carbohydrate stores in the body are small. Carbohydrate in excess of the body's energy needs is stored in limited amounts in the liver and muscle. Most excess is converted to fat and stored as such. Less than one pound is stored as glycogen. This amount can furnish energy for 12 to 24 hours. However, the excess converted to fat can be stored in unlimited amounts in the body.

A carbohydrate deficiency leads to a loss of muscle tissue as protein is burned to meet energy and glucose needs. In addition, fats are incompletely broken down and a condition of ketosis results. Prolonged carbohydrate deficiencies can cause damage to the liver. Low-fiber diets are associated with constipation and are linked to colon cancer. Scientists now recommend that 50%–60% of the daily caloric intake be from carbohydrate foods, especially the complex carbohydrates (starches).

Of the classes of carbohydrate, sugars and sweets are the least desirable. Overconsumption of sugar promotes dental caries and frequently leads to a poor nutritional quality diet. Table 4-3 shows the sugar content of some popular foods. Diabetes mellitus and lactose intolerance are examples of diseases in which carbohydrates are not utilized normally by the body.

TABLE 4-3	Sugar Content of Selected Foods	
Food	**Serving Amount**	**Total Grams Sugar (Sucrose, Glucose, Fructose, Maltose)***
Apple juice	8 oz	25–35
Beer (average of all brands)	12 oz	3–4
Brownie	50 gm	22.5
Carbonated beverages	12 oz	38–41
Chocolate	2 oz	35–43
Granola (average of all brands)	¼ c	7–8
Honey	1 tbsp	14–16
Ketchup	1 tbsp	4–6
Nondairy creamer	1 tbsp	9–11
Pineapple juice	8 oz	28–31
Tomato, red (raw)	1 tomato	4–6
Tomato paste (canned)	½ c	23–27
Yogurt (sweetened)	8 oz	30–40

*Types of sugars in each food not differentiated. Calories for each item may be obtained by multiplying total × 4.
Source: Adapted from Food Nutrients Database, www.usda.gov.

ATHLETIC ACTIVITIES

Except for an increased energy requirement, athletes require the same basic nutrients that all people require. The amount of energy expended in training and competition determines the amount of food needed. The recommended distribution of nutrients for anyone is 50% to 60% of daily caloric intake from carbohydrate, 15% to 20% from protein, and 30% to 35% from fat. If energy needs increase, the distribution should remain the same, with the size of individual portions being increased to meet the requirements.

Carbohydrates are the most efficient energy source for both athletes and nonathletes and, as such, should be used to meet the need for increased energy. Athletes' carbohydrate needs are better met through extensive use of grains, fruits, and vegetables instead of sugary foods. For the body to convert foods into energy, certain vitamins and minerals are necessary. These are found only in nutrient-dense foods, not in candies and other sweets.

Of all athletic activities, endurance performance is most frequently associated with carbohydrate consumption. The premise is simple. A high carbohydrate diet helps increase body glycogen storage and extend the endurance of an athlete. In a process called carbohydrate or glycogen loading, athletes adjust their carbohydrate consumption and practice schedules to maximize their muscle glycogen storage.

There are professional guidelines to help adult athletes to implement a safe and effective carbohydrate loading regimen. Such guidelines are available in some of the books in the references for this chapter. They are also available in training manuals for both amateur and professional athletes engaged in endurance sports such as short- and long-distance running. In general such guidelines revolve around the following premises:

1. Carbohydrate intake before exercise
2. Carbohydrate intake during exercise
3. Carbohydrate intake following exercise
4. Meal plans and menus

The concept of carbohydrate loading is also practiced by athletes in other sports that are not endurance sports such as basketball, football, and soccer. However, it is recommended that the practice of carbohydrate loading should be implemented under the directions of a qualified professional, especially for nonadult athletes.

HEALTH IMPLICATIONS

Health risks are associated with excessive sugar consumption, but it is difficult to make positive correlations between sugar consumption and the development of many diseases that have been linked to it. Included among the associations of sugar and health problems are the following:

1. Obesity—Sugar is often named as being the cause of obesity. If persons are obese, they certainly have consumed excess calories. It is probably an overall excess intake rather than sugar alone. Sugar is usually curtailed in reduction diets along with fats and alcohol because such foods contribute mainly calories.
2. Cardiovascular disease—Except for certain types of lipid disorder, in which an individual exhibits abnormal glucose tolerance along with an elevation of blood triglycerides, research studies cannot prove any correlation between sugar intake and cardiovascular disorder. Obesity is probably more closely related to this disorder than a high sugar consumption.
3. Diabetes—The cause of the malfunction of the pancreas is not known, but heredity plays a role as well as obesity. The chance of becoming diabetic more than doubles for every 20% of excess weight, according to the U.S. National Diabetes Commission. While studies have shown that the incidence of diabetes rose in population groups that "Westernized" and started consuming excess sugary foods, most researchers agree that individuals have become fat from excess calories, not just sugar.
4. Dental caries—Carbohydrates, especially sugar, play a role in tooth decay. Sucrose is especially implicated. The frequency of eating sugar, sweets, and similar snacks is more damaging than the amount eaten in one sitting. Good oral hygiene (brushing after meals) helps prevent dental caries. The general state of health also influences susceptibility to caries.

5. Cancer—Population group studies have not linked nonnutritive sweeteners to cancer. Certain groups with increased susceptibility to bladder cancer include some heavy saccharine users. This correlation is also associated with heavy cigarette smokers. At present, the use of saccharine is in a "suspended" status—that is, if new data show definitive hazards, the use of this substance will be banned.

6. Fiber—Low-fiber diets are believed to play a major role in the onset of diverticulosis and may contribute to appendicitis. The added pressure in the colon caused by a low-fiber intake may increase the occurrence of hemorrhoids, varicose veins, and hiatal hernia. Colon cancer has been linked to low-fiber diets, but the relationship is not clear. There are several theories regarding the cause-and-effect relationships, but the current general recommendation is to maintain a balanced diet with ample intake of fiber and fluids. No RDA has been set for fiber, but 15 g/day is recommended in *Healthy People 2000*.

PROGRESS CHECK ON ACTIVITY 1

SHORT ANSWERS

1. Using meal planning exchange lists in Appendix F, rank the following foods by carbohydrate content, beginning with the food that has the most carbohydrate. If two foods have the same value, give them the same number.

   _____ a. 1 orange
   _____ b. 1 c whole kernel corn
   _____ c. ¹⁄₁₀ of a devil's food cake with icing (from a mix)
   _____ d. 1 slice wheat bread
   _____ e. ½ c zucchini squash
   _____ f. ½ c cooked oatmeal

2. Rank the following vegetables by carbohydrate content, beginning with the one that has the most carbohydrate. If two foods have the same value, give them the same number.

   _____ a. ½ c green beans, cooked
   _____ b. ½ c cooked carrots
   _____ c. 1 baked potato
   _____ d. 1 sweet potato
   _____ e. 1 stalk broccoli
   _____ f. ½ c lettuce, chopped

3. If a person's carbohydrate intake is greater than his or her energy needs, what happens to the excess?

   _____

4. What is the function of fiber in the diet? _____

   _____

5. Name three good food sources of fiber.

   a. _____
   b. _____
   c. _____

6. Name two health problems related to overconsumption of sugar.

   a. _____
   b. _____

7. Why are diets that severely restrict carbohydrates dangerous? _____

   _____

   _____

MULTIPLE CHOICE

Circle the letter of the correct answer.

8. If a 2000 kcal/day diet derives approximately 1000 kcal from carbohydrates, how many grams of carbohydrate does that diet contain?

   a. 150
   b. 200
   c. 250
   d. 400

9. Identify the trend in food consumption in the United States that has occurred since the turn of the century.

   a. Potato consumption has continued to increase.
   b. Consumption of refined sugar and processed sugar products has increased.
   c. Fruit and vegetable consumption has greatly increased.
   d. Consumption of cereals has greatly increased.

10. Cellulose is a _____ carbohydrate.

    a. digestible
    b. nondigestible
    c. disaccharide
    d. processed

11. Which two of the following food groups contain the greatest amounts of cellulose and other food fiber?

    a. meat and dairy products
    b. whole grain cereals
    c. fruit juices
    d. raw fruits and vegetables

12. Which of the following represent blood sugar levels within the normal range?

    a. 30 to 60 mg per 100 ml
    b. 70 to 120 mg per 100 ml

c. 140 to 160 mg per 100 ml

d. 100 to 120 mg per 100 ml

13. Insulin is secreted by the:

    a. alpha cells of the pancreas.

    b. beta cells of the pancreas.

    c. nephron of the kidney.

    d. digestive cells in the intestinal wall.

14. From the items below, choose the snack that produces the least amount of caries.

    a. plain popcorn and an apple

    b. taffy and raisins

    c. noodles with butter

    d. sherbet and 7-Up float

15. Carbohydrates are the raw materials that we eat mainly as:

    a. starches and sugars.

    b. proteins and fats.

    c. plants and animals.

    d. pectin and cellulose.

16. Carbohydrates provide one of the main fuel sources for energy. Which of the following carbohydrate foods provides the quickest source of energy?

    a. slice of bread

    b. glass of orange juice

    c. chocolate candy bar

    d. glass of milk

17. Chemical digestion of carbohydrates is completed in the small intestine by enzymes from the:

    a. pancreas and gallbladder.

    b. gallbladder and liver.

    c. small intestine and pancreas.

    d. liver and small intestine.

18. The refined fuel glucose is delivered to the cells by the blood for production of energy. The hormone controlling use of glucose by the cells is:

    a. thyroxin.

    b. growth hormone.

    c. adrenal steroid.

    d. insulin.

MATCHING

Match the phrases on the right with the terms on the left that they best describe.

19. Insulin   a. hormone that causes the release of glucose into the blood

20. Hyperglycemia   b. glucose in the blood

21. Glycemia   c. low blood glucose levels

22. Hypoglycemia   d. high blood glucose levels

23. Glucagon   e. hormone that affects the uptake of glucose from the blood into various body cells

Match the carbohydrate in Column A to its type in Column B. Terms may be used more than once.

    Column A   Column B

24. Sucrose   a. polysaccharide

25. Glucose   b. monosaccharide

26. Glycogen   c. disaccharide

27. Lactose

28. Grains

29. Fructose

30. Cellulose

ACTIVITY 2:

Fats: Characteristics and Effects on Health

DEFINITIONS AND FOOD SOURCES

Although both fats and carbohydrates contain carbon, hydrogen, and oxygen, fats are entirely different compounds from carbohydrates because of their chemical structures. Foods that contribute fat to the diet include whole milk and milk products containing whole milk or butterfat, such as butter, ice cream, and cheese; egg yolk; meat, fish, and poultry; nuts and seeds; vegetable oils; and hydrogenated vegetable fats (shortenings and margarine).

A fat is classified as saturated, monounsaturated, or polyunsaturated according to the type of fatty acids it contains in greatest quantity. Saturated food fats are generally solid at room temperature and come from animal sources. Saturated fats are found in whole milk and products made from whole milk; egg yolk; meat; meat fat (bacon, lard); coconut oil and palm oil; chocolate; regular margarine; and hydrogenated vegetable shortenings. Unsaturated food fats are generally liquid at room temperature and come from plant sources. They can be monounsaturated or polyunsaturated. Sources of polyunsaturated fats are safflower, sunflower, corn, cottonseed, soybean, and sesame oil; salad dressings made from these oils; special margarines that contain a high percentage of such oils; and fatty fish such as mackerel, salmon, and herring. Sources of monounsaturated fats are olive oil and most nuts. Diets rich in saturated fat and/or cholesterol can lead to elevated blood cholesterol levels. Polyunsaturated and monounsaturated fats appear to lower blood cholesterol level.

Cholesterol is a fatlike substance (lipid) that is a key component of cell membranes and a precursor of bile acids and steroid hormones. Cholesterol travels in the circulation in spherical particles containing both lipids and proteins called lipoproteins. A lipoprotein is made up of fats (cholesterol, triglycerides, fatty acids, etc.), protein, and a small amount of other substances. The cholesterol level in blood plasma is determined partly by inheritance and partly by the fat and cholesterol content of the diet. Other factors, such as obesity and physical inactivity, may also play a role.

Organ meats and egg yolk are very rich sources of cholesterol; shrimp is a moderately rich source. Other sources include meat, fish, poultry, whole milk, and foods made from whole milk or butterfat.

FUNCTIONS AND STORAGE

Fat functions in the body as the following:

1. A source of essential fatty acids
2. The most concentrated source of energy (9 kcals/g)
3. A reserve energy supply in the body
4. A carrier for the fat-soluble vitamins (A, D, E, and K)
5. A cushion and an insulation for the body
6. A satiety factor (satisfaction from a fatty meal)

All fats that are not burned as energy are stored as adipose tissue. Most people have a large storage of fat in the body.

DIET, FATS, AND HEALTH

All information in this section has been modified from official publications distributed by the United States Department of Agriculture (USDA), the National Institute of Health (NIH), and Food and Drug Administration (FDA). There are three major publications:

1. *Dietary Guidelines for Americans*, 2005. (www.healthierus.gov, www.usda.gov). *See also* Chapter 1 and Chapter 16.
2. MyPyramid (www.usda.gov, www.mypyramid.gov). *See also* Chapter 1.
3. National Cholesterol Education Program. *Third Report of the Expert Panel on Detection, Evaluation, and Treatment of High Blood Cholesterol in Adults* (ATP-III), 2001, (www.NIH.gov). *See also* Chapter 16.

Background Information

Fats and oils are part of a healthful diet, but the type of fat makes a difference to heart health, and the total amount of fat consumed is also important. High intake of saturated fats, trans fats, and cholesterol increases the risk of unhealthy blood lipid levels, which, in turn, may increase the risk of coronary heart disease. A high intake of fat (greater than 35% of calories) generally increases saturated fat intake and makes it more difficult to avoid consuming excess calories. A low intake of fats and oils (less than 20% of calories) increases the risk of inadequate intakes of vitamin E and of essential fatty acids and may contribute to unfavorable changes in high-density lipoprotein (HDL) blood cholesterol and triglycerides.

Fats supply energy and essential fatty acids and serve as a carrier for the absorption of the fat-soluble vitamins A, D, E, and K and carotenoids. Fats serve as building blocks of membranes and play a key regulatory role in numerous biological functions. Dietary fat is found in foods derived from both plants and animals. The recommended total fat intake is between 20% and 35% of calories for adults. A fat intake of 30%–35% of calories is recommended for children 2 to 3 years of age, and 25%–35% of calories for children and adolescents 4 to 18 years of age. Few Americans consume less than 20% of calories from fat. Fat intakes that exceed 35% of calories are associated with both total increased saturated fat and calorie intakes.

Considerations for the General Public

Three major classes of lipoproteins can be measured in the serum of a fasting individual: very-low-density lipoproteins (VLDL), low-density lipoproteins (LDL), and high-density lipoproteins (HDL). The LDL are the major culprits in cardiovascular diseases (CVD) and typically contain 60%–70% of the total serum cholesterol. The HDL usually contain 20%–30% of the total cholesterol, and their levels are inversely correlated with risk for coronary heart disease (CHD). The VLDL, which are largely composed of triglycerides, contain 10%–15% of the total serum cholesterol.

To decrease their risk of elevated low-density lipoprotein (LDL) cholesterol in the blood, most Americans need to decrease their intakes of saturated fat and trans fats, and many need to decrease their dietary intake of cholesterol. Because men tend to have higher intakes of dietary cholesterol, it is especially important for them to meet this recommendation. Population-based studies of American diets show that intake of saturated fat is more excessive than intake of trans fats and cholesterol. Therefore, it is most important for Americans to decrease their intake of saturated fat. However, intake of all three should be decreased to meet recommendations. Table 4-4 shows, for selected calorie levels, the maximum gram amounts of saturated fat to consume to keep saturated fat intake below 10% of total calorie intake. This table may be useful when combined with label-reading guidance. Table 4-5 gives a few practical examples of the differences in the saturated fat content of different forms of commonly consumed foods. The contribution of saturated fat intake varies with the type of foods being consumed. Diets can be planned to meet nutrient recommendations for linoleic acid and α-linolenic acid while providing very low amounts of saturated fatty acids.

TABLE 4-4 **Maximum Daily Amounts of Saturated Fat to Keep Saturated Fat Below 10% of Total Calorie Intake**

Total Calorie Intake	Limit on Saturated Fat Intake
1600	18 g or less
2000[a]	20 g or less
2200	24 g or less
2500[b]	25 g or less
2800	31 g or less

Notes:
[a]The maximum gram amounts of saturated fat that can be consumed to keep saturated fat intake below 10% of total calorie intake for selected calorie levels. A 2000-calorie example is included for consistency with the food label. This table may be useful when combined with label-reading guidance.
[b]Percent Daily Values on the Nutrition Facts panel of food labels are based on a 2000-calorie diet. Values for 2000 and 2500 calories are rounded to the nearest 5 grams to be consistent with the Nutrition Facts panel.
Source: Courtesy of the USDA.

Based on 1994–1996 data, the estimated average daily intake of trans fats in the United States was about 2.6% of total energy intake. Processed foods and oils provide approximately 80% of trans fats in the diet, compared to 20% that occur naturally in food from animal sources. Table 4-6 provides the major dietary sources of trans fats listed in decreasing order. Trans fat content of certain processed foods has changed and is likely to continue to change as the industry reformulates products. Because the trans-fatty acids produced in the partial hydrogenation of vegetable oils account for more than 80% of total intake, the food industry has an important role in decreasing trans-fatty acid content of the food supply. Limited consumption of foods made with processed sources of trans fats provides the most effective means of reducing intake of trans fats. By looking at the food label, consumers can select products that are lowest in saturated fat, trans fats, and cholesterol.

TABLE 4-5   Differences in Saturated Fat and Calorie Content of Commonly Consumed Foods

Food Category	Portion	Saturated Fat Content (grams)	Calories
Cheese			
Regular cheddar cheese	1 oz	6.0	114
Low-fat cheddar cheese	1 oz	1.2	49
Ground beef			
Regular ground beef (25% fat)	3 oz (cooked)	6.1	236
Extra-lean ground beef (5% fat)	3 oz (cooked)	2.6	148
Milk			
Whole milk (3.25%)	1 c	4.6	146
Low-fat (1%) milk	1 c	1.5	102
Breads			
Croissant (med)	1 medium	6.6	231
Bagel, oat bran (4")	1 medium	0.2	227
Frozen desserts			
Regular ice cream	½ c	4.9	145
Frozen yogurt, low-fat	½ c	2.0	110
Table spreads			
Butter	1 tsp	2.4	34
Soft margarine with zero trans fats	1 tsp	0.7	25
Chicken			
Fried chicken (leg with skin)	3 oz (cooked)	3.3	212
Roasted chicken (breast no skin)	3 oz (cooked)	0.9	140
Fish			
Fried fish	3 oz	2.8	195
Baked fish	3 oz	1.5	129

Note: This table shows a few practical examples of the differences in the saturated fat content of different forms of commonly consumed foods. Comparisons are made between foods in the same food group (e.g., regular cheddar cheese and low-fat cheddar cheese), illustrating that lower saturated fat choices can be made within the same food group.
Source: ARS/USDA Nutrient Database for Standard Reference, Latest Release (www.ars.usda.gov, www.usda.gov).

TABLE 4-6	Contribution of Various Foods to Trans Fat Intake in the American Diet (Mean Intake = 5.84 g) [a]	
Food Group	**Contribution (percent of total trans fats consumed)**	
Cakes, cookies, crackers, pies, bread, etc.	40	
Animal products	21	
Margarine	17	
Fried potatoes	8	
Potato chips, corn chips, popcorn	5	
Household shortening	4	
Other[b]	5	

[a]The major dietary sources of trans fats listed in decreasing order. Processed foods and oils provide approximately 80 percent of trans fats in the diet, compared to 20 percent that occur naturally in food from animal sources. Trans fats content of certain processed foods has changed and is likely to continue to change as the industry reformulates products.
[b]Includes breakfast cereal and candy. USDA analysis reported 0 grams of trans fats in salad dressing.
Source: Adapted from *Federal Register* notice. Food Labeling; Trans Fatty Acids in Nutrition Labeling; Consumer Research to Consider Nutrient Content and Health Claims and Possible Footnote or Disclosure Statements; Final Rule and Proposed Rule. (2003). 68(133), 41433–41506.

To meet the total fat recommendation of 20% to 35% of calories, most dietary fats should come from sources of polyunsaturated and monounsaturated fatty acids. Sources of omega-6 polyunsaturated fatty acids are liquid vegetable oils, including soybean oil, corn oil, and safflower oil. Plant sources of omega-3 polyunsaturated fatty acids (α-linolenic acid) include soybean oil, canola oil, walnuts, and flaxseed. Eicosapentaenoic acid (EPA) and docosahexaenoic acid (DHA) are omega-3 fatty acids that are contained in fish and shellfish. Fish that naturally contain more oil (e.g., salmon, trout, herring) are higher in EPA and DHA than are lean fish (e.g., cod, haddock, catfish). Limited evidence suggests an association between consumption of fatty acids in fish and reduced risks of mortality from cardiovascular disease for the general population. Other sources of EPA and DHA may provide similar benefits; however, more research is needed. Plant sources that are rich in monounsaturated fatty acids include nuts and vegetable oils (e.g., canola, olive, high oleic safflower, and sunflower oils) that are liquid at room temperature.

Considerations for Specific Population Groups

Evidence suggests that consuming approximately two servings of fish per week (approximately 8 ounces total)

may reduce the risk of mortality from coronary heart disease and that consuming EPA and DHA may reduce the risk of mortality from cardiovascular disease in people who have already experienced a cardiac event.

Federal and state advisories provide current information about lowering exposure to environmental contaminants in fish. For example, methylmercury is a heavy metal toxin found in varying levels in nearly all fish and shellfish. For most people, the risk from mercury by eating fish and shellfish is not a health concern. However, some fish contain higher levels of mercury that may harm an unborn baby or young child's developing nervous system. The risks from mercury in fish and shellfish depend on the amount of fish eaten and the levels of mercury in the fish. Therefore, the Food and Drug Administration (FDA) and the Environmental Protection Agency are advising women of childbearing age who may become pregnant, pregnant women, nursing mothers, and young children to avoid some types of fish and shellfish and eat fish and shellfish that are lower in mercury. For more information, see Chapter 9.

Recommendations

Lower intakes (less than 7% of calories from saturated fat and less than 200 mg/day of cholesterol) are recommended as part of a therapeutic diet for adults with elevated LDL blood cholesterol (i.e., above their LDL blood cholesterol goal [see Table 4-7]. People with an elevated LDL blood cholesterol level should be under the care of a healthcare provider.

Key recommendations for the general public are as follows:

1. Consume less than 10% of calories from saturated fatty acids and less than 300 mg/day of cholesterol, and keep *trans*-fatty acid consumption as low as possible.
2. Keep total fat intake between 20 to 35% of calories, with most fats coming from sources of polyunsaturated and monounsaturated fatty acids, such as fish, nuts, and vegetable oils.
3. When selecting and preparing meat, poultry, dry beans, and milk or milk products, make choices that are lean, low fat, or fat free.
4. Limit intake of fats and oils high in saturated and/or *trans*-fatty acids, and choose products low in such fats and oils.

Key recommendations for specific population groups are:

Keep total fat intake between 30 to 35% of calories for children 2 to 3 years of age and between 25 to 35% of calories for children and adolescents 4 to 18 years of age, with most fats coming from sources of polyunsaturated and monounsaturated fatty acids, such as fish, nuts, and vegetable oils.

TABLE 4-7   Relationship Between LDL Blood Cholesterol Goal and the Level of Coronary Heart Disease Risk[a]

If Someone Has:	LDL Blood Cholesterol Goal Is:
CHD or CHD risk equivalent[b]	Less than 100 mg/dL
Two or more risk factors other than elevated LDL blood cholesterol[c]	Less than 130 mg/dL
Zero or one risk factor other than elevated LDL blood cholesterol[c]	Less than 160 mg/dL

[a]Information for adults with elevated LDL blood cholesterol. LDL blood cholesterol goals for these individuals are related to the level of coronary heart disease risk. People with an elevated LDL blood cholesterol value should make therapeutic lifestyle changes (diet, physical activity, weight control) under the care of a healthcare provider to lower LDL blood cholesterol. *Source:* NIH Publication No. 01-3290, U.S. Department of Health and Human Services, National Institutes of Health, National Heart, Lung, and Blood Institute, National Cholesterol Education Program Brochure, High blood cholesterol: What you need to know, May 2001. www.nhlbi.nih.gov/health/public/heart/chol/hbc_what.htm.
[b]CHD (coronary heart disease) risk equivalent = presence of clinical atherosclerotic disease that confers high risk for CHD events:
1. Clinical CHD
2. Symptomatic carotid artery disease
3. Peripheral arterial disease
4. Abdominal aortic aneurysm
5. Diabetes
6. Two or more risk factors with > 20% risk for CHD (or myocardial infarction or CHD death) within 10 years
[c]Major risk factors that affect your LDL goal:
1. Cigarette smoking
2. High blood pressure (140/90 mmHg or higher or on blood pressure medication)
3. Low HDL blood cholesterol (less than 40 mg/dl)
4. Family history of early heart disease (heart disease in father or brother before age 55; heart disease in mother or sister before age 65)
5. Age (men 45 years or older; women 55 years or older)

PROGRESS CHECK ON ACTIVITY 2

MULTIPLE CHOICE

1. Which of the following is incorrect?

   a. When the total calorie intake is 2200, limit saturated fat intake to 24 g or less.
   b. When the total calorie intake is 2800, limit saturated fat intake to 31 g or less.
   c. When the total calorie intake is 2000, limit saturated fat intake to 18 g or less.
   d. When the total calorie intake is 2500, limit saturated fat intake to 28 g or less.

2. Cholesterol:

   a. in blood is determined by height.
   b. is a key component of cell membranes.
   c. in shrimp is more than that in eggs.
   d. is found in some plant foods.

3. Describe the key recommendations for a specific population group.

   a. Keep total fat intake between 30 to 35% of calories for children 2 to 3 years of age.
   b. Keep total fat intake between 35 to 40% of calories for children 2 to 3 years of age.
   c. Keep total fat intake between 25 to 35% of calories for children 4 to 11 years of age.
   d. Keep total fat intake between 25 to 35% of calories for adolescents 11 to 18 years of age.

TRUE OR FALSE

4. T F Lower intakes (less than 7% of calories from saturated fat and less than 200 mg/day of cholesterol) are recommended as part of a therapeutic diet for adults with elevated LDL blood cholesterol.

5. T F Fat functions in the body as the major protection for the womb and the fetus in a pregnant woman.

6. T F Regular ground beef (3 oz) has three times more fat than extra-lean ground beef (3 oz).

7. T F Smoking cigarettes is a one of the major risk factors that affect a person's LDL goal.

8. T F The risk of CHD increases when one has prostate cancer.

FILL-IN

9. The reading for high blood pressure is

   _____.

10. The level of low HDL blood cholesterol is

    _____.

11. What is highest percentage of total trans fats consumed by Americans? _____

DEFINE

12. LDL: _____

13. Lipoprotein: _____

14. CHD: _____

15. EPA: _____

16. DHA: _____

REFERENCES

Carbohydrates

Aston, L. M. (2006). Glycaemic index and metabolic disease risk. *Proceedings of Nutrition Society, 65*: 125–134.

Bessesen, D. H. (2001). The role of carbohydrates in insulin resistance. *Journal of Nutrition, 131*: 2782s–2786s.

Caballero, B., Allen, L., & Prentice, A. (Eds.). (2005). *Encyclopedia of Human Nutrition* (2nd ed.). Boston: Elsevier/Academic Press.

Cherbut, C. (2002). Insulin and oligofructose in the dietary fiber concept. *British Journal of Nutrition, 87*: s159–s162.

Eastwood, M. (2003). *Principles of Human Nutrition* (2nd ed.). Malden, MA: Blackwell Science.

Flight, I. (2006). Cereal grains and legumes in the prevention of coronary heart disease and stroke: A review of the literature. *European Journal of Clinical Nutrition, 60*: 1145–1159.

Gaesser, G. A. (2007). Carbohydrate quality and quantity in relation to body mass index. *Journal of American Dietetic Association, 107*: 1768–1780.

Gibson, E. L. (2007). Carbohydrates and mental function: feeding or impeding the brain. *Nutrition Bulletin, 32* (Suppl 1): 71–83.

Jones, J. M. (2001). The benefits of eating breakfast cereals. *Cereal Foods World 46*: 461–464, 466–467.

Jones, J. R. (2006). Dietary reference intake: Implications for fiber labeling and consumption. *Nutrition Review, 64*: 31–38.

Livesay, G. (2001). Tolerance of low-digestible carbohydrates: A review. *British Journal of Nutrition, 85*: s7–s16.

Lunn, J. (2007). Carbohydrates and dietary fiber. *Nutrition Bulletin, 32*: 21–64.

Mann, J. & Truswell, S. (Eds.). (2007). *Essentials of Human Nutrition* (3rd ed.). New York: Oxford University Press.

Mussatto, S. I. (2007). Non-digestible oligosaccharides: A review. *Carbohydrate Polymers, 68*: 587–597.

Scheppach, W. (2001). Beneficial health effect of low-digestible carbohydrate consumption. *British Journal of Nutrition, 85*: s23–s30.

Seal, C. J. (2006). Whole grains and CVD risk. *Proceedings of Nutrition Society, 65*: 24–34.

Stipanuk, M. H. (Ed.). (2006). *Biochemical, Physiological and Molecular Aspects of Human Nutrition* (2nd ed.). St. Louis, MO: Saunders Elsevier.

Topping, D. (2007). Cereal complex carbohydrates and their contribution to human health. *Journal of Cereal Science, 46*: 220–229.

Webster-Gandy, J., Madden, A., & Holdworth, M. (Eds.). (2006). *Oxford Handbook of Nutrition and Dietetics*. Oxford, London: Oxford University Press.

Whitney, E. N. & Rolfe, S. R. (2002). *Understanding Nutrition*. Belmont, CA: Wadsworth.

Fats

Akoh, C. C. (2006). *Handbook of Functional Lipids*. Boca Raton, FL: CRC Press.

Akoh, C. C. & Min, D. B. (Eds.). (2007). *Food Lipids: Chemistry, Nutrition and Biochemistry* (3rd ed.). New York: Marcel Dekker.

Caballero, B., Allen, L., & Prentice, A. (Eds.). (2005). *Encyclopedia of Human Nutrition* (2nd ed.). Boston: Elsevier Academic Press.

Chow, C. K. (Ed.). (2008). *Fatty Acids in Foods and Their Health Implications* (3rd ed.). Boca Raton, FL: CRC Press.

Diniz, Y. S. (2004). Diets rich in saturated and polyunsaturated fatty acids: Metabolic shifting and cardiac health. *Nutrition, 20*: 218–224.

Driskell, J. A. (2007). *Sports Nutrition: Fats and Proteins*. Boca Raton, FL: CRC Press.

Eastwood, M. (2003). *Principles of Human Nutrition* (2nd ed.). Malden, MA: Blackwell Science.

Holland, W. L. (2007). Lipid mediators of insulin resistance. *Nutrition Reviews, 65*(pt. 2): s39–s46.

Huang, Y. S., Yanagita, Y., & Krapp, H. R. (Eds.). (2006). *Dietary Fats and Risk of Chronic Disease*. Champaign, IL: AOCS Press.

Hunter, J. E. (2006). Dietary trans fatty acids: Review of recent human studies and food industry response. *Lipids, 41*: 967–992.

Kelly, D. S. (2007). Docosahexaenoic acid supplementation improves fasting and postprandial lipid profiles in hyperglyceridemic men. *American Journal of Clinical Nutrition, 86*: 324–333.

Ma, Y. (2006). Association between carbohydrate intake and serum lipids. *Journal American College of Nutrition, 25*: 155–163.

Mann, J., & Truswell, S. (Eds.). (2007). *Essentials of Human Nutrition* (3rd ed.). New York: Oxford University Press.

Mensink, R. P. (2006). Effects of stearic acid on plasma lipids and lipoproteins in men. *Lipids, 40*: 1201–1205.

Messina, M. J. (2003). Potential public health implications of the hypocholesterolemic effects of soy proteins. *Nutrition, 19*: 280–281.

Okuyama, H. (2007). Dietary lipids impacts on healthy aging. *Lipids, 42*: 821–825.

Parodi, P. N. (2004). Milk fat in human nutrition. *Australian Journal of Dairy Technology, 59*: 31–59.

Rajaram, S. (2001). A monounsaturated fatty acid-rich pecan-rich diet favorably alters the serum lipid profile of healthy men and women. *Journal of Nutrition, 131*: 2275–2279.

Ruano, J. (2007). Intake of phenol-rich virgin olive oil improves the postprandial prothrombotic profile in hypercholesterolemic patients. *American Journal of Clinical Nutrition, 86*: 341–346.

Simopoulos, A. P. (2004). Health effects of eating walnuts. *Food Reviews International, 20*: 91–98.

Stipanuk, M. H. (Ed.). (2006). *Biochemical, Physiological and Molecular Aspects of Human Nutrition* (2nd ed.). St. Louis, MO: Saunders Elsevier.

Webster-Gandy, J., Madden, A., & Holdworth, M. (Eds.). (2006). *Oxford Handbook of Nutrition and Dietetics*. Oxford, London: Oxford University Press.

Whitney, E. N. & Rolfe, S. R. (2002). *Understanding Nutrition*. Belmont, CA: Wadsworth.

CHAPTER

5

Vitamins and Health

Time for completion
Activities: 1½ hours
Optional examination: ½ hour

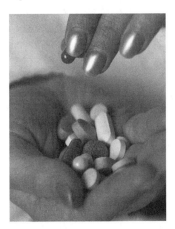

OBJECTIVES

Upon completion of this chapter, the student should be able to do the following:

1. Describe the general characteristics of vitamins.
2. Identify the fat-soluble vitamins and list:
    a. their functions
    b. their food sources
    c. the results of a deficiency or excess
    d. the conditions requiring an increase
    e. the specific characteristics of each
3. Identify the water-soluble vitamins and list:
    a. their functions
    b. their food sources
    c. the results of a deficiency or excess
    d. the conditions requiring an increase
    e. the specific characteristics of each
4. State RDA/DRIs for selected vitamins and discuss amounts of foods needed to meet the requirements.
5. Discuss health risks associated with massive intake of vitamins to prevent or treat disease.
6. Evaluate the effectiveness of megavitamin intake.
7. Indicate population groups for whom vitamin/mineral supplements may be necessary.

GLOSSARY

Carotene: a yellow pigment in plants that can be converted to vitamin A in the intestinal wall.

Cheilosis: a condition in which lesions appear on the lips and the angles of the mouth (cracks).

Coenzyme: a substance such as a vitamin that can attach to the inactive form of an enzyme to make it an active compound or complete enzyme.

Collagen: a gelatin-like protein substance found in connective tissue and bones; a cementing material between body cells.

Dermatitis: inflammation of the skin.

Enzyme: a compound that speeds up the rate of a chemical reaction without itself being changed in the process.

Glossitis: inflammation of the tongue.

Hypervitaminosis: a toxic condition caused by excessive accumulation of a vitamin in the body.

Intrinsic factor: a factor found inside a system. An intrinsic factor is a glycoprotein secreted by the gastric glands necessary for the absorption of vitamin B_{12}.

Megadose: a very large dose of a vitamin, 5 to 100 times or more than the daily recommended allowance.

Organic: (1) containing carbon, a chemical definition; (2) free of chemical fertilizers, pesticides, and additives; a definition used by the lay public. In this chapter, *organic* refers to the first definition.

Osteomalacia: a disease occurring in adults in which bones become softened; caused by a deficiency of vitamin D and calcium. Adult rickets (*see* Rickets).

Osteoporosis: a disease in which calcium is lost from bones, causing them to fracture easily.

Provitamin or precursor: an ingested substance that is converted into a vitamin in the body. For example, carotene is the precursor of vitamin A, and tryptophan is the precursor of niacin.

Rickets: the vitamin D- and calcium-deficiency disease in children; results in bone malformation; equivalent to osteomalacia in adults.

Scurvy: the vitamin C-deficiency disease; characterized by loss of appetite and growth, anemia, weakness, bleeding gums, loose teeth, swollen ankles and wrists, and tiny hemorrhages in the skin.

BACKGROUND INFORMATION

What Are Vitamins?

1. Vitamins are essential organic substances needed daily in very small amounts to perform a specific function in the body. Although they are grouped under one term because they all contain carbon, the essentiality of vitamins for one species may not apply to another.
2. Vitamins cannot be manufactured by the human body; they must be obtained from the diet. Monkeys and guinea pigs need the same outside sources of vitamins as humans do, whereas rabbits, rats, and dogs are able to manufacture some of them in the body.
3. Vitamins are essential for growth and health. An absence or deficiency of vitamins creates specific disorders.
4. The amount of vitamins needed is very small. The total daily requirement is less than 1 tsp.
5. Currently, 13 vitamins are identified as essential. Continued research may identify additional essential vitamins.
6. Synthetic vitamins are nutritionally equivalent to naturally occurring vitamins.

What Can Vitamins Do?

1. In the digestive process, vitamins interact with other vitamins and/or nutrients to enhance absorption.
2. Vitamins can function as coenzymes; that is, they can work with enzymes to speed body chemical reactions. They are used up in the reactions, whereas the enzymes remain unchanged.
3. Vitamins help release energy from biological reactions during metabolism. They do not provide energy.
4. Vitamins are not a structural part of the body.

How Are Vitamins Named?

1. Vitamins are named by letters of the alphabet, sometimes with a number, such as vitamins A, B_1, B_2, C, and D.
2. Vitamins are also given chemical names, for example, retinol, ascorbic acid, thiamin, and riboflavin refer to vitamins A, C, B_1, and B_2, respectively.

How Are Vitamins Classified?

Vitamins are classified into groups with regard to their solubility in either fat or water.

1. The four fat-soluble vitamins are
   a. vitamin A (retinol)
   b. vitamin D (cholecalciferol)
   c. vitamin E (tocopherol)
   d. vitamin K (menadione)
2. The nine water-soluble vitamins are
   a. vitamin C (ascorbic acid)
   b. vitamin B complex:
      vitamin B_1 (thiamin)
      vitamin B_2 (riboflavin)
      niacin
      vitamin B_6 (pyridoxine)
      vitamin B_{12} (cobalamin)
      folacin or folic acid
      pantothenic acid
      biotin

Several vitamins exist in more than one chemical form.

How Is Food Preparation Related to the Solubility of Vitamins?

The solubility of vitamins is directly related to their retention in foods during preparation.

1. Water-soluble vitamins are lost into cooking water. For greater vitamin retention, the following general guidelines apply:
   a. Use only a small quantity of cooking water.
   b. Use leftover cooking water for making gravies, soups, and sauces. Do not discard it.
   c. Minimize cutting food into pieces.
   d. Use the shortest cooking time. Cooking with a lid helps to shorten cooking time.
2. Fat-soluble vitamins are not affected by cooking and preparation in water, but may be destroyed by:
   a. high cooking heat, sun drying, or other forms of dehydration.
   b. oxidation that accompanies rancidity in fat. Fat-soluble vitamins are found in fat.

How Are Vitamins Stored?

1. Excess fat-soluble vitamins are stored in body fat and organs, especially the liver. This storage ability:
   a. can delay deficiency for several months, even if the host does not receive such vitamins in the diet.

b. means that the host needs a dietary supply every other day instead of daily.
   c. does not mean that the host is immune to large doses. Megadoses are toxic to the body.
2. The body does not store excess water-soluble vitamins, but instead excretes them in the urine. As a result:
   a. Vitamin deficiency appears only a few weeks after dietary deprivation.
   b. The vitamins must be consumed daily.
   c. Vitamin supplements do not have extra benefits if a person is consuming an adequate diet. Any excess is lost in the urine.
   d. Some people assume that excess intake of water-soluble vitamins is harmless. However, there are reports documenting the ill effect of excess ingestion of these vitamins.

A summary of the characteristics of the two classes of vitamins is found in Table 5-1.

ACTIVITY 1:

The Water-Soluble Vitamins

REFERENCE TABLES

The water-soluble vitamins, as discussed in the background information, are ascorbic acid (vitamin C) and the B vitamin complex. Tables 5-2 through 5-10 summarize the specific characteristics of each of these vitamins. Study them in preparation for the progress check that follows.

TABLE 5-1   A General Comparison of Water- and Fat-Soluble Vitamins

	Vitamins	
Criteria	Water-Soluble	Fat-Soluble
1. Medium in which soluble	Aqueous, such as water	Nonpolar, organic, such as oil, fat, or ether
2. Number known to be essential to humans	9	4
3. Number human body can synthesize if precursors are provided	1	2
4. Body storage capacity	Minimal	High
5. Body handling of excess intake	Mainly excreted; low toxicity to body	Optimal amount stored; rest excreted; toxicity to body high for two vitamins
6. Means of body disposal	Urine	Bile; if conjugated, urine
7. Urgency of dietary intake	At short intervals, e.g., daily	At longer intervals, e.g., weekly or monthly
8. Rapidity of symptom appearance if deficient	Fast	Slow
9. Chemical constituents	C, H, and O; S, N, and Co in some vitamins	C, H, and O only

TABLE 5-2   Vitamin C (Ascorbic Acid)

Functions	Food Sources[†]	Results of Deficiency or Excess	Conditions Requiring Increase	Specific Characteristics
Essential in formation of collagen, a protein that binds cells together. Needed to heal wounds build new tissue, and provide strength to supporting tissue. Aids formation of bone matrix and tooth dentin. Absorbs iron, which promotes prothrombin formation. Helps maintain elasticity of blood vessels and capillaries. Acts as an antioxidant, protecting the cells from oxidation. Has a sparing effect on several vitamins, especially A, B, and E.	For adults 19–30 years RDA, male: 90 mg/d RDA. female: 75 mg/d *Excellent Sources* chili peppers, green peppers parsley broccoli kale cabbage strawberries papaya oranges (and juice) lemons grapefruit (and juice) guava tangerines cantaloupe watermelon *Good Sources* tomatoes (and juice) white potatoes (with skin on) sweet potatoes honeydew melon pineapple The only animal source of vitamin C is liver.	*Deficiency* acute deficiency—scurvy* delayed wound healing failure to thrive (children) decayed and breaking teeth iron deficient gingivitis anemia (if iron intake is also low) low resistance to infection (especially infants) small vessel hemorrhage seen under skin easy bruising *Excess* (specific effects depend on the individual's tolerance level) rebound scurvy interference with certain drugs gastrointestinal upsets and diarrhea bladder irritations kidney stones interference with anticoagulant drug therapy	Pregnancy and lactation Malnutrition Alcoholism/drug addiction Infections, burns, injuries, fever Certain drug therapies, e.g., isoniazid,[†] OCAs** High stress conditions	1. Vitamin C is easily destroyed by heat, storage, exposure to air, dehydration alkali (such as baking soda), and lengthy exposure to copper and iron utensils. 2. Vitamin C deficiency is rare in developed countries, but can occur in any cases of serious neglect such as psychiatric problems, substance abuse, advanced age, and lack of knowledge about nutrition. 3. Extra care must be taken in preparation of foods containing vitamin C to prevent excessive loss: a. use small amount water b. avoid prolonged cooking c. cut up just before use d. avoid leftovers e. cook quickly, covered or steamed f. use any cooking liquid (do not drain)

*See definition in glossary.
[†]Drug used in treatment of tuberculosis.
**Oral contraceptive agents.
#RDA obtained from Dietary Reference Intakes (DRIs) in Table F-1.

PROGRESS CHECK ON ACTIVITY 1

MULTIPLE CHOICE

Circle the letter of the correct answer.

1. A person on a strict vegetarian diet is most likely to become deficient in which of the following vitamins?

   a. B_{12}
   b. folacin
   c. ascorbic acid
   d. B_6

2. Vitamin B_6 requirements are increased:

   a. with increased energy intake.
   b. with increased protein intake.
   c. when on a reduction diet.
   d. with increased carbohydrate intake.

TABLE 5-3   Vitamin B₁ (Thiamin)

Functions	Food Sources†	Results of Deficiency or Excess	Conditions Requiring Increase	Specific Characteristics
Releases energy from fat and carbohydrate. Helps transmits nerve impulses. Breaks down alcohol. Promotes better appetite and functioning of the digestive tract.	For adults 19–30 years RDA, male: 1.2 mg/d RDA, female: 1.1 mg/d *Excellent Sources* sunflower seeds sesame seeds soybeans wheat germ peanuts animal sources: liver, kidney, pork *Good Sources* enriched cereals enriched pasta enriched or brown rice whole grains oatmeal animal sources: eggs, poultry	*Deficiency* acute: beri-beri* subacute: loss of appetite, vomiting, leg cramps, mental depression, edema, weight loss *Excess* no evidence of toxicity in excess amounts. May create a shortage of other B vitamins if taken exclusively	Any condition that increases metabolic rate Alcoholism Old age (whether elderly are on low-calories diets or not) Pregnancy and lactation growth periods People on fad diets Illness/stress conditions Athletic training (whenever extra need for kcal)	The B vitamins have four common properties: 1. All of them function as coenzymes in biochemical reactions. 2. All are water-soluble. 3. All are natural parts of yeast and liver. 4. All promote the growth of bacteria. If there is a deficiency in one of the B vitamins, there will be deficiencies in the others. The B vitamins function together— excess of one creates greater need for the others. Converted rice contains more thiamin than other types of rice.

*Beri-beri: means "I cannot." Major symptoms are paralysis, heart, and vessel impairment.
†RDA obtained from Dietary Reference Intakes (DRIs) in Table F-1.

3. A deficiency of vitamin B₁₂ produces:

   a. pernicious anemia.
   b. cheilosis.
   c. microcytic anemia.
   d. sickle cell anemia.

4. Research studies have shown that a 1 g dose of vitamin C daily:

   a. will reduce the total number of colds among adults.
   b. is no more effective against cold symptoms than is 75 mg daily.
   c. will lessen the effects of a hangover.
   d. will be stored in the body.

5. Which condition(s) may result in folic acid deficiency?

   a. a strict vegetarian diet
   b. use of contraceptive pills and/or pregnancy
   c. malabsorption syndromes
   d. all of the above

6. The RDA/DRI gives a safe and adequate intake for ascorbic acid a 19–30 year old male as:

   a. 400 IU per day.
   b. 90 mg per day.
   c. 2 to 3 mg per day.
   d. 40 g per day.

7. Risks associated with megadose ascorbic acid intake include all except:

   a. bladder infections.
   b. possible increase in kidney stone formation.
   c. diarrhea.
   d. eye infections.

8. Ascorbic acid plays a major role in the formation of which protein?

   a. histidine
   b. keratin
   c. collagen
   d. mucus

TABLE 5-4   Vitamin B$_2$ (Riboflavin)

Functions	Food Sources†	Results of Deficiency or Excess	Conditions Requiring Increase	Specific Characteristics
Releases energy from fat, carbohydrate, and protein. Essential for healthy skin and growth. Promotes visual health. Functions in the production of corticosteroids* and red blood cells.	For adults 19–30 years RDA, male: 1.3 mg/d RDA, female: 1.1 mg/d *Excellent Sources* milk cheese wheat germ yeast liver and kidney *Good Sources* meat, poultry, fish eggs dark green leafy vegetables dry beans and peas nuts	*Deficiency* lesions around the mouth and nose hair loss scaly skin failure to thrive (children) light sensitivity clouding of the cornea of the eye weight loss glossitis *Excess* no evidence yet that this nutrient is toxic in large amounts	Increase in body size, metabolic rate, or growth rate, such as pregnancy, lactation, and growth Alcoholism Poverty Old age Strict vegetarian diets that prohibit meat, eggs, and milk Stress and malabsorption of nutrients Any condition where there is loss of gastric secretions (achlorhydria) may precipitate a deficiency Following burns or any surgical procedure where there is extensive protein loss	1. No evidence that the requirement for B$_2$ goes up as kcal rise. 2. Few individuals in the U.S. show any deficiency. 3. Foods high in calcium are usually high in B$_2$. 4. Before riboflavin is absorbed it must be phosphorylated (combined with phosphorus). Both are found in milk and cheeses. 5. Is sensitive to light; should be kept in opaque containers. 6. Cooking and drying may enhance the availability. 7. Only partially water-soluble. 8. If a deficiency occurs, multiple B vitamins are given because of their interrelationships. 9. B$_2$ is destroyed by alkaline.

*Hormones of the adrenal cortex that influence or control key body functions.
†RDA obtained from Dietary Reference Intakes (DRIs) in Table F-1.

9. All of the following refer to vitamin B$_{12}$ except which one?

   a. It requires an intrinsic factor for absorption.
   b. A deficiency results in pernicious anemia.
   c. Food sources rich in vitamin B$_{12}$ include asparagus and broccoli.
   d. Vitamin B$_{12}$ is necessary for normal red blood cell formation.

10. Riboflavin is:

   a. added to white flour for enrichment.
   b. found abundantly in milk and cheese.
   c. an essential nutrient.
   d. all of the above

11. Niacin:

   a. can be made by the body from tryptophan, an essential amino acid.

   b. is found in abundance in meats, poultry, and fish.
   c. is fat soluble.
   d. is none of the above.

12. Pyridoxine:

   a. is a coenzyme in protein metabolism and heme formation.
   b. is found in wheat, corn, meats, and liver.
   c. aids functioning of the nervous system.
   d. is all of the above.

13. Cobalamin:

   a. requires an intrinsic factor from the stomach for absorption.
   b. should be supplemented in the average person's diet.
   c. is toxic if taken in excess.
   d. is none of the above.

TABLE 5-5   Vitamin B₆ (Pyridoxine)

Functions	Food Sources*	Results of Deficiency or Excess	Conditions Requiring Increase	Specific Characteristics
Forms reactions that break down and rebuild amino acids. Produces antibodies and red blood cells. Aids functioning of the nervous system and regeneration of nerve tissue. Changes one fatty acid into another.	For adults 19–30 years RDA, male, female: 1.3 mg/d *Excellent Sources* yeast sunflower seeds wheat germ wheat bran avocado banana animal source: liver *Good Sources* meats poultry fish whole grains nuts	*Deficiency* decreased antibody production anemia vomiting failure to thrive (children) skin lesions liver and kidney problems central nervous system abnormalities: confusion irritability depression convulsions *Excess* no toxicity reported with megadoses, but dependency may be induced with large doses	Increased protein intake Pregnancy Use of oral contraceptive agents, isoniazid Advancing age	1. B₆ deficiencies occur almost entirely in wealthy, developed countries. 2. The essential fatty acid, linoleic, is converted to arachidonic acid. 3. Converts tryptophan to niacin. 4. Involved in conversions and catabolism of all the amino acids.

*RDA obtained from Dietary Reference Intakes (DRIs) in Table F-1.

14. Factors that may cause a deficiency of water-soluble vitamins include:

    a. taking no vitamin supplement.
    b. fad diets.
    c. high-fat diets.
    d. none of the above.

15. A deficiency of vitamin C:

    a. causes delayed wound healing.
    b. decreases iron absorption.
    c. increases capillary bleeding.
    d. all of the above.

16. Water-soluble vitamins:

    a. are generally stored by the body.
    b. are destroyed by fats and oils.
    c. are minimally excreted.
    d. none of the above.

17. B complex vitamins:

    a. function as coenzymes.
    b. are best supplied by supplements.
    c. can be synthesized by the body.
    d. are excreted in feces.

18. Which of the following is the poorest source of ascorbic acid?

    a. cheddar cheese
    b. baked potato
    c. strawberries
    d. coleslaw

ACTIVITY 2:

The Fat-Soluble Vitamins

REFERENCE TABLES

The fat-soluble vitamins, as discussed earlier, are vitamins A, D, E, and K. Other than the general characteristics noted, these vitamins bear no resemblance to water-soluble vitamins nor to each other. In Tables 5-11 through 5-14 the specific characteristics of each fat-soluble vitamin are outlined for easy reference. Study them in preparation for this activity's progress check.

ANTIOXIDANTS

Antioxidants are substances that may protect your cells against the effects of free radicals. Free radicals are

TABLE 5-6   Vitamin B₁₂ (Cobalamin)*

Functions	Food Sources†	Results of Deficiency or Excess	Conditions Requiring Increase	Specific Characteristics
Aids proper formation of red blood cells. Part of the RNA-DNA nucleic acids; is therefore essential for normal function of all body cells, especially gastrointestinal tract, nervous system. Bone marrow formation. Used in folacin metabolism. Prevention of pernicious anemia.	For adults 19–30 years RDA, male, female: 2.4 µg/d *Animal products are the main food sources:* clams/oysters organ meats eggs shrimp chicken pork hot dogs	*Deficiency* glossitis anorexia weakness weight loss mental and nervous symptoms abdominal pain constipation/diarrhea macrocytic anemia and if intrinsic factor also missing: pernicious anemia (see #4 under characteristics) *Excess* no toxicity observed; but at high doses, vitamins are considered drugs and often create imbalances in the functioning of other nutrients.	Strict vegetarian diet (vegans) Malabsorption Stomach injury Total gastrectomy Pregnancy and lactation Old age	1. The normal liver will store enough B₁₂ to last for two to five years. 2. B₁₂ is made only by microorganisms in the intestines. 3. Only 30%–70% of what is consumed is absorbed. 4. B₁₂ must bind to the intrinsic factor, which is a protein secreted by the stomach lining. 5. Calcium is also necessary in this reaction. 6. Absorption of B₁₂ is influenced by body levels of B₆. 7. The elderly are at highest risk of developing pernicious anemia. 8. Smooth, bland foods are indicated for megaloblastic and pernicious anemia (the mouth is sore). 9. All foods needed for blood cell production included.

*Folic acid deficiency is frequently associated with B₁₂ deficiency, creating a vicious cycle.
†RDA obtained from Dietary Reference Intakes (DRIs) in Table F-1.

molecules produced when your body breaks down food; they are also produced by environmental exposures such as tobacco smoke and radiation. Free radicals can damage cells, and may play a role in heart disease, cancer, and other disorders. Antioxidants are molecules that can safely interact with free radicals and terminate or prevent the damaging effects of free radicals. Antioxidant substances include the following:

- Beta-carotene
- Lutein
- Lycopene
- Selenium
- Vitamin A
- Vitamin C
- Vitamin E

Antioxidants are found in many foods. These include fruits and vegetables, nuts, grains, and some meats, poultry and fish. Some potential health benefits of antioxidants are:

1. Prevent or neutralize the negative effects of free radicals.
2. Slow the aging process and protect against heart disease and strokes.
3. Prevent or interfere with the development of cancer.
4. Retard induced cell damage from exercise and/or enhance recovery.

Researchers are actively studying the role of antioxidants in many human diseases. However, it will take years before definitive results are available.

TABLE 5-7 Niacin

Functions	Food Sources[†]	Results of Deficiency or Excess	Conditions Requiring Increase	Specific Characteristics
Releases energy from carbohydrates, protein, fat. Synthesizes proteins and nucleic acids. Synthesizes fatty acids from glucose.	For adults 19–30 years RDA, male: 16 mg/d RDA. female: 14 mg/d *Excellent Sources* yeast peanuts and peanut butter soybeans sesame seeds sunflower seeds animal sources: beef, poultry, fish, organ meats especially high *Good Sources* meats nuts wheat germ enriched cereals, bread, pasta	*Deficiency* acute: Pellagra* subacute: weakness, indigestion, anorexia, lack of energy, cracked skin, sore mouth and tongue, failure to thrive (children), insomnia, irritability, mental depression; damage to the skin, gastrointestinal tract, and central nervous system *Excess* (megadose treatment for certain conditions) severe flushing glucose intolerance gastrointestinal disorders irregular heartbeat vision disturbances liver damage	Whenever more kcal are consumed, e.g., pregnancy/lactation illness stress chronic alcoholism intestinal disorders	1. Niacin is synthesized in the body from tryptophan, an essential amino acid. Diets adequate in protein are adequate in niacin. 2. Niacin is stable in foods; it can withstand reasonable periods of heat, cooling, and storage. 3. Niacin is water-soluble; use the cooking liquids (do not drain off).

*The 3 Ds of Pellagra symptoms: 1. Dermatitis (inflammation of the skin); 2. Diarrhea (inflammation of the gastrointestinal tract); 3. Dementia (mental confusion); (if untreated: add death).
[†]RDA obtained from Dietary Reference Intakes (DRIs) in Table F-1.

VITAMINS AND THE PREPARATION AND PROCESSING OF FOOD*

All foods undergo some processing and are subject to varying degrees of vitamin loss in content or bioavailability. Although processing techniques that minimize nutrient loss are used, the vitamin content of foods can decrease when processed.

Other factors that influence the vitamin content of foods are growing conditions, genetic variation, and postharvest or postmortem practices. The factors that influence the vitamin content of vegetables, fruits, and grain crops are soil conditions, including moisture level and fertilizer use. The vitamin content of eggs, meat, and milk is affected by animal breed and strain, health, level of production, as well as the nutrient content of the rations fed.

After harvest, the vitamin C content of fruits and vegetables can dramatically decrease. Moreover, the stage of maturity of the fruit or vegetable will influence the maximum content of vitamin C in the food.

Milling procedures for cereals result in a general loss of vitamin content. To compensate for the loss, food products produced from flours are usually fortified with B vitamins (thiamin, riboflavin, and niacin). A prime example of a food fortified with vitamins is enriched bread. Further, many breakfast cereals are heavily enriched with vitamins.

Another major source of vitamin loss in foods occurs during washing, blanching, and cooking. The extent of vitamin loss is dependent on temperature, amount of water used in the process, and cooking procedure. Usually the loss of vitamin C in foods exceeds that of the B complex and fat-soluble vitamins.

The use of antioxidants (BHT, TBHQ, ascorbic acid, tocopherols) as preservatives significantly protect foods from excessive vitamin loss. Reducing lipid oxidation and oxidative rancidity in foods can prevent destruction of

*The information in this section has been modified from *Food Processing Manual* (2009), by Y. H. Hui. Published and copyrighted by Science Technology System, West Sacramento, California. Used with permission.

TABLE 5-8   Folic Acid (Folacin, Folate)

Functions	Food Sources**	Results of Deficiency or Excess	Conditions Requiring Increase	Specific Characteristics
Synthesizes the nucleic acids (RNA-DNA). Essential for breakdown of most of the amino acids. Necessary for proper formation of red blood cells.	For adults 19–30 years RDA, male, female: 400 µg/d *Excellent Sources* liver/kidney yeast oranges/orange juice* green leafy vegetables asparagus* broccoli wheat germ* nuts *Good Sources* melons sweet potato pumpkin	*Deficiency* slows growth, interferes with cell regeneration *Macrocytic Anemia* (red blood cells are large and too few and have less Hgb than normal) *Megoblastic Anemia* (young red blood cells fail to mature, reduction in white blood cells; also histidine, an amino acid, not utilized) *Excess* no toxic effect from megadose, but will mask pernicious anemias†, vitamin supplements may not contain more than 0.1 mg/folacin (by law)	Whenever the metabolic rate is high: pregnancy/lactation infections/fever growth of malignant tumors hyperthyroidism anemias Excess alcohol intake Use of oral contraceptive agents Malabsorptive disorders Certain other diseases, e.g., leukemia Hodgkin's disease cancer Use of drugs in anticonvulsant therapy When chemotherapy is used for cancer	1. When there is a folic acid deficiency, the diet must include all the other nutrients needed to produce red blood cells, i.e., protein copper iron B_{12}/vitamin C 2. Persons with macrocytic or megoblastic anemia have sore mouths and tongues; soft bland foods or liquids may be needed. 3. Prolonged cooking destroys most of the folacin. 4. Folic acid deficiency is common in the third trimester of pregnancy; the requirement is six times the normal amount.

*Highest in folacin
**RDA obtained from Dietary Reference Intakes (DRIs) in Table F-1.
†Pernicious anemia does not respond to iron and folacin; requires treatment with B_{12}.

vitamins A, C, and E. Changing the pH of foods and reducing lipid oxidation will also help to retard the damage to and loss of carotenoids and oxygen-sensitive vitamins in foods.

The vitamins that are sensitive to heat are vitamin D, vitamin E, thiamin, riboflavin, pyridoxine, pantothenate, and folic acid. Vitamins sensitive to oxygen are the fat-soluble vitamins, ascorbic acid, thiamin, biotin, pantothenate, and folic acid.

Under the laws and regulations governing food additives, vitamins or their derivatives are used as follows:

1. They serve as ingredients in dietary supplements. If so, a separate law on dietary supplement also applies.
2. They serve as ingredients in medical food used under clinical conditions, orally or intravenously.
3. They serve as ingredients in animal feeds.
4. They serve as food additives in fortifying foods. The FDA issues requirements defining which vitamin can be added to what foods and at what levels, accompanied by additional restriction.
5. They serve as antioxidants in food processing.

A brief discussion will be provided here on the last application. The vitamins with antioxidant activities are ascorbic acid, tocopherol, and carotene. Ascorbic acid will serve as an example for discussion. Ascorbic acid (vitamin C) is used extensively in the food industry for two important purposes:

- As a nutritional ingredient
- As a food additive to serve multiple processing functions

Acting as an antioxidant, ascorbic acid can improve the color, palatability, and related quality of many food products. Ascorbic acid in its reduced form becomes the oxidized form, dehydroascorbic acid. It is an effective antioxidant because it can remove available oxygen in its immediate surroundings under most processing conditions.

Beverages

During the manufacture of beverages, especially fruit juices, ascorbic acid is commonly added to improve sensory profiles such as color and palatability.

TABLE 5-9   Pantothenic Acid

Functions	Food Sources*	Results of Deficiency or Excess	Conditions Requiring Increase	Specific Characteristics
Helps release energy from carbohydrates, fat, and protein. Aids in formation of cholesterol, hemoglobin, and other hormones. Assists in synthesizing certain fatty aids.	For adults 19–30 years AI, male, female: 5 mg/d *Richest Sources* liver, kidney fish whole grains Is found in every plant and animal food	*Deficiency* uncommon; not observed under normal conditions Induced deficiencies cause headaches, insomnia, nausea, vomiting, tingling of hands and feet poor coordination *Excess* no toxicity observed	Rare Situations severe malnutrition (e.g., prisoner of war, starving children)	1. Most commonly occurring of all the vitamins 2. Name taken from the Greek and means "everywhere"

*AI obtained from Dietary Reference Intakes (DRIs) in Table F-1.

TABLE 5-10   Biotin

Functions	Food Sources*	Results of Deficiency or Excess	Conditions Requiring Increase	Specific Characteristics
Acts as a coenzyme in metabolism of fat and carbohydrate.	For adults 19–30 years AI, male, female: 30 µg/d *Richest Sources* liver/kidney egg yolk milk yeast Is found in almost all foods	*Deficiency* uncommon; intestinal bacteria produces biotin. can be induced large-scale use of raw eggs as in tube feedings, etc., may cause development of symptoms such as: nausea muscle pain dermatitis glossitis abnormal EKG (electro-cardiogram) elevated cholesterol level	Anyone consuming raw eggs in quantity Some infants under age of 6 mo.	1. Biotin can be bound by avidin, a protein in raw egg, and becomes unavailable to the body.

*AI obtained from Dietary Reference Intakes (DRIs) in Table F-1.

Fruits such as apples, bananas, and peaches show discoloration when cut. When these fruits are processed to produce fruit juices or purees, ascorbic acid may be added during the crushing, straining, or pressing stages to prevent enzymatic browning of the raw fruits.

Meat Products

Ascorbic acid is commonly used as an antioxidant in cured meat processing with the following objectives:

1. To accelerate color development
2. To inhibit nitrosamine formation
3. To prevent oxidation
4. To avoid color fading

Fats and Oils

When fats and oils are exposed to heat, light, and air, their unsaturated long-chain fatty acids readily oxidize. This causes rancid odors and flavors because of the

TABLE 5-11   Vitamin A (Retinol)

Functions	Food Sources*	Results of Deficiency or Excess	Conditions Requiring Increase	Specific Characteristics
Enables eye to adjust to changes in light (formation of rhodopsin in the retina). Helps maintain healthy skin and mucous membranes as well as the cornea of the eye. Develops healthy teeth and bones. Aids reproductive processes. Synthesizes glycogen in the liver. Regulates fat metabolism in formation of cholesterol. Aids formation of cortisone in the adrenal gland.	For adults 19–30 years RDA, male: 900 µg/d RDA. female: 700 µg/d *Excellent Sources* liver eggs carrots cantaloupe sweet potato winter squash pumpkin apricots broccoli green pepper dark green leafy vegetables *Good Sources* tomatoes (and juice) butter margarine peaches	*Deficiency*** night blindness (inability to see in dim light) keratinization (formation of a horny layer of skin, cracking of skin) xerophthalmia (cornea of eye becomes opaque, causing blindness) faulty bone growth, defective tooth enamel, less resistance to decay decreased resistance to infection, impaired wound healing *Excess* highly toxic in excessive doses (1–3,000 µg RE/kg/body weight) accumulates in liver, causing enlargement, vomiting, skin rashes, hair loss, diarrhea, cramps, joint pain, dry scaly skin, anorexia, abnormal bone growth, cerebral edema	Self-neglect due to psychiatric disturbances, old age, alcoholism, lack of nutritional knowledge Pregnancy and lactation Protein-deficient diets Any condition of fat malabsorption Infectious hepatitis Gallbladder diseases Children and pregnant women in poverty	1. Preformed vitamin A (retinol) is found only in animal sources. 2. Provitamin A (beta carotene) is found in plant sources and is a yellow-orange group of pigments. It is called a precursor. 3. Xerophthalmia is an important world health problem: more than 1,000,000 children go blind yearly, especially in developing countries. 4. Very low-fat diets decrease absorption. 5. Vitamin A must be bound to protein for transport. 6. Bile salts must be in the intestine for absorption. 7. Is stable at usual cooking temperatures. Cover pan recommended. 8. Processing and advance preparation cause only minimal loss. 9. Hypervitaminosis is usually from megavitamin supplements. 10. Excess intake of foods with beta carotene may discolor skin but is not harmful. 11. Beta carotene is being considered for prevention of certain types of skin cancer.

*RDA obtained from Dietary Reference Intakes (DRIs) in Table F-1.
**Deficiencies more uncommon in Western countries because of dietary abundance.

TABLE 5-12   **Vitamin D (Cholecalciferol)**

Functions	Food Sources*	Results of Deficiency or Excess	Conditions Requiring Increase	Specific Characteristics
Promotes the absorption of calcium and phosphorus in the intestine. Helps maintain blood calcium and phosphorus levels for normal bone calcification. Aids in formation of bone matrix.	For adults 19–30 years AI, male, female: 5 µg/d *Sources:* irradiated fortified vitamin D milk minimal amounts present in fish, egg yolk, butter *Primary food source* fish, liver (cod liver, halibut liver) oils *Synthetic form* from irradiation of plants; used most in supplements and dairy products *Principal source* sunlight; ultraviolet rays penetrate a cholesterol-like substance in the skin which is converted to active vitamin D in the kidneys	*Deficiency severe* rickets, serious decalcification of bones, osteomalacia (tender, painful bones in adults), tooth decay *Excess* high blood calcium levels kidney damage growth retardation vomiting, diarrhea, weight loss	Invalids (housebound) Individuals who are rarely exposed to sunlight Premature infants Children of strict vegetarians who drink no fortified milk Pregnancy and lactation Early childhood Breast-fed infants Any disease that interferes with fat absorption or vitamin D absorption Chronic renal failure Certain drug therapies that interfere with absorption Dark-skinned people	1. Ultraviolet light is filtered out by smog, fog, smoke, and window glass. 2. Can be classified as a hormone since it can be made by the body. 3. Milk, unless fortified, is a poor source of vitamin D. 4. As much as 95% of ultraviolet rays for conversion to vitamin D may be prevented in dark-skinned races. 5. Vitamin D permits 30 to 35% absorption of ingested calcium: without it only 10% is absorbed.

*AI obtained from Dietary Reference Intakes (DRIs) in Table F-1.

formation of low-molecular weight compounds. Special formula preparation containing ascorbic acid can prevent this undesirable condition.

Dough Products

In the manufacture of bakery products, adding ascorbic acid to the flour improves both bread texture and loaf volume. This ability of ascorbic acid to improve bread dough has been appreciated since the 1930s.

PROGRESS CHECK ON ACTIVITY 2

MULTIPLE CHOICE

Circle the letter of the correct answer.

1. All except _____ are good sources of vitamin A.

   a. egg yolks
   b. potatoes
   c. dark green and deep yellow vegetables
   d. beef liver

2. Toxicity symptoms of vitamin A include all except:

   a. joint pain, loss of hair, jaundice.
   b. anorexia, fatigue, weight loss.
   c. vasodilation, decreased glucose tolerance.
   d. skin rash, edema.

3. Which of the following foods would you recommend in order to increase a person's vitamin A intake?

   a. grapefruit
   b. egg whites
   c. potatoes
   d. pumpkin

TABLE 5-13   Vitamin E (Tocopherol)

Functions	Food Sources*	Results of Deficiency or Excess	Conditions Requiring Increase	Specific Characteristics
The only demonstrated function is as an antioxidant (protects vitamin A and unsaturated fats from destruction; protects red and white blood cells from destruction by preventing oxidation of cell membrane). Protects vitamin C and fatty acids. Believed to enter into biochemical changes that release energy. Assists in cellular respiration. Helps synthesize other body substances. Helps maintain intact cell membranes.	For adults 19–30 years RDA, male, female: 15 mg/d *Best Sources (plant)* vegetable oils margarines shortenings sunflower seeds wheat germ nuts whole grains *Good Sources (animal)* liver codfish butter human milk	*Deficiency* none observed except in premature infants or SGA** infants *Excess* headache nausea fatigue dizziness blurred vision skin changes thrombophlebitis†	Premature infants (or SGA)** Whenever greater amounts of polyunsaturated fats are ingested Possibly in disorders resulting in fat malabsorption	1. Does not travel well across placenta of pregnant women. 2. Is usually given with vitamin A when there is a vitamin A deficiency. 3. Vitamin E content of breast milk is adequate for the infant. 4. Many animal disorders have responded to vitamin E therapy but have not been effective for humans. For this reason, vitamin E is the most controversial of all vitamin therapies. 5. Contrary to popular opinion, excess intake creates side effects. 6. The role of vitamin E as an antioxidant is being linked to retardation of the aging process.

*RDA obtained from Dietary Reference Intakes (DRIs) in Table F-1.
†Blood clots in veins.
**SGA = small for gestational age.

4. Vitamin D is needed by the body to:

   a. digest protein.
   b. absorb amino acids.
   c. absorb calcium.
   d. make collagen.

5. Fat-soluble vitamins:

   a. may be altered by exposure to alkali.
   b. are stable to ordinary cooking.
   c. can store in liver and tissues.
   d. all of the above.

6. Carotene, or provitamin A, is contained in significant amounts in all of these except:

   a. corn, cauliflower.
   b. spinach, collard greens.
   c. apricots, pumpkin.
   d. green pepper, peaches.

7. Vitamin D:

   a. enhances calcium and phosphorus absorption.
   b. enhances mineralization of bones and cartilage.
   c. lowers serum calcium levels.
   d. all of the above.

8. Excess vitamin D:

   a. is stored in adipose tissue and the liver.
   b. can cause calcification of soft tissue such as blood vessels and renal tubules.
   c. is excreted in the urine.
   d. a and b

9. The only demonstrated function of vitamin E in humans is to:

   a. increase sexual prowess.
   b. increase fertility.

TABLE 5-14   Vitamin K (Menadione)

Functions	Food Sources*	Results of Deficiency or Excess	Conditions Requiring Increase	Specific Characteristics
Prothrombin formation (prothrombin is a protein that converts eventually to fibrin, the key substance in blood clotting) Blood coagulation	For adults 19–30 years AI, male: 120 µg/d AI, female: 90 µg/d The two sources are: 1. intestinal bacteria and 2. food sources: dark green vegetables cauliflower tomatoes soybeans wheat bran *small amounts in:* egg yolk organ meats cheese	*Deficiency* hemorrhaging when blood does not clot *Excess* irritation of skin and respiratory tract with the synthetic form, menadione toxicity found only in newborns who are administered doses above 5 mg causes excessive breakdown of red blood cells brain damage	Newborn infants Persons on antibiotics Persons with diseases where there is chronic diarrhea or poor absorption Possibly prior to surgery	1. Deficiency is rare since it is synthesized by intestinal bacteria. Food sources not usually needed by healthy people. 2. The intestinal tract of the newborn may be free of bacteria for several days. 3. Antibiotics kill the natural bacteria in the intestine.

**AI obtained from Dietary Reference Intakes (DRIs) in Table F-1.

c. act as an antioxidant.
d. prevent heart disease.

10. The only known function of vitamin K is its:

a. use in forming blood-clotting factors.
b. antioxidant property.
c. antirachitic property.
d. antibiotic property.

MATCHING

Match the following statements with the letter of their corresponding vitamin.

11. Inadequate intake causes osteomalacia and rickets.
12. Inadequate intake causes poor night vision and skin infection.
13. Promotes normal blood clotting.
14. Prevents destruction of unsaturated fatty acids.

a. vitamin A
b. vitamin D
c. vitamin E
d. vitamin K

RESPONSIBILITIES OF HEALTH PERSONNEL

1. Treat clients' vitamin deficiency diseases by supplying the missing vitamin(s) as drug therapy (through tablets, capsules, or intravenously) as an adjunct to a high-protein, high-calorie balanced diet.

2. Treat borderline vitamin deficiencies by supplying the appropriate diet and including rich sources of the missing vitamin(s).
3. Be aware that some patients may not be able to take food or medication by mouth. Nausea and anorexia, common among people suffering from vitamin-deficiency diseases, may require different forms of ingestion.
4. Be aware that most outright deficiency diseases occur among alcoholics, drug abusers, psychiatric patients, the aged, low-income groups, or people on extreme diets.
5. Be aware that borderline deficiencies cut across all socioeconomic lines, and are caused by poor eating habits and ignorance of essential nutrients.
6. Be prepared to give multivitamin and mineral supplements to allow for the metabolic interrelationships among the vitamins as well as their action as catalysts and coenzymes.
7. Request extra vitamins for clients with conditions that increase the metabolic rate.
8. Be aware that very low-fat diets lead to decreased intake and absorption of the fat-soluble vitamins.
9. Be aware that the fat-soluble vitamins A and D are highly toxic in doses that greatly exceed the DRIs/RDA.
10. Request fat-soluble vitamin supplements in aqueous form any time there is a disease where fat malabsorption occurs, such as celiac disease or cystic fibrosis.

SUMMARY

Vitamins are organic compounds that are required in the diet in very small amounts, but which perform very important functions. They are classified on the basis of solubility in either water or fat.

Fat-soluble vitamins are stored in the fats of foods and in the body. Because of this, humans may not need a daily source. Excess intakes of fat-soluble vitamins can be toxic, especially vitamins A and D. Fat-soluble vitamins can withstand factors such as heat and pressure.

Daily consumption of water-soluble vitamins is necessary because the body does not store them. These vitamins are easily lost from food not properly prepared, stored, or processed. While large doses of water-soluble vitamins are usually not considered toxic, an excess intake of certain vitamins results in adverse side effects.

No vitamin provides energy, but some vitamins are involved in releasing energy from the metabolism of carbohydrate, protein, and fat. Vitamins are considered as coenzymes, and therefore do not undergo changes during biological reactions.

Megavitamin therapy is a controversial topic. Promoters have linked massive doses of vitamins with the prevention and treatment of numerous human diseases, but most of these "cures" remain unproven or have been shown to be dangerous. Nutrients are considered drugs when they are used in large doses for treating any disease. At high doses, vitamins behave differently than at recommended doses. The Food and Drug Administration (FDA) has tried but failed to limit or prohibit the sale of megavitamins without a prescription.

Many people believe that "natural" vitamins are better than synthetic ones, and that natural vitamins are "pure" and contain no chemicals. Both beliefs are untrue. The chemical structure of a synthetic and a natural vitamin is exactly the same, and the body cannot distinguish between them. In addition, "natural" vitamins have synthetic substances holding them together. There is only one difference between a natural and a synthetic vitamin: the natural one costs two to three times more.

Supplementing the diet with vitamins has been another long-standing controversial issue. Most nutritionists are in agreement that you cannot compensate for a poor diet by taking a supplement; many foods contain necessary nutrients not included in commercial supplements. But some population groups are at high risk of vitamin deficiency and probably need a supplement. These groups include the following:

1. Women during pregnancy and lactation
2. Infants
3. Anyone on a diet containing fewer than 1000 calories per day
4. Users of oral contraceptives
5. Alcoholics
6. Smokers
7. Strict vegetarians
8. Many senior citizens
9. Persons with certain illnesses or convalescing from surgery

Other than for the last group, nutrient supplements should not be taken in megadose quantities. They should be administered in quantities that assist the person to fulfill the DRI requirements.

The DRI requirements for males and females of 51 years and over may not be high enough for the elderly. Subclinical deficiencies have been identified in this population. Factors believed to be responsible are decreased intake and impaired metabolism. Health professionals should assist elderly clients in choosing supplements appropriately, however, as many are unaware that some vitamins are toxic in excess doses and that others interfere with medications they may be taking or with diagnostic tests. Self-medicating with megavitamins without directions from qualified health personnel can cause great harm.

PROGRESS CHECK ON CHAPTER 5

MATCHING

Match the vitamin to the letter of the phrase that best describes it.

1. Riboflavin
2. Thiamin
3. Vitamin B_6
4. Vitamin B_{12}
5. Niacin

a. Requirement is based on the amount of carbohydrate in diet
b. May be synthesized from the amino acid tryptophan
c. Deficiency causes cracked skin around the mouth, inflamed lips, and sore tongue
d. Helps change one amino acid into another
e. A cobalt-containing vitamin needed for red blood cell formation

Match the nutrients listed in the left column with the major sources of those nutrients in the right column.

6. Vitamin B_{12} a. orange juice
7. Riboflavin   b. dark green leafy vegetables
8. Vitamin C   c. sunshine
9. Vitamin D   d. meats
10. Beta carotene   e. milk

TRUE/FALSE

Circle T for True and F for False.

11. T F Synthetic vitamins are nutritionally equivalent to naturally occurring vitamins.
12. T F Vitamin losses from fruits and vegetables can occur as a result of poor conditions of harvesting and storage.
13. T F Natural and synthetic vitamins are used by the body in the same way.
14. T F Vitamin K is required for the synthesis of blood-clotting factors.
15. T F B vitamins serve as coenzymes in metabolic reactions in the body.
16. T F There is no DRI/RDA for vitamin K because it is produced by the body.

CLASSIFICATION

Classify the following phrases as descriptive of either water-soluble or fat-soluble vitamins.

Water-soluble vitamins = a

Fat-soluble vitamins = b

17. _____ are stored in appreciable amounts in the body.
18. _____ are excreted in the urine.
19. _____ require regular consumption in the diet because storage in the body is minimal.
20. _____ deficiencies are slow to develop.
21. _____ include the vitamin B complex and vitamin C.
22. _____ include vitamins A, D, E, and K.

MULTIPLE CHOICE

Circle the letter of the correct answer.

23. Which of the following food-preparation methods is most likely to cause large losses of vitamins?

   a. cooking fruits and vegetables whole and unpared
   b. dicing fruits and vegetables into small pieces
   c. cutting fruits and vegetables into medium-size, chunky pieces
   d. cutting just before serving time

24. When cooking vegetables to conserve vitamins, which is preferred?

   a. small amounts of water
   b. large amounts of water
   c. no water
   d. addition of baking soda

25. Which vegetable preparation method tends to conserve the most vitamins?

   a. boiling
   b. simmering
   c. stir-frying
   d. baking

26. Excessive vitamin intake has:

   a. not been demonstrated to be beneficial in humans.
   b. been shown to cause toxicity by some vitamins.
   c. been shown to cause increased excretion of the water-soluble vitamins.
   d. all of the above.

27. An important role of the water-soluble vitamins is to serve as:

   a. enzymes.
   b. hormones.
   c. electrolytes.
   d. coenzymes.

28. Vitamin/mineral supplements are generally recommended for _____ because they are at higher risk of developing deficiencies.

   a. infants
   b. pregnant and lactating women
   c. strict vegetarians
   d. persons with malabsorption diseases

29. One should avoid taking vitamin pills unless especially prescribed by one's doctor because:

   a. they are too expensive.
   b. fat-soluble vitamins are stored in the body and can build up to toxic levels.
   c. water-soluble vitamins in excess of daily requirements may become toxic to the liver.
   d. edema can result from high blood levels of water-soluble vitamins.

30. Good food sources of thiamin include all except:

   a. lean pork, beef, and liver.
   b. citrus fruits.
   c. green leafy vegetables.
   d. sunflower and sesame seeds.

REFERENCES

Ball, G. F. (2004). *Vitamins: Their Role in the Human Body.* Ames, IA: Blackwell.

Bartley, K. A. (2005). A life cycle micronutrient perspective for women's health. *American Journal of Clinical Nutrition, 81*: 1188s–1193s.

Benders, D. A. (2007). *Introduction to Nutrition and Metabolism* (4th ed.). Boca Raton, FL: CRC Press.

Benders, D. A. (2003). *Nutritional Biochemistry of the Vitamins* (2nd ed.). New York: Cambridge University Press.

Beredamier, C. D., Dwyer, J., & Vieldman, E. B. (2007). *Handbook of Nutrition and Food* (2nd ed.). Boca Raton, FL: CRC Press.

Berger, M. M. (2006). Vitamins and trace elements: Practical aspects of supplementation. *Nutrition, 22*: 952–955.

Brown, I. (2004). Does diet protect against Parkinson's disease? Part 4. Vitamins and minerals. *Nutrition and Food Science, 34*: 198–202.

Caballero, B., Allen, L., & Prentice, A. (Eds.) (2005). *Encyclopedia of human nutrition* (2nd ed.). Boston: Elsevier/Academic Press.

Chernoff, R. (2005). Micronutrient requirements in older women. *American Journal of Clinical Nutrition, 81*: 1240s–1245s.

Dani, J. (2005). The remarkable role of nutrition in learning and behavior. *Nutrition and Food Science, 35*: 258–263.

Driskell, J. A. & Wolinsky, I. (Eds.). (2006). *Sports Nutrition: Vitamins and Trace Elements.* Boca Raton, FL: CRC Press.

Fairfield, K. (2007). Vitamin and mineral supplements for cancer prevention: Issues and evidence. *American Journal of Clinical Nutrition, 85*: 289s–292s.

Fawzi, W. (2005). Studies of vitamins and minerals and HIV transmission and disease progression. *Journal of Nutrition, 135*: 938–944.

Food and Agricultural Organization (UN). (2004). *Vitamins and Mineral Requirements in Human Nutrition.* Geneva, Italy: World Health Organization.

Hatchcock, J. N. (2005). Vitamins E and C are safe across a broad range of intakes. *American Journal of Clinical Nutrition, 81*: 736–745.

Higdon, J. (2003). *An Evidence-Based Approach to Vitamins and Minerals-Health Implications and Intake Recommendations.* New York: Thieme.

Huang, H. Y. (2007). Multivitamin/mineral supplements and prevention of chronic disease: Executive summary. *American Journal of Clinical Nutrition, 85*: 265s–268s.

Kelly, F. J. (2005). Vitamins and respiratory disease: antioxidant micronutrients in pulmonary health and disease. *Proceedings of Nutrition Society, 64*: 510–526.

Lesourd, B. (2006). Nutritional factors and immunological ageing. *Proceedings of Nutrition Society, 65*: 319–325.

Mann, J. & Truswell, S. (Eds.). (2007). *Essentials of Human Nutrition* (3rd ed.). New York: Oxford University Press.

Navarra, T. (2004). *The Encyclopedia of Vitamins, Minerals and Supplements* (2nd ed.). New York: Facts on File.

Perrotta, S. (2003). Vitamin A and infancy: Biochemical, functional and clinical aspects. *Vitamins and Hormones, 66*: 457–591.

Rosenberg, I. H. (2007). Challenges and opportunities in the translation of science of vitamins. *American Journal of Clinical Nutrition, 85*: 325s–327s.

Staehelin, H. B. (2005). Micronutrients and Alzeimer's disease. *Proceedings of Nutrition Society, 4*: 543–553.

Stephen, A. I. (2006). A systematic review of multivitamin and multimineral supplementation for infection. *Journal of Human Nutrition and Dietetics, 19*: 179–190.

Vieth, R. (2006). Critique of the consideration for establishing the tolerable upper intake level of vitamin D: Critical need for revision upwards. *Journal of Nutrition, 136*: 1117–1122.

Walter, P., Hornig, D., & Moser, U. (Eds.). (2001). *Functions of Vitamins Beyond Recommended Dietary Allowances.* Basel, NY: Karger.

Webster-Gandy, J., Madden, A., & Holdworth, M. (Eds.) (2006). *Oxford Handbook of Nutrition and Dietetics.* Oxford, London: Oxford University Press.

Wildish, D. E. (2004). An evidence-based approach for dietitian prescription of multiple vitamins and minerals. *Journal of American Dietetic Association, 104*: 779–786.

Woodside, J. V. (2005). Micronutrients: Dietary intake vs. supplement use. *Proceedings of Nutrition Society, 64*: 543–553.

Woodside, M. A. (2004). Micronutrients and cancer therapy. *Nutrition Reviews, 62*: 142–147.

Yethey, E. A. (2007). Multivitamin and multimineral dietary supplements: Definitions, characterization, bioavailability and drug interactions. *American Journal of Clinical Nutrition, 85*: 269s–276s.

Zempleni, J., Rucker, R. B., Suttie, J. W., & McCormick, D. B. (Eds.). *Handbook of Vitamins* (4th ed.). Boca Raton, FL: CRC Press.

CHAPTER

6

Minerals, Water, and Body Processes

Time for completion
Activities: 2 hours
Optional examination: ½ hour

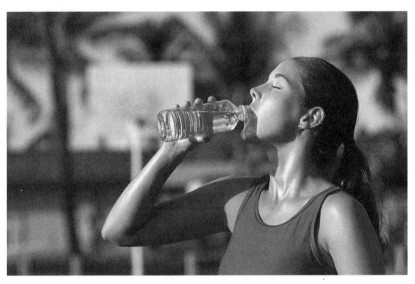

OBJECTIVES

Upon completion of this chapter, the student should be able to do the following:

1. Explain the role of minerals in regulating body processes.
2. List the essential minerals and their major functions.
3. Describe the characteristics of the minerals and the difference between macro- and microminerals.
4. Identify major food sources of each mineral.
5. List the minerals for which there are RDAs and the amounts required to maintain health.
6. Discuss factors that affect the absorption of minerals.
7. Describe the clinical effects of a deficiency or excess of each mineral.
8. Summarize food-handling procedures that minimize mineral loss.
9. Identify the major sources and functions of water in the body.
10. Evaluate the routes by which water is lost from the body.
11. Explain how fluid and electrolyte balance is maintained.
12. Analyze the recommended practices to maintain fluid and electrolyte balance during athletic activity.

Glossary

Minerals

Gram (g): metric measure, 28.3 g = 1 oz.; usually rounded to 30 g for ease of calculation.

Hyper: excess of normal.

Hypo: less than normal.

Inorganic: a compound of inert elements such as minerals.

Macro: involving large quantities.

Micro: involving minute quantities.

Microgram (mcg): 1/1000 of a mg; 1/1,000,000 of a gram.

Milligram (mg): 1/1000 of a gram.

Organic: any compound containing carbon.

pH: degree of acidity or alkalinity of a solution; a pH of 7 is neutral; below 7 is acid; above 7 is alkaline.

Water

Electrolyte: an ionic (charged particle) form of a mineral.

Extracellular: fluids such as blood plasma and cerebrospinal fluid; fluid around and between cells.

Fluid and electrolyte balance: maintenance of a stable internal environment by means of regulation of the water and minerals in solution within and around the cells.

Interstitial: fluid found between the cells. Blood plasma is often considered with it because of similarity in composition.

Intracellular: fluid contained within a cell.

Osmolarity: osmotic pressure difference between pressures across a membrane. Total number of dissolved particles per unit of fluid outside the cell equals the number of dissolved particles inside the cell.

Solute: solid matter in a solution.

Background Information

Mineral Occurrences

Only 4% of human body weight is composed of minerals. The other 96% is composed of water and the organic compounds of carbon, hydrogen, oxygen, and nitrogen that we know as carbohydrates, proteins, and fats. Minerals are inorganic elements. When plant or animal tissue is burned, the ash that remains is the mineral content. Minerals are present in the body as inorganic compounds in combination with organic compounds and alone.

Many minerals have been proven essential to human nutrition, and there are others with unknown essentiality. Still other minerals enter the body as pollutants through contamination of air, soil, and water.

Minerals vary widely in the amounts the body will absorb and excrete. Some minerals require the presence of other minerals in the body to function properly. Some minerals are transported by carriers in the body. Most minerals are toxic when ingested at just slightly higher than the safe and effective levels.

Mineral Classifications

Minerals are divided into two general categories—macrominerals and microminerals—based on the quantity in which they are found in the body.

The macrominerals are calcium (Ca), phosphorus (P), potassium (K), sodium (Na), sulfur (S), magnesium (Mg), and chlorine (Cl). The microminerals are iron (Fe), zinc (Zn), manganese (Mn), fluorine (F), copper (Cu), cobalt (Co), iodine (I), selenium (Se), chromium (Cr), and molybdenum (Mo). Microminerals are frequently referred to as "trace elements" because they are present in the body in such small quantities (less than .005% of body weight). These essential trace elements are required daily in the body in the milligram range.

Mineral Essentiality and Functions

Those microminerals with functions not yet known are not discussed here. The macro- and microminerals essential to human nutrition are the ones discussed. *Essential* refers to those substances the body is unable to manufacture; they must be available from an outside source. Essential minerals improve growth and development and regulate vital life processes.

Minerals are:

1. A part of the structure of all body cells.
2. Components of enzymes, hormones, blood, and other vital body compounds.
3. Regulators of:
   a. acid–base balance of the body.
   b. response of nerves to stimuli.
   c. muscle contractions.
   d. cell membrane permeability.
   e. osmotic pressure and water balance.

Mineral Acidity and Alkalinity

Since the acid–base balance (pH) of the body is regulated by acid- and base- (alkaline) forming minerals, we can group foods according to their predominant acid or base mineral content.

Sodium (Na), magnesium (Mg), potassium (K), iron (Fe), and calcium (Ca) are the minerals that produce an alkaline (base) residue (ash). The foods that are base (alkaline) producing, with high levels of these minerals, include most fruits and vegetables. The exceptions are plums, prunes, and cranberries, which are acid-producing fruits.

The acid-forming elements are sulfur (S), phosphorus (P), and chlorine (Cl). The foods containing the largest amounts of these minerals are the grains and protein foods (milk, cheese, meats, and eggs).

Mineral Absorption and Solubility

Minerals are absorbed best by the body at a specific pH. For instance, neither calcium nor iron will be absorbed in an alkaline medium. They require an acid pH for absorption. The acid and base properties of minerals, then, become an important consideration when planning for maximum absorption of minerals and other nutrients.

Most of the minerals in foods occur as mineral salts, which are generally water soluble. Minerals can be lost in cooking water in much the same way that water-soluble vitamins can. Therefore, foods should be cooked in the smallest amount of water possible for the shortest length of time and covered. Steam cooking and stir-frying methods conserve minerals. The water in which the foods have been cooked should be reused in cooking other foods; this recycles the minerals for the body.

For ease of discussion, Tables F-1 and F-2 in this chapter refer to the tables inside the front cover. NAS refers to the National Academy of Sciences.

WATER: A PRIMER

A meaningful discussion of minerals is not possible without explaining the role of water. A major factor of the internal environment of the body is the fluid and electrolyte balance. The fluid involved is water, and most of the electrolytes are ionic forms of essential minerals. Specifically, these are sodium (Na^+), potassium (K^+), magnesium (Mg^{++}), calcium (Ca^{++}), chloride (Cl^-), sulfate (SO_4^-), and phosphates (HPO_4^- and $H_2PO_4^=$).

Muscle tissue is relatively high in water content, while adipose (fat) tissue is relatively low. Fifty to seventy percent of adult body weight is water, depending on the amount of fat tissue. The water content of the body falls with age, unrelated to body weight. An infant has a higher percentage of body water than an adult. Water beyond one's immediate needs cannot be stored for future use.

In a normal person, daily water intake equals output; the balance is controlled. Thirst usually is a reliable guide to such regulation in a healthy person.

Because minerals and water are so interrelated, there is only one progress check for the two activities in this chapter. This approach permits the student to integrate the knowledge of minerals and water.

ACTIVITY 1:

The Essential Minerals: Functions, Sources, and Characteristics

REFERENCE TABLES

Because each mineral has particular functions, food sources, and specific characteristics, the student should study Tables 6-1 to 6-16, which describe these factors in detail. In this activity, we will specifically discuss only calcium, potassium, sodium, and iron. The student should follow the information in the corresponding tables for these and the other minerals.

CALCIUM

Calcium is the mineral present in the largest amount in the human body. Ninety-nine percent of it is found in the bones and teeth. The remainder (1%) is in body fluids, soft tissue, and membranes. Refer to Table 6-1.

According to Table F-2, the DRI for calcium for an adult is 1000 mg daily for a 30-year-old male or female. The calcium equivalents for 1 c (8 oz) of milk are as follows: (1 c milk = app. 300 mg calcium)

1. 8 oz yogurt
2. 1-½ oz cheddar cheese
3. 2 c cream cheese
4. 2 c cottage cheese
5. 1-¾ c ice cream
6. 4 oz canned salmon with bones
7. 15 to 24 medium oysters

The absorption of calcium depends upon body need, vitamin D, the amount of calcium in the body fluids, ratio of calcium to phosphorus, and the acidity of the gastrointestinal tract. Calcium is stored in the bones and teeth, but is withdrawn and replaced as serum calcium fluctuates, maintaining a steady state. Calcium is excreted via feces and urine. It is prevented from intestinal absorption by a low vitamin D intake, by alkaline, and by binding agents such as oxalic and phytic acid, which are naturally occurring acids in certain vegetables. It is currently suspected that a high protein intake over extended periods of time can decrease the absorption and increase the excretion of calcium. It is believed that the phosphorus content of protein foods upsets the calcium-to-phosphorus ratio in the food, the intestinal system, and the body.

One clinical disorder of calcium metabolism is osteoporosis, which is the thinning of bones through calcium loss. The person with osteoporosis has less bone substance. The bones become thin and brittle, prone to breaking easily. Compressed vertebra fractures are common. Osteoporosis is the most common bone disorder in the United States, affecting women about three times as often as men. Although the disorder is most often seen in older women, it starts in early adulthood without symptoms. The amount of bone an older woman has is influenced by the amount of calcium in her diet throughout her adulthood. Among the reasons women develop osteoporosis more often than men are the following:

1. They have smaller body frames with less bone mass.
2. They eat many nonfattening foods that contribute little calcium.

TABLE 6-1   Calcium (Ca)

Functions	Food Sources	Results of Deficiency or Excess	Conditions Requiring Increase	Specific Characteristics
Aids bone and tooth formation. Maintains serum calcium levels. Aids blood clotting. Aids muscle contraction and relaxation. Aids transmission of nerve impulses. Maintains normal heart rhythm.	AI (mg/d) Male & female (19–30 y): 1000 *Milk Group* milk and cheeses* yogurt *Meat Group* egg (yolk) sardines, salmon† *Vegetable Group* *green leafy vegetables** legumes nuts *Grain Group* whole grains	*Deficiency* rickets (childhood disorder of calcium metabolism from a vitamin D deficiency resulting in stunted growth, bowed legs, enlarged joints, especially legs, arms, and hollow chest) osteomalacia (adult form of rickets: a softening of the bones) osteoporosis (widespread disorder, especially in women, wherein bones become thin, brittle, diminish in size, and break) slow blood clotting tetany (see Specific Characteristics) poor tooth formation *Excess* renal calculi (see Specific Characteristics) hypercalcemia (deposits in joints and soft tissue)	Low intake (any age) Low serum calcium due to: growth pregnancy lactation Any condition that causes excess withdrawal, such as: body casts immobility low estrogen levels	1. Body need is major factor governing the amount of calcium absorbed. Normally 30 to 40% of dietary calcium is absorbed. 2. Presence of vitamin D and lactose (milk sugar) enhance absorption. 3. An acid environment in the gastrointestinal tract enhances absorption (see acid base balance). 4. Calcium in the bones and teeth are constantly withdrawn and replaced to keep the serum level stable. 5. The parathyroid hormone controls regulation. 6. The intake of calcium and phosphorus should be 1:1 ratio for optimal absorption. 7. Tetany is a condition resulting from a deficiency of calcium that causes muscle spasms in legs, arms. 8. Renal calculi are kidney stones. Ninety-six percent of all stones consist of calcium. 9. Overdoses of vitamin D can cause hypercalcemia, as can prolonged intake of antacids and milk. 10. Acute calcium deficiency does not usually occur without a lack of vitamin D and phosphorus also.

AI = Adequate Intakes.
Adapted from Table F-2.
*Best source
**Some contain binding agents
†With bones included

TABLE 6-2   Phosphorus (P)

Functions	Food Sources	Results of Deficiency or Excess	Conditions Requiring Increase	Specific Characteristics
Aids bone and tooth formation. Maintains metabolism of fat and carbohydrates. Part of the compounds that act as buffers to control pH of the blood.	RDA (mg/d) Male & female (19–30 y): 700 *Meat Group** cheeses (especially cheddar), peanuts, beef, pork, poultry, fish, eggs *Milk Group* milk and milk products *Vegetable/Fruit Group*** all foods in this group *Grain*** wheat, oats, barley, rice *Other* carbonated drinks contain large amounts of phosphorus	*Deficiency* rickets osteomalacia osteoporosis slow blood clotting poor tooth formation disturbed acid–base balance *Excess* same as calcium	Low intake, especially of protein foods, due to: growth pregnancy lactation illness	1. Approximately 80% of phosphorus is in bones and teeth in a ratio with calcium of 2:1. 2. Aids in producing energy by phosphorylation. 3. Phospholipids assist in transferring substances in and out of the cells. 4. Phosphorus is more efficiently absorbed than calcium; approximately 70% is absorbed. Some factors that enhance or decrease the absorption of calcium affect phosphorus the same way. 5. Consumption of antacids lowers phosphorus absorption. 6. Both calcium and phosphorus are released from bone when serum levels are low. 7. Diets containing enough protein and calcium will be adequate in phosphorus.

RDA = Recommended Dietary Allowances.
Adapted from Table F-2.
*Best source
**Fair to poor source

3. Their bodies have reduced estrogen levels after menopause. The disappearance of this hormone upsets the balance between deposition and withdrawal of body calcium.

One cause of osteoporosis is reduced calcium intake and absorption. This absorption of calcium is controlled by:

1. Heredity: Osteoporosis tends to run in families.
2. Estrogen: Less calcium will be absorbed and deposited when body estrogen decreases.
3. Dietary factors and exercise.

A low calcium intake after a person reaches adulthood leads to osteoporosis because the body will start "consuming" its own bones. For example, after 25 years on a low-calcium diet, the body can theoretically use up one-third of the body skeleton. As a major body organ, the skeleton is not a static system. Minerals, especially calcium, are constantly removed from the bones and used for other body functions. The bones are an important reservoir for calcium. When there is a chronic shortage of calcium in the diet, it is withdrawn from bones so that the body maintains a normal level of this mineral in the blood.

Although osteoporosis cannot be "cured," its symptoms (such as pain) can be decreased by:

1. a calcium-rich diet
2. exercise

TABLE 6-3   Sodium (Na)

Functions	Food Sources	Results of Deficiency or Excess	Conditions Requiring Increase	Specific Characteristics
Maintains water balance. Normalizes osmotic pressure. Balances acid base. Regulates nerve impulses. Regulates muscle contraction. Aids in carbohydrate and protein absorption.	*Estimated minimum requirement:* 2000 mg for a 24-year-old adult table salt (40% sodium) milk and dairy foods protein foods (fish, shellfish, meat, poultry, eggs) processed foods: any containing baking soda, baking powder, and preservative additives some drinking water is high in sodium some vegetables contain fair sources of sodium: spinach, celery, beets, carrots	*Deficiency* hyponatremia (low serum sodium): nausea headache anorexia muscle spasms mental confusion fluid and electrolyte imbalance *Excess* hypernatremia (high serum sodium) cardiovascular disturbances hypertension edema mental confusion	Excessive loss of body fluids: heavy use of diuretics, vomiting/diarrhea, heavy perspiring, burns Certain diseases: cystic fibrosis Addison's disease	1. More than half the body sodium is in the fluid surrounding the cells. It is the major cation of the extracellular fluid. Its functions are very similar to potassium. 2. Most Americans consume far more sodium than the RDA. 3. Extracellular fluids include fluid in the blood vessels, veins, arteries, and capillaries. 4. Sodium is well conserved by the body. 5. Hyponatremia due to inadequate intake is uncommon. A condition causing excess fluid loss such as described in column 4 (Conditions Requiring Increase) would be necessary. 6. Hypernatremia is related to high incidence of hypertension in the United States. 7. Dietary guidelines for Americans encourage less consumption of sodium, especially for those at high risk of developing high blood pressure. 8. Often a reduction in intake can be done simply by omitting salt added to food in preparation or at the table. Elimination of high-salt snack foods and foods preserved in salt also is helpful.

AI = Adequate Intakes.
Adapted from Table F-2.

3. avoidance of things that decrease the body's ability to absorb calcium

Further, it is believed that such practices can prevent osteoporosis or delay its onset.

POTASSIUM

About 95% of ingested potassium is readily absorbed by the body. Potassium circulates in all body fluids, primarily located within the cell. Excesses are usually efficiently

TABLE 6-4 Potassium (K)

Functions	Food Sources	Results of Deficiency or Excess	Conditions Requiring Increase	Specific Characteristics
Maintains protein and carbohydrate metabolism. Maintains water balance. Normalizes osmotic pressure. Balances acid base. Regulates muscle activity.	AI (g/d); male & female (19–30 y): 4.7 *Milk Group* all foods *Meat Group* all foods (best sources: red meats, dark meat, poultry) *Vegetable/Fruit Group* all foods (especially oranges, bananas, prunes) *Grain Group* especially whole grains *Other* coffee (especially instant)	*Deficiency* hypokalemia (see Specific Characteristics) fluid and electrolyte imbalances tissue breakdown *Excess* hyperkalemia (see Specific Characteristics) renal failure severe dehydration shock	Inadequate intake (starvation, imbalanced diets) Gastrointestinal disorders, especially diarrhea Burns, injuries Diabetic acidosis Chronic use of diuretics Adrenal gland tumors	1. The major cation in the intracellular fluid. 2. Balances with sodium to maintain water balance and osmotic pressure. 3. When there are excess acid elements, potassium combines and neutralizes, thus maintaining acid–base balance. 4. Potassium is poorly conserved by the body. 5. Hypokalemia is a condition where there is low serum potassium. It manifests itself in muscle weakness, loss of appetite, nausea, vomiting, and rapid heart beat (tachycardia). 6. Hyperkalemia is a condition that causes serum potassium to rise to toxic levels. It results in a weakened heart action that causes mental confusion, poor respiration, numbness of extremities, and heart failure.

AI = Adequate Intakes.
Adapted from Table F-2.

excreted. Aldosterone, a hormone secreted by the adrenal gland, signals the kidney to excrete what is not needed.

The average U.S. diet supplies from two to six grams of potassium daily. Its deficiency is not a problem until certain abnormal conditions arise. (Refer to Table 6-4.)

SODIUM

The kidneys, under the influence of aldosterone, normally control sodium excretion according to need and intake. It is excreted via the kidneys, with small amounts lost in the feces. Large amounts can be lost in perspiration during strenuous activity and in a hot environment. Severe vomiting in certain disorders and chronic use of diuretics increase sodium loss. Ninety-five percent of sodium is recirculated through the en-

terohepatic system by kidney reabsorption. If the serum sodium rises, water is retained and blood volume increases. This, in turn, increases blood pressure. (Refer to Table 6-3.)

IRON

Although the total amount of iron needed daily in the human body is small, iron is one of the most important micronutrients. Iron intake, especially in the female, is usually low. Iron-deficiency anemia is a major problem in the United States, especially for those high-risk groups noted under specific Characteristics in Table 6-8. It occurs usually as a result of inadequate intake, impaired absorption, blood loss, or repeated pregnancies. Iron is poorly absorbed in the intestine, with most excreted in

TABLE 6-5   Magnesium (Mg)

Functions	Food Sources	Results of Deficiency or Excess	Conditions Requiring Increase	Specific Characteristics
Assists in regulation of body fluids. Activates enzymes. Regulates metabolism of carbohydrate, fat, and protein. Necessary for formation of ATP (energy production). Component of chlorophyll. Works with Ca, P, and vitamin D in bone formation.	RDA (mg/d) Male (19–30 y): 400 Female (19–30 y): 310 grains, green vegetables, soybeans, milk, meat, poultry	*Deficiency* fluid and electrolyte imbalance skin breakdown *Excess* magnesemia	Alcoholism Inadequate intake of Ca, P, or any disease affecting their use Growth Pregnancy Lactation Prolonged use of diuretics	1. Magnesium deficiencies occur most often in disease states such as cirrhosis of the liver, severe renal disease, and toxemia of pregnant women. 2. American diets may be low in magnesium compared to RDAs if diet is low in calories or contains mostly highly refined and processed foods. 3. Magnesium and calcium share a control system in the kidneys.

RDA = Recommended Dietary Allowances.
Adapted from Table F-2.

TABLE 6-6   Chlorine (Cl)

Functions	Food Sources	Results of Deficiency or Excess	Conditions Requiring Increase	Specific Characteristics
Aids in maintaining fluid electrolyte balance and acid–base balance. Aids in digestion and absorption of nutrients as a constituent of gastric secretion.	AI (g/d); male & female (19–30 y): 2.3 table salt (60% chloride) protein foods: seafood, meats, eggs, milk	Intake is not usually a problem unless a condition as in next column exists.	Excessive vomiting Aging (decreased gastric secretions)	1. Chloride is the chief anion of the fluid outside the cells. 2. The gastric (stomach) contents are primarily hydrochloric acid (HCI). 3. Chloride is a buffer in a reaction in the body known as the chloride shift. This has the effect of maintaining the delicate pH balance of the blood.

AI = Adequate Intakes.
Adapted from Table F-2.

TABLE 6-7   Sulfur (S)

Functions	Food Sources	Results of Deficiency or Excess	Conditions Requiring Increase	Specific Characteristics
Participates in detoxifying harmful compounds. Component of amino acids.	RDA: not established protein foods that contain the amino acids methionine, cysteine, and cystine (cheeses, eggs, poultry, and fish)	No specific descriptions of a deficiency or excess	No specific conditions requiring an increase	1. Much information remains to be learned about the role of sulfur in human physiology. 2. Greatest concentration is in hair and nails.

TABLE 6-8   Iron (Fe)

Functions	Food Sources	Results of Deficiency or Excess	Conditions Requiring Increase	Specific Characteristics

Plays essential role in formation of hemoglobin.
 	
Is found in myoglobin, the iron-protein molecule in muscles.
	RDA (mg/d)
	Male (19–30 y): 8
	Female (19–30 y): 18
	liver, kidneys, lean meats, whole grains, parsley, enriched breads, cereals, legumes, almonds
	dried fruit: prunes (and juice), raisins, apricots
	approximately 2 to 10% of iron in vegetables and grains can be absorbed, compared with 10 to 30% absorption of iron from animal protein
		Deficiency
		iron-deficiency anemia
		
		Excess
		hemosiderosis: a condition where iron is deposited in the liver and body tissues. The cell becomes distorted and dies. The liver is damaged.
			Girls and women of childbearing age due to menstrual losses (about 30 mg per month lost)
			Pregnancy (supplementation with iron and folacin needed)
			Acute or chronic blood loss
			Inadequate protein intake
				1. Approximately ¾ of functioning iron in the body is in hemoglobin.
				2. Hemoglobin is the principal part of the red blood cell, and carries oxygen from the lungs to the tissues. It assists in returning CO_2 (carbon dioxide) to the lungs.
				3. Iron is only absorbed in an acid medium. Absorption is enhanced by ascorbic acid.
				4. Milk is a very poor source of iron, containing only a trace.
				5. Iron is not well absorbed in the body, even under good conditions. Generally about 10% in a mixed diet is absorbed.
				6. Iron is the most difficult nutrient to meet through diet for women.
				7. The following nutrients are essential for the manufacture of red blood cells:
				  a. iron, vitamin B_6, and copper for hemoglobin formation
				  b. protein for globin formation
				  c. vitamin C to aid the absorption of iron
				8. The populations at risk for iron-deficiency anemia are:
				  infants (6–12 months)
				  adolescent girls
				  menstruating women
				  pregnant women

RDA = Recommended Dietary Allowances.
Adapted from Table F-2.

TABLE 6-9   Iodine (I)

Functions	Food Sources	Results of Deficiency or Excess	Conditions Requiring Increase	Specific Characteristics
Basic component of thyroxin, a hormone in the thyroid gland that regulates the basal metabolic rate (BMR). Contributes to normal growth and development of the body.	RDA (μg/d) Male & female (19–30 y): 150 Iodized salt (major source) seafood: salt water fish food additives: dough oxidizers, dairy disinfectants, coloring agents foods containing seaweed	*Deficiency* cretinism (stunted growth, dwarfism) goiter (enlargement of thyroid gland) *Excess* hyperthyroidism (toxic goiter)	Wherever soil is low in iodine In areas where goiter is endemic In pregnant women with deficient diets	1. Certain foods contain substances that block absorption of iodine: cabbage, turnips, rutabagas. 2. Iodine-containing food additives may cause excess intake of iodine in some areas of the United States.

RDA = Recommended Dietary Allowances.
Adapted from Table F-2.

TABLE 6-10   Zinc (Zn)

Functions	Food Sources	Results of Deficiency or Excess	Conditions Requiring Increase	Specific Characteristics
Contributes to formation of enzymes needed in metabolism. Affects normal sensitivity to taste and smell. Aids protein synthesis. Aids normal growth and sexual maturation. Promotes wound healing. May help in the treatment of acne.*	RDA (mg/d) Male (19–30 y): 11 Female (19–30 y): 8 oysters, liver, meats, poultry, legumes, nuts	*Deficiency* associated with extreme malnutrition impairs wound healing decreases taste and smell dwarfism and impaired sexual development in children *Excess* toxicity associated with ingestion of acid foods stored in zinc-lined containers	Following surgery, especially when diet has been inadequate prior to surgery Those with alterations in taste and smell Certain diseases of dark-skinned races, such as sickle cell anemia	Availability of zinc is greater from animal sources; vegetable sources contain phytates, which bind it, causing its excretion.

RDA = Recommended Dietary Allowances.
Adapted from Table F-2.
*Latest studies indicate that zinc supplements can be effective in treating acne in some subjects.

the stool. When iron is absorbed in excess of body needs, it can be stored. Major storage areas are the liver, spleen, and bone marrow. The body has no mechanism for excretion of excess iron. (Refer to Table 6-8.)

Planning an iron-rich diet acceptable to most families is a challenge. If liver and other organ meats are not included in the diet, other foods must be selected to increase dietary iron. Some examples of such foods or food preparation methods include raisin cookies and prune bread (especially with whole wheat flour), casseroles with dried beans and peas, substituting molasses for sugar, and adding parsley to dishes. Slow cooking in an iron pot increases available iron by 50 to 75%.

IMPLICATIONS FOR HEALTH PERSONNEL

Of all the essential minerals, iron probably poses the most clinical problems. All healthcare professionals

TABLE 6-11   Fluoride (F)

Functions	Food Sources	Results of Deficiency or Excess	Conditions Requiring Increase	Specific Characteristics
Protects against dental caries.	AI (mg/d) Male (19–30 y): 4 Female (19–30 y): 3 seafood fluoridated drinking water (1 PPM* added to water)	*Deficiency* 50 to 70% cases of tooth decay from fluoride deficiency *Excess:* fluorosis mottled stains on teeth (children) dense bones mental depression (adults)	Areas where no fluoride available elderly (see Specific Characteristics)	Fluoride is being used to assist in regenerating bone loss due to osteoporosis in selected studies.

AI = Adequate Intakes.
Adapted from Table F-2.
*PPM = parts per million

TABLE 6-12   Copper (Cu)

Functions	Food Sources	Results of Deficiency or Excess	Conditions Requiring Increase	Specific Characteristics
Considered "twin" to iron; aids in formation of hemoglobin and energy production. Promotes absorption of iron from gastrointestinal tract. Aids bone formation. Aids brain tissue formation. Contributes to myelin sheath of the nervous system.	RDA (µg/d) Male & female (19–30 y): 900 liver, kidney, shellfish, lobster, oysters, nuts, raisins, legumes, corn oil	*Deficiency* occurs in association with disease states such as: PEM (protein energy malnutrition) kwashiorkor (extreme protein deficiency) sprue (disease marked by diarrhea) cystic fibrosis kidney disease iron deficiency anemia *Excess* ingestion of large amounts is toxic to humans	Disease states noted under Deficiencies	1. Copper is concentrated in the liver, brain, heart, and kidneys. 2. Absorption takes place in small intestine. 3. Other minerals can interfere with copper absorption. 4. Zinc is an antagonist to copper because it reduces absorption.

RDA = Recommended Dietary Allowances.
Adapted from Table F-2.

TABLE 6-13   Cobalt (Co)

Functions	Food Sources	Results of Deficiency or Excess	Conditions Requiring Increase	Specific Characteristics
Acts as a component of vitamin B$_{12}$.	RDA: not established (see Specific Characteristics) organ meats, muscle meat, vitamin B$_{12}$	No specific deficiency in humans; deficient production of B$_{12}$ noted in animals	No specific conditions requiring an increase	1. RDAs for cobalt not established, but 15 mcg/day is suggested.

RDA = Recommended Dietary Allowances. AI = Adequate Intakes. UL = Upper Limits.
Adapted from Dietary Reference Intakes, National Academic Sciences. See complete tables in Appendix A.
*PPM = parts per million

TABLE 6-14   **Manganese (Mn)**

Functions	Food Sources	Results of Deficiency or Excess	Conditions Requiring Increase	Specific Characteristics
Appears necessary for bone growth and reproduction. Acts as an enzyme activator.	AI (mg/d) Male (19–30 y): 2.3 Female (19–30 y): 1.8 nuts, legumes, tea, coffee, grains	No deficiencies noted in humans except protein energy malnutrition	No specific conditions requiring an increase Protein energy malnutrition	1. Manganese has not been demonstrated to be an essential nutrient in humans

AI = Adequate Intakes.
Adapted from Table F-2.

TABLE 6-15   **Selenium (Se)**

Functions	Food Sources	Results of Deficiency or Excess	Conditions Requiring Increase	Specific Characteristics
Parts of an enzyme that functions as an antioxidant. With vitamin E repairs damage caused by oxygen.	AI (µg/d) Male & Female (19–30 y): 55 *Main sources* meat, eggs, seafoods *Other* vegetables grown in selenium rich soil	*Deficiency* increased risk of cancer causes one type of heart disease *Excess* Selenosis*	Pregnancy and lactation Children living in countries where no selenium exists in soil or water, e.g., parts of China	1. Found in all body cells as part of an enzyme system. 2. Adequate RDA intakes believed to have a role in cancer prevention. 3. Excess selenium toxic. 4. The line between health and overdose is very thin. 5. Daily dose should not exceed 70 µg.

AI = Adequate Intakes.
Adapted from Table F-2.
*Selenium toxicity

should pay special attention to the following information and guidelines:

1. Because iron is a nutrient likely to be deficient in the human body, the following tips will be helpful when instructing a client:
   a. Cooking foods in larger pieces and in smaller amounts of water reduces the amount of iron lost in preparation.
   b. The use of meat drippings and fruit pulp conserves iron.
   c. A diet high in bulk reduces iron absorption; clients at risk of iron deficiency should use only moderate fiber content.
   d. High intake of antacids makes the gastric juices alkaline and reduces iron absorption.
   e. An adequate calcium intake increases iron absorption because the calcium will bind with the phosphates, phytates, oxalates, and cellulose and leave the iron free for absorption.
   f. Spinach is not a good source of iron. It contains a large amount of the oxalates that hinder iron absorption.
   g. Since ascorbic acid promotes iron absorption, eating foods containing iron and vitamin C together produces the best results.
2. Iron-poor foods are pale in color (lack pigment). Iron salts are colored and impart their color to the foods they are in. Examples are milk (iron poor) and liver (iron rich).
3. Because the body cannot excrete excess iron, and it can therefore pose health hazards if consumed in large amounts:
   a. Keep iron medication out of the reach of children (iron poisoning among children is the fourth most common type of poisoning).

TABLE 6-16   Trace Minerals with Newly Defined Functions

Functions	Food Sources	Results of Deficiency or Excess	Conditions Requiring Increase	Specific Characteristics
		Chromium		
Cofactor in insulin metabolism: Improves uptake of glucose Lower LDL cholesterol, increases HDL cholesterol	AI (µg/d) Male (19–30y): 35 Female (19–30y): 25 Liver Cheese Brewers yeast Whole grains Leafy vegetables	*Deficiency:* Impaired glucose tolerance Impaired function of CNS (TPN)* *Excess* No symptoms of excess	Malnutrition Patients on long-term TPN	1. Total body content small (less than 6 mg) 2. Essential component of the complex glucose tolerance factor (GTF) 3. Absorption: Small amounts absorbed in the intestine 4. Excretion: Mainly in the urine
		Molybdenum		
Catalyst in metabolic reactions Cofactor in certain oxidative enzymes	AI (µg/d) Male & Female (19–30y): 45 UL (µg/d) Male & Female (19–30y): 2000 Animal: organ meats (liver, kidney) Milk Legumes Cereal grains	*Deficiency:* Defects in infants, including mental retardation irritability possible coma dislocated lenses *Excess* Toxic: Causes symptoms resembling gout	Malnutrition Patients on long-term TPN	1. Amount in body exceeding small 2. Precise occurrence and clear metabolic role under continuing investigation 3. Is rapidly excreted in urine 4. Genetic defect (inborn error of metabolism) creates deficiency with severe effects

*CNS = Central nervous system. TPN = Total parenteral nutrition.

b. Read labels on over-the-counter preparations (some are high in iron and, when mixed with other iron compounds, may create excess).
4. Iron medications interfere with some antibiotic absorption. Patients taking both preparations need to take them at different times.

The health team should also pay attention to the following information to ensure clients are at their optimal mineral status.

1. Both the quality and quantity of food intake should be monitored.
2. The use of diuretics may lead to alteration in the fluid and electrolyte balance in the body, especially high losses of sodium (hyponatremia) and potassium (hypokalemia).
3. Hypokalemia may become severe in the following disorders: vomiting, diarrhea, wound drainage, diabetic acidosis, and in those taking digitalis for heart conditions.
4. Persons with poor food intake may suffer from multiple mineral deficiencies.

5. Alcoholics, psychiatric patients, drug abusers, the aged, the poverty stricken, and those with malabsorptive disorders are most likely to suffer mineral deficiencies.
6. Certain foods and conditions of the intestinal tract will greatly influence the absorption of minerals. Each mineral should merit separate consideration, since not all react to the same conditions and foods.
7. Calcium deficiency results from insufficient intake, malabsorption, or lack of vitamin D. Acute hypocalcemia causes tetany and may cause death. Hypocalcemia from inadequate intake over long periods of time results in osteoporosis, which occurs in three out of five women over the age of 60, and is a severe disorder.
8. Recognize the factors that promote or inhibit iron absorption. Be able to plan an iron-rich diet that excludes least-liked foods high in iron.
9. Recognize major symptoms that may indicate deficiencies of minerals and follow up with treatment.
10. Be able to list the best food sources of the mineral(s) that the client is deficient in.

11. Find resources for those who have inadequate mineral intake due to lack of money for food or ignorance of nutrition needs.

ACTIVITY 2:

Water and the Internal Environment

Next to oxygen, water is the most important nutrient for the body. Lack of water causes the cells to become dehydrated. A total lack of water can cause death in a few days. Fifty to seventy percent of body weight is water, and an individual's body water content does not vary significantly. The body does not tolerate much fluctuation, since it upsets the delicate balance and concentration of dissolved substances and causes a rapid loss of cell integrity. The major nutrient electrolytes (Na^+, K^+, Cl^-, Mg^{++}, Ca^{++}, HPO_4^-, and $H_2PO_4^=$) have already been discussed in Activity 1. Small changes in diet can cause changes in water content and affect fluid balance. Low carbohydrate intake can increase water loss, as can low protein intake, although for different reasons. The water loss associated with low carbohydrate intake appears much faster than that associated with low protein intake. Omitting sodium from the diet may result in a small fluid loss. Individuals who reduce their sodium intake usually lose a little body weight. This is due, however, to fluid loss, not actual fat loss. The output of water is normally balanced by input. If extra water is ingested, urinary output increases. The body maintains a steady water content state.

FUNCTIONS AND DISTRIBUTION OF BODY WATER

Water serves many important functions. In the human body, water acts as the following:

1. Solvent
2. Component of all body cells, giving structure and form to the body
3. Body temperature regulator
4. Lubricant
5. Medium for the digestion of food
6. Transport medium for nutrients and waste products
7. Participant in biological reactions
8. Regulator of acid–base balance

In the body, water is distributed in the following manner:

1. ECF, or extracellular fluid (surrounding the cells): 20 to 25% of the body water is outside the cells. ECF includes the vascular system.
2. ICF, or intracellular fluid (inside the cells): 40 to 45% of the body water is inside the cells. The ICF contains twice as much water as the ECF.

BODY WATER BALANCE

Water requirements are dependent upon many factors, including the amount of solids in the diet, air humidity, environmental temperature, type of clothing worn, type of exercise performed (amount and energy output), respiratory (breathing) rate, and the state of health. The human body obtains water from these sources:

1. Beverages
2. Foods, including dry ones such as meat and crackers
3. Metabolic breakdown of food for use by the body (oxidation of energy nutrients); this amount of metabolic water is not large, but it is significant, especially in certain disease conditions.

Water is lost from the body in many ways:

1. Most water is lost through the kidneys as urine.
2. Water is lost from skin as perspiration. Some insensible (unnoticed) perspiration occurs because it evaporates rapidly. Sweating, the key means of cooling the body, causes large water loss.
3. Water is lost from the lungs in breathing (water vapor).
4. Water is lost in the feces.
5. Certain disease conditions and injury can result in great water losses, creating a crisis situation if not replaced at once. Some examples are acute diarrhea, burns, and blood losses.

A deficiency or excess of water can produce harmful effects to the body. The major outcome of water deficiency is dehydration. Prolonged dehydration leads to cell death, and multiple cell losses kill the organism. The very young, whose bodies contain a higher percentage of water, and the very old, whose bodies contain less water than younger persons, are the most susceptible to dehydration. In these individuals, it occurs more rapidly and is more severe.

Excessive consumption of liquids is usually not a problem for a healthy body, because the kidneys control the excretion of fluids, balancing intake with output. During kidney or other disorders where the body suffers a fluid imbalance, edema, ascites, and congestive heart failure may result. In these patients, water intake is restricted. Drinking excess liquids with a low mineral content (such as distilled water) may cause a condition known as water intoxication. Mineral replacement will normalize fluid and electrolyte balance.

Maintenance of fluid and electrolyte balance within and between the cells is important for normal health. Control of these shifts is accomplished by complex mechanisms in the body. An extended analysis is not appropriate here, but the following points will help explain the mechanism of body water distribution:

1. Pressure balance: This kind of pressure controls fluid balance and hydrostatic-capillary blood pressure, osmotic pressure, and serum proteins (albumin) movement.
2. Hormonal influence: Antidiuretic hormone (ADH), a hormone from the pituitary gland, and aldosterone from the adrenal gland regulate the excretion of fluid from the kidneys.
3. Thirst or lack of thirst: This response controls how much liquid is ingested.
4. Shifts of electrolytes (Ca^{++}, P^+, Mg^{++}, Na^+): For example, when the shifts move from bone to serum, the concentration of electrolytes in the body fluid is changed.

How much water do we need every day? For an adult with regular physical activity, a recommendation of about 7 glasses a day is most common. This is in addition to the water we consume from foods. However, the actual consumption varies with different individuals. Since we drink water when we are thirsty, the adequacy question is moot under a normal ambient environment.

However, for medical considerations including those for public health, the actual requirements for water for humans at different stages of life are important. According to the DRIs established by the NAP, some scientific data for water requirement from food, beverages, and drinking water are (where 1 liter ~ 4 cups):

- A newborn baby: 0.7 liter a day
- A 30-year-old man: 3.7 liters a day
- A 30-year-old woman: 2.7 liters a day
- A 30-year-old pregnant woman: 3.0 liters a day
- A 30-year-old nursing mother: 3.8 liters a day

Information of this nature is most useful in many clinical conditions such as shock, infection, selected disorders, and so on. The next section discusses the considerations for an athlete.

WATER REQUIREMENTS FOR ATHLETES

Because water is the nutrient most often depleted, its replacement should be of prime concern. Fortunately, it is the most easily restored nutrient of all. Anyone engaged in prolonged activity or enclosed in a hot environment can become dehydrated and should ingest fluids. Athletes are especially prone to dehydration. A fluid loss of up to 2% body weight is harmless, but a 4 to 5% loss is harmful.

Most athletes need to drink fluid during exercise. Long distance runners may lose 8 to 15 pounds of fluid during a race. This is equivalent to 16 to 30 cups of water. They should drink liquids before, during, and after a race. Since sweetened liquids or those with a high mineral content tend to hasten dehydration and cause diarrhea,

plain water, unsweetened fruit juices, tomato or V-8 juice, and diluted colas and ginger ale are preferred. The so-called electrolyte replacements that contain sugar, sodium, and potassium have no special value.

Extra fluids and minerals should be consumed cautiously in long distance events. Small amounts of sugar, for example, consumed every 30 minutes to 1 hour during a long event is the preferred consumption method. Short-term events do not require special replacement other than water. Water can be taken at any time during an event.

Minerals affected by heavy exercise are sodium and potassium. Iron deficiency is common in female athletes. For athletes, mineral supplements are a temporary measure. They should consume foods with a high content of sodium, potassium, and iron.

RESPONSIBILITIES OF HEALTH PERSONNEL

1. Recognize the factors that promote or inhibit adequate fluid intake.
2. Recognize symptoms of dehydration and water intoxication.
3. Be aware that diet can cause changes in the fluid balance of the body, and make adjustments as necessary.
4. Recognize the importance of sodium, potassium, and water in the body's fluid and electrolyte balance.
5. Understand the significance of equal input and output of fluid in maintaining homeostasis by knowing the ways the body gains fluid, loses fluid, and how water is distributed in the body.
6. Question scheduling of tests that require withholding fluids to such an extent that it might lead to dehydration.
7. Be aware that rising blood pressure may indicate retention of fluids.
8. Advise persons engaged in prolonged activity about appropriate replacement of water and body fluids.
9. Watch for symptoms of dehydration and replace lost electrolytes as well as fluids if needed.
10. Provide information to consumers regarding appropriate food and fluid intake.

SUMMARY

The concentration of each electrolyte in the body fluid must be maintained within a narrow range so that the delicate balance will not be disturbed. Changes in electrolyte concentration, acidity, and alkalinity can adversely affect the whole body. The system of body fluid and electrolyte balance is so important that the body provides various mechanisms for regulation. A deficit in water or minerals can rapidly become life threatening.

PROGRESS CHECK ON CHAPTER 6

MULTIPLE CHOICE

Circle the letter of the correct answer.

1. The vitamin most closely related to calcium utilization is:

    a. vitamin A.
    b. vitamin D.
    c. vitamin K.
    d. phosphorus.

2. Three nutrients needed for bone growth are:

    a. ascorbic acid, vitamin D, and magnesium.
    b. calcium, potassium, and vitamin D.
    c. phosphorus, calcium, and vitamin D.
    d. magnesium, manganese, and calcium.

3. Functions of sodium in the human body include:

    a. maintenance of water balance.
    b. maintenance of acid–base balance.
    c. aiding glucose absorption.
    d. all of the above.

4. A mineral important to normal functioning of the heart is:

    a. chlorine.
    b. potassium.
    c. phosphate.
    d. bicarbonate.

5. Calcium is:

    a. used in muscle building.
    b. used to control electrolyte balance.
    c. used in blood clotting.
    d. found in abundance in soft tissues.

6. Phosphorus:

    a. is absorbed best when calcium is present.
    b. is found in many of the same foods as calcium.
    c. is needed in greater amounts during pregnancy.
    d. all of the above.

7. The only known function of iodine in human nutrition is synthesis of the thyroid hormone. Which of the following functions does this hormone perform?

    a. protects the cells from oxidation
    b. controls the basal metabolic rate
    c. lowers the oxygen intake
    d. controls nerve impulses

8. The mineral needed to strengthen the teeth to resist decay is:

    a. calcium.
    b. phosphorus.
    c. iron.
    d. fluoride.

9. Which two items are both rich sources of potassium?

    a. cooked rice and fortified margarine
    b. mashed potatoes and apple juice
    c. bananas and orange juice
    d. cranberry juice and grape juice

10. The two minerals whose major function is regulating the fluid balance of the body inside the cell (ICF) and outside the cell (ECF) are:

    a. calcium and phosphorus.
    b. sodium and potassium.
    c. magnesium and iodine.
    d. chlorine and iron.

11. Sodium intake may need to be increased:

    a. when vomiting, exudating burns, or diarrhea occur.
    b. to regulate acid–base balance and to prevent headaches.
    c. when nausea, anorexia, muscle spasms, or mental confusion occur.
    d. when hypertension and edema occur.

12. Which of the following would be considered the best source of iodine?

    a. baked potato with iodized salt
    b. tossed green salad with iodized salt
    c. baked salmon with iodized salt
    d. broccoli with iodized salt

13. Chloride:

    a. is directly necessary for protein synthesis in cells.
    b. protects bone structures against degeneration.
    c. is the body's principal intracellular electrolyte.
    d. helps maintain gastric acidity.

14. Magnesium functions:

    a. in production of thyroid hormone.
    b. as a catalyst in energy metabolism.
    c. to transport oxygen.
    d. in prevention of anemia.

15. Potassium:

    a. is directly necessary for protein synthesis in cells.
    b. protects bone structures against degeneration.
    c. is necessary for wound healing.
    d. helps maintain gastric acidity.

16. Sulfur is present in all:

    a. carbohydrates.
    b. fatty acids.

c. proteins.
d. vitamins.

17. A high need for calcium, such as during pregnancy:

a. increases calcium absorption.
b. decreases calcium absorption.
c. does not affect calcium absorption.
d. is related to other nutrient intake.

18. Heart failure related to potassium loss may occur except:

a. during fasting.
b. with severe diarrhea.
c. in children with iron-deficiency anemia.
d. in hypokalemia.

19. The food source from which calcium is obtained in the highest concentration and most absorbable form is:

a. dark green vegetables.
b. bone meal.
c. milk.
d. meats.

20. The most reliable food source of chloride is:

a. meats and whole grain cereals.
b. salt.
c. dark green vegetables.
d. public water.

21. Potassium supplements:

a. should always be taken with diuretics.
b. should be taken only under a physician's direction.
c. are necessary because food sources are limited.
d. increase muscle strength.

22. Which of the following contains the least sodium?

a. lemon juice
b. soy sauce
c. canned tomato juice
d. boiled ham

23. Which of the following substances is an electrolyte?

a. water
b. sodium
c. fatty acid
d. amino acid

24. The force that moves water into a space where a solute is more concentrated is

a. caloric energy.
b. osmotic pressure.
c. buffer action.
d. electrolyte imbalance.

25. A mineral found in higher concentrations in hard water than in soft water is:

a. sodium.
b. potassium.
c. calcium.
d. fluoride.

26. A mineral found in higher concentrations in soft water than in hard water is:

a. calcium.
b. magnesium.
c. sodium.
d. potassium.

27. Which of the following minerals is a cofactor in hemoglobin formation?

a. iodine
b. copper
c. sodium
d. calcium

28. Fluoride seems helpful in preventing:

a. osteoporosis.
b. cancer.
c. diabetes.
d. heart disease.

29. Which nutrient enhances iron absorption from the intestinal tract?

a. biotin
b. vitamin C
c. vitamin D
d. calcium

30. Women have a higher RDA than men for:

a. copper.
b. zinc.
c. iron.
d. ergosterol.

31. An iodine deficiency can cause:

a. anemia.
b. hypertension.
c. goiter.
d. gout.

32. Fluoride is added to fluoridate water at a level of:

a. 1 part per million (ppm).
b. 2 ppm.
c. 3 ppm.
d. 4 ppm.

33. Vitamin B$_{12}$ contains:

a. iron.
b. cobalt.

c. molybdenum.
d. zinc.

34. A high-salt diet may cause:

    a. mottling of the teeth.
    b. a high-cholesterol level.
    c. elevated blood pressure.
    d. reduced blood pressure.

35. Iodine is stored in the body in the:

    a. stomach.
    b. thyroid gland.
    c. liver.
    d. muscles.

36. An excellent source of phosphorus is:

    a. vitamin capsules.
    b. meat.
    c. celery.
    d. watermelon.

37. The best sources of zinc are:

    a. shellfish, meats, and liver.
    b. breads, cereals, and grains.
    c. fruits and vegetables.
    d. milk products.

38. Contraction of the heart muscle is regulated by the level of:

    a. iron.
    b. copper.
    c. calcium.
    d. manganese.

39. The best source of iron in the following list is:

    a. egg yolks.
    b. polished rice.
    c. oranges.
    d. coconut.

40. Iron ordinarily is:

    a. reused in the body.
    b. excreted efficiently in the urine.
    c. exhaled through the lungs.
    d. destroyed after it is released from hemoglobin.

41. Copper is needed:

    a. to catalyze the formation of hemoglobin.
    b. to form elastin.
    c. for energy release in metabolic reactions.
    d. to regulate nerve impulses.

42. A valuable source of copper is:

    a. olives.
    b. oranges.
    c. shellfish.
    d. meats.

43. A rich source of magnesium is:

    a. cod liver oil.
    b. milk.
    c. breads and cereals.
    d. liver.

44. Good food sources of potassium include all except:

    a. dried fruits.
    b. instant coffee.
    c. meats.
    d. olives.

TRUE/FALSE

Circle T for True and F for False.

45. T F Adequate calcium, ascorbic acid, and hydrochloric acid from the stomach are necessary for good absorption of iron.
46. T F Iron balance is controlled by urinary excretion.
47. T F The liver is the body's main storage site for iron.
48. T F Most iron is lost from the body whenever old blood cells wear out.
49. T F Hemorrhagic anemia is caused by a dietary deficiency of iron.
50. T F Pregnancy and lactation require supplementary iron.
51. T F Iron is widespread in foods, so a deficiency is rare.
52. T F Hemoglobin formation is the major function of iron.
53. T F The lack of calcium in the diet may cause muscle spasms, particularly in the extremities.
54. T F Growth, including wound healing, could be retarded by a zinc-deficient diet.
55. T F Food sources of zinc include meat, nuts, legumes, and shellfish.
56. T F Using large quantities of table salt may increase the risk of hypertension.
57. T F Foods that are high in protein are usually good sources of sodium.
58. T F Phosphorus is usually adequate in a diet that contains sufficient calcium and protein.
59. T F Most minerals that are essential in trace amounts are toxic in larger amounts.

MATCHING

Match the statements in Column A to their corresponding statements in Column B to complete the sentence.

Column A	Column B
60. A function of water is	a. outside the cells and inside the cells
61. Water is found in the body	b. breathing, perspiring, urinating, defecating
62. Water is gained in the body by	c. drinking, eating, cell metabolism

63. Water is lost from the body by
64. Output of water exceeding intake causes

d. dehydration, cell death
e. maintenance of a stable body temperature

REFERENCES

Abrams, S. A. (2005). Calcium supplementation during childhood: Long-term effects on bone mineralization. *Nutrition Reviews, 63*: 251–255.

Block, A., Maillet, J. O., Winkler, M. F., & Howell, W. H. (2006). *Issues and Choices in Clinical Nutrition and Practice*. Philadelphia: Lippincott, Williams and Wilkins.

Bogden, J. D., & Klevay, L. M. (Eds.). (2000). *Clinical Nutrition of the Essential Trace Elements and Minerals: The Guide for Health Professionals*. Totowa, NJ: Humana Press.

Caballero, B., Allen, L., & Prentice, A. (Eds.). (2005). *Encyclopedia of Human Nutrition* (2nd ed.). Boston: Elsevier/Academic Press.

CRC. (2004). *Handbook of Chemistry and Physics* (85th ed.). Boca Raton, FL: CRC Press.

Deen, D. & Hark, L. (2007). *The Complete Guide to Nutrition in Primary Care*. Malden, MA: Blackwell.

Droke, E. A. (2008). Dietary fatty acids and minerals. In Chow, C. K. (Ed.). *Fatty Acids in Foods and Their Health Implications*. Boca Raton, FL: CRC Press.

Eckhert, C. D. (2006). Other trace elements. In Shils, M. E. (Ed.). *Modern Nutrition in Health and Disease* (10th ed.) (pp. 338–350). Philadelphia: Lippincott Williams and Wilkins.

Escott-Stump, S. (2002). *Nutrition and Diagnosis-Related Care* (5th ed.). Philadelphia: Lippincott, Williams and Wilkins.

Food and Agriculture Organization. (2002). *Human Vitamin and Mineral Requirements: Report of a Joint FAO/WHO Expert Consultation*. Rome, Italy: World Health Organization.

Gupta, V. B., Anitha, S., Hegde, M. L., Zecca, L., Garruto, R. M., Ravid, R., et al. (2005). Aluminum in Alzheimer's disease: Are we still at a crossroad? *Cellular and Molecular Life Sciences 62*(2): 143–158.

Higdon, J. (2003). *An Evidence-Based Approach to Vitamins and Minerals: Health Implications and Intake Recommendations*. New York: Thieme.

Iannotti, L. L. (2006). Iron supplementation in childhood: Health benefits and risks. *American Journal of Clinical Nutrition, 84*: 1261–1276.

Kaplan, R. J. (2006). Beverage guidance system is not evidence-based. *American Journal of Clinical Nutrition 84*: 1248–1249.

Lane, H. W. (2002). Water and energy dietary requirements and endocrinology of human space flight. *Nutrition, 18*: 820–828.

Lopez, M. A., & Martos, F. C. (2004). Iron availability: An updated review. *International Journal of Food Sciences and Nutrition, 55*(8): 597–606.

Mahan, L. K. & Escott-Stump, S. (Eds.). (2008). *Krause's Food and Nutrition Therapy* (12th ed.). Philadelphia: Elsevier Saunders.

Mann, J., & Truswell, S. (Eds.). (2007). *Essentials of Human Nutrition* (3rd ed.). New York: Oxford University Press.

Moore, M. C. (2005). *Pocket Guide to Nutritional Assessment and Care* (5th ed.). St. Louis, MO: Elvesier Mosby.

Navarra, T. (Ed.). (2004). *The Encyclopedia of Vitamins, Minerals, and Supplements* (2nd ed.). New York: Facts on File.

Neilsen, F. H. (2001). Other trace elements. In Bnowman, B.A. & Russell, R. M. (Eds.). *Present Knowledge in Nutrition* (8th ed.) (pp. 384–400). Washington, DC: ILSI Press.

Otten, J. J., Hellwig, P. J., & Meyers, L. D. (Eds.). (2006). *Dietary Reference Intakes: The Essential Guide to Nutrient Requirements*. Washington, DC: National Academy Press.

Papanikolaou, G., & Pantopoulos, K. (2005). Iron metabolism and toxicity. *Toxicology and Applied Pharmacology, 202*(2): 199–211.

Shils, M. E. & Shike, M. (Eds.). (2006). *Modern Nutrition in Health and Disease* (10th ed.). Philadelphia: Lippincott, Williams and Wilkins.

Water, Sanitation, and Health Protection and Human Environment (WHO). (2005). *Nutrients in Drinking Water*. Geneva, Switzerland: World Health Organization.

Webster-Gandy, J., Madden, A., & Holdworth, M. (Eds.). (2006). *Oxford Handbook of Nutrition and Dietetics*. Oxford, England: Oxford University Press.

Yves, R., Mazue, A., & Durlach, J. (2001). *Advances in Magnesium Research: Nutrition and Health*. Eastleigh, England: John Libby.

CHAPTER 7

Meeting Energy Needs

Time for completion
Activities: 1½ hours
Optional examination: ½ hour

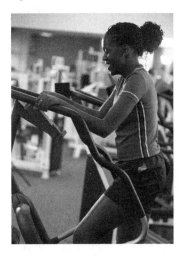

OBJECTIVES

Upon completion of this chapter the student should be able to do the following:

1. Describe how energy is measured.
2. Define energy balance.
3. Identify the energy-producing nutrients and state their fuel value.
4. Calculate the calorie content of foods based on their carbohydrate, protein, fat, and/or alcohol content.
5. Relate food and activity to weight control.
6. List techniques for evaluating body weight.
7. Discuss methods for controlling body weight.
8. Evaluate the effects of under- and overnutrition.
9. State the health implications of being underweight.
10. Differentiate between overweight and obesity.
11. Analyze health problems associated with fad dieting and obesity.
12. Describe the differences between ideal versus healthy weight.
13. Determine weight by using the body mass index (BMI).

GLOSSARY

Anthropometric measurements: measurements of body size and composition, including height, weight, body circumference measurements (midarm, head, abdominal girth), and skin-fold thickness (fat fold). To be valid, these measurements must be obtained in an accurate manner and compared to reference standards.

Basal metabolic rate (BMR): expression of the number of kilocalories used hourly in relation to the surface area of the body. The speed at which fuel is needed to maintain vital body processes at rest, or the amount of energy the body requires to carry out its involuntary maintenance work.

Basal metabolism: the amount of energy required to carry on vital body processes when the body is at rest.

Body composition: the amount of lean muscle mass, water, fat, and minerals that compose the human body.

Body mass index (BMI): the ratio of body fat to muscle mass as measured from body density. An indicator of underweight or overweight conditions.

Caloric density: the number of kilocalories in a unit of weight of a specific food.

Calorie (cal): unit of energy. The amount of heat necessary to raise one gram of water one degree centigrade. The energy released from food is too enormous to be described by these units, so nutritionists use the kilocalorie equivalent of 1000 of these small calories (see Kilocalorie).

Energy metabolism: all the chemical changes that result in the release of energy in the body.

Hyperplasia: increase in the total number of cells.

Hyperthyroidism: excessive secretion of the thyroid gland, increasing the basal metabolic rate.

Hypertrophy: enlargement of cells.

Hypothyroidism: deficiency of thyroid secretion resulting in a lowered basal metabolic rate.

Kilocalorie (kcal): unit of energy. The amount of heat needed to raise one kilogram of water one degree centigrade. Although not technically correct, most consumer and professional literature calls these units *calories*. Nutritionists use a capital *C* when describing a kilocalorie.

Metabolism: the total of all the chemical and biological processes that take place in the body.

Obesity: the clinical term for body weight in excess of 20%–30% above standard weights found in height–weight tables. Not an accurate measure of the amount of excess fat (see Overfat).

Overfat: a more correct term. Clinically, it defines obesity as an excess of body fat that has negative effects on health. It refers to body composition: how much of the body weight is lean muscle mass and how much is fat.

Overweight: clinical term for body weight higher than height–weight standards, but less than the 20%–30% that is designated obesity.

Synthesis: the process of building up; the formation of complex substances from simpler ones.

Thermic effect of food: the increase in metabolism caused by the digestion, absorption, and transportation of nutrients in the body.

BACKGROUND INFORMATION

Weight control has become a 21st-century health problem. Before this century, excess weight was the mark of a healthy body, an affluent family, good mothering, and shapely beauty. Being underweight or what would now be considered normal weight was held in low esteem. These attitudes have since reversed. The terms *overweight*, *overfat*, and *obesity* are common to modern societies. In the United States, 52% of the population is overweight with the following profile:

- 10% of them are school children.
- 33% of them can be classified as obese.

Another third of the population is struggling to keep a stable weight. It should not come as a surprise, then, that repercussions from obsessions about thinness occur.

Health professionals are witnessing cases of eating disorders such as anorexia nervosa and bulimia as a response to the pressures to be thin (refer to Chapter 22). At the same time, the opposite end of these disorders, obesity, is escalating. Due to psychogenic overtones, many scientists now believe that obesity and anorexia nervosa are conditions on a continuum of the same disorder. The manifestations of either appear to result in the same kinds of clinical disturbances.

Students in a health profession should be familiar with weight control in order to assist clients to achieve their optimal weight goals.

ACTIVITY 1:

Energy Balance

Energy balance occurs when an individual's total caloric expenditure equals the individual's total caloric intake. Factors over which we have control are our intake and expenditure. There are some variables that influence our energy balance over which we have little or no control.

ENERGY MEASUREMENT

The energy value of a food is measured in kilocalories (kcals). Much work has been devoted to developing reference tables of foods' caloric values for use in estimating our energy intake. A food's caloric value is determined by its content of protein, fat, and carbohydrate. These are the only nutrients that produce energy; vitamins and minerals do not. Protein provides 4 kcal per gram (g), carbohydrate 4, and fat 9. For example, 1 tsp of sugar (carbohydrate) equals 5 g and 20 kcal, and 1 tsp salad oil equals 5 g and 45 kcal. Alcohol, while not a basic nutrient, provides 7 kcal/g and can create problems in weight control as well as other undesirable effects. Carbohydrates and fats are the preferred energy sources. Proteins are used for energy if carbohydrates are not available in the diet. If carbohydrate supplies are limited, fat and protein stores will be used for energy and may result in a buildup of toxic by-products (ketones) in the blood.

Total energy needs are measured in three major areas: the basal metabolic rate, activity or voluntary energy expenditure, and the thermic effect of food.

BASAL METABOLIC RATE

Basal metabolism, the energy required for the vital life processes, is measured in terms of basal metabolic rate (BMR) and is affected by several factors:

1. Body composition and surface—The BMR of a body is higher for a person with more muscle than fat. Muscle is the lean body mass of the body. Also, the larger a person's amount of skin area, the higher the BMR.
2. Sex—Women have lower BMR values than men because of the difference in activity of sex hormones and women's generally lower lean body mass.
3. Age—A person's BMR is highest during infancy. After adolescence, the BMR begins a gradual decline of about 2% each decade after the age of 20 years.
4. Body temperature—A cold external temperature raises the BMR as the body tries to keep warm. However, a high internal temperature (fever) also significantly increases BMR.
5. Physiological status—Conditions such as malnutrition, hypothyroidism, and starvation decrease the BMR. Diseases such as cancer, hypertension, or emphysema increase the BMR, as does hyperthyroidism.

ENERGY AND PHYSICAL ACTIVITY

Voluntary energy expenditure affects the energy balance. Muscular exercise burns calories, but mental activity or paperwork does not. The energy needed for various activities increases as the weight of the person increases, but overweight persons usually make up for this by becoming less active. Table 7-1 provides a partial listing of various activities and the amount of kilocalories needed for each.

THERMIC EFFECT OF FOOD

A person's BMR increases for about 12 hours after eating a meal. The digestion, absorption, transportation, and metabolism of nutrients all require energy. The produc-

TABLE 7-1   Approximate Energy Cost of Different Forms of Activities for a 70-kg (154 lb) Man*

Activity	Kcal/min
Basketball	9.0–10.00
Boxing	9.0–10.00
Cleaning	4.0–4.5
Coal mining	6.0–8.0
Cooking	3.0–3.5
Dancing	3.5–12.5
Eating	1.0–2.0
Fishing	4.0–5.0
Gardening	3.5–9.0
Horse riding	3.0–10.0
Painting	2.0–6.0
Piano playing	2.5–3.0
Running	9.0–21.0
Scrubbing floors	7.0–8.0
Standing	1.5–2.0
Swimming	4.0–12.0
Typing, electric	1.5–2.0
Walking	1.5–6.0
Writing	2.0–2.5

*The data in this table have been collected from many sources. Because of large variation among the results of different investigators, ranges of values are used so as to give a general idea of the relationship between types of activity and the energy cost.

tion of heat following a meal is known as the thermic effect of food. This effect varies with the kind and amounts of food eaten and the person's metabolic needs. The use of nutrients to build new tissue requires more energy than the breakdown of nutrients to provide energy. The thermic effect of food varies from about 10 to 15% of total energy needs.

ENERGY INTAKE AND OUTPUT

Energy balance results when the number of kilocalories consumed equals the number used for energy. The body weight is an index of this relationship of intake to output. Exercise is a valuable aid in achieving energy balance. If consistently more calories are consumed than used for energy, the result will be a weight gain. Excess calories are stored in the form of fat. If less is eaten than the body needs, the result will be weight loss. Energy must come from somewhere, so calories needed but not provided by food are withdrawn from body stores.

A pound of body fat represents 3500 kcal. For every 3500 kcal lacking in the diet, 1 lb of body weight will be lost, and for every 3500 kcal excess, 1 lb of weight will be gained. It does not matter whether the excess or shortage occurs over a period of a week or a year.

Examples

Every calorie absorbed by the body must be used as energy or stored as fat. This principle is illustrated by the following examples:

1. Robert has an office job where he sits constantly programming a computer. He has been out of college for four years. Although he has tried to control his weight, his weight has still escalated. Let us compare his conditions during 1990 and 1994.

   In 1990, Robert's daily kcal intake from food was 2250. He played racquetball daily with his roommate. This, combined with other activities and his BMR, expended 2250 kcal energy daily. He weighed 160 pounds when he graduated.

   In 1994, Robert's food intake is still 2250 kcal per day. He plays only one game of racquetball a week. This, combined with his other activities and BMR, expends 2000 kcal of energy per day. All other variables have remained the same, including his eating habits. He now weighs 264 lb.

   The equation is simple:
   a. 250 kcal/day excess = 1750 kcal excess per week
   b. 1750 kcal = ½ lb body fat per week
   c. ½ lb weight gain every week = 26 lb per year
   d. 26 lb per year × 4 years = 104 lb weight gained

2. Jane is attending a wellness class at her local college and finds she is roughly 40% above her ideal body weight of 130 lb. Her average 24-hour food intake yields 1800 kcal. Jane gets counseling from a health educator. They work out a program whereby Jane substitutes her daily late-afternoon snack of 250 calories for a 2-½ mile brisk walk. The walk uses approximately 250 calories. At the end of a year Jane has reached her ideal weight of 130 lb without "suffering" and feels much better physically and mentally. The equation is simple:
   a. 250 calorie deficit from food plus 250 calorie deficit from exercise = 500 calorie deficit per day
   b. 500 calories × 7 days a week = 3500 calories or 1 lb weight loss per week
   c. 1 × 52 weeks per year = 52 lb weight loss per year
   d. 130 lb (ideal body weight) × 40% = 182 lb (starting weight)
   e. 182 lb – 52 lb = 130 lb (ideal body weight) at end of one year

   Skin-fold measurements following the successful loss of 52 lb. revealed that total percentage of body fat was 20%, well within the 18 to 25% normal range for females. This confirmed that body fat, not muscle and water, was lost. This pattern of weight loss is highly recommended for its value in maintaining a lower body weight once the goal is reached. It provides ample time to modify eating habits and lifestyles.

   The difficulty people have balancing their intake and output of energy nutrients is clearly demonstrated by the fact that obesity is a major health problem in the United States. It is believed to cause or complicate many of the chronic disorders of later life.

BODY ENERGY NEED

Release of energy in the cells is a complex process requiring the activity of vitamins and minerals as well as enzymes and hormones. A person's total energy needs are based on basal metabolism, voluntary physical activity, and the thermic effect of food. The BMR is the speed at which fuel is spent to maintain the vita body processes at rest. It is influenced by body composition, sex, age, body temperature, and various other physical conditions. The effect of physical activity on total caloric need depends on the type of activity, the length of time over which it is performed, and the size of the person doing it.

Foods vary in energy value in proportion to the energy-producing nutrients they contain. Foods that contain fat or alcohol or have a low water content tend to have a relatively high energy value; lean meats, cereal foods, and starchy vegetables are intermediate in energy value; and fruits and vegetables are relatively low in energy value.

All essential nutrients should be provided within the calorie level required to maintain ideal weight. The more calories a person obtains from sugars, fats, and alcohol, the more likely he or she is to be poorly nourished.

Quick weight loss, usually obtained by extreme fad dieting, reflects loss of protein (muscle), tissue, and water rather than fat loss. In addition, very low-calorie diets decrease the BMR.

The scientific method of estimating our body energy need is presented in Activity 2.

CALCULATING ENERGY INTAKE

There are several ways to calculate caloric intake. For the general public, the easiest way is to find out how much calories we eat by using the following steps:

1. Write down what we eat for breakfast.
2. Use a standard food composition table to identify the foods and their caloric contribution.
3. Add the calories from the list of foods consumed.
4. Repeat the same for lunch and dinner.
5. The total calories of the three meals are an approximation of calories consumed that day.

To estimate the caloric values of foods, we need a reference table. Caloric and nutrient values of foods are found in many publications, both government and commercial. Using a government source, Table 7-2 provides some examples.

Beginning in 1960, most Western and many other countries started compiling the nutrient contents of food into food composition table. Each country has its

TABLE 7-2   Energy Value of Selected Foods Compared

Foods from Food Groups	Portion	Kcal
Meat and Alternates		
1. Beef (lean and fat)	3 oz	245
(lean only)	3 oz	140
2. Chicken, no skin, broiled	3 oz	115
skin and flesh broiled	3 oz	155
3. Fish, haddock, fried	3 oz	135
shrimp, canned	3 oz	100
tuna, in oil, drained	3 oz	170
Vegetables and Fruits		
1. Beans, lima, cooked, drained	½ c	95
green, snap	½ c	15
2. Beets, cooked, diced	½ c	25
3. Corn, canned	½ c	85
4. Onions, cooked	½ c	30
5. Carrots, grated	½ c	20
6. Peas, green, cooked	½ c	58
7. Grapes, raw	½ c	32
8. Applesauce, unsweetened	½ c	50
9. Apricots, unsweetened, cooked	½ c	120
10. Orange juice	½ c	55
11. Pineapple, canned, in juice	½ c	40
Grains (Bread, Cereal)		
1. Bagel	1	165
2. Biscuit, baking powder, 2″ dia.	1	90
3. Bran flakes (40%)	1 c	105
4. Bread, white or wheat	1 slice	70
5. Cake		
a. angel food, ½₂ of 10″ diameter	1 piece	135
b. devils food, ½₆ of 9″ diameter	1 piece	235
6. Cookies		
a. chocolate chip (small)	1	50
b. brownies (small)	1	85
7. Pies		
a. apple, ½ of 9″ diameter	1 piece	350
b. pecan, ½ of 9″ diameter	1 piece	490
8. Pizza (cheese), 5-½″	1 piece	185
9. Popcorn, plain	1 c	20
Milk and Alternates		
1. Milk, fluid, whole	1 c	160
skim	1 c	90
buttermilk from skim	1 c	90
2. Cheese, cheddar	1 oz	115
cottage, creamed	½ c	130
creamed	1 cu inch	60
3. Ice cream, vanilla	1 c	255
4. Ice milk, regular hardened	1 c	200
soft serve	1 c	265
5. Yogurt, whole milk	1 c	150
low fat	1 c	125

Source: Adapted from USDA Web site at www.ars.usda.gov/ba/bhnrc/ndl.

common foods processed and prepared according to its culture. The United States Department of Agriculture prepared and distributed for public use a number of useful publications on food composition from 1960 to 2005.

A list of such books is available at www.usda.gov. The key words for searching are *food composition tables*.

Most of the publications are in one volume, and some are in series. Once the computer was invented, the USDA started electronic databases to store food composition data. With the introduction of the Internet, the USDA National Nutrient Database for Standard Reference has become the largest food (raw, processed, and prepared) composition database in the world. It can be, among other useful properties, accessed, searched, downloaded, copied, and so on. Of course, its use and application is free to citizens of the world. Officially, the suggested citation for this database is:

> U.S. Department of Agriculture, Agricultural Research Service. (2005). USDA National Nutrient Database for Standard Reference, Release #. Nutrient Data Laboratory Home Page, http://www.ars.usda.gov/ba/bhnrc/ndl.

"Release #" represents each new release as it becomes available. As of summer 2008, Release 18 was the latest.

Another method of estimating the caloric intake is familiarization with the foods and serving sizes contained in each of the groups in the Food Exchange Lists for weight loss, diabetes, and kidney diseases. Chapters 18 and 20 and Appendix F provide more details.

PROGRESS CHECK ON ACTIVITY 1

FILL-IN

1. What are the three factors that determine a person's total energy needs? Describe each of these factors.

   a. _____
   b. _____
   c. _____

2. A ½-cup serving of New England clam chowder contains 4 g protein, 5 g fat, and 7 g carbohydrate. Using this information, calculate the energy value of this food serving:

   EXAMPLE: ½ c whole milk contains 4.2 g protein, 6 g carbohydrate, and 4.2 g fat. The calorie content of this milk is:

4.2 g protein × 4 kcal/g	= 16.8 kcal
6.0 g carbohydrate × 4 kcal/g	= 24.0 kcal
4.2 g fat × 9 kcal/g	= 37.8 kcal
Total	= 78.6 kcal

3. What is the guide for determining whether your caloric intake is in balance with your energy needs? Explain. _____

   _____

   _____

   _____

What happens to excess calories?

_____

_____

_____

_____

4. Explain the error in the statement: "Potatoes are fattening."

   _____

   _____

   _____

5. A 25-year-old woman who is 5'2" tall and weighs 125 lb consumes 1800 calories a day to maintain her weight. She wants to lose 3 lb of weight per week.

   a. To lose this 3 lb of weight per week, how many calories per day could she eat?

      _____

      _____

   b. Is a weight loss of 3 lb per week realistic for this woman? Explain.

      _____

      _____

      _____

6. Identify the exchange group to which the following energy values belong (values are rounded).

   a. 90 kcal _____
   b. 60 kcal _____
   c. 80 kcal _____
   d. 25 kcal _____
   e. 45 kcal _____
   f. 55 kcal _____

MATCHING

Match the phrases on the right to the items on the left that best describe them.

7. Fever   a. basal metabolic rate
8. BMR   b. amount of energy needed to raise one g water one degree centigrade
9. Calorie c. causes a significant increase in BMR

ACTIVITY 2:

The Effects of Energy Imbalance

DEFINITIONS

Malnutrition is a general term indicating an excess, deficit, or imbalance in one or more of the essential nutrients. It is also used to describe an excess or deficit of calories. Physical, psychosocial, and economic factors can contribute to the development of malnutrition.

Malnutrition is classified as either primary or secondary. Primary malnutrition is due to poor food choices or inadequate food supply. Secondary malnutrition refers to faulty body functioning, such as the inability to digest certain essential foods. It may also be a result of certain drug therapies.

Two other terms that are used to describe malnutrition are *undernutrition* and *overnutrition*. These terms are frequently identified in the underweight or overweight individual, indicating either inadequate or excessive caloric intake. Both types can interfere with body processes and affect health.

Underweight is generally accepted as being below 10% of ideal body weight, and overweight is defined as 10 to 20% above ideal body weight.

HOW TO DETERMINE YOUR WEIGHT

At first, it seems like an easy question to answer. However, defining overweight and obesity proves more difficult than might be expected. At what point do the extra pounds cease to be an annoyance and become a serious threat to health? As Americans become heavier and heavier, the toll of obesity-related diseases such as diabetes and cardiovascular disease becomes greater. To appreciate the impact of excess weight on disease, one must realize that overweight and obesity are conditions that are defined by more than just total body weight as shown on a bathroom scale. Because of this, several methods to measure body mass and body fat have been developed.

Among health care professionals, perhaps the best known method for assessing body size is the body mass index, or BMI. BMI is a value derived from a person's height divided by his weight. Specifically, weight in kilograms is divided by height in meters, squared. Persons with a BMI of between 25 and 30 are considered to be overweight, while those with a BMI greater than 30 are classified as obese. For example, a person who is 6' tall and weighs 175 lb has a BMI of 23.7, a value that is within normal range. If a person of the same height weighed 200 lbs, his BMI would rise to 27.1, indicating overweight. At 230 pounds, his BMI would be 31.2, indicating obesity. BMI represents a valuable and easy-to-calculate manner of determining whether a person is obese, and BMI may be used by both men and women to estimate their relative risk of developing disease. Table 7-3 presents the body mass index.

A healthy weight is key to a long, healthy life. If you are an adult, follow the directions in Table 7-3 to evaluate your weight in relation to your height, or BMI. Not all adults who have a BMI in the range labeled "healthy" are at their most healthy weight. For example, some may have lots of fat and little muscle. A BMI above the healthy range is less healthy for most people, but it may be fine if you have lots of muscle and little fat. The further your BMI is above the healthy range, the higher your weight-related risk.

If your BMI is above the healthy range, you may benefit from weight loss, especially if you have other health risk factors.

BMIs slightly below the healthy range may still be healthy unless they result from illness. If your BMI is below the healthy range, you may have increased risk of menstrual irregularity, infertility, and osteoporosis. If you lose weight suddenly or for unknown reasons, see a healthcare provider. Unexplained weight loss may be an early clue to a health problem. Keep track of your weight and your waist measurement, and take action if either of them increases. If your BMI is greater than 25, or even if it is in the "healthy" range, at least try to avoid further weight gain. If your waist measurement increases, you are probably gaining fat. If so, take steps to eat fewer calories and become more active.

BODY COMPOSITION

Body composition is a much more accurate indicator of ideal body weight than are weight and height tables in determining the fatness or leanness of a person.

The adult body is approximately 65% water. This proportion is higher in lean persons because muscle tissue contains more water than fat tissue. Minerals account for about 6% of body weight, most of which is in the bones, and lean body mass can range from 40% to 70%, depending upon size and activity. Lean body mass decreases with age. Body fat also fluctuates. In adult males it ranges from 15% to 30%; in women 20% to 35%. Again, these percentages change with age and degree of fitness. Some older people maintain a lower body fat ratio through exercise and weight maintenance. For survival, some fat is needed to insulate the body from environmental temperature fluctuation, regulate the body's internal temperature, and protect the body against shock. The ideal range of body fat varies with survival needs.

Some accurate measurements of body composition that are used to determine body weight include the following:

TABLE 7-3   How to Evaluate Your Weight (Adults)

• Weigh yourself and have your height measured.
• Find your BMI category in the table. The higher your BMI category, the greater the risk for health problems.
• Measure around your waist, just above your hip bones, while standing. Health risks increase as waist measurement increases, particularly if waist is greater than 35 inches for women or 40 inches for men. Excess abdominal fat may place you at greater risk of health problems, even if your BMI is about right.

The higher your BMI and waist measurement, and the more risk factors you have, the more you are likely to benefit from weight loss.

NOTE: Weight loss is usually not advisable for pregnant woman.

Body Mass Index (BMI) Table																	
BMI	19	20	21	22	23	24	25	26	27	28	29	30	31	32	33	34	35
Height	Weight (in pounds)																
4'10" (58")	91	96	100	105	110	115	119	124	129	134	138	143	148	153	158	162	167
4'11" (59")	94	99	104	109	114	119	124	128	133	138	143	148	153	158	163	168	173
5' (60")	97	102	107	112	118	123	128	133	138	143	148	153	158	163	168	174	179
5'1" (61")	100	106	111	116	122	127	132	137	143	148	153	158	164	169	174	180	185
5'2" (62")	104	109	115	120	126	131	136	142	147	153	158	164	169	175	180	186	191
5'3" (63")	107	113	118	124	130	135	141	146	152	158	163	169	175	180	186	191	197
5'4" (64")	110	116	122	128	134	140	145	151	157	163	169	174	180	186	192	197	204
5'5" (65")	114	120	126	132	138	144	150	156	162	168	174	180	186	192	198	204	210
5'6" (66")	118	124	130	136	142	148	155	161	167	173	179	186	192	198	204	210	216
5'7" (67")	121	127	134	140	146	153	159	166	172	178	185	191	198	204	211	217	223
5'8" (68")	125	131	138	144	151	158	164	171	177	184	190	197	203	210	216	223	230
5'9" (69")	128	135	142	149	155	162	169	176	182	189	196	203	209	216	223	230	236
5'10" (70")	132	139	146	153	160	167	174	181	188	195	202	209	216	222	229	236	243
5'11" (71")	136	143	150	157	165	172	179	186	193	200	208	215	222	229	236	243	250
6' (72")	140	147	154	162	169	177	184	191	199	206	213	221	228	235	242	250	258
6'1" (73")	144	151	159	166	174	182	189	197	204	212	219	227	235	242	250	257	265
6'2" (74")	148	155	163	171	179	186	194	202	210	218	225	233	241	249	256	264	272
6'3" (75")	152	160	168	176	184	192	200	208	216	224	232	240	248	256	264	272	279

Source: Evidence Report of Clinical Guidelines on the Identification, Evaluation, and Treatment of Overweight and Obesity in Adults, 1998. NIH/National Heart, Lung, and Blood Institute (NHLBI).

1. Water displacement and determination of specific gravity—This method is accurate, but requires special equipment. Most medical centers and hospitals have the equipment and will charge a nominal fee for a standard measurement. Many persons participating in fitness and conditioning programs have this type of assessment performed prior to and at intervals during the program.
2. Skin-fold thicknesses measured by calipers at specific body sites—These measurements should be taken by a skilled person and assessed by comparing to reference standards.
3. Anthropometric measurements including skeletal, head, muscle, and body contour circumferences—These measurements are useful at any age, but especially for evaluating growth in children.
4. Radiological and laboratory studies to identify signs of malnutrition—Tests such as measuring an individual's radioactive potassium content are useful in determining lean body mass. A high potassium count indicates little fat tissue.

ESTIMATE ENERGY OR CALORIC REQUIREMENTS

In the last decade, research data have transformed the method of estimating energy requirements (EER) for men and women. For many years, the method was simple. Tables were available to show the energy need of a person according, sex, age, height, and weight. Tables further divided this caloric need into BMR (basal metabolic rate) and physical activity.

At present the scientific method of obtaining EER is complicated. To do so we need the following information:

• Sex
• Height
• BMI table for body weight

- BMR
- Physical activity level (PAL) (sedentary, low activity, active, very active) for men and women of a specific height and body weight
- Specific mathematical regression equations to establish the EER for men or women with all the variables

The NAS has established EER for selected groups of men and women (age, height, and so on) that includes all the above variables. EER is part of a series of DRIs. Two examples are provided below showing only three variables (age, height, and weight):

For a man with the following criteria and who is physically activite, the EER is about 2800–3200 kcal per day depending on the BMI:

- Age: 30 years
- Height: 5'11"
- Weight: 135 lb

For a woman with the following criteria and who is physically activite, the EER is about 2250–2500 kcal per day depending on the BMI:

- Age: 30 year
- Height: 5'5"
- Weight: 110 lb

Thus, it is no longer easy or convenient to identify one's real energy need. However, currently, at the levels of the consumers, health providers still use many tables that show the energy requirement once the patient's weight is known. This is obviously not as accurate as those developed by the NAS for our DRIs. In research and clinical patient care, healthcare providers use the DRIs developed by the NAS to estimate the energy requirement.

It is expected that in the near future, computerized tables for EER will be available for all individuals in all stages of life with consideration for sex, weight, height, BMI, BMR, and PAL (physical activity level).

UNDERNUTRITION

When an individual is undernourished, nutrient reserves dwindle, tissues become deprived of essential nutrients, and medical disorders result. Protein stores are depleted as muscle tissue is used as a source of energy. Antibody production against invasions of bacteria and viruses becomes limited. Lack of nutrient reserves may lead to more severe forms of malnutrition, such as marasmus and kwashiorkor, or the mixed condition of protein energy malnutrition (PEM). These conditions are discussed further in Chapter 3.

A woman who is underweight during pregnancy is at high obstetric risk. Newborn infants of such women are also likely to have problems, such as being small for gestational age (SGA, underweight through full term) and/or premature.

The most severe form of undernutrition is anorexia nervosa, a condition due largely to psychological problems. It manifests as a physiological disorder where signs of starvation are evident. It requires psychiatric treatment before and during nutritional rehabilitation. This disorder is life threatening and can recur after recovery. Chapter 22 has a detailed discussion of this disorder.

OBESITY

Overview

Being overweight may be more of a social than a medical problem. The overweight individual may develop a distorted body image manifested in low self-esteem, embarrassment, and social isolation. Counseling the obese individual toward a regular exercise routine and an accurate perception of body weight and composition is beneficial.

The average American who is overweight to mildly obese is likely to have gained the extra weight over a period of several years. The grossly obese individual usually gains several hundred pounds in the teens to early twenties. The term *overweight* usually refers to body weight in excess of some standard, and does not indicate the degree of fatness. See earlier discussion.

Adopting a regular exercise program and a controlled diet will permit the overweight individual to reduce to a normal weight. There appears to be a significant difference between the overweight and the obese individual in terms of percentage of body fat and the appearance of body systems changes that accompany the deposition of adipose tissues.

Fat Cells

The fundamental characteristics of adipose tissue are determined in the last three months of gestation, the first three years of life, and during adolescence. The adipose cell is 72% lipid (fat), 23% water, and is very active. It recycles its lipids. The total amount of body fat depends upon the size of the cells (hypertrophy) and the number of cells (hyperplasia). All obese people show enlargement of fat cells, but the obese individual who has three to five times the number of fat cells as the nonobese will be more resistant to weight loss. This is usually the case in juvenile onset obesity. These individuals remain resistant to significant weight loss throughout life, and constitute a population group with high health hazards.

Health Risks

Beyond the social, psychosocial, and aesthetic problems that must be dealt with by the obese, there are also a number of serious health problems caused or accelerated by obesity. Among these problems are:

1. Hernias: abdominal and hiatal hernias are especially common. Hiatal hernias are displacement of part of the stomach into the chest cavity.
2. Varicose veins and osteoarthritis: extra load on the weight-bearing joints creates a high incidence of these two conditions.
3. Winter coughing and bronchitis: common because of fat surrounding the diaphragm.
4. Decreased tolerance for exercise: poor breathing ability lowers oxygen intake.
5. Cholelithiasis (gallbladder stones): 96% of these stones are composed of cholesterol derived from the saturated fats of the body.
6. High blood lipids: both triglyceride and cholesterol levels tend to rise in the obese, leading to a higher risk of heart disease.
7. Hypertension (high blood pressure) and kidney diseases: common conditions among the obese due to the increased workload and the building of additional capillary systems to nourish the fat cells and move the additional weight. Newest studies implicate obesity rather than excess sodium intake as the major contributor to high blood pressure.
8. Type II diabetes: common among the obese. Many scientists believe that this disorder is a result of long-term obesity, as well as genetic predisposition.
9. Increased cancer risk: breast, uterine, pancreatic, and gallbladder carcinomas are being studied in regard to their relationship to obesity.
10. Sexuality and the obese:
    a. Sexual response diminishes due to both aesthetic reasons and physical barriers.
    b. Folds of fatty tissue around the scrotum raise local temperature and can lead to infertility in the male.
    c. Skin infections and irritations, especially around the genital areas, occur because of heat and moisture and folds of fat that make it difficult to clean the areas.
    d. Menstrual disorders are common in obese females.
    e. Obese women experience difficult pregnancies, and infants are likely to suffer fetal distress. There is also a higher stillborn rate among obese women.
11. Premature aging has been noted among the obese. It is estimated that the life span of an obese individual is reduced by 15 years.

Questions to Ask

The health practitioner should consider a variety of factors that may make a client vulnerable to obesity. Some assessments the health practitioner should make are:

1. What are the cultural practices? The main staples of the diet may be calorie dense with a small variety of other foods.
2. What is the income level? People in a low income level tend to eat filling and cheap foods (usually high in fats, sugars, and starches). Intake of protein foods, fruits, and vegetables may be low.
3. What does the client believe about weight in relation to health? In Western society thinness is a fetish, and large amounts of time and money are spent attaining it. At the same time, obesity is rampant. This is a paradox. Among some ethnic groups living in the United States, overweight and obesity are acceptable and perhaps even desirable conditions.
4. What is the emotional status? For what reasons do clients eat? What is their general mood? Are they dependent or independent? How do food and activity fit their daily living patterns? How do they adapt to stress?

Summary

Obesity is a multifaceted problem involving physiological, psychological, and cultural factors, all of which are resistant to current therapeutic efforts. *Obesity* is the precise term to use in referring to a gain of excess fat. *Overweight* is a more general term referring to increased weight gain in all body parts (fat, water, cells). The obese person is overweight, but the overweight person is not necessarily obese, and being overweight is not always undesirable. However, the public usually does not distinguish between the two terms.

Obesity may occur in two ways: existing adipocytes (fat cells) may enlarge or hypertrophy, or the number of fat cells may increase in a process called hyperplasia. All obese individuals experience hypertrophy, but not all have abnormal amounts of fat cells. Hyperplastic obesity is also called "juvenile onset" because development of extra adipocytes occurs during early or late childhood. Adult onset obesity is strictly hypertrophic. Once hyperplastic obesity has developed, weight can be lost from the cells, but the number of cells is not reduced.

The exact mechanism that causes obesity is not known, but the main factor appears to be overeating combined with inadequate levels of activity. Metabolic and glandular disorders, heredity, basal metabolic rate, and body type all influence the development of obesity.

Obesity has not been shown to cause disease, but it may predispose and complicate numerous serious health problems, including diabetes, digestive disease, arthritis, cerebral hemorrhage, difficulty in breathing, angina pectoris, circulatory collapse, varicose veins, hypertension, kidney disease, infertility, and dermatologic problems. Obesity lowers sexual drive and is connected with complications of pregnancy and premature aging. Obesity accounts for many psychological and social problems, such as low self-esteem and discrimination in sports, school, and jobs.

PROGRESS CHECK ON ACTIVITY 2

TRUE/FALSE

Circle T for True and F for False.

1. T F The term *obesity* is used to indicate excess body weight of 15% or more above ideal body weight.
2. T F Increasing the amount of energy expended for physical activity is a means of weight control.
3. T F The energy value of a weight-reduction diet usually ranges between 1000 and 1500 calories, depending on individual size and need.
4. T F In the Food Exchange Lists of dietary control, foods listed in one group may be exchanged freely with foods listed in another group.
5. T F Between-meal snacks should never be eaten on a weight-reduction diet.

For someone giving practical suggestions for persons on reduction diets, which of the following statements are true and which are false?

6. T F Purchase special low-calorie foods and eat separately from the rest of the family.
7. T F Eat only from the Food Guide Pyramid to lose weight.
8. T F Even when the diet plan is followed carefully, some weeks you will not show any weight loss.
9. T F Do not eat more than three meals per day.
10. T F Avoid dependence on appetite suppressants.
11. T F Personal adaptation to the diet plan is mandatory.
12. T F When eating in a restaurant, order single items instead of combinations.
13. T F Eat as much meat as you wish, but never eat carbohydrates.
14. T F As the body weight gets heavier and heavier, the toll of obesity-related diseases such as diabetes and cardiovascular disease becomes greater.
15. T F Body mass index (BMI) is the ratio of weight to height.
16. T F With a BMI of 25, a person is considered obese.
17. T F Unexpected weight loss may be an early clue to a health problem.
18. T F An increase in waist line is an indication of gaining fat.

MULTIPLE CHOICE

Circle the letter of the correct answer.

19. Obesity as a health hazard increases the risk in which of the following diseases or conditions? (Circle all that apply.)

    a. hypertension
    b. diabetes
    c. heart disease
    d. cancer

20. A reduction of 1000 calories in an obese person's daily diet would enable the individual to lose weight at which of the following rates?

    a. 1 lb per week
    b. 2 lb per week
    c. 3 lb per week
    d. 4 lb per week

21. Which of the following food portions has the lowest caloric value?

    a. 4 oz lean meat
    b. ½ c orange juice
    c. 1 slice bread
    d. 8 oz of 2% milk

22. In the exchange system of diet management, which of the following foods may be exchanged for one slice of bread?

    a. 1 scoop cottage cheese
    b. ½ avocado
    c. 3 c of popcorn (popped)
    d. 1 egg

23. In the exchange system, which one of the following food items is "free" and therefore can be eaten as desired?

    a. mustard
    b. carrots
    c. salsa
    d. lean meat
    e. orange juice

24. Which of the following foods is not a member of any of the meat exchange groups?

    a. ½ c pinto beans
    b. 1 c soy milk
    c. 1 tbsp peanut butter
    d. 1 hot dog

25. To maintain healthy body weight, the energy value of the daily diet should (circle all that apply):

    a. be equal to the energy used by the body at rest.
    b. include the energy used in activities of daily living.

c. be controlled by appetite.

d. be controlled by medication.

26. A pound of adipose tissue has an energy value of

    a. 1750 calories.
    b. 3500 calories.
    c. 4000 calories.
    d. 9000 calories.

27. Sue's intake for a 24-hour period contained 190 g carbohydrate, 75 g protein, and 50 g fat. The energy value of her diet (rounded to nearest number) is

    a. 2000 calories.
    b. 1750 calories.
    c. 1500 calories.
    d. 1200 calories.

28. Sue's basal metabolic rate used 1350 calories in 24 hours and her daily activities used 400 calories. If her energy intake (from question 27) remained the same for a week, and her energy output remained the same for a week, Sue should:

    a. lose ½ lb.
    b. gain ½ lb.
    c. maintain her present weight.
    d. lose 2 lb.

29. John has an 8 oz glass of cola (which contains 100 calories) each day, in excess of his energy needs. If he continues this practice for one year, how much weight will he gain? (Round to nearest whole number.)

    a. 2 lb
    b. 6 lb
    c. 10 lb
    d. none

SITUATION

30. On October 1 Joe decides that he must lose 20 lb before the next tennis meet scheduled for December 7. He begins a diet of 700 kcal per day reduction and plays an hour of active tennis every day (count active tennis as using 300 kcal per hour). Answer the following questions regarding this situation.

    a. How many pounds per week will Joe lose if he continues his diet and exercise program?
    b. Will Joe lose 20 lb in time for the tennis meet?
    c. How many pounds a week would Joe lose if he only increased his exercise to one hour per day and did not diet?
    d. Would Joe lose 20 lb in time for the meet by exercise alone?

ACTIVITY 3:

Weight Control and Dieting

The best advice that one can give clients regarding weight control is to prevent the excess accumulation. The recommended approach is a controlled, but not deficient, eating pattern, combined with a regular exercise program. Weight problems are easier to correct when they begin to develop. Waiting until excess weight accumulates over the years presents great difficulties. Simple monitoring of one's body weight and attention to the fit of clothing through the years can assist with weight control. Weighing should be done on the same scale weekly at the same time of day, without clothing on, so that the variables, and therefore excuses, are minimized. The practice of keeping some clothing (such as a uniform or other correctly fitted garment) and trying it on for size twice each year is another monitoring device.

CALORIES, EATING HABITS, AND EXERCISE

Weight gain comes from eating more food energy (kcalories) than is expended. It will be gained as body fat if the person is not exercising, but weight may also be gained as lean tissue. Newer research findings show that there are different types of obesity, and these influence the kinds of approaches that are useful in determining treatment.

The factors that are receiving the most attention now have changed many of the preconceived ideas about obesity and dieting that have prevailed for years. For instance, the assumption that obesity was 98% caused by external behaviors is being challenged. Researchers are finding genetic differences that contribute to obesity. The set-point theory that was introduced in the 1980s continues to be studied. This theory holds that the body is programmed to choose a certain weight and to hold on to it by regulating eating behaviors and hormones.

These theories are substantiated by studies of individuals who had obese parents. If one parent was obese, the offspring had a 60% chance of becoming obese. If both parents were obese, the percentage rose to 90. Evidently genetic makeup contributes to how much fat is stored, as well as how much energy is consumed. There is strong evidence that the enzyme that enables excess fat to be stored is inherited; thus obesity runs in families. Studies of identical and fraternal twins who have been reared apart have also contributed to the studies on inherited obesity. Simple obesity is not as simple as was once believed.

This ongoing research does not negate the critical environment factors that contribute to obesity. The family's cultural and social attitudes toward food and appearance have a strong influence on how food is prepared and eaten and what is considered desirable body weight. Overweight and obesity are certainly not strictly genetic. Healthy body weights can be obtained and maintained by the majority of the population, although for most this does require some lifestyle changes.

Calories (Kilocalorie)

As discussed previously, the fuel value of foods provides the energy that keeps the body engine running, and the body is a more efficient engine than man-made machines. Activity 1 provided the fuel value of the energy-producing nutrients: 4 kcal/g of carbohydrate, 4 kcal/g of protein, and 9 kcal/g of fat. Alcohol also contributes 7 kcal/g and, although alcohol is considered a drug, it is listed with foods because of its energy production, which can provide excess calories. The ways in which the body breaks down the nutrients provides the rationale for decided changes in diet modification for weight reduction.

Carbohydrates of all kinds (except fiber) are broken down to sugars to be absorbed. Excess carbohydrate is converted to glycogen and stored in the liver and muscle, or converted to fat and stored in adipose tissue. Fats are broken down to fatty acids and glycerol for use by the body, and the excess stored as fat in adipose tissue. Fats are stored with greater efficiency in the body than are proteins or carbohydrates. A high-fat diet, therefore, is a strong predictor of excess body fat, even when the total caloric intake is not excessive. Protein is broken down to amino acids. These essential components of the body should be used to replace, repair, or maintain lean body tissues and protein fluids. Excess amino acids will lose their nitrogen component and be stored as fat, and they cannot be recovered by the body to form proteins.

These energy-producing nutrients are discussed in detail in the following chapters. This brief explanation serves to help the student understand the basis for calculating the amounts of carbohydrates, protein, and fat when planning weight-reduction diets.

Although alcohol is not really a nutrient, since it does produce kcalories when consumed it causes more fat to be stored in the body, especially in the abdomen (the "beer belly" effect) and other parts of the body where excess fat can be stored. It must be considered when planning weight control.

Eating Habits

Chapter 2 discussed how food habits are formed. They are extremely difficult to change. Eating behaviors are the only thing that is under individual control, so in order to achieve a healthy body weight and appropriate body composition, one must use some of the guidelines that have been developed by competent health professionals. These include knowledge of the way foods are broken down and used by the body, an exercise plan, using acceptable guidelines for dieting, and behavior modification.

Behavior modification can be a useful tool in achieving and maintaining weight control. Reasons for weight fluctuation can be identified and measures taken to change the situations or alter the behaviors that cause the problems. Behavior modification is also useful in weight maintenance once the desired weight has been reached, since a change in eating behaviors and activity is achieved over a long period of time and thus can give the dieter a chance to gain permanent control. An exercise program that is enjoyable is more likely to remain a part of the individual's lifestyle. While rewarding oneself for satisfactory weight loss or gain is recommended (positive reinforcement) in behavioral programs, the satisfaction that comes from improved appearance and attitude about self can be sufficiently motivating to require no additional reinforcement. The habit of daily exercise may require encouragement, support, and coercion to get started, but if the exercise program is done long enough, it becomes self-enforcing.

Exercise

In any type of weight-management program, exercise plays an important role. In addition to the benefits of decreasing excess body fat and increasing lean muscle mass, many other positive outcomes occur with regular exercise.

Certain types of exercise (aerobic) can produce dramatic changes in body composition. Jogging, brisk walking, jumping rope, and bicycling are examples of this type of exercise. Also, aerobic exercise can increase cardiovascular fitness, raise basal metabolic rate, and decrease appetite (contrary to popular belief). It lowers cholesterol levels and provides a healthy way to release tension. Coping with stress through exercise rather than overeating is a major means of weight control. Additional benefits of exercise include improved appearance as muscles are firmed and enhanced confidence and self-esteem. People who exercise regularly suggest that their thought processes and overall efficiency are improved.

Exercise should be undertaken slowly and, for the older person, with medical supervision. Exercise should never hurt; the axiom "no pain, no gain" is inaccurate. If exercise hurts, it is too strenuous and may cause injury. Mild, regular exercise at a steady pace can be as effective as strenuous exercise, which can be traumatic for some. The former may become enjoyable as well as therapeutic.

People who exercise and are moderately active live longer than those who are sedentary, and they enjoy a better quality of life far into their later years.

GUIDELINES FOR DIETING

Portion control, balanced menus meeting the RDAs, and judicious food preparation are the keys to successful dieting. Weight loss is most satisfactorily achieved by planning meals around nutritionally sound food guides, such as the Food Exchange Lists for meal planning. These were discussed in Chapter 1, and the complete Food Exchange Lists appear in Appendix F. Table 7-4 (a and b) uses these lists to prepare menu plans at four different calorie levels. Table 7-5 provides a sample menu for a 1200-kcal diet using the Food Exchange Lists in Appendix F and Table 7-4. Other diet planning strategies that can be used, for yourself as well as in counseling others, are found at the end of this chapter in the Responsibilities of Health Personnel section.

THE BUSINESS OF DIETING

In spite of massive efforts on the part of government agencies and nutrition specialists to promote a healthy lifestyle and educate the public regarding the advantages of correct methods of obtaining and maintaining desirable body composition, it appears that Americans are not listening. The latest surveys indicate that overweight and obesity are higher than before and still gaining. It is not that people aren't diet conscious, but the tried-and-true methods take time and a change in lifestyle. In today's fast-paced world Americans are looking for a quick fix. This has given credence to a proliferation of diet scams, fads, and products.

It would be nice to believe that some of these combinations and concoctions could increase longevity, improve sexual prowess, prevent aging, and promote glamorous body images, but they do not. Many entertainers have capitalized on these hopes by implying that

TABLE 7-4a   Using the Food Exchange Lists to Prepare Menu Plans at Four Different Calorie Levels (Caloric Distribution: 50% Carbohydrate, 20% Protein, and 30% Fat)

| Daily Food Distribution | | | | |
Food Group (Total/Day)	1000 kcal	1200 kcal	1500 kcal	1800 kcal
Carbohydrate Group				
Starch/Bread	4	5	6	9
Vegetable	3	3	4	4
Fruit	3	3	4	4
Milk (skim)	2	2	2	2
Meat and Meat Substitute Group				
Meat (lean)	4	4	5	6
Fat				
Polyunsaturated	1	1	2	2
Monounsaturated	1	1	2	2
Saturated	1	1	1	1

TABLE 7-4b   Using the Food Exchange Lists to Prepare Menu Plans at Four Different Caloric Levels (Caloric Distribution: 50% Carbohydrate, 20% Protein, and 30% Fat)

| Meal Pattern (Exchanges per meal) | | | | |
Food Group (Total/Day)	1000 kcal	1200 kcal	1500 kcal	1800 kcal
Breakfast				
Carbohydrates				
Starch/Bread	1	1	2	2
Fruit	1	1	1	1
Milk	½	½	½	½
Meat	0	0	1	1
Fat	1	1	1	1
Lunch/Dinner				
Carbohydrates				
Starch/Bread	1	2	2	3
Vegetable	1	1	2	2
Fruit	1	1	1	1
Milk	½	½	½	½
Meat	2	2	2	2
Fat	1	1	2	2
Dinner/Supper				
Carbohydrates				
Starch/Bread	1	1	1	3
Vegetable	2	2	2	2
Fruit	1	1	1	1
Milk	½	½	½	½
Meat	2	2	2	2
Fat	1	2	2	2
Snack				
Carbohydrates				
Starch/Bread	1	1	1	1
Milk	½	½	½	½
Fruit	0	0	1	1
Meat	0	0	0	1

purchasing and using their health and beauty books or aids will fulfill all one's fantasies about looking good. The quacks and charlatans of the past were the first to discover the gullibility of the public and prey upon their superstitions and susceptibility. Lack of education regarding actual body needs and the utilization of foods has created a fertile field for misinformation. Some of this information is merely misleading and costly; some of it is dangerous. The amount of money (over $10 billion per year) spent on these books and products could be used to educate the public and purchase nutritious foods, thereby helping to truly alleviate weight problems.

TABLE 7-5   Sample Menu for a 1200 Kcal Diet Using Meal Pattern from Table 7-4b

Breakfast

½ c orange juice
1 slice raisin toast with 1 tbsp cream cheese
2 tsp sugar-free jelly, if desired
½ c skim milk
Coffee or tea

Lunch/Dinner

2 oz broiled chicken breast
½ c mashed potatoes
½ c green beans
1 small roll with 1 tsp margarine
⅓ 5" cantaloupe
½ c skim milk
Coffee or tea

Dinner/Supper

1 c bouillon
2 oz roast pork
⅓ c wild rice
½ c ea. mushrooms and pea pods sautéed in 2 tsp oil
1 large kiwi
½ c skim milk
Coffee or tea

Snack (afternoon or evening)

½ c bran flakes
½ c skim milk
Sugar-free gelatin, if desired

TABLE 7-6   Rating the Weight Loss Diets

Criteria

Acceptable

1. Not less than 1200 kcal, at least 100 g carbohydrate
2. Meets, but not exceeds, the RDA for protein
3. Approximately 30% of total kcal from fat; types of fat to use recommended
4. Provides variety: can select from a large number of foods
5. Can buy the foods at a local grocery store
6. Offers foods from all the food groups
7. Provides for slow but steady weight loss
8. Instructions include regular exercise and behavior modification tips
9. Comes from a reliable source
10. Has no unproven weight-loss aids or devices

Some examples:

Weight Watchers diet plans

The American Heart Association Diet

Individual plans by qualified nutrition specialists

Unacceptable

1. Kcals may range as low as 300 per day
2. Low in carbohydrate (less than 100 g)
3. Protein exceeds or is less than RDA
4. Only certain, specified foods used; may be formulas
5. Foods bought from one source only; usually expensive
6. Nutritionally inadequate
7. Extremely low fat (< 20% total kcal)
8. Promotes rapid weight loss
9. Eliminates food decisions
10. "Counselors" unqualified
11. Does not inform clients of any risks
12. May require signing a long-term contract
13. May cause long-term health problems
14. Frequently has "other products/devices" that are supposed to speed up the process

Some examples:*

Atkins Diet Revolution

The Pritikin Diet

Herbalife

Drinking Man's Diet

*Not an all-inclusive list; there are many, many more with new ones arriving daily.

and wish to attain their weight goals in the shortest possible time.

Eating disorders have proliferated, starting at the elementary school level. Anorexia nervosa, bulimia nervosa, and other eating disorders are discussed in Chapter 22.

Health practitioners need to be able to judge the myriad diet plans available and help clients choose ones that conform to good nutrition standards. Table 7-6 lists some things to look for when assessing the suitability of diet schemes.

SUMMARY

A sedentary lifestyle for most Americans has decreased energy needs to the point where, if weight is to remain stable, total caloric intake should not exceed the BMR by more than a few hundred calories. The continual consumption of more calories than are expended results in obesity. It is necessary for people to understand that obesity is not a problem of fattening foods, but of total overconsumption of foods that contain calories. Weight control can be achieved by maintaining a balance between total calories consumed and those expended.

Eating a balanced diet of moderate proportions and exercising regularly are valuable for maintaining energy balance, once the balance has been achieved. The consequences of either excess or deficit energy can be severe and create or complicate conditions and disorders that shorten the life span.

Diets to achieve weight control need to be varied; foods should meet acceptable criteria for essential nutrients as well as psychological and aesthetic criteria. They should be lifetime diets. For optimum health, weight control should be established from early childhood. Crash diets, fraudulent, and fad diets may be hazardous to one's health and should be avoided, and regular exercise should become a part of the plan to control body weight.

Although the disease continuum of obesity–anorexia nervosa is a complex phenomenon, the measures for promoting a healthy, stable, normal weight throughout the life span are simple and practical, once these principles are understood and practiced.

RESPONSIBILITIES OF HEALTH PERSONNEL

1. Follow and teach the principle that a balanced diet contains adequate nutrients and calories and maintains a stable weight.
2. Make accurate assessments and judgments regarding appropriate use of food and diets used for weight loss.
3. Recognize that malnutrition, whether due to an excess or deficit in nutrients and calories, must be resolved.
   a. Substitute appropriate foods if malnutrition is caused by poor food choices.
   b. Be prepared to find resources when an inadequate food supply is the problem.
   c. Recognize the effects of faulty body function or intake of drugs on nutrient intake and recommend appropriate steps.
4. Recognize the differences among overweight, overfat, and obese, and be prepared to explain to others. Use a variety of tools to determine body fat.
5. Know the health risks of being underweight, and be prepared to teach others how to gain weight while maintaining a quality diet.
6. Recognize the symptoms of anorexia nervosa and bulimia and seek appropriate referrals. Nursing personnel may be specially trained in this area and can work with psychiatrists and psychologists in the treatment of severe eating disorders.
7. Use techniques from the behavioral sciences to assist clients in controlling weight.
8. Explain the use of exercise in promoting stable body weight and relaxing tensions. Demonstrate some helpful exercises for different age groups.
9. Use and teach acceptable diet-control methods that include use of a balanced diet, proper food preparation, portion control, and sound food guides for selection.
10. Educate yourself and others to the dangers and health hazards of the fad diets on the market today.
11. Evaluate all literature regarding reduction diets and the actual diets using scientific criteria.
12. Teach and practice basic principles of weight maintenance.
13. Evaluate all reduction diets carefully. Realize that there are countless diets for weight loss, and that

most popular diets promise weight loss without deprivation.
14. Educate yourself and others to approved diets that are balanced and provide optimum nutrients for maintenance of health.
15. Encourage individuals who wish to lose weight to increase exercise at the same time as they reduce the quantity of food intake.
16. Advise clients that successful diet plans require adaptation to a new lifestyle that includes altered food intake and exercise.
17. Be aware that the best prescription for obesity is diet modification. The use of drugs and surgical procedures is dangerous and a last resort.
18. Promote low-calorie diets that contain the essential nutrients in proper proportions. Diets should do the following:
   a. Be based on the daily food guide
   b. Contain a minimum of 1200 kcal for women and 1500 kcal for men
   c. Follow the dietary guidelines for distribution of nutrients: 50% of total calories as complex carbohydrate, 20% as protein, and 30% as fat, with approximately half of the fat being unsaturated
   d. Provide weight loss of 1 to 2 lb per week
19. Advise clients to weigh themselves once per week. If exercise is undertaken, measurements may be more accurate than weighing.
20. Encourage the attitude that clients are adopting a more healthful diet instead of giving up certain foods.
21. Recognize the plateau periods in weight reduction, and encourage the dieter to stay with the diet until the body readjusts.
22. Become familiar with behavior modification techniques for changing eating habits, and assist clients to use those that work for them.

PROGRESS CHECK ON ACTIVITY 3

MULTIPLE CHOICE

Circle the letter of the correct answer.

1. Behavior modification is an educational tool used to
   a. change people's eating habits.
   b. achieve weight control.
   c. maintain desired weight.
   d. all of the above.

2. Mary lost 10 lb in six weeks and rewarded herself with a new blouse. This is an example of
   a. pampering oneself.
   b. negative reinforcement.

c. positive reinforcement.

d. self-gratification.

3. Aerobic exercise is defined as

a. exercise performed inside a building.

b. exercise that causes sweating.

c. exercise that increases oxygen intake.

d. exercise that is strenuous.

FILL-IN

4. List three potential health hazards of unbalanced diet regimes.

a. _____

b. _____

c. _____

TRUE/FALSE

Circle T for True and F for False.

5. T F Although the grapefruit diet is unbalanced, Dr. Stillman's "Inches Off" diet should be all right for weight reduction.

6. T F Entertainers cannot afford to offer poor nutrition advice for fear of lawsuits.

7. T F The major reason for misinformation is lack of education.

8. T F It is possible to lose weight without dieting if you exercise regularly.

REFERENCES

Bendich, A. & Deckelbaum, R. J. (Eds.). (2005). *Preventive Nutrition: The Comprehensive Guide for Health Professionals* (3rd ed.). Totowa, NJ: Humana Press.

Caballero, B., Allen, L., & Prentice, A. (Eds.) (2005). *Encyclopedia of Human Nutrition* (2nd ed.). Boston: Elsevier/Academic Press.

Eastwood, M. (2003). *Principles of Human Nutrition* (2nd ed.). Malden, MA: Blackwell Science.

Food and Agriculture Organization. (2001). *Human Energy Requirements: Report of a Joint FAO/WHO/ UNU Expert Consultation.* Rome, Italy: Food and Agriculture Organization of the United Nations.

Haas, E., & Levin, M. (2006). *Staying Healthy with Nutrition: The Complete Guide to Diet and Nutrition Medicine* (21st ed.). Berkeley, CA: Celestial Arts.

Hargove, J. L. (2006). History of the calorie in nutrition. *Journal of Nutrition, 136*: 2957–2961.

Hark, L., & Morrison, G. (Eds.). (2003). *Medical Nutrition and Disease* (3rd ed.). Malden, MA: Blackwell.

Klein, S. (2007). Waist circumference and cardiometabolic risk: A consensus statement from Shaping America's Health: Association for Weight Management and Obesity Prevention: NAASO, The Obesity Society: The American Society for Nutrition; and The American Diabetes Association. *American Journal for Nutrition, 85*: 1197–1202.

Knukowski, R. A. (2006). Consumers may not use or understand calorie labeling in restaurants. *Journal of American Dietetic Association, 106*: 917–920.

Lane, H. W. (2002). Water and energy dietary requirements and endocrinology of human space flight. *Nutrition, 18*: 820–828.

Mahan, L. K., & Escott-Stump, S. (Eds.). (2008). *Krause's Food and Nutrition Therapy* (12th ed.). Philadelphia: Elsevier Saunders.

Mann, J., & Truswell, S. (Eds.). (2007). *Essentials of Human Nutrition* (3rd ed.) New York: Oxford University Press.

Moore, M. C. (2005). *Pocket Guide to Nutritional Assessment and Care* (5th ed.). St. Louis, MO: Elvesier Mosby.

Ormachigui, A. (2002). Prepregnancy and pregnancy nutrition and its impact on women health. *Nutrition Reviews, 60* (5, pt. 2): s64–s67.

Otten, J. J., Pitzi, J., Hellwig, L., & Meyers, D. (Eds.). (2006). *Dietary Reference Intakes: The Essential Guide to Nutrient Requirements.* Washington, DC: National Academy Press.

Park, M. I. (2005). Gastric motor and sensory functions in obesity. *Obesity Research 13*: 491–500.

Payne-James, J., & Wicks, C. (2003). *Key Facts in Clinical Nutrition* (2nd ed.). London: Greenwich Medical Media.

Sardesai, V. M. (2003). *Introduction to Clinical Nutrition* (2nd ed.). New York: Marcel Dekker.

Shils, M. E., & Shike, M. (Eds.). (2006). *Modern Nutrition in Health and Disease* (10th ed.). Philadelphia: Lippincott, Williams and Wilkins.

Stewart-Knox, B. (2005). Dietary strategies and update of reduced fat foods. *Journal of Human Nutrition and Dietetics, 18*: 121–128.

Stover, P. J. (2006). Influence of human genetic variation on nutritional requirements. *American Journal of Clinical Nutrition, 83*: 436s–442s.

Temple, N. J., Wilson, T., & Jacobs, D. R. (2006). *Nutrition Health: Strategies for Disease Prevention* (2nd ed.). Totowa, NJ: Humana Press.

Thomas, B. & Bishop, J. (Eds.). (2007). *Manual of Dietetic Practice* (4th ed.). Ames, IA: Blackwell.

United States Department of Health and Human Services and United States Department of Agriculture. (2005). *Dietary Guidelines for Americans* (6th ed.). Washington, DC: Government Printing Office.

Webster-Gandy, J., Madden, A., & Holdworth, M. (Eds.). (2006). *Oxford Handbook of Nutrition and Dietetics.* Oxford, England: Oxford University Press.

PART II

Public Health Nutrition

CHAPTER

8

Nutritional Assessment

Time for completion
Activities: 1½ hours
Optional examination: ½ hour

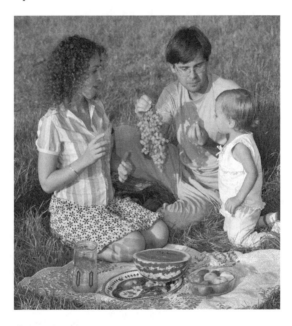

OBJECTIVES

Upon completion of this chapter the student should be able to do the following:

1. Identify some physical signs of malnutrition.
2. Describe tools used in the assessment of nutritional status, such as:
   a. diagnostic tests (radiologic/laboratory data).
   b. anthropometric measurements.
   c. dietary history and recalls.
   d. physical findings and sociological data.
3. Recognize some common nutrition problems, and propose corrective measures.
4. Be familiar with the responsibilities of health personnel in educating clients about nutritional needs.

GLOSSARY

Anthropometrics: measurement of the physical body, such as height and weight, chest and head circumferences.

Assessment: gathering of data about a person in order to logically identify his or her physical, psychological, social, and economic assets and liabilities.

Malnutrition: general term indicating an excess, deficit, or imbalance of one or more of the essential nutrients. May be used to describe an excess or deficit of calories. Psychosocial, economic, geographic, and physical factors can contribute to the development of malnutrition.

Nutrient: chemical substance in food that is needed by the body.

Nutritional status: the condition of the body as it relates to the consumption and utilization of food. *Good nutritional status* refers to the intake of a balanced diet containing all the essential nutrients to meet the body's requirements for energy, maintenance, and growth. *Poor nutritional status* refers to an inadequate intake (or utilization) of nutrients to meet the body's requirements for energy, maintenance, and growth.

Serum: the watery portion of the blood that remains after the cells and clot-forming material (fibrinogen) have been removed; plasma is unclotted blood. In most cases serum and plasma concentrations are similar to one another. The serum sample often is preferred because plasma samples occasionally clog the mechanical blood analyzers.

BACKGROUND INFORMATION

Health professionals, healthcare workers, and the client or patient comprise the health team in institutions and public health facilities. However, there are many types and kinds of noninstitutionalized health services, accompanied by an increasing number of private health practitioners.

The role of healthcare professionals is defined by law and based on educational preparation. Healthcare professionals are required to receive certification, registration, licensing, or a combination of these.

An independent health practitioner may or may not be credentialed. However, as increasing numbers of people want to be responsible for their own health, these independent practitioners often serve as health resources. Through their counseling, health practitioners can influence the attitudes and health of many people. But, the practice of self-care must be preceded by the acquisition of information about health; that is, both the healthcare worker and the client need a solid background in the assessment of nutritional status, the techniques of health promotion, and accurate nutrition information.

This chapter is designed to assist the student to understand how to assess the nutritional status of clients or patients. The student will also learn the tools necessary to assist a healthcare professional to restore and promote health. Finally, the chapter teaches a student the problem-solving process used in many healthcare systems.

ACTIVITY 1:

Assessment of Nutritional Status

In this activity we will explore four major techniques to assess nutritional status: (1) physical findings, (2) anthropometric measurements, (3) laboratory data, and (4) health and diet history.

PHYSICAL FINDINGS

There are many clinical signs of good and poor nutrition. Although some of these signs are not related to a person's nutritional status, they serve as a general indicator of health. Data from a physical assessment are considered objective data and helpful to the health practitioner. Table 8-1 summarizes these findings.

ANTHROPOMETRIC MEASUREMENTS

These measurements are relatively objective and are usually an important part of nutrition assessment. They are valuable in evaluating protein energy malnutrition (PEM). Figure 8-1 illustrates such measurements.

Approximately half the fat in our bodies is located directly below the skin (subcutaneous). In some parts of the body, this fat is more loosely attached, and can be pulled up between the thumb and forefinger. Such sites can be used for measuring fat-fold thickness. Since fat stores decrease slowly even with an inadequate energy intake, a depletion of subcutaneous fat can reflect either long-term undernutrition or successful weight loss through dieting and exercise. Actual diagnostic tests used to determine nutritional status are usually made in the laboratory from blood and urine samples.

LABORATORY DATA

Laboratory tests are generally used to determine internal body chemistry. Although determined with great care and accuracy, these tests are influenced by many factors and are subject to different interpretations.

The most common and useful biochemical techniques in evaluating malnutrition employ measurements of hemoglobin, blood cell counts (hematocrit), nitrogen balance, and creatinine excretion. The measurements are obtained from serum and plasma samples.

Laboratory tests valuable in assessing vitamin, mineral, and trace element status are listed in Table 8-2.

DIET HISTORY AND METHODS OF EVALUATING DATA

The type of data needed for health and diet history is subjective and involves interviews and food records. The accuracy of both approaches depends on the skill of the interviewer and the client's memory, perception, and cooperation. From an interview, information can be obtained on the client's food intake history, presence of

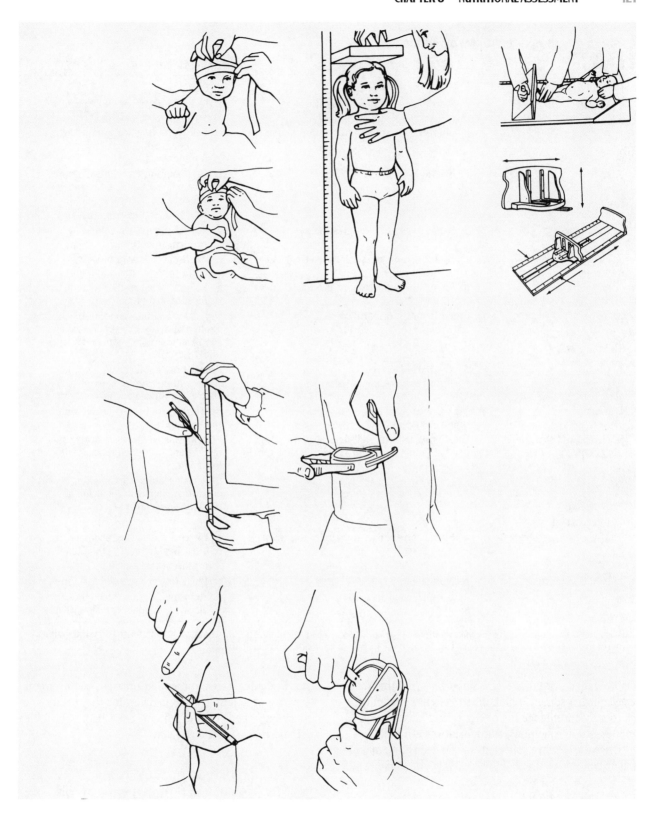

FIGURE 8-1   Anthropometric Measurements

Assessment of growth and development by studying anthropometric measurements (physical measurements of the human body) provides important information about the nutritional status of infants, children, adolescents, and pregnant women. Standard measurements include weight, height, head circumference, midarm circumference, chest circumference, and skin-fold thickness. These data provide developmentally significant ratios, including weight:height, midarm circumference:head circumference, chest circumference:head circumference, and midarm circumference:height. Data obtained over a period of time are especially helpful.

TABLE 8-1   Physical Indicators of Nutritional Status

Body Area	Signs of Good Nutrition	Signs of Malnutrition
1. Head to neck		
a. Hair	a. Shiny, lustrous; smooth healthy scalp	a. Dull, dry, thin, wirelike, sparse, brittle; scalp rough, flaky
b. Face	b. Skin smooth, moist, with uniform color	b. Pale or mottled, dark under eyes, swollen, scaling or flakiness, lumpiness
c. Eyes	c. Bright, clear, moist	c. Dry membranes, redness, fissures at corners, red rimmed, fine blood vessels or scars at cornea
d. Lips	d. Smooth, pink	d. Red, swollen, lesions or fissures
e. Tongue	e. Deep red, slightly rough surface	e. Scarlet or purplish color; raw, swollen, smooth
f. Teeth	f. Straight; none missing, no overlap, without cavities	f. Cavities, black or gray spots, erupting abnormally, missing
g. Gums	g. Firm, pink, smooth, no bleeding	g. Spongy, bleed easily, inflammation, receded, atrophied
2. Skin	2. Smooth, moist, uniform color	2. Dry, flaky, scaling, "gooseflesh," swollen, grayish, bruises due to capillary bleeding under skin, no fat layer under skin
3. Glands	3. No thyroid enlargement: No lumps at parotid juncture	3. Front of neck and cheeks become swollen lumps visible at parotid; goiter visible if advanced hypothyroidism
4. Nails	4. Pink nail beds, smooth, firm, flexible, uniform shape	4. Brittle, ridged, pale nail beds, clubbed, spoon shaped
5. Muscle and skeletal system	5. Good posture, firm, well-developed muscles, good mobility; no malformations of skeleton	5. Flaccid, wasted muscles, weakness, tenderness, decreased reflexes, difficulty in walking. Children: beading ribs, swelling at end of bones, abnormal protrusion of frontal or parietal areas
6. Internal systems		
a. Gastrointestinal	a. Flat abdomen, liver not tender to palpate, normal size	a. Distended, enlarged abdomen, ascites, hepatomegaly (enlarged liver). Children: "potbelly"
b. Cardiovascular	b. Normal pulse rate. Normal blood pressure	b. Pulse rate exceeds 100 beats/min, abnormal rhythm, blood pressure elevated, mental confusion, edema

While physical appearances give us clues to internal problems, they can be misleading. They may not be nutrition related. Physical findings must be coupled with other indications (lab test, anthropometrics, etc.) in order to validate them.

disorder, and drug usage. It is important that the interviewer learn something about the client's life and the factors that influence his or her eating habits (such as money, storage facilities, transportation, ethnicity).

Once the data are collected, we can determine the nutrient content of the diet and evaluate the person's dietary intake using available references such the *Dietary Guidelines*. At present this is easily done with computer software designed for that purpose. To interpret the information, we use the following basic tools, among others:

DRIs

One method compares a person's nutrient intake to the DRIs (RDA/AI) values. The result gives a quantitative base of a person's dietary adequacy. You will also need to know that individual's recommended nutrient requirements to arrive at a definitive conclusion for the dietary adequacy and needs of this person. See Chapter 1, Tables F-1 and F-2, and www.nas.edu.

MyPyramid, Dietary Guidelines for Americans, Healthy People, and National Cholesterol Education Program

These four tools have already been discussed in Chapter 1. They are online tools for assessment of dietary intake. A consumer or a nutritional professional can use the *MyPramid* tracker at the Web site to compare a typical day's intake to the recommendations of these four tools. Though not specific, the results can give answers to the following:

TABLE 8-2   Selected Blood Tests Useful for Determining Nutritional Status

Nutrient	Laboratory Test	Acceptable Limits
1. Carbohydrate	Plasma glucose	70–120 mg[1]/100 ml[2]
2. Fat	a. Serum cholesterol	140–220 mg/100 ml
	b. Serum triglycerides	60–150 mg/100 ml
3. Protein	a. Visceral serum protein	above 6.5 g[3]/100 ml
	b. Immune functions:	
	(Total lymphocyte count)	above 1200
4. Fat-Soluble Vitamins		
Vitamin A	a. Serum vitamin A	20–45 μg[4]/100 ml
	b. Serum carotene	40–300 μg/100 ml
Vitamin D	a. Serum alkaline phosphatase	35–145 IU[5]/l[6]
	b. Plasma 25 hydroxy cholecalciferol	10–40 IU/l
Vitamin E	Plasma vitamin E	above 0.6 mg/100 ml
Vitamin K	Prothrombin time	12 seconds
5. Water-Soluble Vitamins		
a. Vitamin C	Serum ascorbic acid	above 0.3/100 ml
b. B complex:		
1. Thiamin	Red blood cell transketolase	0–15%
2. Riboflavin	Red blood cell glutathione	below 1.2
3. Niacin	Urinary nitrogen*	above 0.6 mg/g creatinine
4. Vitamin B_6	Tryptophan load*	below 50 μg/24 hrs.
5. Vitamin B_{12}	Serum B_{12}	above 200 pg[7]/100 ml
6. Folacin	Serum folacin	above 6.0 ng[8]/100 ml
6. Minerals		
Iodine	Serum protein bound iodine (PBI)	4.8–8.0 μg/100 ml
Iron	a. Hemoglobin	male 14 mg/100 ml
		female 12 mg/100 ml
	b. Hematocrit	male 44%
		female 33%
Calcium	Serum calcium	9.0–11.0 mg/100 ml
Phosphorus	Serum phosphorus	2.5–4.5 mg/100 ml
Magnesium	Serum magnesium	1.3–2.0 mEq[7]/l[8]
Sodium	Serum sodium	130–150 mEq/l
Potassium	Serum potassium	3.5–5.0 mEq/l
Chloride	Serum chloride	99–110 mEq/l
Zinc	Plasma zinc	80–100 μg/100 ml

*Urine analysis rather than blood sampling
NOTE:
Measurement terminology:
[1]mg (milligram) 1000 mg = 1 g (gram)
[2]ml (milliliter) 1 ml = 1 cc (cubic centimeter)
[3]g (gram) 1000 mg or 0.0001 kg (kilogram)
[4]μg (microgram) 1000 = 1 mg or 0.001 gm
[5]IU (International Unit) not a metric measure
[6]l (liter) 1000 ml or 1,000 cc
[7]pg (picogram) 10^{-12} gm
[8]ng (nanogram) 10^{-9} gm

1. Is the person consuming high or low saturated fat?
2. Is the subject's consumption of fruits, vegetables, and whole grains adequate?

Table 8-3 gives a simple illustration of the discussion above.

Assessment Conclusion

We have the following data:

- Anthropometric measures
- Biochemical tests
- Clinical exams
- Dietary evaluation

- Family history, socioeconomic status, and other personal information

These data may lead to recommendation such as the following:

- Changes to lose weight or to lower blood cholesterol
- Using vitamin or mineral supplements for various reasons
- Measures to correct growth in infants
- Others

RESPONSIBILITIES OF HEALTH PERSONNEL

The general responsibilities of health practitioners include recognizing a problem when it exists; correcting

Table 8-3   Nutritional Assessment and Diet History

Identification and Activity

1. Personal Data:

    Identifying number or name _____

    Age _____ Sex _____ Marital status _____

    Race _____ Religious preference _____ Ethnic origin _____

    Education _____ (Highest completed grade/degree)

    Employment: type _____ hours _____ approximate income _____

    Unemployed _____ Public assistance _____ Other _____

    Family composition (all living at one residence, ages and relationships) _____

    Person(s) most responsible for purchase, preparation of food _____

    Housing: type _____ facilities for storage, preparation of food _____

2. Health Data:

    A. Anthropometric: Height _____

    Present weight _____ (lb) _____ (kg)

    Usual weight _____ (lb) _____ (kg)

    Recent changes in weight _____

    Planned change? _____

    Triceps skin fold _____ (mm) Standard _____

    Midarm circumference _____ (cm) Standard _____

    B. Physical: Appearance of:

1. Skin _____	8. Teeth: Dentures _____
2. Hair _____	Edentulous _____
3. Eyes _____	Chews well _____
4. Ears _____	Chews with difficulty _____
5. Nails _____	9. Swallowing good _____ poor _____
6. Posture _____	10. Any other pertinent physical data _____
7. Mouth, tongue, lips _____	

    C. Laboratory: CBC _____ Hbg _____ Hct _____

    Serum levels of albumin/transferrin _____

    Urinary values _____

    Creatinine clearance _____

    Other _____

    D. Habits:

1. Meals: number per day _____	Snacks: number per day _____
2. Alcohol: amount daily _____	type _____
3. Smoking: amount daily _____	type _____ (include cigars, pipes, and marijuana)
4. Drugs: amount daily _____	specific kinds _____
5. Exercise: kind _____	frequency _____ amount of time _____

    E. Other

    1. Gastrointestinal function:

        Appetite: good _____ fair _____ poor _____ recent changes _____

        Taste/smell: good _____ fair _____ poor _____ recent changes _____

        Indigestion: often _____ seldom _____ never _____

        If yes, list foods that cause _____

        List any foods that cause nausea/vomiting _____

        List any foods that cause diarrhea _____

        Bowel elimination: frequency _____ consistency _____

    2. Emotional state:

        calm _____ agitated _____ anxious _____ depressed _____

        Other: (Explain) _____

Table 8-3   (continued)

24-Hour Intake Record

3. Dietary History:

A. Food Preferences   Foods Acceptable   Food Dislikes   Food Allergies   Other

B. Meals: Usual   Serving Size   Time   Where   Special occasions
                                                     weekends/holidays

    Breakfast

    Lunch/dinner

    Dinner/supper

    Snacks

C. Vitamin, mineral supplements taken: kind _____ amount _____
   Reason for taking _____
D. Usual preparation method (bake, boil, broil, fry, etc.)
   1. Meats _____
   2. Vegetables _____

Analysis

Nutritional Diagnosis/Planning (for nurse's use)

1. Review the assessment and diet history and list the potential needs for nutrition education.
2. Questions to guide the beginning practitioner:
a. Was daily intake adequate in kcal, nutrients, kinds and amounts of food?
   If no, indicate:
   1. Which food groups have been omitted or are in inadequate amounts?

   2. Which of the RDAs for major nutrients have not been met?

   3. Does the caloric intake provide for maintenance of normal weight?
   Too low? _____ Too high? _____ For recovery from illness/injury? _____
b. What foods will need to be added/subtracted/substituted to meet the assessed needs of this person and maintain individuality?

c. Identify areas of patient teaching that need to be included as you plan your nursing care and interventions.

Explanatory Notes

The nutritional assessment should be a part of every health practitioner's relationship to the client. It is one of the tools that provide information to identify and meet client needs.

The purpose of nutritional assessment is to provide an essential part of the overall nursing assessment. Some people, because of their nutritional status at the time of disease or injury, may be at high risk for nutritional problems that affect the outcome of the disease process. This assessment may become critical in the overall recovery.

Some forms of food survey/intake should be obtained for every client at admission. If the client is unable to respond, information should be obtained from family or others who know the client's eating patterns, in order to individualize the diet. Some of the data may be collected from other recorded observations and tests.

The nutritional assessment and diet history can be used as a basis for planning a diet with a patient that will speed recovery, as well as for teaching sound nutrition principles and promoting health maintenance.

the problem if experience permits; and, most importantly, referring the client to another health professional if special expertise is needed. This responsibility can only be appropriately met if the health practitioner is familiar with and advises clients with accurate information on the following?

1. The kinds of nutrients the body needs
2. The estimation of nutrients a person needs
3. The body's method of obtaining and maintaining adequate supplies of nutrients
4. The functions of various nutrients in the body
5. The relationship between nutrition and health
6. the relationship between food, exercise, and health
7. Resources needed to facilitate nutritional education of the public
8. Skill in applying the problem-solving process
9. Use of anthropometric, physical, biochemical, and historical data to do the following:
   a. Assess growth, weight changes, fat stores, muscle mass, and skeletal development.
   b. Plan a nutrition program suitable to individual needs.
   c. Cooperate fully with other health professionals.

SUMMARY

Many parameters are useful in assessing nutrition status, including anthropometric, laboratory, physical, and historical data. These data form the basis for interpreting nutrient needs and determining how they will be met. Each client's individual needs in all the areas must be considered. Needs can change as people change—aging, recovering from diseases, or adopting different lifestyles are some of the important changes that require different nutritional patterns. Health practitioners should employ any or all of the tools described to assist them in determining the nutritional status of a person.

PROGRESS CHECK ON ACTIVITY 1

FILL-IN

1. List and define the four factors generally used for assessment data:

   a. _____

   b. _____

   c. _____

   d. _____

2. This progress check contains exercises that will help the student apply the information just covered. List the areas identified in the Practices

below that will require health education (use a separate sheet of paper to answer Practices A through D).

Practice A
Using the Nutritional Assessment and Diet History (Table 8-3), interview a family member or friend and try to determine his or her nutrient intake.

Practice B
Using Table 8-1, Physical Indicators of Nutritional Status, observe the person you are interviewing closely. Try to determine if he or she meets any of the physical criteria for malnutrition.

Practice C
Using a scale and tape measure, weigh and measure your subject.

Practice D
Compile the data and determine what kind of health education this person may need to improve his or her nutritional status.

3. List one indicator of good nutritional status for each of the following areas:

   a. hair _____

   b. skin _____

   c. eyes _____

   d. lips and tongue _____

   e. teeth and gums _____

   f. nails _____

   g. muscles _____

4. List five laboratory tests that are useful in assessing deficiencies, and one finding associated with each:

   a. _____
      _____

   b. _____
      _____

   c. _____
      _____

   d. _____
      _____

   e. _____
      _____

MATCHING

Match the data listed on the left to the data type listed on the right.

5. 5'6", 154 lb
6. 30% above ideal body weight
7. "I don't eat very much."
8. "I receive Social Security benefits."
9. "I think food is for enjoying."
10. "My stomach hurts when I eat spinach."

a. objective data
b. subjective data

REFERENCES

American Dietetic Association. (2006). *Nutrition Diagnosis: A Critical Step in Nutrition Care Process.* Chicago: American Dietetic Association.

Beham, E. (2006). *Therapeutic Nutrition: A Guide to Patient Education.* Philadelphia: Lippincott, Williams and Wilkins.

Bendich, A. & Deckelbaum, R. J. (Eds.). (2005). *Preventive Nutrition: The Comprehensive Guide for Health Professionals* (3rd ed.). Totowa, NJ: Humana Press.

Buchman, A. (2004). *Practical Nutritional Support Technique* (2nd ed.). Thorofare, NJ: Slack.

Caballero, B., Allen, L., & Prentice, A. (Eds.). (2005). *Encyclopedia of Human Nutrition* (2nd ed.). Boston: Elsevier/Academic Press.

Chamey, P. & Malone, A. (Eds.). (2004). *ADA Pocket Guide to Nutritional Assessment.* Chicago: American Dietetic Association.

Coulston, A. M., Rock, C. L., & Monsen, E. L. (Eds.). (2001). *Nutrition in the Prevention and Treatment of Disease.* San Diego, CA: Academic Press.

Deen, D. & Hark, L. (2007). *The Complete Guide to Nutrition in Primary Care.* Malden, MA: Blackwell.

Driskell, J. A. & Wolinsky, I. (Eds.). (2002). *Nutritional Assessment of Athletes.* Boca Raton, FL: CRC Press.

Gershwin, M. E., Netle, P., & Keen, C. (Eds.) (2004). *Handbook of Nutrition and Immunity.* Totowa, NJ: Humana Press.

Gibson, R. S. (2005). *Principles of Nutritional Assessment.* New York: Oxford University Press.

Haas, E. & Levin, M. (2006). *Staying Healthy with Nutrition: The Complete Guide to Diet and Nutrition Medicine* (21st ed.). Berkeley, CA: Celestial Arts.

Hark, L. & Morrison, G. (Eds.). (2003). *Medical Nutrition and Disease* (3rd ed.). Malden, MA: Blackwell.

Katz, D. L. (2001). *Nutrition in Clinical Practice* (2nd ed.). Philadelphia: Lippincott, Williams and Wilkins.

Keller, H. H. (2005). Validity and reliability of SCREEN II (Senior in the Community: Risk evaluation for eating and nutrition). *European Journal of Clinical Nutrition, 59*: 1149–1157.

Krester, A. J. (2003). Effects of two models of nutritional intervention on homebound older adults at nutritional risk. *Journal of American Dietetic Association, 103*: 329–336.

Lagua, R. T. & Qaudio, V. S. (2004). *Nutrition and Diet Therapy: Reference Dictionary* (5th ed.). Ames, IA: Blackwell.

Lee, R. D. & Nieman, D. C. (2003). *Nutritional Assessment* (3rd ed.). Boston: McGraw-Hill.

Mahan, L. K. & Escott-Stump, S. (Eds.). (2008). *Krause's Food and Nutrition Therapy* (12th ed.). Philadelphia: Elsevier Saunders.

Mann, J. & Truswell, S. (Eds.). (2007). *Essentials of Human Nutrition* (3rd ed.). New York: Oxford University Press.

Marian, M. J., Williams-Muller, P., & Bower, J. (2007). *Integrating Therapeutic and Complementary Nutrition.* Boca Raton, FL: CRC Press.

Moore, M. C. (2005). *Pocket Guide to Nutritional Assessment and Care.* St. Louis, MO: Elsevier Mosbey.

Sardesai, V. M. (2003). *Introduction to Clinical Nutrition* (2nd ed.). New York: Marcel Dekker.

Thomas, B. & Bishop, J. (Eds.). (2007). *Manual of Dietetic Practice* (4th ed.). Ames, IA: Blackwell.

Webster-Gandy, J., Madden, A., & Holdworth, M. (Eds.). (2006). *Oxford Handbook of Nutrition and Dietetics.* Oxford, England: Oxford University Press.

CHAPTER **9**

Nutrition and the Life Cycle

Time for completion
Activities: 1½ hours
Optional examination: ½ hour

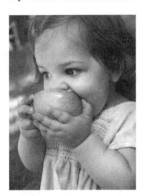

OBJECTIVES

Activity 1: Maternal and Infant Nutrition

Upon completion of the activity, the student should be able to do the following:

1. Identify factors that influence the course and outcome of pregnancy, with special reference to the client's health history, nutritional status, and food habits.
2. Describe the nutritional needs of women during pregnancy and lactation.
3. Explain the recommended weight-gain pattern for a pregnant woman.
4. List health concerns during pregnancy and lactation.
5. Summarize the nutritional needs of the neonate/infant.
6. Compare the advantages and disadvantages of breastfeeding.
7. Discuss the introduction of solid foods to an infant's diet in relation to the sequence, process, and need for supplements.
8. Analyze the health concerns of the infant.

Activity 2: Childhood and Adolescent Nutrition

Upon completion of the activity, the student should be able to do the following:

1. Describe the body changes that occur in the stages of:
   a. Early childhood: toddler, preschooler
   b. Middle childhood: school age to adolescence
   c. Adolescence

2. Identify the nutritional needs of children and adolescents.
3. Discuss the health problems that often occur during childhood and adolescence.
4. Analyze areas of concern regarding eating behaviors of children and adolescents.
5. List ways to promote sound nutritional practices among children and adolescents.

Activity 3: Adulthood and Nutrition

Upon completion of the activity, the student should be able to do the following:

1. Describe the body changes that occur during the span of the adult years.
2. Identify the nutritional needs during early, middle, and late adulthood.
3. Explain the health concerns of early, middle, and late adulthood.
4. Analyze the psychosocial, physiological, and economic influences on eating behaviors.
5. Evaluate the importance of maintaining a regular exercise program throughout the adult years.
6. List the effects of drugs, including alcohol, on nutrients and health.
7. Propose measures to promote healthful eating habits during adulthood, especially the later years.

Activity 4: Exercise, Fitness, and Stress-Reduction Principles

Upon completion of the activity, the student should be able to do the following:

1. Describe the major health concerns of adulthood.
2. Identify the nutritional components of keeping fit.
3. Describe the key elements of an exercise program.
4. Discuss the effects of nutrition and controlled exercise.
5. Describe an effective dietary regime for a person interested in staying healthy into old age.
6. Recognize the biological, psychological, and sociological factors that promote stress.
7. Counsel patients on techniques of stress reduction, relaxation, exercise, and optimal nutrition at any stage of the life cycle.
8. Follow the principles of a healthy lifestyle.

GLOSSARY

Angina pectoris: intense chest pain resulting from myocardial anoxia.
Congenital anomalies: birth defects; abnormally formed organs or body parts.
Course and outcome of pregnancy: the absence or presence of complications.

Fetus: the developing baby during the third trimester.
Hypertension: blood pressure elevated above normal limits.
Intrauterine device (IUD): birth control device consisting of plastic or copper coils placed in the uterus for long periods of time to prevent conception.
Lactation: secretion of milk.
Low birth weight (LBW): weight of baby lower than normal for calculated age.
Miscarriage: interrupted pregnancy prior to seventh month.
Mortality: death.
Myocardial infarction: technical term for a heart attack.
Neonate: a newborn child, from birth to 28 days old.
Oral contraceptive agent (OCA): oral medication (hormones) that can prevent conception.
Pica: the practice of eating nonfood items, such as laundry starch and clay.
Placenta: the structure that develops on the wall of the uterus during pregnancy and through which the fetus is attached by the umbilical cord to receive nourishment and excrete waste.
Premature: birth of a baby prior to 38-week gestational age.
Psychomotor: mind-directed muscle movements.
RBCs: red blood cells.
Small for gestational age (SGA): same as low birth weight (LBW).
Toxemia: a life-threatening condition associated with the presence of toxic substances in the blood. The term *toxemia* recently has been changed to pregnancy-induced hypertension (PIH). Its symptoms include abnormal edema, albuminuria, and very high blood pressure. In severe cases there may be coma, convulsions (eclampsia), or even death.
Triglyceride: a form of fat found in food and blood.
Trimester: a 3-month period during pregnancy; the 9-month pregnancy is divided into three trimesters.
Women, Infants, and Children (WIC): special supplemental food program for women, infants, and children (up to age five).

BACKGROUND INFORMATION

The life cycle is the course of life from birth to death. Each stage in this cycle has effects upon the succeeding stages. In turn, each childbearing couple leaves its mark upon succeeding generations. The kind of nutrition a woman receives before and during pregnancy affects the growth and development of her child, as well as her own health. The nourishment that infants and children receive affects them as adults, and affects any offspring they may have.

Health practitioners must recognize that there are many different approaches to planning a diet for a pregnant woman, depending on factors such as culture, ethnicity, folklore, and others. The changing American lifestyle, with its distinct eating patterns and sedentary habits, is evaluated by health practitioners in terms of its health implications.

Every effort should be made to help people meet their nutritional needs at each stage of life. The health practitioner should develop approaches and knowledge appropriate to the various stages of life in order to promote sound nutritional practices for clients of all ages.

Every health practitioner should have a working knowledge of the interrelated effects of exercise, nutrition, and stress on the human body and practical applications to assist clients in healthy lifestyle changes.

ACTIVITY 1:

Maternal and Infant Nutrition

PREGNANCY: DETERMINING FACTORS

A healthy, well-nourished woman whose nutritional status was good prior to becoming pregnant has a very good chance of delivering a healthy, full-term baby of normal birth weight.

Food intake during pregnancy is important, but entering pregnancy with nutrient reserves has many advantages. It provides a margin of safety if food intake is interfered with during the early stages of pregnancy—for example, morning sickness (nausea and vomiting). The amount of each nutrient that can be stored in the body varies from small to large. However, a well-nourished body usually has a small surplus of all nutrients. This surplus can be crucial in the first trimester of pregnancy, when the ability to eat is impaired by the hormonal shifts, and the tissues and organs of the embryo are being differentiated. This is the time when adequate nutrition is believed to help protect against some birth defects.

Good prepregnancy nutritional status also is an indicator of reasonably good eating practices. A woman who depends on a reliable food guide for regular meal planning will find it easy to adapt her diet to the higher requirements imposed during pregnancy. Because diet affects the course and outcome of pregnancy so greatly, the woman contemplating becoming pregnant in the near or distant future should learn to follow the principles of good nutrition. The adolescent female whose diet is considered to be unsatisfactory should be strongly encouraged to alter her nutritional habits before a planned pregnancy.

Teenage pregnancies are associated with many social and medical problems. The pregnant teenager under 17 years of age is at particularly high risk. Nearly one third of all teenage mothers are under the age of 16. The teenage mother faces two major concerns: her own development and that of the child, both of whom are likely to suffer. The course and outcome of teenage pregnancy are at risk and include the following complications: a higher incidence of maternal and infant mortality, premature or SGA (small for gestational age) infants, congenital anomalies, stillborns, and PIH. While these complications are potential hazards for any pregnant and malnourished mother, their severity increases with the decreasing age of the mother. The teenager often fails to eat an adequate diet because she does not want to gain weight. Since a normal recommended pattern of weight gain is a major criterion in evaluating a healthy pregnancy, it is not surprising that diet counseling for a pregnant teenager is very important.

PREGNANCY: NUTRITIONAL NEEDS AND WEIGHT GAIN

The recommended pattern of weight gain is illustrated in Figure 9-1. This pattern is recommended even if the woman is overweight or obese at the beginning of pregnancy. While the pattern of weight gain is important, if a woman gains more during a trimester than was planned, she should not be advised to reduce caloric intake in the remaining weeks.

The recommended total weight gain during pregnancy is 25 to 35 lb for normal adult women and 15 to 25 lb for overweight women. The underweight woman will need to gain more weight: 28–40 lb. Usually a first-time pregnancy will sustain a higher net gain, especially in younger women. Of this weight, approximately 7 to 10 lb is fetus, 1-½ to 2 lb placenta, 2 lb uterus, 8-½ lb increase in blood volume and fluids, and 3 to 4 lb increase in breast tissue and fat reserves. The increase in breast tissue and fat reserve is in preparation for breastfeeding.

Table 9-1 depicts the increased need for nutrients during pregnancy and lactation according to the DRIs of the National Academy of Sciences (NAS) and other sources. Following this recommendation should result in the recommended weight increase. The nutrients needed by

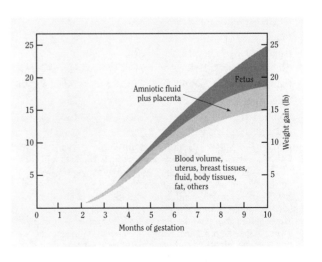

FIGURE 9-1   Weight Gain During Pregnancy

pregnant women are the same as for nonpregnant women, but the amounts are sharply increased.

The pattern of weight gain is more important than the total amount gained. The desirable weight-gain pattern is approximately 3 lb during the first trimester of pregnancy and 1 lb per week for the remainder of the pregnancy. A sharp increase in weight gain after the 20th week may signal excess fluid retention, a sign of the potential development of PIH. Rapid weight gain from water is an effect, not a cause, of PIH. Women who gain too much weight (fat) usually find it difficult to return to normal weight after pregnancy. Their babies may be fat, with an excess weight problem later in life.

TABLE 9-1   DRI (RDA/AI) for a 25-Year-Old Woman at Three Physiological Stages

Nutrient	Daily Amount Needed	Pregnancy	Lactation
Energy (kcal)	2400	2740–2800[a]	2800–3200[a]
Protein (g)	44–48	70–73	70–73
Vitamin A (mg RE)	700	770	1300
Vitamin D (mg)	5	5	5
Vitamin E (mg)	15	15	19
Vitamin K (mg)	90	90	90
Vitamin C (mg)	75	85	120
Vitamin B_1 (mg)	1.1	1.4	1.4
Vitamin B_2 (mg)	1.1	1.4	0.6
Niacin (mg)	14	18	17
Vitamin B_6 (mg)	1.3	1.9	2.0
Folate (mg)[b]	400	600	500
Vitamin B_{12} (mg)	2.4	2.6	2.8
Pantothenic acid (mg)	5	6	7
Biotin (mg)	30	30	35
Choline (mg)	425	450	550
Calcium (mg)	1000	1000	1000
Phosphorus (mg)	700	700	700
Magnesium (mg)	310	350	310
Flouride	3	3	3
Iron (mg)	18	27	9
Zinc (mg)	8	11	12
Iodine (mg)	150	220	290
Selenium (mg)	55	60	70
Sodium (mg)	1500	1500	1500
Chloride (mg)	2300	2300	2300
Potassium (mg)	4700	4700	5100

Source: Adapted from Tables F-1 and Table F-2 except the requirements for protein and calories.
NOTE: Energy requirement varies with the stage of pregnancy and lactation. The numbers given are of general applications. The protein requirements are provided in ranges from multiple sources. Specific recommendations for public health application must be calculated according to individual energy and protein requirements based on variations such as height, weight, activity, and resting metabolic rates.

All nutrients for the developing fetus must be supplied by the mother's diet or her body reserves. In addition, nutrients and energy must be available for increases in the mother's tissues and blood.

The 30-gram increase in protein intake is important for a satisfactory pregnancy. Studies confirm that infants born to mothers with adequate protein intake are taller, have better brain development, and can resist diseases better. In addition, PIH is more common in women with a low protein intake. Since protein will be used for energy if dietary energy is low, any diet below 1800 calories may also negatively influence the outcome of pregnancy.

Even with a diet adequate in other respects, an iron supplement may be recommended for pregnant women. Usually this is prescribed by the woman's physician, along with vitamins and minerals as a margin of safety. Some women misinterpret this to mean that if they take the supplements, they do not have to plan a careful diet. This is a dangerous interpretation, since the supplements contain no protein and usually only 25% to 30% of the recommended calcium. The prescription of a supplement by a doctor does not mean that megadoses of vitamins and minerals during pregnancy will guarantee better health. The opposite is true. The excess is stored in fetal tissues and can be toxic. High doses of vitamins A and D have been known to cause birth defects. Tables 9-2 and 9-3 summarize information related to vitamin intake during pregnancy. Although folic acid is not listed in these tables, it should be supplemented for all women of childbearing age to protect against megaloblastic anemia and neural tube defects. Folic acid and vitamin C are usually given along with the iron supplement to improve absorption.

A sample meal plan and menu suitable for an adequate diet for a pregnant woman are given in Tables 9-4 and 9-5.

In the last decade, the U.S. Food and Drug Administration (FDA) has issued an advisory for the consumption of fish related to the presence of mercy. This is especially significant for pregnant women. The precaution includes:

1. Do not eat shark, swordfish, king mackerel, or tilefish because they contain high levels of mercury.
2. Eat up to 12 oz (2 average meals) a week of a variety of fish and shellfish that are lower in mercury.
   a. Five of the most commonly eaten fish that are low in mercury are shrimp, canned light tuna, salmon, pollock, and catfish.
   b. Another commonly eaten fish, albacore ("white") tuna has more mercury than canned light tuna. So, when choosing your two meals of fish and shellfish, you may eat up to 6 oz (one average meal) of albacore tuna per week.
3. Check local advisories about the safety of fish caught by family and friends in your local lakes, rivers, and coastal areas. If no advice is available, eat up to 6 oz (one average meal) per week of fish you catch from

TABLE 9-2   Water-Soluble Vitamins and Pregnancy

Vitamin	Remarks
C	Requirement increases during pregnancy; can cross placenta freely. Deficiency during pregnancy may lead to easy rupture of fetal membrane and increased newborn mortality rate. Excessive intake during pregnancy is suspected to lead to a higher requirement in the newborn.
B_1	Requirement increases during pregnancy because of a higher consumption of calories; a woman can retain more B_1 in the tissues. There is a claim that a large dose of this vitamin can alleviate the symptoms of morning sickness.
B_2	Requirement increases during pregnancy. Deficiency in a pregnant animal can cause birth defects in the offspring.
B_6	Requirement increases during pregnancy. Blood level decreases when some brands of oral contraceptive pills are used. Pregnant women who used these pills may have a low storage of the vitamin. Supplementation during pregnancy has been recommended, although the practice is not common. There is a claim that a large dose of this vitamin can alleviate the symptoms of morning sickness.
B_{12}	Although absorption increases during pregnancy, the fetus uses up a large amount. An inadequate intake reduces the blood level of this vitamin, which returns to normal after pregnancy. A woman who smokes has a smaller body storage than nonsmokers. The fetus can draw from its mother's minimal storage even if she is deficient in this vitamin, and a newborn baby has a fair storage of this vitamin. There is a suggestion that the baby may be premature if the mother's body storage is very low.

TABLE 9-3   Fat-Soluble Vitamins and Pregnancy

Vitamin	Remarks
A	In animals, deficiency or excess of this vitamin during pregnancy can produce adverse effects in newborns, including birth defects. In humans, a pregnant woman deficient in this vitamin may give birth to a child with arrested bone growth. It is claimed that excess intake during pregnancy may produce birth defects.
D	The intake of vitamin D during pregnancy must be carefully evaluated, since most foods are relatively low in this vitamin unless they are fortified. Deficiency or excess of this vitamin during pregnancy can be harmful to the newborn and may cause birth defects.
E	Although much is known about this vitamin concerning animal reproduction, little information is available concerning human pregnancy. By eating a well-balanced diet, the pregnant woman receives an adequate intake. Because very little vitamin E can cross the placenta, the infant has very little storage.
K	Hemorrhage in some mothers and newborns is caused by a lack of vitamin K. Vitamin K in the appropriate form and dosage can alleviate the bleeding problems. The wrong form and dosage of the vitamin can harm an infant.

local waters, but don't consume any other fish during that week.

PREGNANCY: HEALTH CONCERNS

Most of the health problems that occur during pregnancy can be reduced or prevented by nutritional adjustments. Among these problems are nausea, constipation, anemia, pica, heartburn, urinary urgency, muscle cramps, bloating, toxemia, and excessive alcohol consumption. While it is not possible in this chapter to discuss the probable causes, a brief summary of the nutritional adjustments designed to correct these conditions is given below:

1. Nausea: Eat dry toast or crackers before arising; drink fluids between meals only; eat no fats and oils; use skim milk.
2. Constipation: Eat high-fiber foods such as fresh fruits, vegetables, prunes, and whole grain breads and cereals.
3. Anemias: Increase intake of iron and the vitamins associated with red blood cell formation (folacin, B_6, B_{12}, and C).
4. Pica (the practice of eating nonfood items such as laundry starch and clay): Educate the patient about the need to discontinue the practice.
5. Heartburn: Eat bland foods; take antacids if prescribed; plan small and frequent meals.
6. Urinary urgency: Generally avoid consuming tea, coffee, spices, and alcoholic beverages.
7. Muscle cramps: Increase calcium and decrease phosphorus intake.
8. Bloating/cramping: Plan frequent and small meals; eat no greasy foods; reduce roughage and cold beverages.
9. Excessive alcohol intake: Consume few or no alcoholic beverages in view of documented birth defects from alcohol consumption.

LACTATION AND EARLY INFANCY: AN OVERVIEW

Breastfeeding is a preferred method of feeding infants and has advantages over other methods of feeding, but the mother, after consulting her physician, makes the decision on how to feed her infant. Many infants have been successfully fed by other methods. In some cases, it is detrimental to the infant to be breastfed. These cases will be discussed later.

Lactation requires more energy and produces more stress on the body than does pregnancy. The mother must consume an adequate diet to replenish her reserves and produce enough milk for the baby.

The nutrient increases for lactation are described in Table 9-1. A nursing mother's diet is nearly the same as that of a pregnant woman, although her nutritional needs increase as the child's demand for milk increases. The nursing mother needs more protein, vitamins, minerals, and calories than she did during pregnancy.

TABLE 9-4   Sample Meal Plan for a Pregnant Woman

Breakfast	Lunch	Dinner
Milk or milk products, 1 serving	Milk or milk products, 1 serving	Milk or milk products, 1 serving
Fruits or vegetables rich in vitamin C, 1 serving	Other fruits and vegetables, 2 servings	Green leafy vegetables, 2 servings
Grain products, 1 serving	Protein products, 1 serving	Protein products, 2 servings
Snack*	Grain products, 2 servings	
Milk or milk products, ½ serving	Snack*	
Protein products, 1 serving	Milk or milk products, ½ serving	

*The snacks may be consumed at any time of the day.

TABLE 9-5   Sample Menu for a Pregnant Woman, Including Protective (Basic) and Supplemental Foods

Breakfast	Lunch	Dinner
Orange juice, 4 oz	Sandwich	Roast beef, 6 oz
Oatmeal, ½ c	whole wheat bread, 2 slices	Egg noodles, ½ c with sautéed
Brown sugar, 1–2 tsp	tuna fish, ½ c	poppy seeds
Milk, 8 oz	diced celery with onion	Cut asparagus, ¾ c
Coffee or tea	mayonnaise	Salad
Snack	lettuce	torn spinach, 1 c
Salted peanuts, ½ c	Banana, 1 small	sliced mushrooms
Milk, 4 oz	Milk, 8 oz	radishes
	Coffee or tea	oil
	Snack	vinegar
	Oatmeal raisin cookies, 2	Milk, 8 oz
	Milk, 4 oz	Coffee or tea

Lactation is more stressful and requires more energy than pregnancy. The fat reserves in a woman's body will provide 200 to 300 calories and the remaining calories must be derived from the diet. Two to three months after childbirth, the mother should be back to her prepregnancy weight, although she will still be eating 500 to 1000 calories more per day. If the food supply is adequate, the woman will usually eat well, lose weight, and maintain her figure while adequately nourishing her infant. Tables 9-6 and 9-7 describe an acceptable menu plan and sample menu for lactation.

Hormones that stimulate milk production are suppressed by anxiety and fatigue. These psychological conditions rather than any physical problem usually deter women from successful breastfeeding. When counseling new mothers, the health practitioner should discuss these factors as well as dietary considerations.

The first year of life for an infant is marked by rapid growth. Birth weight triples and length increases by approximately 50%. Nutrition plays a major role in the rate of growth, although overall height will be genetically determined.

The period of the neonate, from birth to 28 days, is one of rapid adjustment. Stomach capacity triples and kidneys become more efficient. In the first 48 hours, an infant must coordinate its breathing, sucking, and swallowing. It must also adjust its temperature control and regulation. The premature infant has very limited abilities to do these things and is likely to have immature liver and respiratory functions as well.

During the first two years of life, an infant will grow approximately 20 deciduous teeth and calcify its permanent teeth buds. The brain undergoes its most rapid growth period, increasing in cell size and number. The brain will have reached 80% of its growth by age two. Muscles and skeletal structures will strengthen and increase in size. Adequate nutrition is critical during the stage of infancy.

BREASTFEEDING

The advantages of breastfeeding are discussed below.

Nutritional Benefits

Breastmilk offers some nutritional benefits not available in a formula. A higher level of lactose in breastmilk creates a better intestinal environment in the infant, permitting better bowel movements as well as better absorption of calcium, protein, and magnesium. Some formulas contain added lactose.

The fat in breastmilk is high in linoleic acid, an essential fatty acid. The milk is also relatively high in cholesterol,

TABLE 9-6   **Sample Meal Plan for a Lactating Woman**

Breakfast	Lunch	Dinner
Milk or milk products, 1 serving	Milk or milk products, 1 serving	Milk or milk products, 1 serving
Fruits or vegetables rich in vitamin C, 1 serving	Other fruits and vegetables, 2 servings	Green leafy vegetables, 2 servings
Grain products, 1 serving	Protein products, 2 servings	Protein products, 2 servings
Snack*	Grain products, 2 servings	
Milk or milk products, 1 serving	Snack*	
Protein products, 1 serving	Milk or milk products, 1 serving	

*The snacks may be consumed at any time of the day.

TABLE 9-7   **Sample Menu for a Lactating Woman, Including Protective (Basic) and Supplemental Foods**

Breakfast	Lunch	Dinner
Orange juice, 4 oz	Sandwich	Roast beef, 6 oz
Oatmeal, ½ c	whole wheat bread, 2 slices	Egg noodles, ½ c with sauteed poppy seeds
Brown sugar, 1–2 tsp	tuna fish, ½ c	Cut asparagus, ¾ c
Milk, 8 oz	diced celery	Salad
Coffee or tea	mayonnaise	torn spinach, 1 c
Snack	lettuce	sliced mushrooms
Salted peanuts, ½ c	Banana, 1 small	radishes
Milk, 8 oz	Milk, 8 oz	oil
	Snack	vinegar
	Oatmeal raisin cookies, 2	Milk, 8 oz
	Milk, 8 oz	

which is essential for the structures and functions of cell membranes, nerve tissue, and other compounds.

If the mother's diet is adequate, vitamin stores, even though small, are well utilized. If the diet is inadequate, the water-soluble vitamins may be low in her milk. Vitamin D and fluoride are not provided in adequate amounts in breastmilk.

In the first few days after childbirth, the woman secretes a yellowish fluid called colostrum. It cannot be duplicated by any modern formula. It has an anti-infection property and provides immunity against several undesirable factors. The colostrum-fed infant has less diarrhea and constipation, since some factors in colostrum inhibit the growth of bacteria. Colostrum contains antibodies that protect the infant from intestinal infections. Some reports indicate that colostrum can also protect against nonintestinal infections. Breastfed babies have fewer respiratory infections and fewer allergies than nonbreastfed babies.

Psychological Benefits

Breastfeeding is believed to assist in establishing the bond between the woman and her child, but this claim receives mixed responses. The father may experience better bonding if the infant is bottle-fed. A relaxed feeding atmosphere appears to be more important than the feeding method.

Other Considerations

Some research indicates that bottle-fed babies are more likely to become obese than breastfed ones. The caloric content of both types of milk is the same (20 calories per ounce), but a breastfeeding mother is not as likely to overfeed the infant as the one who is bottle-feeding. Bottle-fed infants are also more likely to be given solid foods at an earlier age.

One of the hormones released when a woman is breastfeeding causes the uterus to contract and return to normal size. This helps the mother to regain her prepregnancy figure. Breastfeeding also helps delay ovulation, and while it has been used as a birth control method, it is not a sure method.

BOTTLE-FEEDING

Some advantages of bottle-feeding are listed below:

1. For those women who have an aversion to breastfeeding or whose spouses object, bottle-feeding may be a wise choice.
2. Bottle-feeding is not as restrictive as breastfeeding. For mothers who work outside the home, this can be a major reason for bottle-feeding.
3. When the mother suffers chronic conditions such as heart disease, tuberculosis, or kidney disorder, bottle-feeding is the preferred method.

4. Whenever a mother is on prescribed or illegal drugs or has been sick during the pregnancy, bottle-feeding is preferred. Many drugs pass from the mother into the milk and enter the infant. The infant is unable to detoxify and eliminate drugs. Even a small amount of drugs can result in overdose for the infant.

5. A bottle-fed child grows equally as well as a breastfed one. If a woman wishes to bottle-feed, she should do so. The cost, types, and techniques of formula-feeding should be taught by health personnel, and emphasis should be placed on cleanliness. The problem of poor sanitation is especially common among families of low socioeconomic status.

For mothers who have decided to use infant formulas, note the following types:

Cow's Milk-Based Infant Formulas

Manufacturers use the guidelines distributed by the American Academy of Pediatrics, and the U.S. FDA enforces these recommendations. These formulas have the following profiles:

1. Use cow's milk as a base.
2. Milk fat is replaced with vegetable oils.
3. May be fortified with vitamins and minerals.

Soy-Based Infant Formulas

When infants react negatively to cow's milk (diarrhea, vomiting, colic, etc.), pediatricians may recommend formulas based on soy milk, which may be fortified stronger than regular infant formulas.

Specialty Infant Formulas

These refer to all infant formulas with special features such as prematurity, genetic disorders, and so on.

HEALTH CONCERNS OF INFANCY

Some health concerns of infancy are the following:

1. For infants allergic to milk, soybean preparations are used. They should be supplemented with the essential amino acid methionine to make them complete protein. Milk allergies are not the same as abnormal body protein metabolism from genetic predisposition. Infants with the latter type of trouble require special formulas.

2. Overfeeding infants is common in the United States, and obesity becomes a major concern. Overfeeding during this period can result in an excess formation of fat cells. The child will develop an overeating pattern, resulting in lifelong obesity problems. The use of skim or low-fat milk for infants, to prevent obesity, however, is to be avoided. These products are not appropriate for infants since they do not contain essential linoleic acid or the cholesterol necessary for building body compounds. Some infants develop diarrhea from a low fat intake. Preferred methods of preventing obesity include not introducing solid foods too early, not adding sugar to foods, and not offering formula to a fully fed child.

3. Inadequacy of dietary iron and the onset of anemia are more common in infants after their fourth month when iron stores are depleted and birth weight has increased. If the prenatal diet of the mother was poor, and iron stores are lacking in the infant, anemia can begin earlier.

INTRODUCTION OF SOLID FOODS

The decision on when to add solid foods to the infant's diet should be based on three factors: appropriate physical and physiological development, nutritional requirements, and the need to begin teaching lifelong dietary habits.

The ability to eat solid foods is a developmental task. Between three to six months of age, an infant can recognize a spoon and swallow nonliquid foods.

The enzyme system in the intestine must be ready to digest starches and nonmilk proteins before these foods are added. Usually starches can be digested after two to three months of age, but four to six months are required before infants acquire enzymes to digest nonmilk proteins.

When foods are added to a baby's diet, they should be introduced one at a time to detect allergic reactions. Only small amounts should be given. Mixtures of foods should be avoided. The use of sugar, salt, and other seasonings should generally be avoided. A wide variety of foods should be given to teach good eating habits, and the child should not be forced to eat more than he or she wants.

Baby food can be made at home, but the caretaker should be instructed about the type of foods to puree, and to omit foods high in spices, salt, and sugar. When the infant begins to eat table foods, the health practitioner should determine what the family diet is like. The child could begin receiving nutritionally inadequate foods if the family's diet is inadequate. Table 9-8 illustrates suitable supplemental foods that can be added to an infant's diet, and the usual age for introduction.

RESPONSIBILITIES OF HEALTH PERSONNEL

The pregnant woman should be counseled by the health professional to do the following:

1. Select her diet with the help of a reliable food guide.
2. Include good food sources of folic acid.
3. Avoid skipping breakfast.
4. Eat to gain weight at the recommended pattern even if she is overweight.
5. Not reduce food intake or avoid gaining the recommended weight.

TABLE 9-8   Suitable Supplemental Food for Infants During the First Year

Foods	Usual Age When Food Supplemented
Well-cooked cereals (iron fortified)	4–6 months
Strained or pureed vegetables	6–8 months
Strained meats	6–8 months
Fruit juice	6–8 months
Crackers, zwieback	6–8 months
Egg yolk	9–10 months
Well-cooked, soft, bite-sized pieces of meats, fruits, and vegetables, soft breads, and other finger foods	9–10 months
Egg white	12 months or later

6. Use a moderate amount of iodized salt and extra liquids.
7. Call her physician immediately if weight increases suddenly.
8. Limit or quit smoking.
9. Avoid alcoholic beverages.
10. Avoid all drugs unless prescribed by a physician familiar with her pregnancy status.
11. Take nutrient supplements prescribed by a physician or nurse practitioner.
12. Adjust foods to minimize common problems, but without interfering with recommended intake.
13. Avoid fasting to reduce weight before a prenatal appointment. Fasting can lead to acidosis, which can cause fetal damage.

The lactating woman should be counseled by the health professional to do the following:

1. Consume more food than during pregnancy and continue to do so as the infant eats more.
2. Continue to follow a reliable food guide.
3. Consume 400 IU of vitamin D daily from food or supplements.
4. Continue to take prenatal iron supplements for two to three months.
5. Drink at least three liters of fluid daily.
6. Rest and relax so that breastfeeding can be successful.
7. Consult the physician about the use of coffee, alcohol, and drugs, since they are excreted in the breast milk. (For more information about the effects of drugs on pregnancy and lactation, see Chapter 10, Activity 2.)

If bottle-feeding, the caregiver should be counseled by the health professional to do the following:

1. Follow the directions exactly.
2. Not force the baby to drink every drop.
3. Practice aseptic technique when making formula.

4. Recognize developmental stages indicating when an infant should be started on solid foods.
5. Follow a reliable guide for addition of solid foods.
6. Offer single foods and note any allergies.
7. Introduce a variety of foods.
8. Reintroduce once-rejected food items at another time.
9. Avoid allowing the child to drink more than one quart of milk a day, to prevent refusal of other foods.
10. Make mealtimes for the infant a pleasurable, special time.

The health practitioner should also offer the following advice to the caretaker:

1. Continue close physical contact with infant after breast- or bottle-feedings have been discontinued.
2. Note the following when using commercial baby foods:
   a. Items such as baby soups and mixed or prepared dinners have high water content and little meat. When meats and vegetables are selected separately, they provide better nutrition.
   b. Commercial baby foods are safe, and most contain little sugar or salt.
   c. Items such as desserts contain extra sugar and should not be used frequently. Some may choose to avoid them completely.
3. Note the following when feeding toddlers:
   a. Allow toddlers their rituals during mealtime.
   b. Do not permit arguments at mealtime.
   c. Do not use rewards and reprimands to increase food consumption.

In general, a health practitioner should be aware of special problems of nutrition and provide information and service when needed.

PROGRESS CHECK ON ACTIVITY 1

MULTIPLE CHOICE

Circle the letter of the correct answer.

1. A recommended pattern of weight gain during pregnancy is:
   a. 8 pounds (first trimester), 8 pounds (second trimester), 8 pounds (last trimester) = 24 pounds
   b. 5 pounds (first trimester), 5 pounds (second trimester), 14 pounds (last trimester) = 24 pounds
   c. 3 pounds (first trimester), 10 pounds (second trimester), 11 pounds (last trimester) = 24 pounds
   d. 0 pounds (first trimester), 12 pounds (second trimester), 12 pounds (last trimester) = 24 pounds

2. When are caloric needs during pregnancy the highest?

   a. first trimester
   b. second trimester
   c. third trimester
   d. same each trimester

3. What is the RDA energy allowance for the pregnant woman?

   a. 2600 kcal
   b. 2780 kcal
   c. 2500 kcal
   d. 2900 kcal

4. What is the RDA allowance for the lactating woman?

   a. 3300 kcal
   b. 2730 kcal
   c. 2850 kcal
   d. 2600 kcal

5. In addition to dietary sources, what mineral is recommended to be supplemented during pregnancy?

   a. potassium
   b. iron
   c. iodine
   d. zinc

6. What vitamin may need to be supplemented during pregnancy to prevent a type of megaloblastic anemia?

   a. folacin
   b. ascorbic acid
   c. riboflavin
   d. niacin

7. The factor(s) thought to assist the pregnant woman in meeting her calcium requirement include(s) all except:

   a. absorption of calcium is increased during pregnancy.
   b. extra servings from the meat group are recommended.
   c. supplemental vitamins are prescribed.
   d. ascorbic acid is provided to increase absorption.

8. What mineral intake is no longer thought generally beneficial to restrict during pregnancy?

   a. iron
   b. sodium
   c. calcium
   d. potassium

9. Increased risks for the pregnant teenager include:

   a. prematurity.
   b. toxemia.
   c. anemia.
   d. all of the above.

10. The most common dietary complaints during pregnancy include all except:

    a. diarrhea.
    b. nausea and vomiting.
    c. constipation.
    d. indigestion.

11. Colostrum is needed by the infant to provide:

    a. extra protein.
    b. antibodies.
    c. extra lactose.
    d. antigens.

12. Two nutrients for which supplementation is recommended to meet the increased requirements for pregnancy are:

    a. iron and folacin.
    b. iron and phosphorus.
    c. zinc and folacin.
    d. iodine and calcium.

13. The mineral that is most related to the expansion of blood volume in pregnancy is:

    a. magnesium.
    b. iron.
    c. sodium.
    d. calcium.

14. All but which of the following increases a pregnant woman's chances of having a low birth weight infant?

    a. consuming a high-protein diet during pregnancy
    b. having the first baby before age 17 years
    c. smoking cigarettes
    d. failing to gain the recommended amount of weight while pregnant

15. Which of the following statements about breast-milk is true?

    a. It is lower in protein than cow's milk.
    b. It is generally less nourishing for infants than baby formula.
    c. It is more likely to cause allergy than formula.
    d. All of the above.

16. If a mother finds she cannot breastfeed, the baby should be weaned onto:

    a. whole milk.
    b. low-fat milk.

c. formula.

d. cereal gruel.

17. When the baby is eating solid foods, which food should be introduced first?

a. fruits

b. vegetables

c. cereals

d. eggs

18. To meet the food groups, a pregnant woman needs:

a. 4 glasses of milk a day.

b. 6 servings of vitamin C-rich foods a day.

c. 2 servings of breads and cereals a day.

d. 1 fruit or vegetable serving.

19. Behavior by the mother that may be harmful to an unborn child is:

a. smoking.

b. protein deprivation.

c. drinking alcohol.

d. all of the above.

20. Toxemia during pregnancy may be due to:

a. excessive sodium intake.

b. excessive water intake.

c. a low-protein diet.

d. a high-protein diet.

21. An unnatural taste ("craving") for clay, ice, cornstarch, and other nonnutritious substances is:

a. a need for support, understanding, and love.

b. called pica.

c. a psychological abnormality.

d. the body's signal for needed nutrients.

22. If a baby is thirsty, you should give it a bottle of:

a. fruit juice.

b. sweetened water.

c. formula.

d. water.

23. Close physical contact after breast- or bottle-feeding:

a. will create an overly dependent child.

b. will cause the infant to dislike others.

c. is needed for the infant to thrive.

d. is nice but not necessary.

TRUE/FALSE

Circle T for True and F for False.

24. T F The pattern of weight gain is more important than the total weight gain during pregnancy.

25. T F If a pregnant woman gains 25 lbs in her first trimester, she should avoid any further weight gain during the second and third trimesters.

26. T F The highest growth rate for an individual occurs during infancy.

27. T F An overweight or obese woman should try to gain little or no weight during pregnancy.

28. T F It is not possible to become pregnant while breastfeeding.

29. T F Breast milk is high in vitamin D.

30. T F Introducing solids to an infant will help it sleep through the night.

ACTIVITY 2:

Childhood and Adolescent Nutrition

The basic social unit to which a child belongs, the family, is the primary source from which the child learns culturally acceptable food behaviors. In turn, these food habits are passed on to the next generation. Families can establish good nutrition by doing the following:

1. Practicing good eating habits
2. Providing wholesome, acceptable foods that promote good health
3. Establishing eating patterns that are socially enjoyable and satisfying

Childhood and adolescence are the growth periods from infancy to the beginning of adulthood and are marked by many body changes. Childhood spans the period from birth to prepuberty, with the period of the toddler (ages one to three years) as a transition. Adolescence ends when sexual organ development and physical maturity are complete.

This activity examines the nutritional needs of the toddler, early and late childhood, and adolescence.

TODDLER: AGES ONE TO THREE

Children, ages one to three, should be introduced to good foods and healthy eating habits. Growth and development of children progress in an orderly manner. After the first year of life, the rate of growth slows. Early and middle childhood is marked by slow but steady growth increases. A toddler gains from 5 to 10 lbs per year and grows about three inches in height. The toddler has a reduced appetite and requires less food. He or she has cut 20 deciduous teeth generally by the age of two-and-a-half to three. Foods that require more chewing can be added at this time. The toddler's psychomotor skills have improved, making use of utensils for eating possible. However, the toddler spills his or her food frequently and may appear clumsy. Time and practice will improve eating skills.

Because of their short attention spans, toddlers usually cannot stay seated to finish a meal. The developmental task of the toddler is to strive for autonomy and is reflected in eating behavior. Children between the ages of two to three want to feed themselves; their favorite words are "want" and "no." They may say no even to foods they like to establish their own authority. This period is known as the "terrible twos" and it can be a frustrating experience for parents, especially new ones. Parents should recognize that offering a toddler choices between equally appropriate foods is acceptable and may increase desired eating habits.

PRESCHOOLER: AGES THREE TO FIVE

Children continue to develop new food behavior patterns while their growth continues at a slow rate. The preschool-aged child gains three to five pounds and grows two to three inches a year. Children between the ages of three and five are usually lean, raising concerns in their parents. An awareness of body changes will alleviate this concern.

The preschooler is energetic, active, and restless and has a high caloric need. Nutritious snacks that supply extra calories and essential nutrients should be offered. As muscle control improves, the child is better able to handle eating utensils. By age four or five, the child may be able to cut some of his or her own food.

Because preschoolers are inquisitive and learn by imitation, they will learn readily from the people with whom they are in contact. The food habits of the parents, such as food likes and dislikes, will be noted. Media and television capture preschoolers' attention. From the information so acquired they will form concepts about food. This is an ideal time to start teaching simple nutrition concepts such as equating foods that taste the best with those that are nutritious. However, children in this age group will request those foods preferred by their peers. Check the foods and snacks that are served preschoolers when they are away from home. Children cannot distinguish between good and bad foods at this stage. Tables 9-9 and 9-10 evaluate nutritious meals and snacks for toddlers and preschoolers.

EARLY CHILDHOOD: HEALTH CONCERNS

The feeding of young children poses a number of concerns, including low food intake, manipulative behavior, food jags, and pica. With the exception of pica, all such concerns are easily remedied. Studies have shown that some children with pica are also anemic, and most of them are from poor families in unclean environments. The greater concern, however, is lead poisoning that sometimes accompanies pica. Many children eat peeling paint from wall plaster because it has a slightly sweet taste. Lead poisoning adversely affects the nervous system, kidney, and bone marrow and may lead to death.

TABLE 9-9   Daily Food Needs for Toddlers
Breads and Cereals
4 servings
Whole grain, enriched, or restored: cornmeal, crackers, breads, flour, macaroni and spaghetti, rice, rolled oats
Vegetables and Fruits
4 servings
Include foods rich in vitamin A and C
Vitamin A-rich foods: (dark yellow or leafy green foods) apricots, broccoli, cantaloupe, carrots, pumpkin, spinach, sweet potatoes
Vitamin C-rich foods: oranges, grapefruit, cantaloupe, raw strawberries, broccoli, Brussels sprouts, green peppers, lemon, asparagus tips, raw cabbage, potatoes and sweet potatoes (boiled in skins), tomatoes
Milk and Dairy Products
3 servings
Milk, cheese, ice cream, yogurt
Meat, Fish, and Nuts
2 servings
Beef, lamb, pork, liver, poultry, eggs, fish, shellfish, dry beans, dry peas, lentils, nuts, peanut butter

Source: Idaho Department of Health and Welfare.

Healthcare workers need to assist caretakers to prevent young children from playing near potential lead sources.

The four common health problems of young children in the United States are anemia, dental caries, obesity, and allergies.

Iron-Deficiency Anemia

Iron-deficiency anemia is a problem for all ages, but especially so for children. Many iron-deficient children come from low-income families with poor diets. However, some studies indicate that cultural traditions and ignorance of nutrition requirements are also factors contributing to iron deficiencies. Low blood-iron levels affect the child's resistance to disease, attention span, behavior, and intellectual performance. Iron-rich foods that children usually like include enriched breads, cereals and tortillas, eggs, dried fruit, molasses, lentils, and baked beans.

Dental Caries

Dental caries is a widespread problem for all age groups. It is easily prevented by a balanced diet and assisted by self-care oral hygiene. A daily intake of fluoride, either through water, tablets, or supplements, also reduces the incidence of cavities by 50%–60%. Fluoridated toothpaste is not recommended for children under the age of three because they may ingest excess fluoride from swallowing the toothpaste.

TABLE 9-10   A Guide to Snacks for Toddlers

Planning Snacks

Choose snacks that are appropriate for the age of the child. Some foods are too hard for young children (3 years and under) to chew and may even be dangerous.

In general, small, round foods (peanuts, cherry tomatoes, peas, raisins), or chunky and crunchy foods (carrots, celery, and other raw vegetables) should not be given to the young child.

Select Basic Foods

Almost everyone snacks. Snacks give us a lift when we need it and can help meet daily energy and growth needs. A good guideline for snacks is to avoid high-sugar foods and choose from the basic food groups: vegetables and fruits; breads and cereals; milk and dairy products; meat, fish, and nuts.

Why Not Sugar Snacks?

Foods high in sugar content contribute to tooth decay and gum disease. Examples include:

jams and jellies	dried fruits	cake	pastries
honey	canned fruit	cookies	pie
syrups	gum	candy	carbonated drinks
sugar-coated cereals	breath mints	doughnuts	Jell-O

Try to limit high-sugar food to mealtimes.

Beware of Hidden Sugars

Many foods that we do not think of as sugar-foods may, in fact, contain sugar. For example:

peanut butter	chili sauce	salad dressings	lunch meats
soup	canned vegetables	white bread	flavored yogurt
catsup	crackers	snack bars	ice cream

When shopping, read food labels and select foods with little or no sugar. Ingredients are listed on labels in descending order according to their percentage of the total product. Sugar may be listed as sugar, sucrose, corn syrup, honey, dextrose, maltose, and so on (look for the *ose* ending). In general, avoid foods that contain sugar as a main ingredient.

Good Foods for Children

Juicy		Hungry	
apples	pears	cottage cheese	Vienna sausages
blackberries	pineapple	meat cubes:	sardines
cantaloupe	plums	chicken	shrimp
cherries	raspberries	beef	cheese cubes
dill pickle	strawberries	ham	eggs—hard cooked or deviled
grapefruit	tangerines	lamb	peanuts and other nuts
grapes	tomatoes	lunch meat	plain yogurt with fruit added
oranges	watermelon	pork	
peaches		turkey	

Crunchy		Thirsty	
cabbage wedges	lettuce wedges	white milk	juices—no sugar added:
carrots	popcorn	buttermilk	orange juice
cauliflower flowerets	radishes	tomato juice	grapefruit juice
celery	peppers, raw slices		pineapple juice
cucumber strips	sunflower seeds		apple juice
green onions			other fruit juices

Source: Idaho Department of Health and Welfare.

Obesity

Between the ages from birth to four years and seven to eleven years, the incidence of obesity is high. Most studies confirm that a fat child ingests the same number of calories as a lean child, but the fat child is less active. Some fat children have emotional problems. Some imitate family eating habits, and each member in the family is usually overweight. A controlled caloric intake that permits growth and a regular exercise program are recommended. Behavior modification and a strong support system are useful in retraining the child's eating pattern. The whole family should participate in this effort.

Allergies

Many childhood allergies are caused by food. In youngsters, milk allergy is common, followed by egg white, citrus, chocolate, seafood, wheat, and nut allergies. Symptoms can be respiratory difficulties or some forms of skin rash. The preferred and usually easiest treatment is to remove the offending food or foods. Frequently, an allergic reaction to one food will trigger a reaction to others. Some allergies run in families, and the parent should note any reaction as new food is introduced to a child. The health worker should counsel parents on how to substitute an offending food with a nonoffending one of equal nutritional value. Chapter 27 contains detailed information about food allergies.

EARLY CHILDHOOD: NUTRITIONAL REQUIREMENTS

When one considers the protein and calorie requirements for infants and children, one must understand the following premises:

1. There are scientific requirements such as those recommended by the National Academy of Sciences (e.g., DRIs), university researchers, and care providers at modern medical facilities. In general, the implementation of such recommendations requires calculations using variables such as sex, weight according to BMI, height, physical activity level, resting metabolic rate, and so on. At present, the application of such a process at the consumer level is severely limited until comprehensive charts generated by computer databases are available.
2. There are legal requirements for infant formulas promulgated by the U.S. Food and Drug Administration (FDA).
3. There are recommendations from the medical and health communities such as physicians, nurses, dietitians, pharmacists, and so on. Most of them still use charts that indicate the age and the amount required.
4. Most consumers still use charts that indicate the age and the amount required.

The following are recommended allowances to be individualized by recording to a child's growth rate.

Calories and Proteins

The estimated energy requirements (EER) derived from the DRIs based on the variables mentioned above (sex, age, height, weight and activity levels) will not be discussed her. If interested, one should consult such DRIs and their calculations at www.nas.edu. Many healthcare providers and the general public use the following guides.

The requirements for calories:

- 1 to 3 years: 102 kcal per kg of body weight
- 4 to 6 years: 90 kcal per kg of body weight
- 7 to 10 years: 70 kcal per kg of body weight

The requirements for protein:

- 1 to 3 years: 16 g for a 13-kg child
- 4 to 6 years: 24 g for a 20-kg child
- 7 to 10 years: 28 g for a 28-kg child

The quality of protein ingested influences the growth rate and other nutritional requirements of the child. If inadequate amounts of carbohydrate and fat are ingested, the protein will be used for energy needs, and growth will be arrested. The legal requirements for protein promulgated by the FDA for infant formulas are a safety net for most infants on a regular diet of formula. The FDA requires the following:

- A minimum of 1.8 g/100 kcal of formula
- A maximum of 4.5 g/100 kcal of formula

Obviously, individual planning is needed as growth rates will vary. Estimation of the caloric and protein needs of children is usually done by referring to a chart using the appropriate age, weight, height, activity and other variables, without calculation.

However in research centers and for children with clinical conditions or special needs, the health team may use a special formula to estimate the nutrition needs of these children.

Fat

All children need fat in their diet. Thirty to forty percent of daily calories should come from fat.

Vitamins and Minerals

The requirements for these two nutrients are high for children. If a varied diet is consumed, supplements are unnecessary. If anemia is present, iron may be prescribed, along with other supplements. A diet deficient in one nutrient is likely to be deficient in others. Frequently, children's diets are low in calcium and vitamins A and C. Vitamin C is important for iron absorption. The RDAs/DRIs for early childhood are presented in Tables F-1 and F-2.

MIDDLE CHILDHOOD: GENERAL CONSIDERATIONS

The physical changes that occur in the middle childhood years are not dramatic. Deciduous teeth are shed and permanent teeth are cut. The slow and steady increase in height and weight continues. Children in this age group spend more time away from home, as friends become important to them. Weekday school lunch meals are nutritionally adequate. However, many children complain of the appearance, taste, and texture of foods to which they are not accustomed. Although some lunches are not appetizing, generally it is peer-group pressure that fosters children's attitudes toward school lunches.

The nutritional concerns of middle childhood are characterized by obesity from overeating "empty" calories, insufficient exercise, skipping meals, and adopting negative eating behaviors. Stress from schoolwork and activities influences appetite and the overall eating habits of this group.

Tables 9-11, 9-12, and 9-13 describe various meal plans and sample menus for children ages 1 through 12.

ADOLESCENCE: NUTRITION AND DIET

It is difficult to determine exactly the age at which adolescence begins. The boundaries marking the change vary among individuals. For example, there are marked differences in the rate and amount of physical changes, as well as psychological and social development, among individuals. Some researchers divide adolescence into early and late stages. The preteen or pubescence stage covers ages 10 to 12 and puberty covers ages 12 to 18.

Adolescence is a transition period in the life cycle of individuals and carries many labels or names. There is a dearth of scientific data regarding adolescents' growth, development, and nutritional needs. It is the second greatest growth spurt in the life cycle. Girls begin sooner than boys, usually between the ages of 10 to 12, while boys begin this growth between the ages of 12 to 14.

During the period of adolescence (10 to 18 years), the average male doubles in weight, gaining approximately 70 pounds and 13 to 14 inches in height. Girls gain approximately 50 pounds and nine inches in height. Adequately nourished girls develop permanent layers of adipose or fat tissue. This is normal and desirable, but the fat creates panic in the young girl wishing to be thin and fashionable.

The nutrient needs and energy requirements are very high during adolescence. The basal metabolic rate (BMR) is the highest in any life stage except during pregnancy. More food is needed, and girls need to increase their intake earlier than boys.

Eating habits of the adolescent are generally poor, especially the eating habits of girls. The developmental aspect of adolescence urges them to separate from the family and establish their own identity. One way they assert themselves is to deviate from a normal food habit. Social acceptance by the peer group is more important than family approval, and only peer approval is valued.

The adolescent's diet tends to be low in calcium, iron, and vitamins A and C. Meals are skipped, particularly breakfast, since more time is spent on appearance than eating. Body weight, skin, and hair problems, either real or imagined, take precedence over nutritional concerns.

TABLE 9-11   Suggested Meal Plan and Sample Menu for 1- and 2-Year-Olds*

Meal Plan	Sample Menu
Breakfast	*Breakfast*
Juice or fruit	Orange juice
Cereal (hot or dry) with milk	Hot oatmeal with milk
Toast or egg (soft-boiled)	Whole wheat toast
Butter or margarine	Butter
Milk	Milk
Snack	*Snack*
Milk or juice	Apple juice
Lunch	*Lunch*
Meat, cheese, egg, or alternate	Grilled cheese sandwich
Potato, bread, crackers, or alternate	Peas
Vegetable	Milk
Butter or margarine	Ice cream
Milk	
Dessert	
Snack	*Snack*
Milk, juice, pudding, or crackers with cheese, or alternate	Rice pudding
Dinner	*Dinner*
Meat, cheese, poultry, or alternate	Meat loaf
Vegetable or salad	Spinach or carrots
Potato, bread, roll, or alternate	Roll
Butter or margarine	Butter
Dessert	Applesauce
Milk	Milk

*Serving size varies with the child. Other nutritious items not shown may be used (e.g., jams, oatmeal, cookies, peanut butter). Their inclusion must be integrated into the child's overall daily intake of calories and nutrients.

Health does not play a role in the adolescent's food choices. Among teenagers in parts of the country, the incidence of tuberculosis and other respiratory illness is high, probably due to severe nutrient deficiencies that lower resistance in these individuals. Adolescents, preoccupied as they are with self, do not seem to relate nutrition to body function. They do not think that what they eat today will reflect their health status in the future.

ADOLESCENCE: HEALTH CONCERNS

The major health concerns of adolescence are discussed in the following sections.

TABLE 9-12	Suggested Meal Plan and Sample Menu for 3- through 6-Year-Olds*
Meal Plan	**Sample Menu**
Breakfast	*Breakfast*
Juice or fruit	Applesauce
Cereal (hot or dry)	Bran flakes with milk
Egg, meat, or toast	Egg (soft-boiled) with
Milk	whole wheat toast
	Milk
Snack	*Snack*
Dry fruits or sweet	Dates or
breads	carrot cake
Lunch	*Lunch*
Meat, egg,	Peanut butter and jelly
or alternate	sandwich
Potato, bread,	Vegetable soup with rice
or alternate	Margarine
Vegetable	Milk
Butter or margarine	Custard pudding
Milk	
Dessert	
Snack	*Snack*
Milk or juice	Orange juice
Crackers, pudding, or	Apple wedges with
dried fruits	peanut butter
Dinner	*Dinner*
Meat, cheese, poultry,	Fish sticks
or alternate	Sweet corn
Vegetable or salad	Baked potato
Potato, bread, roll,	Butter
or alternate	Fruit pudding
Butter or margarine	Milk
Dessert	
Milk	

*Serving size varies with the child. Other nutritious items not shown may be used (e.g., granola, oatmeal, cookies, yogurt or ice cream). Their inclusion must be integrated into the child's overall daily intake of calories and nutrients.

TABLE 9-13	Suggested Meal Plan and Sample Menu for 7- through 12-Year-Olds*
Meal Plan	**Sample Menu**
Breakfast	*Breakfast*
Juice or fruit	Orange juice
Cereal (hot or dry) with	Cornflakes or rice cereal
milk	with milk
Toast	Toast, whole wheat
Egg, meat, or alternate	Egg, poached
Butter or margarine	Margarine
Milk	Milk, 2%
Lunch	*Lunch*
Meat, cheese,	Vegetable soup/crackers
or alternate	Macaroni and cheese
Potato, bread,	Coleslaw
or alternate	Milk, 2%
Vegetable	Fresh peaches
Butter or margarine	
Milk	
Dessert	
Snack	*Snack*
Dried fruits or	Banana bread
nutritious breads	Apple juice
Milk or juice	
Dinner	*Dinner*
Meat, cheese, or alternate	Hamburger
	Carrots or peas
Vegetable	Sliced tomato/
Salad	onion
Potato or alternate	Baked potato
Bread or alternate	Bread
Butter or margarine	Margarine
Dessert	Ice cream
Milk	Milk, 2%

*Serving size varies with the child. Other nutritious items not shown may be used (e.g., jams, oatmeal, cookies, peanut butter). Their inclusion must be integrated into the child's overall daily intake of calories and nutrients.

Smoking, Alcohol, and Drugs

Experiments with these substances often begin in the early teens. They affect the nutritional status in different ways: they can lessen the sense of taste and smell, decrease appetite, and reduce vitamin C level in the body. Some adolescents overdose on vitamin or mineral supplements in an effort to "get more energy" or "look better." Poisoning from excess vitamins A and D has been documented.

Physical Development

With the exception of young athletes who maintain a good physique, the majority of preteens and teens are physically poorly developed. Their muscle mass is less dense, with poor tone and endurance. Good physical fitness programs and appropriate nutrition classes in the curriculum should be mandated from kindergarten to grade 12.

Obesity

Teenagers who are obese usually have been overweight or obese since childhood. Since adjusting sexual roles, planning careers, and beginning adult lifestyles create great stress at this time, food is sometimes overused as a comfort and security measure, and the teen can become obese. Their favorite food is usually high-fat, high-calorie food with little nutritional value. Obese adolescents tend to eat less food than their lean counterparts, but they also exercise less. Girls particularly often adopt bizarre eating behaviors because of fad dieting.

If the adolescent needs to diet, it must not be so restricted as to delay growth and maturation. Teenage boys require 45–55 kcal per kg of body weight per day, while girls require 40–47 kcal per kg of body weight a day. The RDA for other nutrients for this group is higher than for others except pregnant and nursing mothers. A diet should be only mildly limited in calories, and the adolescent's activity should increase. Realistic goals to lose weight should be established. Teenagers should be taught that a body cannot lose more than one or two pounds a week without starving. Emotional and peer support is essential, but careful monitoring is also important. If a teenager is not given guidance or follows an unsound fad diet practiced by adults, there may be severe weight loss with associated health problems.

Studies have indicated that teenagers do not consume adequate amounts of iron, calcium, and vitamins A and C.

Anemia

A number of surveys indicate that iron-deficiency anemia is a widespread problem beginning in childhood and continuing through adolescence, particularly among girls. Iron requirements are high because blood volume increases with the rapid growth increases in both sexes. The onset of the menses in the female adds to the need. Poor dietary habits are responsible for this problem and improved habits can eliminate iron deficiencies.

Dental Caries

Cavities occur mainly from the consumption of too much fermentable carbohydrates (sugars and sweets, especially the sticky type) and from poor hygiene (inadequate brushing and flossing). However, an adequate total diet that includes a source of fluoride is also necessary for good teeth and oral tissues.

Acne

Acne may or may not be related to certain foods, such as fats and chocolate. Some scientists suggest that a low zinc intake and increased consumption of alcoholic beverages may be responsible for acne.

Cardiovascular Concerns

Because of the excess fat and salt in the preferred foods of teenagers, the blood cholesterol and triglycerides levels and blood pressure in these individuals may be adversely affected. They may have a higher risk of coronary heart disease later in life. The National Cholesterol Education Program has addressed this concern. More

details are provided in Chapters 4 and 16. Those chapters discuss dietary fats and recommendations for children and adults to decrease the risk of heart and blood diseases.

Teenage Pregnancy

A major health problem for teenage girls is pregnancy. In this country there are one million teenage pregnancies every year. One hundred thousand pregnancies occur in women under the age of 18, and 30,000 pregnancies occur in females under 15 years of age. Nearly one-third of the pregnant teenagers in the United States are under the age of 16. Many become pregnant again within a year.

Pregnant teenagers are at great risk of developing toxemia and delivering stillborn, premature, or low birth weight (LBW) babies. Fetal-maternal mortality rates of this group are higher than those for the adult woman. A young mother's nutritional status has a profound effect on the course and outcome of her pregnancy. A pregnant teenager has the unusually high nutrient demands of pregnancy superimposed over a rapid growth spurt. Without careful planning and support, the results can be hazardous.

Nutrition Education

Adolescents desperately need nutrition education. While health concerns are not effective in motivating good eating habits, some guidelines that relate to their concerns can be used to help adolescents.

1. Emphasize immediate effects, such as improved vitality, increased endurance, and better hair, nails, complexion, and general appearance.
2. Give basic facts so they can make informed choices.
3. Encourage them to eat breakfast and more meals with the family, try new foods, select nutrient-dense snacks, and recognize self-responsibility.
4. Stock only foods that are nutrient dense and preferred.
5. Set a good example. The use of fad diets and the practice of skipping breakfast are noted by the teenager as acceptable eating patterns.

Effective nutrition education is possible only if teenagers realize and accept responsibility for their health. Examples include the following:

1. Emphasizing that teens are responsible for their own health.
2. Acquiring a knowledge of body changes and nutrient requirements.
3. Recognizing teen health problems and understanding that the immediate consequences (appearance, vitality) are more pertinent to the teenager than long-term consequences.

4. Understanding that pregnancy is a time for special support and requires counseling, assistance, and resources.
5. Realizing that peers, coaches, heroes, media idols, and other similar individuals are more influential in a teen's life than parents or caretakers. Examples, suggestions, and encouragement from these individuals through personal contacts or public messages can result in better eating habits.
6. Knowing that nutrient requirements for the teen years are higher because of rapid development.
7. Accepting snacking as a part of teen life. It can contribute to good nutrition if good food choices are made.
8. Recognizing that the use of alcohol and other drugs has negative effects on eating habits.

RESPONSIBILITIES OF HEALTH PERSONNEL

A health practitioner has the following responsibilities:

1. Provide adequate knowledge of the adolescent phase of the life cycle to the caretakers.
2. Practice good eating habits as a role model for children.
3. Relate the use of food to developmental tasks.
4. Relate nutritional requirements to adolescents' stage of the life cycle.
5. Describe body changes to caretakers and children.
6. Be aware of nutritional health problems that can develop during the life cycle, and attempt to prevent them.
7. Identify changing food behaviors at each stage, and take measures to accommodate them.
8. Emphasize safety in handling and eating food, such as washing hands, avoiding touching food, not eating and drinking from others' plates or utensils, returning food to the refrigerator, and the like.
9. Promote healthy eating behaviors by beginning a child's nutrition education early and continuing throughout the formative years.
10. Share guidelines for promoting sound nutrition habits at every opportunity.

PROGRESS CHECK ON ACTIVITY 2

MULTIPLE CHOICE

Circle the letter of the correct answer.

1. Which of these characteristics is not typical of the toddler?

   a. slow but steady growth rate
   b. very big appetite
   c. food jags
   d. has 20 teeth

2. Which of these characteristics is not typical of the preschooler?

   a. develops self-control
   b. is energetic, restless
   c. imitation and inquiry are learning methods
   d. food habits learned now last throughout life

3. The most common health problem(s) of young children in the United States is/are:

   a. anemia.
   b. dental caries.
   c. obesity.
   d. all of the above.

4. Lead poisoning often affects young children with pica. This occurs because they eat:

   a. laundry starch.
   b. peeling paint from wall plaster.
   c. clay.
   d. mud.

5. Iron-deficiency anemia may be caused by all except:

   a. poor dietary intake.
   b. cultural traditions.
   c. ignorance of requirements.
   d. hemorrhage.

6. The iron-rich foods that children usually like include:

   a. spinach, prunes, and liver.
   b. green beans, chicken, and milk.
   c. baked beans, eggs, and dried apricots.
   d. all of the above.

7. From the following list, choose the one factor most likely to cause obesity in childhood:

   a. too much food
   b. not enough supervision
   c. not enough exercise
   d. too much pressure/stress

8. Dental caries can be prevented by:

   a. regular brushing and flossing.
   b. regular checkups with a dentist.
   c. a balanced diet.
   d. all of the above.

9. The nutrients most likely to be low in children's diets are:

   a. iron, calcium, and vitamins A and C.
   b. iron, thiamin, riboflavin, and niacin.
   c. calcium, phosphorus, and vitamin D.
   d. iron, fluoride, and vitamins B_1 and B_2.

10. If a mother is trying to follow the basic food group pattern in feeding her three-year-old child, what would be an appropriate amount for a serving of meat, fruits, and vegetables?

    a. 2 tbsp
    b. 3 tbsp
    c. ½ c
    d. ¾ c

11. The school lunch is intended to provide what part of the child's daily nutrient needs?

    a. one fourth
    b. one third
    c. one half
    d. 15%

12. Which of the following are health concerns of the school-age child?

    a. skipping meals
    b. stress/exhaustion
    c. anorexia
    d. all of the above

13. Just before adolescence, the growth patterns of girls and boys are:

    a. the same.
    b. different, in that girls have a larger percentage of fat.
    c. different, in that boys have a smaller lean body mass.
    d. different, in that boys start out taller.

14. During the period of adolescence, the average boy:

    a. gains approximately 50 lb and 10 inches in height.
    b. gains approximately 10 lb and 1 foot in height.
    c. gains approximately 70 lb and 13–14 inches in height.
    d. gains approximately 1 lb for every 1 inch of height.

15. To educate teenagers about nutrition:

    a. encourage them to eat breakfast.
    b. emphasize health effects when they grow old.
    c. stock both nutrient-dense and nutrient-light foods at home.
    d. advise supplementation of diet.

16. Teenagers should not:

    a. be responsible for their own health.
    b. snack indiscriminately.
    c. be concerned about physiological changes in the body.
    d. be influenced by others.

17. Which of the following are common health problems of teenagers?

    a. tuberculosis
    b. anemia
    c. dental caries
    d. all of the above

18. Pregnant teenagers are at high risk for all except:

    a. delivering stillborns.
    b. delivering premature infants.
    c. developing toxemia.
    d. developing heart disease.

TRUE/FALSE

Circle T for True and F for False.

19. T F A toddler can be expected to gain 10 lb a year and grow 2 inches in height.
20. T F Preschoolers gain approximately 3–5 lb and about 2–3 inches per year.
21. T F Young children do not practice manipulative behavior.
22. T F Young children who are overweight should be put on skim milk.
23. T F A diet that is deficient in one nutrient is likely to be deficient in others as well.
24. T F Adolescence is the second greatest growth spurt in life.
25. T F Pregnant teenagers are less likely to have problem pregnancies than women in their twenties.
26. T F Smoking decreases the sense of taste and smell.
27. T F Obesity affects a significant number of teenagers.
28. T F Teenage girls' eating habits are better when compared to boys the same age.
29. T F Teenage girls require 2200–2400 calories daily, but boys need twice that amount.

FILL-IN

30. Name four of the most common food allergies in young children:

    a. _____
    b. _____
    c. _____
    d. _____

ACTIVITY 3:

Adulthood and Nutrition

EARLY AND MIDDLE ADULTHOOD

The chronological ages of early and middle adulthood differ among expert opinions. For this discussion, the early adult stage covers 18 to 40 and the middle adulthood period covers ages 40 to 65.

During all stages of adulthood, body changes occur. In early adulthood, physical growth ceases. During the adult years, nutrients are mainly used for body repair and maintenance. Body composition changes include a decrease in lean mass, an increase in fat, and a reduction in bone density. Osteomalacia and arthritis may occur. With a reduction in basal metabolic rate (BMR), body functions and the capacity to perform physical work decline with advancing years. The fall in BMR and activity necessitates a decrease in caloric intake. Also, the lifestyles adopted by a person influence food habits and nutrient needs.

Nutrient needs during adulthood may be analyzed as follows:

1. The diet should be optimal in all essential nutrients except for calories. Energy needs decline because of a decrease in activity and BMR.
2. Calcium needs remain high during adulthood as calcium in bones is removed and replenished constantly.
3. Iron needs remain high in women until menopause.
4. Social development continues through adulthood, and nutritional status affects the quality of life.
5. Many factors that adversely affect the health of the adult require a modification of the adult's dietary habits.
6. A regular exercise program benefits nutritional status.

The RDAs for the early and middle years are found in the appendix. The following health concerns and problems of early and middle years should be noted:

1. Psychological stress and sedentary lifestyles are social factors that can create health problems.
2. Alcohol, drug, and tobacco use negatively affect health and nutritional status.
3. Chronic exposure to environmental pollutants is a health hazard, especially in large cities.
4. Obesity, arthritis, and osteomalacia are common disorders of middle age. Osteoporosis is especially common in women.
5. Cardiovascular diseases and cancer are leading causes of death in the adult population.

Some concerns that specifically affect women in the adult years should be noted:

1. Pregnancy, lactation, and menopause change a woman's nutrient requirements.
2. Certain contraceptives can create health problems. The use of the intrauterine device (IUD) as a birth control measure causes a heavy menstrual flow and a greater need for iron. Oral contraceptive agents (OCAs), because they are hormones, affect the body's metabolism of nutrients. The changes mimic the nutritional status of pregnancy; that is, a higher nutritional intake is required. Protein metabolism is

altered and serum cholesterol and glucose levels rise when OCAs are used. Requirements for vitamin C, vitamin B_6, and folacin are increased in these women.
3. Abortions affect iron status of women, as heavy blood loss usually accompanies the process.
4. Menopause decreases the need for iron, but calcium needs are increased in women of childbearing age to retard or prevent osteoporosis.

THE ELDERLY: FACTORS AFFECTING NUTRITION AND DIET

Aging individuals often face major adjustments in social and economic status as well as physical changes. The physical body changes caused by old age greatly affect dietary habits.

Gastrointestinal Tract

Many changes occur in the gastrointestinal tract, including loss of teeth, reduced production of saliva, diminished taste and smell, and decreased ability to digest foods. When these changes occur, chewing may become painful, and a diet with soft foods is preferred. Eating pleasure declines when taste and smell are impaired. Some adults prefer strongly flavored foods, while others avoid food because it does not taste good any more. The decrease of gastric secretions may interfere with the absorption of iron and vitamin B_{12}. Fat digestion may be impaired if the liver produces less bile or the gallbladder is nonfunctional.

Neuromuscular System

Neuromuscular coordination decreases with age and conditions such as arthritis may hamper food preparation and the use of eating utensils. Muscles in the lower gastrointestinal tract become weaker with advancing age and constipation is a common problem. Many of the elderly turn to laxatives, which can interfere with nutrient absorption. Kidney repair and maintenance deteriorates with age, and renal function is impaired in some individuals. Fluid and electrolyte balance is difficult to maintain, especially during illness.

Eyes

Elderly persons may have difficulty in reading recipes or labels on foods.

Personal Factors

Apart from the physical changes just discussed, personal factors affect an elderly person's dietary and nutritional status, including fixed income, loneliness, and susceptibility to health claims. Often the elderly are existing on a fixed income that prevents an adequate food supply. This income deficit also affects housing and facilities, limiting cooking frequency and food storage. Without transportation, the elderly often purchase food from a nearby store or one that will deliver groceries. Such stores usually charge more for foods.

Social isolation affects the eating behaviors of the aged to a great extent. Elderly persons living alone lose their desire to cook or eat. Lonely people become apathetic, depressed, and fail to eat. They are more susceptible to illnesses and other stresses.

Many of the elderly purchase foods and supplements from health food stores because of advertisements claiming that the foods have curative power and may in fact retard the aging process.

Table 9-14 contains a week's sample of menus for older people.

THE ELDERLY: HEALTH PROBLEMS

Many of the health problems of the elderly are nutrition related. Some examples are discussed below.

1. Nutrient deficiencies—Recent studies have shown that the elderly are often deficient in protein, iron, calcium, and vitamins A and C. This increases the incidence of iron-deficiency anemia and osteoporosis, decreases resistance to infections, and lowers overall health status.
2. Alcoholism—This is a major problem among the elderly, especially for those living alone. Other drugs, either prescribed or illegally obtained, also interfere with the body's use of nutrients. Alcohol-drug interactions influence the entire life span, as does the abuse of prescription drugs. (See Chapter 10.)
3. Obesity—This results from reduced activity and caloric need and can complicate any existing problems as well as increase the development of others. Obesity also reduces mobility, increasing risk of falling accidents. As respiratory and cardiovascular functions deteriorate and arthritis conditions worsen, the quality of life is generally diminished. Lack of exercise is a factor in obesity throughout the life span. Exercise is discussed later in this chapter.
4. Osteoporosis—This disorder (see also Chapter 6) remains a major health problem among the elderly, especially women past the age of 60. Although the symptoms appear after menopause, researchers agree that the disorder begins as early as age 30. The 1989 RDAs reflect the young woman's increased needs. At present, no known preventive measure exits, but symptoms can be minimized with an adequate diet and regular exercise. Some believe that limited alcohol and caffeine consumption and a moderate fiber intake can also help. Extra calcium may be helpful, and some studies indicate that fluoride may increase bone density and relieve some symptoms.

Refer to Current Research Updates in Chapter 6 for more information on the role of calcium and fluoride in osteoporosis in the elderly.

5. Diabetes—Noninsulin-dependent diabetes is a common problem among middle-age and elderly people. Approximately 75% of those with diabetes of this type are overweight or obese. In most patients, the disease can be controlled by diet alone, and the most effective treatment is to reduce to and maintain a normal body weight. (See Chapter 18.)
6. Diverticulosis—This widespread problem is characterized by a weakening of the intestinal walls, resulting in diverticulosis. Low-fiber diets, along with weakened muscle tissue, are believed to be a causative agent in this disease.
7. Hypertension—This is a common disorder in the United States and tends to increase with age in many adults. Two nutritional factors believed to play a role in hypertension are salt and body fat. Excessive weight or obesity appears to be a more important factor than a high intake of salt. Recent studies indicate that a calcium deficit may also contribute to the incidence of hypertension.
8. Atherosclerosis—This is a leading medical problem in the elderly and can result in heart attack or stroke. Coronary heart disease is the leading cause of death in the United States. Diet is one of the risk factors involved in the development of the plaque that narrows the lining of the arteries and blocks the blood flow. This subject is discussed in more detail in Chapter 16.
9. Cancer—The second leading cause of death in the United States is cancer. Cancer has been the subject of much research in recent years, especially in the areas of pollutants, food additives, smoking, and diet. While the debate continues, the American Cancer Society's committee on diet and nutrition has issued four guidelines as preventive measures:
   a. Limiting fat intake to 30% of total (calories).
   b. Assuring an adequate (but not excessive) fiber intake to include fresh fruits, vegetables, and whole grains. Fruits and vegetables high in vitamin A are especially encouraged.
   c. Limiting intake of cured, smoked, and charcoal-broiled meats.
   d. Limiting intake of alcohol.

Three other major issues related to food habits and nutritional status are nutrition quackery; drug and nutrient interactions, including alcohol; and an appropriate exercise program. Chapter 10 is devoted entirely to drugs and nutrient interactions. A brief summary of nutrition quackery follows.

NUTRITION QUACKERY

Many people fall prey to claims made by medical quacks, especially people who are trying to cope with aging,

TABLE 9-14   A Week's Sample Menus for Older People

Snacks: Some suggested items are fresh fruit; soft, dried prunes; whole wheat crackers with cheese; cheese sticks; juices; peanut butter on toast; and yogurt. Snacks may be served in midmorning, midafternoon, and/or before bedtime. Five to six oz wine before meals may improve appetite.

Monday

Breakfast
½ c orange juice
1 poached egg
Whole wheat toast/
   margarine
½ c skim milk
Coffee or tea

Lunch
1 c braised beef tips on
   noodles
Celery or carrot sticks
Rye bread/margarine
1 c skim milk
1 orange, sliced

Dinner
Chicken breast, broiled
½ c buttered spinach
½ c wild rice
Hot roll/margarine
Fresh fruit: banana,
   melon, other
Decaffeinated coffee

Tuesday

Breakfast
½ c grapefruit juice
½ c cooked oatmeal, sugar,
   and skim milk
English muffin, 1 oz
   cheese

Lunch
Vegetable soup/crackers
Cottage cheese with
   pineapple salad
Banana
Toasted raisin bread with
   butter
Tea or decaffeinated coffee

Dinner
3 oz broiled fish/lemon
Boiled new potato/parsley
½ c creamed peas
Green onions
Whole wheat bread/mar-
   garine
Gingerbread, 1 square
Decaffeinated coffee

Wednesday

Breakfast
Sliced banana and milk
2 bran muffins/margarine/
   jelly
Cottage cheese
Coffee or tea

Lunch
1 c split pea soup/whole
   wheat crackers
Tomato and shredded
   lettuce salad/dressing
Skim milk
1 pear

Dinner
1 c beef and vegetable
   stew/cornbread sticks,
   margarine
½ c cabbage coleslaw
½ c rice pudding with
   raisins
Decaffeinated coffee/iced tea

Thursday

Breakfast
2 stewed prunes
2 French toast slices with
   butter and syrup
8 oz skim milk
Decaffeinated coffee/tea

Lunch
1 hamburger with
   onions/catsup/mus-
   tard/mayonnaise
Pickles, lettuce
French fries/catsup
Ice cream or sherbet
Skim milk

Dinner
Roast beef
½ c mashed potatoes
½ c buttered broccoli
1 sliced tomato with
   dressing
2 oatmeal cookies
Fruit cup

Friday

Breakfast
Sliced orange
1 c puffed rice with skim
   milk and sugar
Scrambled egg/wheat
   toast/margarine
Hot tea/coffee

Lunch
Tomato and rice
   soup/crackers
⅔ c potato salad with 2 oz
   turkey/ham
Celery or green pepper
   sticks
½ c strawberries/whip
   topping
Skim milk

Dinner
1 c tuna noodle casserole
½ c mixed lettuce salad
1 slice angel food cake
   with fruit cocktail
Decaffeinated coffee

Saturday

Breakfast
Melon or fresh fruit
2 hot
   cakes/margarine/syrup
1 sausage patty
8 oz skim milk
Coffee/tea

Lunch
Chicken nuggets
½ c green peas with mush-
   rooms
½ c carrot and raisin salad
Whole wheat bread/mar-
   garine
Banana pudding
Skim milk

Dinner
1 c spaghetti and meat-
   balls in tomato
   sauce/garlic bread
½ c string beans
½ c fruit gelatin
Decaffeinated coffee

Sunday

Breakfast
3 stewed figs
½ c hot cream of
   wheat/sugar
Skim milk
Cinnamon roll/margarine
2 slices crisp bacon
8 oz hot chocolate made
   with skim milk
Coffee or tea if desired

Lunch
2-egg cheese omelet
½ c steamed rice
½ c asparagus
Celery or carrot sticks
Toast/margarine/jelly
Peach halves
8 oz skim milk

Dinner
1 baked pork chop with
   applesauce
½ c buttered carrots
Mashed potatoes
Lettuce wedge/dressing
½ c custard
Decaffeinated coffee

Note: Each day's caloric contribution is about 1800 kcal. The amount can be increased or decreased by adjusting the serving sizes. Thus, the serving sizes of some items are not provided. To provide adequate RDAs, use the snacks to complete the foundation diet as discussed else-where. If there is concern about the cholesterol in eggs, replace some egg servings with lean meat (e.g., turkey, fish) or use cholesterol-free egg substitutes.

clinical disorders, or psychological problems. Individuals who buy these products because of their claims for cures, longevity, youthful appearance, and painless weight loss are uselessly spending billions of dollars per year. They pay high prices for worthless and unnecessary products. Such products are sometimes actually harmful, and many people delay seeking competent medical advice until it is too late.

It is important to distinguish between valid nutritional or health claims and false advertisements designed to sell ineffective and potentially harmful products. Recognizing valid claims from false ones can be aided by noting the following characteristics of faddist publications and products:

1. Citing research from bogus healthcare facilities (such as Granada Institute for Scientific Research and Holistic Health), or renowned ones (such as Mt. Sinai)
2. Making undocumented claims of success through testimonial evidence
3. Advertising unsubstantiated or unproven claims for products and services. Such advertising includes such wrongful claims as:
   a. "Most people are poorly nourished."
   b. "Sugar is a deadly poison."
   c. "All people need megavitamin Brand X because modern processing has taken all the nutrients from food."
   d. "All food additives and preservatives are poisonous."
   e. "Natural vitamins are better than synthetic ones."
   f. "It's easy to lose weight; lose seven pounds overnight."
   g. "Most diseases are due to faulty diet."
4. Promising quick dramatic cures. Examples include the following:
   a. "The medical community will not use these products because they would lose business."
   b. "Thousands cured of _____ (cancer, arthritis, balding) by using Pangamic Acid."
5. Selling certain substances as "vitamins," although scientifically they are not vitamins. Examples include the following:
   a. Vitamin P—Claims include curing ulcers, inner ear disorders, and asthma; preventing miscarriages, bleeding gums, acne, hemorrhage, rheumatic fever, hemorrhoids, and muscular dystrophy; and protecting the body from the danger of X-rays.
   b. Vitamin B_{15}—Claims include curing high blood pressure, asthma, rheumatism, alcoholism, atherosclerosis, and cancer.
   c. PABA—Claims include preventing hair from graying, delaying aging, restoring depigmented skin.
   d. Vitamin T—Claims include curing hemophilia, memory loss, and anemia.
   e. Vitamin B_{13}—Claims include curing multiple sclerosis, cancer, and hypertension.
   f. Vitamin F—Claims include curing cancer, eczema, psoriasis, dermatitis, and preventing heart disease.

Scientists identify the substances listed in Item 5 as follows:

   a. Vitamin P—A bioflavinoid of a group of substances from citrin, found in the white segment of citrus fruits. Gives characteristic taste, but is not a vitamin. Gives citrus fruit its flavor and holds the segments together.
   b. Vitamin B_{15}—No known composition; no vitamin activity; unknown safety. Not legally recognized as food or drug in the United States and Canada.
   c. PABA—A water-soluble substance found with folacin (a vitamin). Body makes its own PABA, and it is not recognized as a vitamin.
   d. Vitamin T—A product made from sesame seeds; not a vitamin.
   e. Vitamin B_{13} (orotic acid)—Unknown activity and not a vitamin.
   f. Vitamin F—An unsaturated fatty acid and not a vitamin.

The dietary supplement law of 1994 should help to alleviate some of the false health claims (see Chapter 1), but the problem remains for products already in the market. They were not covered under this law.

PROGRESS CHECK ON ACTIVITY 3

MULTIPLE CHOICE

Circle the letter of the correct answer.

1. The basic biological changes in old age center on:

   a. an increased basal metabolic rate.
   b. a gradual loss of functioning cells and reduced cell metabolism.
   c. an increased drug–nutrient absorption rate.
   d. all of the above.

2. Fewer calories are needed in the later years because:

   a. the aged tend to have less appetite.
   b. work will be reduced for the body processes.
   c. there is a gradual decrease in the rate of body metabolism.
   d. there is a decrease in the need for body repair.

3. Feelings (mental attitude) common in the aging process that may affect the nutritional status are:

   a. a sense of rejection and loneliness.
   b. weakness and insecurity.

c. disgust at the inability to chew foods thoroughly.
d. discomfort from poor digestion.

4. The increased use of salt and sugar as an individual grows older is because:

   a. of a special liking for very sweet or salty foods.
   b. of the development of poor food habits.
   c. such seasonings are familiar ones and are not expensive.
   d. of a decreased sense of taste and smell.

5. The nurse who works closely with elderly patients should recognize that the resistance to new foods, or to the familiar foods prepared in a different way, is one evidence of:

   a. feelings of insecurity.
   b. selfishness.
   c. decreased judgment.
   d. their reluctance to eat.

6. Which of the following food lists should be emphasized in planning a diet for an older person?

   a. whole grain breads and cereals, meat, potatoes, and other vegetables
   b. bread, jelly, fruits, butter, milk, and eggs
   c. fresh fruits, vegetables, milk, eggs, lean meat, and whole grain breads/cereals
   d. bland soft-cooked foods

7. An aged patient may best be helped to keep up an interest in food by:

   a. urging the patient to eat everything on the plate or tray.
   b. offering sweets between meals occasionally.
   c. including at least one food that the patient especially likes.
   d. explaining that the body needs that food to keep well.

8. Mrs. A tells you that she has trouble with constipation and that when she was at home she took mineral oil several times a week. Your best response to her would be based on the awareness that mineral oil:

   a. has 5 calories per gram which are "empty calories."
   b. is an ineffective laxative.
   c. increases the problem of constipation.
   d. interferes with the absorption of fat-soluble vitamins.

9. Mrs. A, because of her age and need for good nutrition with minimal caloric intake, should avoid "empty calories" found in:

   a. carbonated drinks.
   b. black coffee.

c. tomato juice.
d. iced tea.

10. To help you, your family, or patients, which one of these statements offers the best guide to good nutrition?

    a. Eating large amounts of food is one of the surest ways of being well nourished.
    b. Reading and following the latest information on diets is a good plan to follow to attain good nutrition.
    c. Eating a variety from the food groups is one of the surest ways to achieve good nutrition.
    d. Taking vitamin and mineral supplements in recommended amounts is the surest way to a well-nourished body.

11. In selecting the protein food for Mr. O, who is on a fat-restricted diet, which of these groups is the best?

    a. pork, cheese, and veal
    b. chicken, legumes, and ham
    c. eggs, cold cuts, and lean beef
    d. chicken, fish, and lean beef

12. A person with a decline in neuromuscular coordination or severe arthritis may find difficulty in:

    a. food preparation.
    b. use of eating utensils.
    c. shopping for food.
    d. all of the above.

13. The RDA for a 50-year-old for calcium is:

    a. 500 mg.
    b. 700 mg.
    c. 800 mg.
    d. 1000 mg.

14. To prevent the development of osteoporosis one needs to:

    a. have a lifelong adequate supply of calcium.
    b. have a lifelong adequate intake of fluoride.
    c. schedule physical workouts as part of a regular routine.
    d. all of the above.

15. The group of foods most neglected by the elderly is the:

    a. milk group.
    b. meat group.
    c. fruit and vegetable group.
    d. bread and cereal group.

16. Malnutrition among the elderly is most often caused by:

    a. loneliness.
    b. lack of education.

    c. poor housing.

    d. multiple disabilities.

17. Drugs commonly used that may interfere with nutrition include:

    a. laxatives.

    b. diuretics.

    c. vitamin/mineral megadoses.

    d. all of the above.

18. Women who take OCAs may have low levels of:

    a. B vitamins and vitamin C.

    b. vitamin C and iron.

    c. calcium and magnesium.

    d. vitamin A and calcium.

19. Women who use an IUD may be low in:

    a. B vitamins and vitamin C.

    b. vitamin C and iron.

    c. calcium and magnesium.

    d. vitamin A and calcium.

TRUE/FALSE

Circle T for True and F for False.

20. T F There is about a 7.5% increase in the need for calories in each decade past the age of 25 years.

21. T F The simplest basis for judging adequacy of caloric intake is the maintenance of normal weight.

22. T F Most elderly persons require additional supplements of vitamins and minerals.

23. T F Older persons are frequent victims of food faddists' claims.

24. T F Obesity may be considered a form of malnutrition.

25. T F Chronologically, the aging process begins after age 65.

26. T F The elderly person is likely to experience reduced body functioning due to physiological changes, disease, and/or psychological factors.

27. T F Taste and smell acuity decreases with advancing age.

28. T F The need for essential amino acids lessens considerably during the aging process.

FILL-IN

29. Why may an elderly person find it necessary to shop for food at markets that may be higher in cost but close to his or her home?

    _____

    _____

30. What are two contributing factors in the reduced caloric needs of elderly persons?

    a. _____

    b. _____

31. Nutrient needs for the elderly _____ compared to younger adults (remain the same/decrease).

32. Obesity is an increased risk for many elderly persons, especially women. What are three problems experienced by obese elderly persons?

    a. _____

    b. _____

    c. _____

33. What might be one factor contributing to iron-deficiency anemia in the elderly? _____

    _____

34. What three nutrients besides iron are often found deficient in the diets of elderly persons?

    a. _____

    b. _____

    c. _____

35. What are two unique benefits of food supplementation through the Nutrition Program for the Elderly?

    a. _____

    b. _____

ACTIVITY 4:

Exercise, Fitness, and Stress-Reduction Principles

Adulthood covers a broad chronological span in which many physical and physiological changes occur. Clearly, genetic factors play a large part in longevity, but recent research indicates that regular exercise, fitness, especially cardiovascular fitness, and reduction of stress lead to extended life spans. The quality of life is also enhanced.

One major concern of adults of any age is physical appearance. Physical appearance is largely a matter of genetics, having inherited the general size and shape that we now possess. However, a determination of body fat may reveal that size and shape can be altered. Since there is a national disdain for fat and since poor body image contributes to social stigma as well as health problems, it is desirable to attain and maintain a healthy body weight.

The role of exercise in maintaining positive body image and physical fitness cannot be overlooked. It is especially beneficial when combined with a healthy eating pattern.

PHYSICAL FITNESS

Although recent polls show that well over half of the adults in the United States participate in some form of exercise, most people are not educated to physical fitness requirements. The key elements to physical fitness include frequency of activity, duration of activity, intensity of activity, and type of activity. The first step in beginning a quest for physical fitness involves program selection. To become physically fit, a program must be selected to reach individual goals. This is important for continued good health.

Exercise testing can calculate the functional capacity of the cardiovascular system, a measurement important to exercise program selection. The goal in such testing is to determine predicted heart rate without causing chest pain.

EXERCISE AND NUTRITIONAL FACTORS

The effects of controlled exercise are clearly beneficial. Experts believe that the recent decline in cardiovascular mortality is a result of increased health consciousness throughout society and the practice of a regular exercise regimen combined with proper nutrition.

Most studies have shown that exercise decreases blood pressure in hypertensive patients, though such findings have not been conclusive. Similar studies have demonstrated that active men have blood pressure lower than inactive men. Exercise has been shown to decrease smoking. Numerous studies have confirmed that exercise lowers the levels of triglycerides in the blood. The blood levels of HDL cholesterol, thought to provide protection against heart disease, increase with exercise. In response to such findings, exercise has become a basic part of the rehabilitation program for patients who have undergone bypass surgery, as well as for those who have angina pectoris or who have suffered a myocardial infarction. Except for patients with certain diseases, such as congestive heart failure, acute myocarditis, or unstable angina pectoris, exercise programs can decrease morbidity and mortality.

AN IDEAL PROGRAM

The ideal physical fitness program must be suited to both health considerations and goals. For example, certain programs will yield increased strength; others will yield increased flexibility; yet others will increase cardiac and respiratory endurance. Although all these goals are worthwhile and can be achieved simultaneously if desired, the most important goal is stimulating the heart and circulatory system. A physical fitness training session is characterized by a warm-up period, an endurance phase, occasional competition, and finally a cooling-down period. Typically the session will last up to an hour in total. Patients undergoing rehabilitation will normally be limited to about half that time.

Frequency and intensity vary according to the individual's medical and exercise history, but three sessions weekly, performed at 70% or greater of a person's maximum heart rate, usually provides sufficient exercise to keep the body conditioned. Three days per week allows ample time for recovery, so the body in general, and critical organs in particular, do not become stressed. The duration of a physical fitness program depends on the body's condition when training is begun. For flexibility and strength programs, exercise must continue after the goal is attained to prevent loss of what has been achieved. An effective program includes good dietary habits that provide optimal nutrition and adequate calories, a diet low in fat but high in energy foods, such as complex carbohydrates.

CALORIC COSTS AND RUNNING

Exercise spends calories. For example, studies of running have determined that pace has little effect on calorie expenditure. Two men of equal body weight who run the same distance will expend about the same number of calories, regardless of whether one is in top physical condition and the other is a neophyte runner. Put another way, a 150-lb man will utilize approximately 1 kcal per pound in running 1-½ miles in 10 minutes. The same man would utilize about 140 calories in covering the same distance in 16 minutes.

When caloric costs are known, exercise can be used to control weight. If 100 extra calories per day are expended, a weight loss of 10 lb per year can be expected. Or, an individual who eats 3000 calories per day and expends 200 calories per day through exercise can eat an additional 200 calories per day without gaining weight.

The key to physical fitness lies in tailoring a program to meet individual needs. If exercise uses more calories than are consumed, weight loss results. Attempts to gain or lose weight can affect both health and performance and should therefore be under supervision. Attempts to gain or lose weight should follow certain basic health guidelines, and nutritious foods from all the food groups should be included. Supplements should not be necessary, except for female athletes, who may require iron and folic acid. Sufficient time to achieve weight loss should be allowed.

A GOOD SPORTS BEVERAGE

The following factors regulate the desirable and recommended ingredients, apart from water, in a sports beverages:

1. Desirable forms of carbohydrate added include some forms that are familiar to us (glucose, sucrose) and

some that are not so familiar (maltodextrin and high fructose corn syrup).

2. For a 6% carbohydrate drink, one should consume about 2–4 c.

3. The carbohydrate concentration should not exceed 10% since it can slow stomach emptying.

4. Electrolytes are of importance for events longer than 4 hours. Sodium, potassium, chloride, and phosphorus loss in the sweat can be replaced by a drink with these electrolytes added.

5. The taste of a drink can be a determining factor in the amount of fluid consumed.

6. Carbonation is discouraged because it may lower fluid intake.

STRESS AND SPECIAL POPULATIONS

The developmental tasks at each stage of the life span offer different stresses and challenges. Successfully completing these tasks is a form of growth. Failure to meet the tasks results in stress, which has multiple effects on the body systems.

Stressors can be biological, psychological, or sociological. Some of the effects of stress at different stages in the life cycle are included in the following examples.

Parents of newborns often find that their lifestyles have been disrupted in many ways they had not expected. Parents of toddlers are stressed by the inquisitiveness shown by children this age. As children grow, their parents' stress increases. Adolescence, the age at which children begin to assert their independence, is particularly painful. Adults who are responsible for the care of their aging parents also experience distress at this added responsibility.

Working adults experience overload and burnout, and the symptoms become progressively more serious over time unless stress reduction can be achieved. Older adults moving from the workforce to retirement encounter many stresses. They may feel a loss of productivity and thus a loss of usefulness. Loneliness and boredom may also be present in those who make no attempt to alleviate these feelings. Primary losses of the aging are losses of physical capacity to care for oneself, lapses of memory, diminished physique, and the death of old friends.

Adults who develop good coping mechanisms such as aerobic exercise, positive nutritional habits, and planned relaxation can stop the progression of symptoms and reverse extreme stages of stress. A word of caution: although stress management is a popular topic, some of the advertised products to fight stress, such as special "stress" vitamins, cassette recordings, and machines of various kinds, may, in fact, cost the consumer much more financially than the consumer will receive in benefits, and thus may increase stress. The prudent course is still to follow proven avenues for health maintenance. Health maintenance refers to measures that will enable an individual to stay young and healthy in body and mind for as many years as possible. These measures include becoming aware of the consequences of imprudent dieting, and often, changing a lifetime of poor eating habits. It also means educating oneself to refute invalid claims for quick fixes and to recognize valid basic factors. It includes paying attention to body signals and learning in what ways and how to relax, when and how to exercise, and, best of all, how to make healthy choices and enjoy the rest of life.

PROGRESS CHECK ON ACTIVITY 4

FILL-IN

1. Name the key elements of establishing a physical fitness regime.

   a. _____

   b. _____

   c. _____

   d. _____

2. An exercise testing is done primarily to make the following determination:

   _____

3. List three beneficial effects of regular exercise.

   a. _____

   b. _____

   c. _____

4. Name the components of a physical fitness training session.

   a. _____

   b. _____

   c. _____

   d. _____

5. An effective fitness program includes good dietary habits. Describe the eating pattern that will meet this criterion.

   _____

   _____

   _____

   _____

   _____

6. Situation: If Mary drinks 6 oz of regular soda pop per day, and it contains approximately 100 calories more than her caloric output of 2000 calories, what will be the outcome if she does this each day for one year? Choose an answer from below and give your rationale.

   a. Nothing will happen; 100 calories extra per day shouldn't count.
   b. She'll probably lose weight, as her diet is unbalanced.
   c. She'll gain about 10 pounds over the year's time.
   d. It will increase her fluid intake, which is healthy.
   e. She will have higher energy levels.

7. Identify four health problems brought about by unrelieved stress.

   a. _____

   b. _____

   c. _____

   d. _____

8. Name three ways to help alleviate some of the stress encountered by adults of all ages.

   a. _____

   b. _____

   c. _____

9. "Stress Tabs" are a popular vitamin supplement on the market and a lot of people buy them. They contain primarily vitamin C and the B complex. Evaluate this product designed for stress management based on your previous knowledge.

   _____

   _____

10. Define health maintenance.

   _____

   _____

SUMMARY

Nutrition plays an important role throughout all phases of the life span. The information following summarizes the key points discussed in Activities 1, 2, 3, and 4 of this chapter.

Optimal nutrition during pregnancy is critical. New tissue is formed at this time, including the developing baby, materials for nourishing the embryo and fetus, and the mother's own body. Pregnancy is divided into three trimesters with each trimester covering three months. Each trimester requires more nutrients than the last. When the fetus's cells are dividing rapidly, the mother's intake of unhealthy food or other substances can have dramatic and sometimes tragic consequences. The desirable weight gain for a healthy pregnant woman ranges between 24 and 30 pounds. The pattern of weight gain and the foods eaten to achieve the gain are most important. The diet should be chosen for nutrient density and balance and must be carefully planned. Certain supplements are usually recommended and should be prescribed.

The first year of life is the most rapid growth period of all and, consequently, the infant has the highest nutrient needs. A healthy full-term infant will have some reserve supplies of some nutrients, but will need replenishing after four to six months.

Both breast- and bottle-feeding can produce a healthy child, each having advantages and disadvantages. While breast milk is uniquely suited to infant needs, formulas can be satisfactory. Psychological, cultural, safety, and health factors need to be considered before choosing the feeding method. Infants need solids added to their diet at about four to six months of age. Developmental readiness is a consideration. Solid foods should be added one at a time and the child observed for reactions.

The food intake of young children is erratic. While their growth has slowed, muscle and skeletal tissue is developing. Their nutrient needs remain high, although caloric intake may decrease. During these years, the most important thing a caregiver can do for a child is to provide a basis for sound eating habits. This is sometimes difficult and always challenging, as advertising, peer pressure, and poor examples influence the child as well as his or her own developmental tasks. Understanding childhood behavior patterns is necessary in order to cope with the growing child. Obesity and iron-deficiency anemia are nutritional problems in this age group.

The second greatest growth spurt of life happens in the adolescent years. Again, nutrient demands are high. Many factors, except concern for the state of health, influence a teenager's eating habits. There is an intense obsession with physical appearance, especially as it relates to weight for girls and athletic performance for boys. The bizarre eating habits of the teenage girl not only make her the least well-nourished of any group in the United States but may also precipitate eating disorders, such as anorexia nervosa and bulimia.

Teenage pregnancies present many medical and nutritional problems, putting both mother and baby at great risk. Since one in five babies is born to a teenage mother, these young women should receive nutrition counseling, government support, and some form of health monitoring by health agencies. Common health problems among teenagers include anemia, calcium deficiency, vitamin C deficiency, alcohol and drug abuse, and obesity.

Having completed the growth cycle of adolescence, the adult settles into maturity, which requires consuming adequate nutrients to maintain and repair body tissue, maintaining a normal weight, getting regular exercise, and avoiding excess stress. These health maintenance measures are believed to prevent or delay the onset of chronic degenerative diseases and improve the quality of later life. The loss of tissue and organ functioning that accompanies the aging process takes place gradually. Generally, scientists believe that the aging process is genetically determined, but most agree that a lifelong commitment to good eating habits and adequate exercise can modify health and longevity. No studies have shown that any special foods or supplements can prolong life any longer than can a regular balanced diet. Nutrition status in the later years is affected not only by food intake and physiological factors but also by stress, poverty, loneliness, and low self-esteem. Middle-aged and older adults are especially susceptible to nutritional quackery.

Drugs and alcohol affect the nutrition of the adult and many drug-nutrient reactions are harmful. Cardiovascular, renal, hepatic, and neuromuscular disorders often develop in these years.

Adults of all ages can get the nutrients they need by following the guidelines for a balanced diet, such as the *Dietary Guidelines for Americans*, the daily food guides, and other guides as described in Chapter 1.

Nutrition plays a role in each stage of the life cycle. Good eating habits should be developed on a continuum throughout life, so that each stage meets the current needs and passes on good nutritional status to the next stage.

The quality of life is enhanced throughout the life cycle whenever principles of optimum nutrition, physical fitness, a healthy weight, and positive mechanisms for coping with stress are recognized, understood, and followed. All of these principles can be learned, thus changing behavior patterns and contributing to a long, healthy, and happy life.

RESPONSIBILITIES OF HEALTH PERSONNEL

A health worker should impart the following information to clients:

1. Young adults who use oral contraceptives should be informed that they need extra folacin, riboflavin, and vitamins C, B_6, and B_{12}.
2. Young women who use IUDs should be informed that they need to compensate for extra menstrual losses with extra iron and vitamin C.
3. A basic food guide should be followed by adults of all ages for optimum nutrition. The only nutritional decrease should be in the caloric intake as aging occurs. The RDA for energy for ages 50 to 75 is 90% of that for the young adult. The RDA for energy for ages over 75 is approximately 75% of that for the young adult.

4. The older adult may need to avoid foods that are difficult to chew.
5. Older adults should be discouraged from overusing laxatives.
6. Adults should be aware that both physiological and psychological factors affect their nutritional well-being.
7. Drugs (including alcohol) can adversely affect nutritional status and foods can interfere with some drug therapies.
8. Adults benefit from using foods that are good sources of fiber.
9. Consuming more high-calcium foods may help to alleviate osteoporosis, a leading disorder in later adulthood.
10. People should not delay adopting good dietary habits until middle age. The dietary guidelines are sensible eating guides and should be followed from adolescence to old age.
11. People on medication should ascertain from their healthcare professional if nutrient supplements are needed to counteract adverse effects of a drug.
12. People treated for a disease requiring a modified diet should seek assistance from a professional, preferably a registered dietitian.
13. Various programs are designed to help adults meet their nutritional requirements.
14. Elderly people cope better with changes brought on by aging if they are advised or assisted to do the following:
    a. Select nutrient-dense foods that are low in fat, permitting adequate nutrients without weight gain.
    b. Drink plenty of liquids, two to three quarts a day. Water is good for the body and has no calories.
    c. Accommodate chewing problems by cutting, chopping, or grinding food when necessary.
    d. Follow a modified diet, if one is prescribed.
    e. Avoid excess salt and try new spices to make food taste better.
    f. Find and use outside resources to improve social interactions and eating habits, such as senior centers, neighborhood groups, exercise groups, Meals on Wheels, extension services, voluntary community services for elders (e.g., free transportation, discounts).
    g. Interact with family and friends, stay in touch, and not become isolated.
    h. Keep physically fit.
15. Many acceptable exercise and fitness programs are designed for people of all ages and various states of health and mobility. The health worker should encourage selecting and following a suitable plan.
16. Stress-reduction techniques and materials should be provided whenever the client indicates need.

REFERENCES

American Dietetic Association. (2006). *Nutrition Diagnosis: A Critical Step in Nutrition Care Process.* Chicago: American Dietetic Association.

Bartley, K. A. (2005). A life cycle micronutrient perspective for women's health. *American Journal of Clinical Nutrition 81*: 1188s–1193s.

Bendich, A., & Deckelbaum, R. J. (Eds.). (2005). *Preventive Nutrition: The Comprehensive Guide for Health Professionals* (3rd ed.). Totowa, NJ: Humana Press.

Branca, F. (2002). Impact of micronutrients deficiencies on growth: The stunting syndrome. *Annals of Nutrition & Metabolism, 46*(Suppl. 1): 8–17.

Deen, D., & Hark, L. (2007). *The Complete Guide to Nutrition in Primary Care.* Malden, MA: Blackwell.

Devine, C. M. (2005). A life course perspective: Understanding food choices in time, social location, and history. *Journal of Nutrition Education and Behavior, 37*: 121–128.

Eastwood, M. (2003). *Principles of Human Nutrition* (2nd ed.). Malden, MA: Blackwell Science.

Escott-Stump, S. (2002). *Nutrition and Diagnosis-Related Care* (5th ed.). Philadelphia: Lippincott, Williams and Wilkins.

Fernandez-Ballart, J. (2001). Preventive nutritional supplementation throughout the reproductive life cycle. *Public Health Nutrition, 4*: 1363–1366.

Garrow, J. S. (2000). *Human Nutrition and Dietetics* (10th ed.). New York: Churchill Livingston.

Gershwin, M. E., Netle, P., & Keen, C. (Eds.). (2004). *Handbook of Nutrition and Immunity.* Totowa, NJ: Humana Press.

Haas, E., & Levin, M. (2006). *Staying Healthy with Nutrition: The Complete Guide to Diet and Nutrition Medicine* (21st ed.). Berkeley, CA: Celestial Arts.

Hark, L., & Morrison, G. (Eds.). (2003). *Medical Nutrition and Disease* (3rd ed.). Malden, MA: Blackwell.

Holick, M. F. (2001). The influence of vitamin D on bone health across the life cycle. *Journal of Nutrition, 135*: 2726s–2727s.

Jackson, A. A. (2005). Integrating the ideas of life course across cellular, individual, and population levels in cancer causation. *Journal of Nutrition, 135*: 2927s–2933s.

Katz, D. L. (2001). *Nutrition in Clinical Practice* (2nd ed.). Philadelphia: Lippincott, Williams and Wilkins.

Mahan, L. K., & Escott-Stump, S. (Eds.). (2008). *Krause's Food and Nutrition Therapy* (12th ed.). Philadelphia: Elsevier Sauders.

Mayo Clinic. (2004). *Mayo Clinic Guide to a Healthy Pregnancy.* Rochester, MN: Mayo Clinic.

Moore, M. C. (2005). *Pocket Guide to Nutritional Assessment and Care* (5th ed.). St. Louis, MO: Elvesier Mosby.

Payne-James, J., & Wicks, C. (2003). *Key Facts in Clinical Nutrition* (2nd ed.). London: Greenwich Medical Media.

Shils, M. E., & Shike, M. (Eds.). (2006). *Modern Nutrition in Health and Disease* (10th ed.). Philadelphia: Lippincott, Williams and Wilkins.

Temple, N. J., Wilson, T., & Jacobs, D. R. (2006). *Nutrition health: Strategies for Disease Prevention* (2nd ed.). Totowa, NJ: Humana Press.

Thomas, B., & Bishop, J. (Eds.). (2007). *Manual of Dietetic Practice* (4th ed.). Ames, IA: Blackwell.

Wethington, E. (2005). An overview of the life course perspective: Implications for health and nutrition. *Journal of Nutrition Education and Behavior, 37*: 115–120.

CHAPTER **10**

Drugs and Nutrition

Time for completion
Activities: 1½ hours
Optional examination: ½ hour

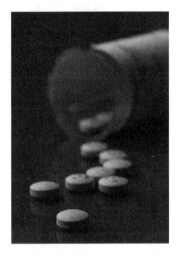

OBJECTIVES

Upon completion of this chapter the student should be able to do the following:

1. Describe the effects of drugs on the utilization of nutrients.
2. Describe the effects of nutrients on the utilization of drugs.
3. Identify food and drug incompatibilities.
4. Accurately assess a client's response to food and drug interactions.
5. Provide specific instructions to clients regarding their diet and drug therapy.

GLOSSARY

Actions: drug actions are grouped according to the body system for which they are specific. The student should consult a physicians' desk reference (PDR) or pharmacopoeia for details. General actions of drugs are listed here.
  1. **Additive:** effects of two drugs are equal to the sum of each.
  2. **Cumulative:** concentration of a drug in the body increases with each successive dose.
  3. **Synergistic:** combined effects of certain drugs are greater than that of the individual drugs.

4. **Tolerance:** drug must be increased to produce the same effect.

5. **Toxicity:** potentially harmful side effects from the use of a drug.

Anti: against. Many drugs work against diseases or disorders. Examples include antibiotics (against infections), antidepressants (against depression), and so on.

Bioavailability: degree to which a drug or other substance becomes available for body use after administration.

Chelate (*kee-late*): form a chemical compound (with another drug or food).

CNS: central nervous system.

MAO: monoamine oxidase, a drug used to treat psychiatric illness.

OCA: oral contraceptive agent.

OTC: over the counter.

PDR: physicians' desk reference.

pH: acidity or alkalinity of fluids and compounds.

Teratogen: agent capable of producing adverse effects.

BACKGROUND INFORMATION

General Considerations

Only in the past decade has the multiple effect of the interactions of drugs and nutrients been recognized. Many drugs and nutrients that are prescribed produce a different effect than was originally intended. Drugs affect taste, appetite, intestinal motility, absorption, and metabolism of nutrients. Many of these interactions compromise nutritional status and health.

The effect of nutrients on drugs is equally important. Food may delay drug absorption, alter drug metabolism by enzyme induction or inhibition, or alter the rate of drug excretion and drug response.

Most people are tremendously concerned about the relationship between drug usage and nutrition. This concern involves not only illicit drugs such as cocaine or marijuana, but many prescription and over-the-counter drugs as well.

The effects of drugs on the body can vary widely. Numerous factors produce these varying results. Consider, for example, the usage difference that can occur. The drug can vary; the dosage can vary; time and frequency of consumption can vary. Reactions also vary according to the health status of the drug user. If body nutrition is good, the body can effectively deal with a larger drug dose than it could otherwise handle. Conversely, a malnourished person may require a higher dosage to produce a desired therapeutic effect. Finally, the ability to absorb drugs and nutrients varies; for example, because of age or differences in digestive juice production, drug response can vary.

Nutritional status can be affected by single or multiple drug therapy. Effects may be short term or long term. In the digestive system, effects such as diarrhea, constipation, nausea and vomiting, and altered taste and smell sensitivity may occur, changing intestinal absorption, utilization, storage, synthesis, and metabolism of nutrients. Of special concern is how drugs can affect the body's ability to manufacture and metabolize nutrients.

The effects of drugs on nutrients are profound. They may directly destroy or change the nutrient, damage intestinal walls, and/or lower absorption. Drugs can directly destroy, displace, or change the nutrients themselves.

Inside the human body, a drug can join with a nutrient, rendering the nutrient incapable of being utilized normally. When this occurs, the nutrient will simply be excreted by the kidney.

Drugs affect all nutrients-carbohydrates, fat, protein, vitamins, minerals-to varying extents. For example, drugs can cause fat to be deposited in the liver, can cause blood insulin levels to fluctuate, can reduce body vitamin storage, and can increase excretion of minerals in the urine.

Ingestion

Drugs affect nutrient ingestion by causing changes in appetite, taste, and smell. Common side effects of many medications administered orally or parenterally are nausea and vomiting, resulting in decreased food intake. Some drugs, such as antidepressants, antihistamines, and oral contraceptives increase appetite. A small amount of alcohol before meals will increase saliva and gastric secretions and stimulate the taste buds.

Drugs that decrease food intake include amphetamines, cholinergic agents, some expectorants, and narcotic analgesics. In the elderly patient, tranquilizers often cause a decrease in food intake because of slow metabolism and disinterest in food and surroundings.

Bulk-forming medications may reduce appetite by creating a feeling of fullness. Some may decrease appetite by inhibiting gastric emptying.

Drugs that affect taste or have offensive odors decrease intake. Examples include penicillamine, streptomycin, potassium chloride, vitamin B complex liquids, and some chemotherapies.

Nausea and vomiting may occur with many drugs, causing a decrease in food intake. Examples include oral hypoglycemic agents, cancer chemotherapeutic agents, and many antibiotics given orally.

Patients on diets with sugar or sodium restrictions should be monitored for intake of drugs containing glucose and sodium or other restrictive nutrients. Cough syrups, expectorants, and elixirs contain large amounts of glucose. Many antibiotics and parenteral solutions contain large amounts of sodium.

Absorption

The most frequently reported diet-drug interaction involves alteration of the bioavailability of the drug because of concurrent food ingestion. At the same time, the drug may alter the absorption of various nutrients.

Absorption of drugs and nutrients occurs by different means. Drug absorption is governed by its physical form, particle size, gastrointestinal pH, and solubility in fats. Nutrient absorption, on the other hand, depends upon an intact enzyme system and gastrointestinal secretions. The small intestine is the major site for drug and nutrient interactions.

Drugs causing malabsorption induce diarrhea, steatorrhea, and weight loss. Abdominal pain, flatulence, and nutrient deficits may also occur.

Metabolism

Alterations in metabolism can be caused by drug interference with the enzyme system or drug-induced vitamin antagonists.

Nutritional imbalances are known to affect the metabolism of drugs. To handle a drug properly, the body requires many nutrients: niacin, riboflavin, pantothenic acid, ascorbic acid, folic acid, vitamin B_{12}, protein (amino acids), fat, glucose, iron, copper, calcium, zinc, and magnesium. If any nutrient is lacking, normal drug metabolism can be diminished. The toxicity of the drug may be increased or decreased by the metabolic alteration. In effect, the altered metabolism yields a change in the dosage's planned therapeutic effect, rendering the dosage either too high or too low under the circumstances.

In humans, an extreme nutrient deficiency or an extreme nutrient excess can be expected to unbalance drug metabolism. When protein is lacking, manufacture of important enzymes involved in drug metabolism is reduced. For example, many protein-deficient children are infested with hookworms. The drug used to combat hookworms, tetrachloroethylene, is known to be toxic in high doses, yet undernourished children do not exhibit toxic effects when given large doses of the drug. It is thought that because of the depressed quality of the enzymes involved, the drug forms fewer of the usual toxic by-products.

Excretion

Drugs affect nutrient excretion by altering reabsorption or transport. It may also alter the kidneys' ability to concentrate. Some drugs affect specific nutrients more than others. Examples include the effect that diuretics have on calcium and potassium excretion, and the increased excretion of ascorbic acid due to aspirin therapy. Aspirin in large doses also depletes potassium.

Foods affect drug excretion by changing urine pH and causing the precipitation of certain drugs. Retention of salt and fluids is another undesirable effect associated with drug-nutrient interactions. Examples include steroids, antihypertensives, and estrogens.

PROGRESS CHECK ON BACKGROUND INFORMATION

FILL-IN

Define:

1. Cumulative _____

2. Synergistic _____

3. Toxicity _____

4. Antibiotic _____

5. Chelate _____

6. OCA _____

7. OTC _____

8. Teratogen _____

9. Drugs profoundly affect nutrient utilization. List five ways in which this effect is accomplished.

   a. _____
   b. _____
   c. _____
   d. _____
   e. _____

10. Describe the most common symptoms exhibited by the digestive tract in response to drug therapy.

    a. _____
    b. _____
    c. _____

11. Drug effects on the body depend on five major variances. Name them.

    a. _____
    b. _____
    c. _____
    d. _____
    e. _____

12. Metabolism alterations may be due to what two major factors?

    a. _____

    b. _____

13. The body requires 14 nutrients in adequate amounts in order to properly metabolize a drug. Name five of them.

    a. _____

    b. _____

    c. _____

    d. _____

    e. _____

14. Drugs affect nutrient excretion by altering _____ and _____.

15. Foods affect drug excretion by causing _____ or _____.

ACTIVITY 1:

Food and Drug Interactions

EFFECTS OF FOOD ON DRUGS

Food can make a drug more or less effective. Just as drugs can interfere with our food utilization, so too can foods and nutrients affect the action of drugs. Foods can change drug absorption, neutralize drug effects, interact with drugs, and influence their excretion rate.

Doctors prescribe drugs for maximum therapeutic effect. Yet, it has long been assumed that the presence of food in the intestinal tract, the primary absorption site, affects the absorption of most drugs. The extent of this effect remains unclear. Food can increase or decrease acidity, digestive secretions, and intestinal motility. Such effects directly determine whether a drug will be easily destroyed, how long it will stay in the intestine, whether a drug will become crystals, whether a drug will be absorbed at all, and other technical changes.

Dietary minerals such as iron, magnesium, calcium, and aluminum salts demonstrate how food chemicals or nutrients can affect drug absorption. These minerals can chemically join with tetracycline, a commonly used antibiotic, to form tiny solid particles (insoluble precipitate). Simultaneous ingestion of these minerals and tetracycline causes the drug to lose its therapeutic value, requiring a large dose to offset the loss. This example shows that the common practice of taking such drugs with food or liquids to mask the drug taste may be questionable. Patients should be given specific directions about combining drugs with meals or snacks, including the rationale for them.

Vitamins are considered drugs if they are used for pharmacological effects. For example, if a person has a bladder infection and a megadose of vitamin C is prescribed, the vitamin C is not being used for its characteristics as a vitamin but rather is being prescribed to acidify the urine. Such use is pharmacological rather than nutritional. Niacin, a B vitamin, is similarly used to lower blood cholesterol.

Administering medications with meals is a common practice to reduce gastrointestinal side effects, but this practice can also result in reduced, delayed, or altered drug action. Using food as a vehicle to administer crushed tablets or to disguise taste can also affect the drug's action if the food alters the pH or chelate of the drug. Oral medications are affected by food in the gastrointestinal tract, the pH of the stomach and small intestine, and the motility of the gastrointestinal tract.

Fatty foods and high-fat, low-fiber meals slow the emptying of the stomach by as much as two hours. The action of a drug administered with or after such a meal would be similarly slowed. High-protein meals increase gastric blood flow and increase the absorption of some drugs. Meals high in glucose cause a slight, transient decrease in blood flow to the gastrointestinal tract, which tends to decrease drug absorption.

EFFECTS OF DRUGS ON FOOD

There is increasing evidence that drug and food interactions can compromise a patient's nutritional status and ultimately a patient's health.

Impaired absorption is a common mechanism by which drugs interfere with vitamin homeostasis. Mineral oil, the first agent found to cause malabsorption, forms an insoluble complex in which the fat-soluble vitamins (A, E, D, and K) pass through the gut before absorption takes place. Elderly patients who are chronic users of mineral oil may be at risk for developing rickets due to malabsorption of vitamin D.

Certain drugs induce enzyme systems that require vitamin cofactors. This may increase vitamin needs. Some drugs compete with vitamins for the sites of action. Additionally, some drugs decrease endogenous nutrient synthesis. For example, the broad spectrum antibiotics interfere with vitamin K synthesis by microorganisms normally present in the colon.

It is now firmly established that oral contraceptives definitely result in a deficiency of vitamin B_6 in about 10%–30% of pill users. The high incidence of headache and depression among these patients is now traced to a lack of this vitamin. Apparently, reduction of vitamin B_6 participation in body metabolism of brain chemicals indirectly causes the depression and headache.

Various efforts have been made to remedy the adverse effects of the pill on the patient's nutritional status. Including vitamins and minerals in the pill has been suggested. Regular blood and urine checking for the levels of vitamins and minerals is another alternative. However, medical politics, clinical philosophies, technical uncertainties, and other factors have prevented any major health policy from being adopted.

Even common aspirin can cause nutritional problems. Chronic salicylate therapy has been shown both to decrease uptake of vitamin C in leukocytes and impair the protein-binding ability of folate.

The more common drug-induced deficiencies that are known have been presented here. Very likely many drug-nutrient interactions that have not yet been recognized take place in acute or chronic therapy, and more data are needed about the interactions that are known.

Both preventive and corrective measures are needed to ensure that therapeutic drug use will not harm a patient's nutritional status. More clinical studies are needed, as are long-range programs, since the complexities regarding the relationship between drugs and nutrition require careful study. Further study is especially needed among populations who take drugs for long periods; for example, women taking oral contraceptives and older Americans.

FOOD AND DRUG INCOMPATIBILITIES

Certain foods and beverages are known to be incompatible with therapeutic drugs. These incompatible reactions occur as the result of pharmacologically active ingredients in the food, notably ethyl alcohol and various amines. These food ingredients react especially with drugs for treating psychiatric illness (monoamine oxidase inhibitors) and alcohol abuse (disulfiram).

Cheese and other foods contain the chemical tyramine (and its related amines). Drugs such as these are often prescribed for treating depression. Tyramine can react with procarbazine to create a "hypertensive crisis" in a patient. Reaction can occur within one-half to one hour after consuming the incompatible substance.

Alcohol, hot beverages, and antacids should not be given with sustained-release tablets or capsules because these substances can cause premature erosion of the pH-sensitive coating on the drug. Enteric-coated tablets should not be given with alkaline meals or antacids.

Many drugs, particularly central nervous system depressants, should not be taken in conjunction with alcohol because of a cumulative depressant effect. Other drugs combined with alcohol intake produce an effect similar to disulfiram (Antabuse), with an acute onset of facial flushing, dyspnea, nausea and vomiting, palpitation, headache, and hypotension. Alcohol consumed with some drugs increases the potential for gastric irritation and bleeding.

The severity of reaction depends on the drug dosage, amount of food ingested, patient susceptibility, and the interval between drug and food consumption. The severity of reaction can also be affected by the condition of the food.

Practicing physicians and all health professionals are encouraged to be familiar with drug-nutrition relationships. They are also encouraged to be at the forefront of efforts to reduce drug-induced malnutrition.

CLINICAL IMPLICATIONS

Patient instructions that appear on all drugs, prescription or OTC, include warnings of possible interactions with food and beverages, and many packaged food products bear warning labels regarding possible interactions with certain drugs as well. While this activity does not have space to list them, for your reference, Appendix D reproduces a brochure distributed by the U.S. Food and Drug Administration and the National Consumers League. The material contained is a helpful tool for your own information as well as for patient teaching. Appendix D describes various drugs and their interactions with nutrients in foods. Here, we will describe four examples of clinical interventions to reduce or eliminate such interactions.

1. Anticonvulsants are used to treat such conditions as seizures. Since they interfere with the absorption of nutrients in food, they should not be taken with foods or feedings, especially in children.
2. Antifungal agents are used to treat fungal infections. Since they increase kidney excretions, especially electrolytes, supplementation with electrolytes (e.g., minerals) is usually needed.
3. Antiarrhythmia agents are used to treat arrhythmia or abnormal heart beats. Since they can result in intestinal distress or discomfort, the drugs should be taken with a small amount of food.
4. Corticosteroids are used to treat many clinical disorders including arthritis, pain, and swelling. Since they can increase the breakdown of muscle protein, the intake of protein and urinary nitrogen output may need to be monitored.

In general, the prescription of medications for patients, especially children at home or in a hospital, usually has the following clinical implications for the patient:

1. What is the nutritional status: weight loss, weight gain, etc.?
2. Is there any previous experience with the prescribed drugs (e.g., dosage, length of treatment)?
3. Can we separate drug response from manifestations of the clinical disorders?
4. Is the effectiveness of the drugs long term or short term?

5. After intake, where does the drug act and where is it absorbed?
6. Will the level of the drugs in the blood be monitored?
7. Can the drug cause diarrhea as diarrhea may have a powerful effect on the absorption of nutrients?

In general, if a patient, especially a child, is receiving a prescription of medications at home or in a hospital, the qualified care provider should implement the following:

1. Keep medication history, using a standard clinical format.
2. When changing prescribed feedings, ascertain if any change in medication is indicated.
3. Use supplements accordingly if prescribed drugs are known to cause nutrient deficiencies, especially if blood chemistry is available for confirmation.
4. Follow up treatment and record patient response to drug and oral feeding preparations.
5. Follow specific protocol for nutrition intervention when a drug prescription is accompanied by enteral and parenteral feedings.

PROGRESS CHECK ON ACTIVITY 1

FILL-IN

1. Name four changes food and nutrients can cause on a drug.

    a. _____
    b. _____
    c. _____
    d. _____

2. Incompatibility of food and drugs results from what two major active ingredients in food?

    a. _____
    b. _____

3. Use of MAOs in treating depression has declined due to what major reaction?

    _____

4. The severity of drug reactions with food is due to five factors. Name them.

    a. _____
    b. _____
    c. _____
    d. _____
    e. _____

5. Cocaine ingestion affects nutritional status by what method? _____

6. Anticholinergics, useful for treating peptic ulcers, will affect nutritional status by causing: _____

7. In taking medications, the two most important precautions are:

    a. _____
    b. _____

8. Name 12 negative effects that can occur when medications are not taken according to directions.

    a. _____
    b. _____
    c. _____
    d. _____
    e. _____
    f. _____
    g. _____
    h. _____
    i. _____
    j. _____
    k. _____
    l. _____

MULTIPLE CHOICE

Circle the letter of the correct answer.

9. Vitamins are considered drugs if/when:
    a. they are prescribed.
    b. they are recommended.
    c. they are used for pharmacological effects.
    d. vitamins are not drugs; they are nutrients.

10. Administering drugs with meals is a common practice used to:
    a. reduce GI side effects.
    b. disguise taste.
    c. chelate the drug.
    d. a and b.
    e. all of the above.

11. Oral medications are affected by food in the GI tract in which of the following ways?
    a. pH of the stomach
    b. motility of the gut
    c. chelate of the medication
    d. all of the above

12. A fatty meal affects passage of a drug by:
    a. absorbing it so that it is unable to pass.
    b. delaying it by as much as two hours.
    c. speeding it by as much as two hours.
    d. a and b.

13. A meal high in protein affects drug therapy by:
    a. increasing absorption of the drug.
    b. decreasing absorption of the drug.
    c. delaying passage of the drug.
    d. neutralizing the effects of the drug.

TRUE/FALSE

Circle T for True and F for False.

14. T F Manufacturers now include vitamins and minerals in oral contraceptives.
15. T F Drugs often require extra vitamins because they use vitamins as cofactors.
16. T F Broad spectrum antibiotics interfere with vitamin K synthesis.
17. T F Headache and depression among OCA users have been traced to a deficiency of vitamin B_6.
18. T F Vitamin E is an essential nutrient, and it can be taken without precaution.
19. T F Potassium is an essential mineral, and foods rich in this mineral can be taken without precaution.

ACTIVITY 2:

Drugs and the Life Cycle

EFFECTS ON PREGNANCY AND LACTATION

A number of drugs, some of which are also classified as food components, have shown harmful effects on the course and outcome of pregnancy. These include alcohol, caffeine, some food additives, and food contaminants.

Alcohol

Alcohol consumption has many adverse effects on fetal development. Infants born to alcoholics exhibit anomalies of the eyes, nose, heart, and central nervous system, as well as mental retardation (fetal alcohol syndrome: FAS). More moderate consumption of alcohol leads to what is termed fetal alcohol effect. These effects include less severe but similar symptoms to FAS. The women also demonstrate higher rates of spontaneous abortion, abruptio placenta, and low birth weight delivery. Deficiencies of folic acid, magnesium, and zinc also may occur in the pregnant female and may play an important role in FAS.

Caffeine

Data is very limited in relation to human pregnancy and ingestion of caffeine, although it has been shown to be teratogenic in rats. A general warning is issued to pregnant women regarding limitation of caffeine intake.

Additives

Food additives, such as saccharin and aspartame, show no ill effects on the developing fetus, although moderation in the use of these substances during pregnancy (as well as nonpregnancy) is encouraged. Women who carry the PKU heterozygous gene should limit (or avoid) their intake of aspartame during pregnancy, as aspartame contains phenylalanine.

Contaminants

Mercury poisoning poses severe risks to the fetus including neurological problems and permanent brain damage. Other heavy metals, such as nickel, cadmium, and selenium, also pose heavy risks to the fetus and infant. Fetal growth retardation is seen in offspring of cigarette smokers due to effects from carbon monoxide, nicotine, and the decreased supply of oxygen transport to the fetus.

Other Food Components

Often overlooked for being potentially threatening, or most often believed to be beneficial rather than harmful, is the use of excessive amounts of vitamins and minerals. Congenital renal anomalies, multiple CNS malformations, cleft palate, and other severe defects have been reported in infants whose mothers took large doses of vitamin A during pregnancy. Other fat-soluble vitamins exhibit toxicity symptoms to the developing fetus and newborn when taken in large doses, though not as severe as that with hypervitaminosis A. An excess of zinc given to pregnant women appears to cause premature delivery and possible incidence of stillbirth.

Recreational and Medicinal Drugs

Recreational and medicinal drugs exert negative and damaging effects to the fetus. The effects are especially severe in the first trimester. Barbituates, hydantoin, anticonvulsants, and anticoagulants are chemicals known to be associated with fetal abnormalities, as well as over-the-counter drugs. All "street" drugs are extremely dangerous. A great spurt in brain growth occurs in the third trimester. Damage to the CNS at this critical stage of development potentially alters later brain functions (see Chapter 29: Diet Therapy for Constipation, Diarrhea, and High-Risk Infants).

Drugs and Breastfeeding

For centuries, breastmilk has been considered the perfect food for infants. But long-standing jokes about infants rejecting breast milk because the mother gorged on garlic, onion, or other strong foods are now gaining credence through clinical findings. Chemical ingredients in onion, garlic, and chocolate apparently produce an unpleasant reaction in nursing babies. A greater concern is that drugs can also appear in breastmilk and affect nursing infants. Doctors are justifiably concerned about the possibility that therapeutic drugs and nondrug chemicals can make their way from mother to infant.

Several factors have contributed to the heightened concern in the medical community. First, breastfeeding has regained popularity and is steadily on the increase. Second, drug use is also on the increase. Numerous new drugs are available, and the number of over-the-counter (OTC) drugs has substantially increased. In addition, more women are taking oral contraceptives while nursing, and industrial and household chemicals have contaminated the environment. For example, pesticides have been found in breastmilk.

Drug Passage to Breastmilk

The amount of a drug appearing in the milk primarily depends on the type of drug consumed, the concentration of the drug, and the time elapsed between drug ingestion and breastfeeding. Contrary to popular belief, the quantity of milk secreted has little to do with the amount of the drug passing to breastmilk. Method of drug administration does affect passage, since injected drugs appear faster than oral doses. The amount appearing in the milk may range from high to insignificant. For various reasons, the drug's presence may be harmless. For example, it may be nontoxic or ineffective, may be destroyed by the infant's system, or may not be absorbed by the infant. Certain drugs may be harmless unless they reach the infant in large quantities, whereas others may be harmful in small quantities.

Physicians must be especially careful when prescribing drugs for a nursing mother and must also determine whether the patient is using OTC drugs and whether environmental chemicals are inadvertently present. If the mother has a recognizable disease such as high blood pressure, edema, diabetes, or arthritis, she must be informed of the potential risk to the child. Of course, physicians can recommend interruption of breastfeeding if a drug that passes to breastmilk must be used. Other professionals such as nurses, dietitians, and nutritionists should be equally familiar with the drugs that can pass to breastmilk.

EFFECTS ON ADULTS

As consumers of many types of OTC and prescription drugs, as well as recreation drugs, young adults are at great risk for overmedicating. They are also prone to use several kinds of drugs at the same time. Prescription medications are not necessarily safer just because they are physician supervised. A person is at high risk whenever OTC drugs are taken along with prescription medication. Add to this the frequent use of alcohol and the combination is life threatening. The many reactions and contraindications from these habits are beyond the scope of this chapter, but the health professional must be aware of all such practices because they are commonplace in our society.

Probably the most common of the chronically used drugs that can profoundly affect nutrition are the estrogen-containing oral contraceptives. Women using these drugs are at risk of a clinical folate deficiency if they have marginal stores of this vitamin. Moreover, certain oral contraceptives reduce pyridoxine levels, a fact that may be associated with the common complaints of depression heard from some women on the pill. In some cases, impaired glucose tolerance related to OCA use has responded to pyridoxine supplementation. And, although no clinical significance has been attached, many users of oral contraceptives are found to have low vitamin C levels.

Oral contraceptives are known to affect the metabolism of virtually all nutrients. Such effects are subject to variables such as dosage, length of time used, prior nutritional status, nutrient intake, and individual susceptibility.

EFFECTS ON THE ELDERLY

The use of multiple drugs by the elderly poses many problems, yet more drugs are prescribed for them than for any other segment of the population. Ninety-nine percent of nursing home patients are multiple drug users, averaging four to six different drugs per day, depending on which surveys are reported. This author has observed as many as 20 different drugs on the chart of one nursing home patient. Elderly people living outside a facility also take many prescription drugs, although in lesser quantities as a usual rule.

The aged commonly have adverse reactions to many drugs, possibly because of deficiency of vitamin C, an important nutrient necessary for the normal process of drug metabolism. The elderly cannot metabolize and excrete drugs as well as younger adults. Therefore, the action of the drug may last longer. In addition, drugs can interact, resulting in toxic and other undesired effects.

Nutrient absorption and metabolism are particularly affected by drug therapies in the elderly. The ability to digest, absorb, and metabolize nutrients decreases with aging without the additional burden of drug usage, yet many of the drugs may be necessary.

Further study is especially needed among populations who take drugs for long periods; for example, women taking oral contraceptives and older Americans need further study.

Practicing physicians are encouraged to be familiar with drug-nutrition relationships. They are also encouraged to be at the forefront of efforts to reduce drug-induced malnutrition. Such efforts include legislation to bring certain nonprescription drugs under tighter control, constraints on excessive use of prescription drugs, and educational efforts. Although nurses, nutritionists, dietitians, and other allied health professionals do not prescribe drugs, their concerned participation in these efforts is obviously important.

AN EXAMPLE OF SIDE EFFECTS FROM MEDICATIONS FOR HYPERACTIVITY

There are potential side effects of medications used to treat attention deficient hyperactivity disorder (ADHD) in adults and children. The most common medications are divided into groups based on their length of action.

Once a day, long-acting, lasting 8–12 hours:

- Adderall XR
- Concerta
- Methodate CD
- Ritalin LA

Short acting, lasting 3–8 hours:

- Ritalin
- Ritalin SR
- Aletadate ER
- Aletvlin
- Methylin ER
- Focalin
- Dexedrine
- Dextorstat
- Adderall

The following are the most common side effects of the stimulant medications:

- Decreased appetite
- Weight loss
- Stomachaches
- Headaches
- Trouble getting to sleep
- Jitteriness and social withdrawal

Manage these side effects by adjusting the dosage or time of day when the medication is given. Other side effects may occur in children on too high a dosage or those that are overly sensitive to stimulants, which might cause them to be overfocused while on the medication or appear dull or overly restricted.

Another medication used for the treatment of ADHD is Strattera, which is not a stimulant and has not been shown to have the appetite dampening effect.

If two or three stimulants do not work, physicians may prescribe the following:

- Tricyclic antidepressants (Imipramine or Desipramine)
- Bupropion (Wellbutrin)
- Clonidine

Clinical care providers suggest the following to manage problems derived from the drugs previously shown.

If the patient suffers from appetite and weight loss, the following guides may help:

1. Give the medication with the meal rather than prior to the meal.
2. Make sure that high-calorie items are offered to children if they are at risk of losing weight.
3. Encourage healthy snacks such as cereal and milk, energy bars, healthy shakes, and so on. Encourage an evening snack when appetites are often maximized.
4. Change dinnertime to a later time so the effects of the stimulant have worn off.
5. Promote a consistent meal schedule.
6. Monitor growth.
7. The symptoms may be due to the medication or other factors such as the child's appetite, which often changes according to the caloric needs of growth.

Other suggestions include the following:

1. If the patient suffers from stomachaches, try to take the medications with food.
2. For insomnia, establish a bedtime routine, including relaxation techniques. Avoid caffeine. Caffeine has a 5-hour half-life. Cocoa and many teas contain caffeine.
3. For jitteriness, avoid caffeine. Counsel with the client and/or family about caffeine content in many sodas and energy drinks children are consuming.

PROGRESS CHECK ON ACTIVITY 2

FILL-IN

1. Describe the most severe effects of hypervitaminosis A on an infant. _____

_____

_____

2. The amount of drugs appearing in breastmilk depends upon three primary factors. Name them.

   a. _____

   b. _____

   c. _____

3. Describe the FAS infant.

_____

_____

4. Describe the effects of alcohol on the pregnant woman. _____

_____

_____

5. The effects of OCAs depend upon four characteristics of the user. What are the four characteristics?

    a. _____

    b. _____

    c. _____

    d. _____

6. List the three most important reasons that the elderly have adverse reactions to drugs.

    a. _____

    b. _____

    c. _____

7. Give three examples of the most common drug-nutrient interactions among the elderly.

    a. _____

    b. _____

    c. _____

MULTIPLE CHOICE

Circle the letter of the correct answer.

8. Zinc taken during a pregnancy can cause:

    a. premature deliveries.
    b. liver damage.
    c. stillbirths.
    d. a and b.
    e. a and c.

9. Pregnant women who are carriers, or who have phenylketonuria, should avoid aspartame ingestion because it:

    a. makes the infant hyperactive.
    b. causes birth defects.
    c. contains phenylalanine.
    d. contains caffeine.

10. The effects of recreational and/or medicinal drugs are most severe in the:

    a. third trimester of pregnancy.
    b. first trimester of pregnancy.
    c. second trimester of pregnancy.
    d. entire pregnancy.

TRUE/FALSE

Circle T for True and F for False.

11. T F Prescription medications are safer than OTC medications.
12. T F Overmedicating means taking a larger dose than prescribed.
13. T F Drug-induced malnutrition is not a problem since so many supplements are available.
14. T F Education is the best method of preventing drug-induced malnutrition.
15. T F Some drugs are harmless to infants.
16. T F The physician is the person who must provide patient education regarding drug use.

NURSING RESPONSIBILITIES

Nurses should be aware that generalities cannot assure proper administration, but knowledge of general principles may assist them in determining the many interactions.

1. Dietary nutrients affect drug actions, altering the pH, chelating, or changing the motility of the GI tract.
2. Drugs profoundly affect the action of the nutrients, interfering with absorption time and depleting body stores of essential nutrients.
3. Some diet and drug interactions create severe adverse side effects.
4. Some drug-nutrient interactions are synergistic.
5. Nutrients affect the distribution process by which drugs are delivered from the site of absorption to areas throughout the body. This process is also true for the effect of drugs on nutrients.
6. Drug-nutrient interactions profoundly affect digestion, absorption, metabolism, and elimination.
7. Many foods and drugs given together are totally incompatible, especially psychotropic drugs.
8. Since these processes are complicated, be prepared to repeat instructions to patients many times.
9. Effects of specific diet-drug reactions should be observed and documented. The patient should be informed.
10. Diet-drug interactions must be assessed on an individual basis for each drug and each individual.

REFERENCES

Alonso-Aperte, E. (2000). Drugs-nutrient interactions: A potential problem during adolescence. *European Journal of Clinical Nutrition, 54*: s69–s74.

Beham, E. (2006). *Therapeutic Nutrition: A Guide to Patient Education.* Philadelphia: Lippincott, Williams and Wilkins.

Boullata, J. I., & Amenti, V. T. (Eds.). (2004). *Handbook of Drug-Nutrient Interactions.* Totowa, NJ: Humana Press.

Couris, R. R. (2000). Assessment of healthcare professionals' knowledge about warfarin-vitamin K drug-nutrient interactions. *Journal of American College of Nutrition, 19*: 439–445.

Deen, D., & Hark, L. (2007). *The Complete Guide to Nutrition in Primary Care.* Malden, MA: Blackwell.

Drug Information for Health Care Professionals (USP-DI, I). (2001). In *United States Pharmacopeia.* (Vol. 1). Rockville, MD: Pharmacopeia Convention.

Escott-Stump, S. (2002). *Nutrition and Diagnosis-Related Care* (5th ed.). Philadelphia: Lippincott, Williams and Wilkins.

Hardman, J. F., & Limbird, L. E. (Eds.). (2001). *Goodman and Gilman's the Pharmacological Basis of Therapeutics* (10th ed.). New York: McGraw-Hill.

Hark, L., & Morrison, G. (Eds.). (2003). *Medical Nutrition and Disease* (3rd ed.). Malden, MA: Blackwell.

Katz, D. L. (2001). *Nutrition in Clinical Practice* (2nd ed.). Philadelphia: Lippincott, Williams and Wilkins.

Mahan, L. K., & Escott-Stump, S. (Eds.). (2008). *Krause's Food and Nutrition Therapy* (12th ed.). Philadelphia: Elsevier Sauders.

Marian, M. J., Williams-Muller, P., & Bower, J. (2007). *Integrating Therapeutic and Complementary Nutrition.* Boca Raton, FL: CRC Press.

McCabe, B. J., Frankel, E. H., & Wolfe, J. J. (Eds.). (2003). *Handbook of Food-Drug Interactions.* Boca Raton, FL: CRC Press.

McEvoy, G. K. (ed.). (2003). *AHFS drug information.* Bethesda, MD: American Society of Health System Pharmacists.

Meckling, K. A. (2007). *Nutrient-Drug Interactions.* Boca Raton, FL: CRC Press.

Payne-James, J., & Wicks, C. (2003). *Key Facts in Clinical Nutrition* (2nd ed.). London: Greenwich Medical Media.

Shils, M. E., Shike, M. (Eds.). (2006). *Modern Nutrition in Health and Disease* (10th ed.). Philadelphia: Lippincott, Williams and Wilkins.

Taketomo, C. K., Hodding, J. H., & Kraus, D. M. (Eds.). (2001). *Pediatric Dosage Handbook* (8th ed.). Hudson, OH: Lexi-Comp.

Watson, R. R., & Predy, V. R. (Eds.). (2004). *Nutrition and Alcohol: Linking Nutrient Interactions and Dietary Intake.* Boca Raton, FL: CRC Press.

Zucchero, F. J., Hogan, M. J., Sonmer, C. D., & Curran, J. P. (Eds.). (2002). *Evaluations of Drug Interactions.* (Vols. 1, 2) St. Louis, MO: First DataBank.

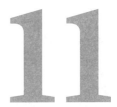

CHAPTER

Dietary Supplements

Time for Completion
Activities: 1½ hours
Optional examination: ½ hour

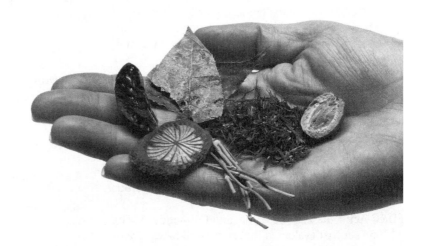

OBJECTIVES

Upon completion of this chapter the student should be able to do the following:

1. Describe how the 1994 Dietary Supplements Health and Education Act (DSHEA) changed the regulation of dietary supplements.
2. List the five criteria that define a supplement according to the DSHEA.
3. Explain the difference in a traditional dietary supplement and the present dietary supplement.
4. List three examples of a structure-function claim.
5. Describe how the FDA regulates claims made for advertising dietary supplements.
6. Identify at least five health claims made for ginseng, and five side effects that may be encountered from its use.
7. Identify the major uses of *Ginkgo biloba* and three possible side effects.
8. Describe five major health claims and five possible side effects of saw palmetto.
9. List five proposed benefits for valerian, and five possible side effects that can occur when valerian is taken for more than 2–3 weeks, or in large doses.
10. Discuss the interactions of supplements with medications.
11. Recognize fraudulent products.

12. Provide clients with information on reputable Web sites for information on supplements, and how to recognize unreliable sources.
13. Become familiar with the FDA's enforcement in dealing with manufacturers of dietary supplements that make illegal health claims and pose danger to the consumers who use their products.

GLOSSARY

Adulterated: the addition of inactive ingredients to a food that cause the food to have toxic effects when ingested.

Dietary supplement: a product used to provide nutritional support to the human diet.
  a. **Traditional definition:** a product composed of essential nutrients, such as vitamins, minerals, and protein.
  b. **Expanded definition:** product containing not only essential nutrients, but also may be composed of herbs and other botanicals, amino acids, glandulars, metabolites, enzymes, extracts, or any combination of these.

DSHEA: Dietary Supplement Health and Education Act. The 1994 amendment to the FD&C Act that included provisions that apply only to dietary supplements and dietary ingredients of supplements.

FDA: Food and Drug Administration. Agency responsible for enforcement of federal regulations regarding manufacture and distribution of food, drugs, and cosmetics as protection against sale of impure or dangerous substances.

FD&C Act: Federal Food, Drug, and Cosmetic Act. The 1958 act that evaluated the safety of all new ingredients, excluding dietary supplements and dietary ingredients of supplements.

Food additive: a new ingredient added to another food. Requires government approval if the ingredient has not been recognized as safe.

GMP for the FD&C Act: Good Manufacturing Practices for the FD&C Act. They are umbrella regulations governing the production of safe food, drugs, and cosmetics.

GMP for the DSHEA: Good manufacturing practices for the DSHEA. They are umbrella regulations governing the production of safe dietary supplements.

Health claims:
  a. **Unapproved:** one that claims to prevent, mitigate, treat, or cure a specific disease, for example, "cures cancer."
  b. **Approved:** one that, if the product substantiates the claim, may be said to improve health status, such as "may lower cholesterol" or "may reduce risk of osteoporosis."

GRAS: Generally recognized as safe: Substances used in foods that have been proven safe to use over a period of time.

BACKGROUND INFORMATION

All information in this chapter is based on documents published by the U.S. Food and Drug Administration, unless otherwise qualified.

Set between a Chinese restaurant and a pizza and sub sandwich eatery, a Rockville health food store offers yet another brand of edible items: bottled herbs such as cat's claw, dandelion root, and blessed thistle; vitamins and minerals in varying doses; and herbal and nutrient concoctions whose labels carry claims about relieving pain, "energizing" and "detoxifying" the body, or providing "guaranteed results."

This store sells dietary supplements, some of the hottest selling items on the market today. Surveys show that more than half of the U.S. adult population uses these products. In 1996 alone, consumers spent more than $6.5 billion on dietary supplements, according to Packaged Facts, Inc., a market research firm in New York City. But even with all the business they generate, consumers still ask questions about dietary supplements: Can their claims be trusted? Are they safe? Does the Food and Drug Administration (FDA) approve them?

Many of these questions come in the wake of the 1994 Dietary Supplement Health and Education Act, or DSHEA, which set up a new framework for FDA regulation of dietary supplements. It also created an office in the National Institutes of Health to coordinate research on dietary supplements, and it called on President Clinton to set up an independent dietary supplement commission to report on the use of claims in dietary supplement labeling.

Dietary Supplement Health and Education Act of 1994

For decades, the Food and Drug Administration regulated dietary supplements as foods, in most circumstances, to ensure that they were safe and wholesome, and that their labeling was truthful and not misleading. An important facet of ensuring safety was FDA's evaluation of the safety of all new ingredients, including those used in dietary supplements, under the 1958 Food Additive Amendments to the federal Food, Drug, and Cosmetic Act (FD&C Act). However, with passage of the Dietary Supplements Health and Education Act of 1994, Congress amended the FD&C Act to include several provisions that apply only to dietary supplements and dietary ingredients of dietary supplements. As a result of these provisions, dietary ingredients used in dietary supplements are no longer subject to the premarket safety evaluations required of other new food ingredients or for new uses of old food ingredients. They must, however, meet the requirements of other safety provisions.

The provisions of DSHEA define dietary supplements and dietary ingredients; establish a new framework for assuring safety; outline guidelines for literature displayed where supplements are sold; provide guidelines for use of claims and nutritional support statements; require ingredient and nutrition labeling; and grant the FDA the authority to establish good manufacturing practice (GMP) regulations. The law also requires formation of an executive-level Commission on Dietary Supplement Labels and an Office of Dietary Supplements within the National Institutes of Health.

These specific provisions of the DSHEA are summarized in Activity 1.

PROGRESS CHECK ON BACKGROUND INFORMATION

TRUE/FALSE

Circle T for True and F for False.

1. T F A traditional definition of dietary supplement is a product composed of essential nutrients, such as vitamins, minerals, and/or proteins.
2. T F The Food and Drug Administration (FDA) is an agency responsible only for enforcement of federal regulations regarding manufacture and distribution of food, drugs, and cosmetics as protection against sale of impure or dangerous substances.
3. T F A food additive is a new ingredient added to another food without government approval.
4. T F A food or supplement is adulterated with the addition of inactive ingredients to a food that cause the food to have toxic effects when ingested.

MULTIPLE CHOICE

Circle the letter of the correct answer.

5. Dietary supplements may be which of the following:

   a. essential nutrients
   b. herbs and other botanicals
   c. amino acids
   d. glandulars
   e. metabolites
   f. enzymes
   g. extracts
   h. any combination of above

FILL-IN

6. The purpose of the 1994 Dietary Supplement Health and Education Act, or DSHEA was to:

   a. _____

   b. _____

   c. _____

7. Define these acronyms:

   a. GRAS _____

   b. GMP _____

   c. DSHEA _____

   d. FD&C _____

ACTIVITY 1:

DSHE Act of 1994

DEFINITION OF DIETARY SUPPLEMENT

The FDA traditionally considered dietary supplements to be composed only of essential nutrients, such as vitamins, minerals, and proteins. The Nutrition Labeling and Education Act of 1990 added "herbs, or similar nutritional substances," to the term *dietary supplement*. Through the DSHEA, Congress expanded the meaning of the term *dietary supplements* beyond essential nutrients to include such substances as ginseng, garlic, fish oils, psyllium, enzymes, glandulars, and mixtures of these ingredients.

The DSHEA established a formal definition of *dietary supplement* using several criteria:

1. A dietary supplement is a product (other than tobacco) that is intended to supplement the diet and which bears or contains one or more of the following dietary ingredients: a vitamin, a mineral, an herb or other botanical; an amino acid; a dietary substance for use by humans to supplement the diet by increasing the total daily intake; or a concentrate, metabolite, constituent, extract, or combinations of these ingredients.
2. A dietary supplement is intended for ingestion in pill, capsule, tablet, or liquid form.
3. A dietary supplement is not represented for use as a conventional food or as the sole item of a meal or diet.
4. A dietary supplement is labeled as a "dietary supplement."
5. A dietary supplement includes products such as an approved new drug, certified antibiotic, or licensed biologic that was marketed as a dietary supplement or food before approval, certification, or license (unless specifically waived).

Dietary supplements come in many forms, including tablets, capsules, powders, softgels, gelcaps, and liquids. Though commonly associated with health food stores, dietary supplements also are sold in grocery, drug, and national discount chain stores, as well as through mail-order catalogs, TV programs, the Internet, and direct sales.

One thing dietary supplements are not is drugs. A drug, which sometimes can be derived from plants used as traditional medicines, is an article that, among other things, is intended to diagnose, cure, mitigate, treat, or prevent diseases. Before marketing, drugs must undergo clinical studies to determine their effectiveness, safety, possible interactions with other substances, and appropriate dosages, and the FDA must review these data and authorize the drugs' use before they are marketed. The FDA does not authorize or test dietary supplements.

A product sold as a dietary supplement and touted in its labeling as a new treatment or cure for a specific disease or condition would be considered an unauthorized—and thus illegal—drug. Labeling changes consistent with the provisions in DSHEA would be required to maintain the product's status as a dietary supplement.

Another thing dietary supplements are not are replacements for conventional diets, nutritionists say. Supplements do not provide all the known—and perhaps unknown—nutritional benefits of conventional food.

NUTRITIONAL SUPPORT STATEMENTS

The DSHEA provides for the use of various types of statements on the label of dietary supplements, although claims may not be made about the use of a dietary supplement to diagnose, prevent, mitigate, treat, or cure a specific disease (unless approved under the new drug provisions of the FD&C Act). For example, a product may not carry the claim "cures cancer" or "treats arthritis." Appropriate health claims authorized by the FDA—such as the claim linking folic acid to reduced risk of neural tube birth defects and the claim that calcium may reduce the risk of osteoporosis—may be made in supplement labeling if the product qualifies to bear the claim. Under the DSHEA, firms can make statements about classical nutrient deficiency diseases—as long as these statements disclose the prevalence of the disease in the United States. In addition, manufacturers may describe the supplement's effects on "structure or function" of the body or the "well-being" achieved by consuming the dietary ingredient. To use these claims, manufacturers must have substantiation that the statements are truthful and not misleading, and the product label must bear the statement "This statement has not been evaluated by the Food and Drug Administration. This product is not intended to diagnose, treat, cure, or prevent any disease." Unlike health claims, nutritional support statements need not be approved by the FDA before manufacturers market products bearing the statements; however, the agency must be notified no later than 30 days after a product that bears the claim is first marketed.

INGREDIENT AND NUTRITION INFORMATION LABELING

Like other foods, dietary supplement products must bear ingredient labeling. This information must include the name and quantity of each dietary ingredient or, for proprietary blends, the total quantity of all dietary ingredients (excluding inert ingredients) in the blend. The label must also identify the product as a "dietary supplement" (e.g., "Vitamin C Dietary Supplement"). Labeling of products containing herbal and botanical ingredients must state the part of the plant from which the ingredient is derived. If a supplement is covered by specifications in an official compendium and is represented as conforming, it is misbranded if it does not conform to those specifications. Official compendia include the U.S. Pharmacopeia, the Homeopathic Pharmacopeia of the United States, or the National Formulary. If not covered by a compendium, a dietary supplement must be the product identified on the label and have the strength it is represented as having.

Labels also must provide nutrition labeling. This labeling must first list dietary ingredients present in "significant amounts" for which the FDA has established daily consumption recommendations, followed by dietary ingredients with no daily intake recommendations. Dietary ingredients that are not present in significant amounts need not be listed. The nutrition labeling must include the quantity per serving for each dietary ingredient (or proprietary blend) and may include the source of a dietary ingredient (for example, "calcium from calcium gluconate"). If an ingredient is listed in the nutrition labeling, it need not appear in the statement of ingredients. Nutrition information must precede ingredient statements on the product label.

An example on the statement of identity (e.g., "ginseng")

1. Net quantity of contents (e.g., "60 capsules")
2. Structure-function claim and the statement "This statement has not been evaluated by the Food and Drug Administration. This product is not intended to diagnose, treat, cure, or prevent any disease."
3. Directions for use (e.g., "Take one capsule daily.").
4. Supplement Facts panel (lists serving size, amount, and active ingredient).
5. Other ingredients in descending order of predominance and by common name or proprietary blend.
6. Name and place of business of manufacturer, packer, or distributor. This is the address to write for more product information.

NEW DIETARY INGREDIENTS

Supplements may contain new dietary ingredients—those not marketed in the United States before October 15, 1994—only if those ingredients have been present in the food supply as an article used for food in a form in which the food has not been chemically altered or there is a history of use, or some other evidence of safety exists that establishes that there is a reasonable expectation of safety when the product is used according to recommended conditions of use. Supplement manufacturers must notify the FDA at least 75 days before marketing products containing new dietary ingredients, providing the agency with the information on which the conclusion that a dietary supplement containing the new dietary ingredient "will reasonably be expected to be safe" was based. Any interested party, including a manufacturer of a dietary supplement, may petition the FDA to issue an order prescribing the conditions of use under which a new dietary ingredient will reasonably be expected to be safe.

MONITORING FOR SAFETY

The FDA oversees safety, manufacturing and product information, such as claims in a product's labeling, package inserts, and accompanying literature. The Federal Trade Commission regulates the advertising of dietary supplements.

As with food, federal law requires manufacturers of dietary supplements to ensure that the products they put on the market are safe. But supplement manufacturers do not have to provide information to the FDA to get a product on the market. FDA review and approval of supplement ingredients and products is not required before marketing.

Unlike dietary supplements, food additives not generally recognized as safe must undergo the FDA's premarket approval process for new food ingredients. This requires manufacturers to conduct safety studies and submit the results to the FDA for review before the ingredient can be used in marketed products. Based on its review, the FDA either authorizes or rejects the food additive.

Under DSHEA, once a dietary supplement is marketed, the FDA has the responsibility for showing that a dietary supplement is unsafe before it can take action to restrict the product's use. This was the case when, in June 1997, FDA proposed, among other things, to limit the amount of ephedrine alkaloids in dietary supplements (marketed as ephedra, Ma huang, Chinese ephedra, and epitonin, for example) and provide warnings to consumers about hazards associated with use of dietary supplements containing the ingredients. The hazards ranged from nervousness, dizziness, and changes in blood pressure and heart rate to chest pain, heart attack, hepatitis, stroke, seizures, psychosis, and death. The proposal stemmed from the FDA's review of adverse event reports it had received, scientific literature, and public comments. The FDA has received many comments on the 1997 proposal and was reviewing them at press time.

Also in 1997, the FDA identified contamination of the herbal ingredient plantain with the harmful herb *Digitalis lanata* after receiving a report of a complete heart block in a young woman. FDA traced all use of the contaminated ingredient and asked manufacturers and retailers to withdraw these products from the market.

UNDERSTANDING CLAIMS

Claims that tout a supplement's healthful benefits have always been a controversial feature of dietary supplements. Manufacturers often rely on them to sell their products, but consumers often wonder whether they can trust them. Under the DSHEA and previous food labeling laws, supplement manufacturers are allowed to use, when appropriate, three types of claims: nutrient-content claims, disease claims, and nutrition support claims, which include "structure-function claims."

Nutrient-content claims describe the level of a nutrient in a food or dietary supplement. For example, a supplement containing at least 200 milligrams of calcium per serving could carry the claim "high in calcium." A supplement with at least 12 mg per serving of vitamin C could state on its label, "Excellent source of vitamin C."

Disease claims show a link between a food or substance and a disease or health-related condition. The FDA authorizes these claims based on a review of the scientific evidence. Or, after the agency is notified, the claims may be based on an authoritative statement from certain scientific bodies, such as the National Academy of Sciences, that shows or describes a well-established diet-to-health link. As of this writing, certain dietary supplements may be eligible to carry disease claims, such as claims that show a link between the following:

1. The vitamin folic acid and a decreased risk of neural tube defect-affected pregnancy, if the supplement contains sufficient amounts of folic acid
2. Calcium and a lower risk of osteoporosis, if the supplement contains sufficient amounts of calcium
3. Psyllium seed husk (as part of a diet low in cholesterol and saturated fat) and coronary heart disease, if the supplement contains sufficient amounts of psyllium seed husk

Nutrition support claims can describe a link between a nutrient and the deficiency disease that can result if the nutrient is lacking in the diet. For example, the label of a vitamin C supplement could state that vitamin C prevents scurvy. When these types of claims are used, the label must mention the prevalence of the nutrient—deficiency disease in the United States.

These claims also can refer to the supplement's effect on the body's structure or function, including its overall effect on a person's well-being. These are known as structure—function claims.

The following are examples of structure-function claims:

1. Calcium builds strong bones.
2. Antioxidants maintain cell integrity.
3. Fiber maintains bowel regularity.

Manufacturers can use structure-function claims without FDA authorization. They base their claims on their review and interpretation of the scientific literature. Like all label claims, structure-function claims must be true and not misleading. Structure-function claims are easy to spot because, on the label, they must be accompanied with the disclaimer "This statement has not been evaluated by the Food and Drug Administration. This product is not intended to diagnose, treat, cure, or prevent any disease."

Manufacturers who plan to use a structure-function claim on a particular product must inform the FDA of the use of the claim no later than 30 days after the product is first marketed. While the manufacturer must be able to substantiate its claim, it does not have to share the substantiation with the FDA or make it publicly available. If the submitted claims promote the products as drugs instead of supplements, the FDA can advise the manufacturer to change or delete the claim.

Because there often is a fine line between disease claims and structure-function claims, the FDA has established criteria under which a label claim would or would not qualify as a disease claim. Among label factors are these:

1. The naming of a specific disease or class of diseases
2. The use of scientific or lay terminology to describe the product's effect on one or more signs or symptoms recognized by healthcare professionals and consumers as characteristic of a specific disease or a number of different specific diseases
3. Product name
4. Statements about product formulation
5. Citations or references that refer to disease
6. Use of the words *disease* or *diseased*
7. Art, such as symbols and pictures
8. Statements that the product can substitute for an approved therapy (for example, a drug)

If shoppers find dietary supplements whose labels state or imply that the product can help diagnose, treat, cure, or prevent a disease (for example, "cures cancer" or "treats arthritis"), they should realize that the product is being marketed illegally as a drug and as such has not been evaluated for safety or effectiveness.

The FTC regulates claims made in the advertising of dietary supplements, and in recent years, that agency has taken a number of enforcement actions against companies whose advertisements contained false and misleading information. The actions targeted, for example, erroneous claims that chromium picolinate was a treatment for weight loss and high blood cholesterol. An action in 1997 targeted ads for an ephedrine alkaloid supplement because they understated the degree of the product's risk and featured a man falsely described as a doctor.

PROGRESS CHECK ON ACTIVITY 1

FILL-IN

1. The label of a dietary supplement should include:

   a. _____

   b. _____

   c. _____

   d. _____

   e. _____

   f. _____

2. Under the DSHEA and previous food labeling laws, supplement manufacturers are allowed to use, when appropriate, which three types of claims:

   a. _____

   b. _____

   c. _____

3. Labels of dietary supplement include two portions:

   a. _____

   b. _____

MULTIPLE CHOICE

Circle the letter of the correct answer.

4. An official compendium applicable to dietary supplements can be which of the following:

   a. U.S. Pharmacopeia
   b. Homeopathic Pharmacopeia of the United States
   c. National Formulary
   d. All of the above

5. A supplement that carries the claim "high in calcium" should have, per serving, at least:

   a. 100 milligrams of calcium
   b. 200 milligrams of calcium
   c. 400 milligrams of calcium

TRUE/FALSE

Circle T for True and F for False.

6. T F The FDA is authorized to test dietary supplements.
7. T F Under the DSHEA, firms cannot make statements about classical nutrient deficiency diseases—even though these statements disclose the prevalence of the disease in the United States.

8. T F Manufacturers using health claims must have substantiation that the statements are truthful and not misleading and the product label must bear the statement "This statement has not been evaluated by the Food and Drug Administration. This product is not intended to diagnose, treat, cure, or prevent any disease."

9. T F Ingredient and nutrition information labeling of dietary supplements are strictly regulated.

10. T F Ingredients listed in the nutrition label of a dietary supplement must also appear in the ingredient label.

11. T F Supplement suppliers have the burden to show that new ingredients in their dietary supplements are reasonably safe.

12. T F The Federal Trade Commission regulates the advertising of dietary supplements.

13. T F FDA review and approval of supplement ingredients and products is not required before marketing.

14. T F Food additives not generally recognized as safe must undergo the FDA's premarket approval process for new food ingredients.

15. T F Under the DSHEA, once a dietary supplement is marketed, the FDA has the responsibility for showing that a dietary supplement is unsafe before it can take action to restrict the product's use.

16. T F Calcium can be claimed to have a link with a lower risk of osteoporosis, if the supplement contains sufficient amounts of calcium.

17. T F Nutrient-content claims describe the level of a nutrient in a food or dietary supplement.

18. T F When nutrition support claims are used, the label must mention the prevalence of the nutrient-deficiency disease in the United States.

19. T F Structure-function claims refers to the supplement's effect on the body's structure or function, including its overall effect on a person's well-being.

ACTIVITY 2:

Folate or Folic Acid

For basic information on this vitamin, consult Chapter 5. The information in this activity has been modified from fact sheets distributed by the Office of Dietary Supplements, National Institutes of Health.

Folate and folic acid are forms of a water-soluble B vitamin. Folate occurs naturally in food. Folic acid is the synthetic form of this vitamin that is found in supplements and fortified foods. Folate gets its name from the Latin word *folium* for *leaf*. A key observation of researcher Lucy Wills nearly 70 years ago led to the identification of folate as the nutrient needed to prevent the anemia of pregnancy. Dr. Wills demonstrated that the anemia could be corrected by a yeast extract. Folate was identified as the corrective substance in yeast extract in the late 1930s and was extracted from spinach leaves in 1941. Folate is necessary for the production and maintenance of new cells. This effect is especially important during periods of rapid cell division and growth such as infancy and pregnancy. Folate is needed to make DNA and RNA, the building blocks of cells. It also helps prevent changes to DNA that may lead to cancer.

Both adults and children need folate to make normal red blood cells and prevent anemia. Leafy greens such as spinach and turnip greens, dry beans and peas, fortified cereals and grain products, and some fruits and vegetables are rich food sources of folate. Some breakfast cereals (ready-to-eat and others) are fortified with 25% or 100% of the Daily Value (DV) for folic acid.

NEED FOR EXTRA FOLIC ACID

Women of childbearing age, people who abuse alcohol, anyone taking anticonvulsants or other medications that interfere with the action of folate, individuals diagnosed with anemia from folate deficiency, and individuals with malabsorption, liver disease, or who are receiving kidney dialysis treatment may benefit from a folic acid supplement. Folic acid is very important for all women who may become pregnant. Adequate folate intake during the periconceptual period, the time just before and just after a woman becomes pregnant, protects against a number of congenital malformations including neural tube defects. Neural tube defects result in malformations of the spine (spina bifida), skull, and brain (anencephaly). The risk of neural tube defects is significantly reduced when supplemental folic acid is consumed in addition to a healthful diet prior to and during the first month following conception. Women who could become pregnant are advised to eat foods fortified with folic acid or take supplements in addition to eating folate-rich foods to reduce the risk of some serious birth defects. Taking 400 micrograms of synthetic folic acid daily from fortified foods and/or supplements has been suggested.

VITAMIN B$_{12}$ AND FOLIC ACID

Folic acid supplements can correct the anemia associated with vitamin B$_{12}$ deficiency. Unfortunately, folic acid will not correct changes in the nervous system that result from vitamin B$_{12}$ deficiency. Permanent nerve damage can occur if vitamin B$_{12}$ deficiency is not treated. Intake of supplemental folic acid should not exceed 1000 micrograms (mcg) per day to prevent folic acid from masking symptoms of vitamin B$_{12}$ deficiency. It is very important for older adults to be aware of the relationship between folic acid and vitamin B_{12} because they are at greater risk of having a vitamin B_{12} deficiency. Persons 50 years of age or older should ask their physicians to check B_{12} status before taking a supplement that contains folic acid.

FOLIC ACID, HEART DISEASE, AND CANCER

A deficiency of folate, vitamin B_{12}, or vitamin B_6 may increase the level of homocysteine, an amino acid normally found in your blood. There is evidence that an elevated homocysteine level is an independent risk factor for heart disease and stroke. The evidence suggests that high levels of homocysteine may damage coronary arteries or make it easier for blood clotting cells called platelets to clump together and form a clot. However, there is currently no evidence available to suggest that lowering homocysteine with vitamins will reduce the risk of heart disease. Clinical intervention trials are needed to determine whether supplementation with folic acid, vitamin B_{12}, or vitamin B_6 can lower the risk of developing coronary heart disease.

Some evidence associates low blood levels of folate with a greater risk of cancer. Folate is involved in the synthesis, repair, and functioning of DNA, our genetic map, and a deficiency of folate may result in damage to DNA that may lead to cancer. Several studies have associated diets low in folate with increased risk of breast, pancreatic, and colon cancer. Findings from a study of over 121,000 nurses suggested that long-term folic acid supplementation (for 15 years) was associated with a decreased risk of colon cancer in women aged 55 to 69 years of age. However, associations between diet and disease do not indicate a direct cause. Researchers are continuing to investigate whether enhanced folate intake from foods or folic acid supplements may reduce the risk of cancer. Until results from such clinical trials are available, folic acid supplements should not be recommended to reduce the risk of cancer.

FOLIC ACID AND METHOTREXATE FOR CANCER

Folate is important for cells and tissues that rapidly divide. Cancer cells divide rapidly, and drugs that interfere with folate metabolism are used to treat cancer. Methotrexate is a drug often used to treat cancer because it limits the activity of enzymes that need folate. Unfortunately, methotrexate can be toxic, producing side effects such as inflammation in the digestive tract that make it difficult to eat normally. Leucovorin is a form of folate that can help "rescue" or reverse the toxic effects of methotrexate. It is not known whether folic acid supplements can help control the side effects of methotrexate without decreasing its effectiveness in chemotherapy. It is important for anyone receiving methotrexate to follow a medical doctor's advice on the use of folic acid supplements.

FOLIC ACID AND METHOTREXATE FOR NONCANCEROUS DISEASES

Low-dose methotrexate is used to treat a wide variety of noncancerous diseases such as rheumatoid arthritis, lupus, psoriasis, asthma, sarcoidosis, primary biliary cirrhosis, and inflammatory bowel disease. Low doses of methotrexate can deplete folate stores and cause side effects that are similar to folate deficiency. Both high-folate diets and supplemental folic acid may help reduce the toxic side effects of low-dose methotrexate without decreasing its effectiveness. Anyone taking low-dose methotrexate for the health problems listed here should consult with a physician about the need for a folic acid supplement.

HEALTH RISK

The risk of toxicity from folic acid is low. The Institute of Medicine has established a tolerable upper intake level (UL) for folate of 1000 mcg for adult men and women, and a UL of 800 mcg for pregnant and lactating (breastfeeding) women less than 18 years of age. Supplemental folic acid should not exceed the UL to prevent folic acid from masking symptoms of vitamin B_{12} deficiency.

PROGRESS CHECK ON ACTIVITY 2

TRUE/FALSE

1. T F Folate and folic acid are forms of a fat-soluble B vitamin.
2. T F Folate does not occur naturally in food.
3. T F Folate was identified as the corrective substance in yeast extract in the late 1930s and was extracted from spinach leaves in 1941.
4. T F Folate is not needed to make DNA and RNA, the building blocks of cells, but it helps prevent changes to DNA that may lead to cancer.
5. T F Breakfast cereals (ready-to-eat and others) are required to be fortified with folic acid.
6. T F Folic acid is only important for all women who may become pregnant.
7. T F The risk of neural tube defects is significantly reduced when supplemental folic acid is consumed in addition to a healthful diet prior to and during the first month following conception.
8. T F Folic acid supplements can correct the anemia associated with vitamin B_{12} deficiency but not correct changes in the nervous system that result from vitamin B_{12} deficiency.
9. T F Intake of supplemental folic acid should not exceed 1000 micrograms (mcg) per day to prevent folic acid from masking symptoms of vitamin B_{12} deficiency.

10. T F There is evidence that an elevated homocysteine level is a dependent risk factor for heart disease and stroke.

11. T F Folic acid supplements can help control the side effects of methotrexate without decreasing its effectiveness in chemotherapy.

12. T F Low doses of methotrexate can deplete folate stores and cause side effects that are similar to folate deficiency.

13. T F A megadose of folic acid may be toxic.

FILL-IN

14. List seven groups of people who may benefit from folic acid supplementation.

   a. _____

   b. _____

   c. _____

   d. _____

   e. _____

   f. _____

   g. _____

15. Neural tube defects caused by folate deficiency result in malformations of the:

   a. _____

   b. _____

   c. _____

16. The recommended daily intake of folic acid either from fortified foods and/or supplemented (synthetic) folic acid is _____

   _____.

ACTIVITY 3:

Kava Kava, *Ginkgo Biloba*, Goldenseal, Echinacea, Comfrey, and Pulegone

Currently, there are thousands of botanicals being sold as dietary supplements. This chapter is not the proper forum to discuss all of them. Rather, six popular ones are discussed here. To make sure that the information is based on science and not testimony, the data have been derived from the following government documents:

1. National Institutes of Health, Office of Dietary Supplements
2. National Institutes of Health, National Toxicology Program
3. National Institutes of Health, National Institute of Aging

The six commercial dietary supplements discussed in this activity are kava kava, *Ginkgo biloba*, goldenseal, echinacea, comfrey, and pulegone.

KAVA KAVA

On March 25, 2002, the Food and Drug Administration (FDA) issued the following warning:

> The FDA is advising consumers of the potential risk of severe liver injury associated with the use of kava-containing dietary supplements. Kava *Piper methysticum* is a plant indigenous to the islands in the South Pacific where it is commonly used to prepare a traditional beverage. Supplements containing the herbal ingredient kava are promoted for relaxation (e.g., to relieve stress, anxiety, and tension), sleeplessness, menopausal symptoms, and other uses. The FDA has not made a determination about the ability of kava dietary supplements to provide such benefits.

> Liver-related risks associated with the use of kava have prompted regulatory agencies in other countries, including those in Germany, Switzerland, France, Canada, and the United Kingdom, to take action ranging from warning consumers about the potential risks of kava use to removing kava-containing products from the marketplace. Although liver damage appears to be rare, the FDA believes consumers should be informed of this potential risk.

> Kava-containing products have been associated with liver-related injuries—including hepatitis, cirrhosis, and liver failure—in over 25 reports of adverse events in other countries. Four patients required liver transplants. In the United States, the FDA has received a report of a previously healthy young female who required liver transplantation, as well as several reports of liver-related injuries.

> Given these reports, people who have liver disease or liver problems, or people who are taking drug products that can affect the liver, should consult a physician before using kava-containing supplements.

> Consumers who use a kava-containing dietary supplement and who experience signs of illness associated with liver disease should also consult their physician. Symptoms of serious liver disease include jaundice (yellowing of the skin or whites of the eyes) and brown urine. Nonspecific symptoms of liver disease can include nausea, vomiting, light-colored stools, unusual tiredness, weakness, stomach or abdominal pain, and loss of appetite.

> The FDA urges consumers and their healthcare professionals to report any cases of liver and other injuries that may be related to the use of kava-containing dietary supplements. Adverse events associated with the use of dietary supplements should be reported as soon as possible.

The presence of kava in a supplement should be identified on the product label in the Supplement Facts box. The following are commonly used names for kava:

ava
ava pepper
awa
intoxicating pepper
kava
kava kava
kava pepper
kava root
kava-kava
kawa
kawa kawa
kawa-kawa
kew
Piper methysticum
Piper methysticum Forst.f.
Piper methysticum G. Forst.
rauschpfeffer
sakau
tonga
wurzelstock
yangona

The FDA will continue to investigate the relationship, if any, between the use of dietary supplements containing kava and liver injury. The agency's investigation includes attempting to determine a biological explanation for the relationship and to identify the different sources of kava in the United States and Europe. The agency will alert consumers, and if warranted, take additional action as more information becomes available.

GINKGO BILOBA

Introduction

Ginkgo biloba, a readily available natural product, has been the focus of recent media reports as a potential treatment for Alzheimer's disease. Although a 1997 study in the United States suggests that a ginkgo extract may be of some help in treating the symptoms of Alzheimer's disease and vascular dementia, there is no evidence that *Ginkgo biloba* will cure or prevent Alzheimer's disease.

In addition, some recent case studies imply that daily use of *Ginkgo biloba* extracts may cause side effects, such as excessive bleeding, especially when combined with daily use of aspirin. Much more research is needed before scientists will know whether and how *Ginkgo biloba* extracts benefit people.

Research Outside of the United States

For centuries, extracts from the leaves of the ginkgo tree have been used as Chinese herbal medicine to treat a va-riety of medical conditions. In Europe and some Asian countries, standardized extracts from ginkgo leaves are taken to treat a wide range of symptoms, including dizziness, memory impairment, inflammation, and reduced blood flow to the brain and other areas of impaired circulation. Because *Ginkgo biloba* is an antioxidant, some claims have been made that it can be used to prevent damage caused by free radicals (harmful oxygen molecules). Although Germany recently approved ginkgo extracts (240 mg a day) to treat Alzheimer's disease, there is not enough information to recommend its broad use.

Research in the United States

Researchers at the New York Institute for Medical Research in Tarrytown, New York, conducted the first clinical study of *Ginkgo biloba* and dementia in the United States. Their findings were published in the *Journal of the American Medical Association* (October 22/29, 1997). These scientists examined how taking 120 mg a day of a *Ginkgo biloba* extract affected the rate of cognitive decline in people with mild to moderately severe dementia caused by Alzheimer's disease and vascular dementia. At the end of the study, they reported a small treatment difference in people given the *Ginkgo biloba* extract.

Three tests were used to measure changes in the condition of participants. First, participants showed a slight improvement on a test that measured their cognitive function (mental processes of knowing, thinking, and learning). Second, participants showed a slight improvement on a test that measured social behavior and mood changes that were observed by their caregivers. Third, participants showed no improvement on a doctor's assessment of change test.

Because 60% of the people did not complete the study, findings are difficult to interpret and may even be distorted. In addition, this study did not address the effect of *Ginkgo biloba* on delaying or preventing the onset of Alzheimer's disease or vascular dementia. The researchers recommend more investigation to accomplish the following: determine if these findings are valid, understand how *Ginkgo biloba* works on brain cells, and identify an effective dosage and potential side effects.

The extract of the ginkgo leaf contains a balance of flavone glycosides (including one suspected high-dose carcinogen, quercetin) and terpene lactones. Other claims are as follows: Ginkgo acts as a blood thinner; it improves circulation and is therefore used to treat migraine headaches, depression, and a range of lung and heart problems.

People should consult with their family doctors before using *Ginkgo biloba* extracts. This recommendation is especially true for those with disorders in blood circulation or blood clotting and those taking anticoagulants such as aspirin. Many different preparations of *Ginkgo biloba* extract are available over the counter. They vary in content and active ingredients. Because not enough research has been done, no specific daily amount of a *Ginkgo biloba* extract can be recommended as safe or effective at this time.

GOLDENSEAL

The root of the goldenseal plant is traditionally used to treat wounds, ulcers, digestive problems, and eye and ear infections. Today, the herb is also used as a laxative, tonic, and diuretic. Goldenseal is used in feminine products such as vaginal douches and is claimed to help with menstrual disorders such as irregular cycle and excessive bleeding. Berberine, one of the chief active components in goldenseal, has antimicrobial and vasodilatory properties and may also be effective in preventing the growth of cancer cells. The other major component of goldenseal, hydrastine (which can be made from berberine), has abortifacient effects and has been shown to induce labor in pregnant women when taken orally. Large internal doses of goldenseal may cause convulsions and irritation of the mouth, throat, and stomach, tingling of the skin, paralysis, respiratory failure, and possibly death at very high doses. Chronic use may inhibit vitamin B absorption.

At present goldenseal is being studied by the federal health authorities and clinical experts to determine its effectiveness, safety, and toxicology.

ECHINACEA

This member of the daisy family is one of the top medicinal herb sellers in the United States. Although once used for everything from snakebites to typhoid, echinacea as a dietary supplement is most commonly used today as an immunostimulant to treat the common cold, sore throat, and flu. Echinacea is not known to have any serious adverse side effects, although there have been reports of skin rash and insomnia among users. The herb is available in many forms-dried root or leaf, liquid extract, powder, capsules, tablets, creams, gels, and injections (outside of North America). It has yet to be determined how echinacea is best administered or exactly how—or if—the plant's complex mixture of polysaccharides, flavonoids, essential oils, and other compounds actually produces beneficial effects. Again, this dietary supplement is being studied for its clinical effect and safety.

COMFREY

Certain dietary supplements contain the herbal ingredient comfrey *Symphytum officionale* (common comfrey), *S. asperum* (prickley comfrey), and *S. x uplandicum* (Russian comfrey). Claims have been made about comfrey.

Applied externally, comfrey acts as an anti-inflammatory to promote healing of bruises, sprains, and open wounds. The roots and leaves of the plant contain the protein allantoin, which stimulates cell proliferation. Comfrey is said to help wounds to heal and broken bones to knit. It is also taken internally as an herbal tea to treat gastric ulcers, rheumatic pain, arthritis, bronchitis, and colitis. This ingestion is a matter of some concern because comfrey contains several pyrrolizidine alkaloids, primarily symphytine, which have been linked to liver and lung cancer in rats. The hepatotoxic effects of pyrrolizidine alkaloids are well established in both animals and humans.

The use of comfrey in dietary supplements is a serious concern to the FDA. These plants contain pyrrolizidine alkaloids, substances that are firmly established to be hepatotoxins in animals. Reports in the scientific literature clearly associate oral exposure of comfrey and pyrrolizidine alkaloids with the occurrence of veno-occlusive disease (VOD) in animals. Moreover, outbreaks of hepatic VOD have been reported in other countries over the years, and the toxicity of these substances in humans is generally accepted. The use of products containing comfrey has also been implicated in serious adverse incidents over the years in the United States and elsewhere. However, while information is generally lacking to establish a cause-effect relationship between comfrey ingestion and observed adverse effects humans, the adverse effects that have been seen are entirely consistent with the known effects of comfrey ingestion that have been described in the scientific literature. The pyrrolizidine alkaloids that are present in comfrey, in addition to being potent hepatotoxins, have also been shown to be toxic to other tissues as well. There is also evidence that implicates these substances as carcinogens. Taken together, the clear evidence of an association between oral exposure to pyrrolizidine alkaloids and serious adverse health effects and the lack of any valid scientific data that would enable the agency to determine whether there is an exposure, if any, that would present no harm to consumers, indicates that this substance should not be used as an ingredient in dietary supplements.

Since 2000, the position of the FDA is as follows:

1. The FDA believes that the available scientific information is sufficient to firmly establish that dietary supplements that contain comfrey or any other source of pyrrolizidine alkaloids are adulterated under the act.
2. The FDA strongly recommends that firms marketing a product containing comfrey or another source of pyrrolizidine alkaloids remove the product from the market and alert its customers to immediately stop using the product.
3. The FDA is prepared to use its authority and resources to remove products from the market that appear to violate the act.

4. The FDA believes that manufacturers need to take adequate steps to identify and report adverse events, especially adverse events that may include liver disorders, associated with any product that has an ingredient that may contain pyrrolizidine alkaloids.

Further, since 2000, the Federal Trade Commission (FTC) has also taken action against unsafe products containing comfrey. The FTC is against the marketing of any comfrey-containing product intended for internal use or use on open wounds and requires a warning on comfrey products marketed for external uses.

PULEGONE

Pulegone is the active ingredient in pennyroyal and is also found in several other species of mint. Pennyroyal is traditionally used as a carminative, insect repellent, emmenagogue, and abortifacient. Prior studies have demonstrated hepatic, renal, and pulmonary toxicity in humans, as well as central nervous system toxicity resulting in seizure, coma, and death. Pulegone is toxic to the developing fetus.

PROGRESS CHECK ON ACTIVITY 3

FILL-IN

1. Name five commercial dietary supplements:

   a. _____

   b. _____

   c. _____

   d. _____

   e. _____

2. Name five commonly used names for *Piper methyleticum*:

   a. _____

   b. _____

   c. _____

   d. _____

   e. _____

TRUE/FALSE

Circle T for True and F for False.

3. T F Kava has been used by Pacific islanders for centuries. Therefore kava-containing supplements have no side effects.

4. T F Supplements containing kava are effective for relaxation, sleeplessness, and menopausal symptoms.

5. T F Dietary supplements are considered as safe by manufacturers. Therefore, consumers do not need to consult a physician before using them.

6. T F *Ginkgo biloba* is effective in preventing Alzheimer's disease.

7. T F Daily use of *Ginkgo biloba* extracts is safe when used with other medications.

8. T F *Ginkgo biloba* is an antioxidant, and can prevent damage caused by free radicals.

9. T F Taking 120 mg a day of a *Ginkgo biloba* extract may affect the rate of cognitive decline in people with mild to moderately severe dementia caused by Alzheimer's disease and vascular dementia.

10. T F Goldenseal root should not be taken by pregnant women.

11. T F Goldenseal root has antimicrobial properties and is therefore useful in treating eye and ear infections.

12. T F Echinacea as a dietary supplement is most commonly used today as an immunostimulant to treat the common cold, sore throat, and flu.

13. T F Comfrey is safe when it is used for external treatment of wounds.

14. T F The main pyrrolizidine alkaloid in comfrey, symphytine, is hepatotoxic and carcinogenic.

15. T F Ingestion of pennyroyal can be fatal as it affects the central nervous system resulting in seizure and coma.

16. T F Pennyroyal should not be taken by pregnant women as it is toxic to a developing fetus.

ACTIVITY 4:

An Example of Side Effects from Medications for Hyperactivity

In the March–April 2002 issue of the *FDA Consumer* magazine, the FDA published an article titled "Tips for the savvy supplement user: Making informed decisions." A slightly modified version is presented here.

The choice to use a dietary supplement can be a wise decision that provides health benefits. However, under certain circumstances, these products may be unnecessary for good health, or they may even create unexpected risks.

Clearly, people choosing to supplement their diets with herbals, vitamins, minerals, or other substances want to know more about the products they choose so that they can make informed decisions about them. Given the abundance and conflicting nature of information now available about dietary supplements, you may need help to sort the reliable information from the questionable. The FDA has prepared these tips and resources to help you become a savvy dietary supplement user. The principles underlying these tips are similar to those principles a savvy consumer would use for any product.

Do I need to think about my total diet?

Yes. Dietary supplements are intended to supplement the diets of some people but not to replace the balance of the variety of foods important to a healthy diet. While you need enough nutrients, too much of some nutrients can cause problems. You can find information on the functions and potential benefits of vitamins and minerals, as well as upper safe limits for nutrients from many nonprofit organizations such as government agencies (e.g., the FDA), university extension offices, American Dietetic Association, and so on, including Chapters 3 to 7 in this book.

Should I check with my doctor or healthcare provider before using a supplement?

This is a good idea, especially for certain population groups. Dietary supplements may not be risk-free under certain circumstances:

- If you are pregnant, nursing a baby, or have a chronic medical condition, such as diabetes, hypertension or heart disease, be sure to consult your doctor or pharmacist before purchasing or taking any supplement.
- While vitamin and mineral supplements are widely used and generally considered safe for children, you may wish to check with your doctor or pharmacist before giving these or any other dietary supplements to your child.
- If you plan to use a dietary supplement in place of drugs or in combination with any drug, tell your healthcare provider first. Many supplements contain active ingredients that have strong biological effects, and their safety is not always assured in all users.
- If you have certain health conditions and take these products, you may be placing yourself at risk.
- Some supplements may interact with prescription and over-the-counter (OTC) medicines. Taking a combination of supplements or using these products together with medications (whether prescription or OTC drugs) could, under certain circumstances, produce adverse effects, some of which could be life threatening.

Be alert to advisories about these products, whether taken alone or in combination. For example, Coumadin (a prescription medicine), *Ginkgo biloba* (an herbal supplement), aspirin (an OTC drug), and vitamin E (a vitamin supplement) can each thin the blood, and taking any of these products together can increase the potential for internal bleeding. Combining St.-John's-wort with certain HIV drugs significantly reduces their effectiveness. St.-John's-wort may also reduce the effectiveness of prescription drugs for heart disease, depression, seizures, certain cancers, or oral contraceptives.

Some supplements can have unwanted effects during surgery. It is important to fully inform your doctor about the vitamins, minerals, herbals, or any other supplements you are taking, especially before elective surgery. You may be asked to stop taking these products at least 2 to 3 weeks ahead of the procedure to avoid potentially dangerous supplement/drug interactions-such as changes in heart rate and blood pressure or increased bleeding-that could adversely affect the outcome of your surgery.

Who is responsible for ensuring the safety and efficacy of dietary supplements?

Under the law, manufacturers of dietary supplements are responsible for making sure their products are safe before they go to market. Manufacturers are also responsible for determining that the claims on their labels are accurate and truthful. Dietary supplement products are not reviewed by the government before they are marketed, but the FDA can take action against any unsafe dietary supplement product that reaches the market. If the FDA can prove that claims on marketed dietary supplement products are false and misleading, the agency may take action against these products.

When searching the Web for information about dietary supplements, try using directory sites of respected organizations, rather than doing blind searches with a search engine. Ask yourself the following questions:

- Who operates the site?
- Is the site run by the government, a university, or a reputable medical or health-related association (such as the American Medical Association, American Diabetes Association, American Heart Association, American Dietetic Association, National Institutes of Health, National Academy of Sciences, or the FDA)?
- Is the information written or reviewed by qualified health professionals, experts in the field, academia, government, or the medical community?
- What is the purpose of the site?
- Is the purpose of the site to objectively educate the public or just to sell a product?

Be aware of practitioners or organizations whose main interest is in marketing products, either directly or through sites with which they are linked. Commercial sites should clearly distinguish scientific information from advertisements. Most nonprofit and government sites contain no advertising, and access to the site and materials offered are usually free.

- What is the source of the information and does it have any references?
- Has the study been reviewed by recognized scientific experts and published in reputable peer-reviewed scientific journals, such as the *New England Journal of Medicine*?
- Does the information say "some studies show . . ." or does it state where the study is listed so that you can check the authenticity of the references? For example, can the study be found in the National Library of Medicine's database of literature citations?
- Is the information current? Check the date when the material was posted or updated. Often new research or

other findings are not reflected in old material, for example, side effects or interactions with other products or new evidence that might have changed earlier thinking. Ideally, health and medical sites should be updated frequently.

- How reliable are the Internet and e-mail solicitations? While the Internet is a rich source of health information, it is also an easy vehicle for spreading myths, hoaxes, and rumors about alleged news, studies, products, or findings. To avoid falling prey to such hoaxes, be skeptical and watch out for overly emphatic language with UPPERCASE LETTERS and lots of exclamation points!!!! Beware of such phrases such as: "This is not a hoax" or "Send this to everyone you know."

MORE TIPS AND TO-DO'S

Ask yourself:

- Does it sound too good to be true?
- Do the claims for the product seem exaggerated or unrealistic?
- Are there simplistic conclusions being drawn from a complex study to sell a product?

While the Web can be a valuable source of accurate, reliable information, it also has a wealth of misinformation that may not be obvious. Learn to distinguish hype from evidence-based science. Nonsensical lingo can sound very convincing. Also, be skeptical about anecdotal information from people who have no formal training in nutrition or botanicals, or personal testimonials (from store employees, friends, or online chat rooms and message boards) about incredible benefits or results obtained from using a product. Question these people on their training and knowledge in nutrition or medicine.

Think twice about chasing the latest headline. Sound health advice is generally based on a body of research, not a single study. Be wary of results claiming a "quick fix" that depart from previous research and scientific beliefs. Keep in mind science does not proceed by dramatic breakthroughs, but by taking many small steps, slowly building towards a consensus. Furthermore, news stories about the latest scientific study, especially those on TV or radio, are often too brief to include important details that may apply to you or allow you to make an informed decision.

Check your assumptions about the following:

Questionable Assumption 1: "Even if a product may not help me, at least it won't hurt me." It's best not to assume that this will always be true. When consumed in high enough amounts, for a long enough time, or in combination with certain other substances, all chemicals can be toxic, including nutrients, plant components, and other biologically active ingredients.

Questionable Assumption 2: "When I see the term 'natural,' it means that a product is healthful and safe." Consumers can be misled if they assume this term assures wholesomeness, or that these foodlike substances necessarily have milder effects, which makes them safer to use than drugs. The term *natural* on labels is not well defined and is sometimes used ambiguously to imply unsubstantiated benefits or safety. For example, many weight-loss products claim to be "natural" or "herbal," but this doesn't necessarily make them safe. Their ingredients may interact with drugs or may be dangerous for people with certain medical conditions.

Questionable Assumption 3: "A product is safe when there is no cautionary information on the product label." Dietary supplement manufacturers may not necessarily include warnings about potential adverse effects on the labels of their products. If consumers want to know about the safety of a specific dietary supplement, they should contact the manufacturer of that brand directly. It is the manufacturer's responsibility to determine that the supplement it produces or distributes is safe and that there is substantiated evidence that the label claims are truthful and not misleading.

Questionable Assumption 4: "A recall of a harmful product guarantees that all such harmful products will be immediately and completely removed from the marketplace." A product recall of a dietary supplement is voluntary, and, while many manufacturers do their best, a recall does not necessarily remove all harmful products from the marketplace. Contact the manufacturer for more information about the specific product that you are purchasing. If you cannot tell whether the product you are purchasing meets the same standards as those used in the research studies you read about, check with the manufacturer or distributor. Ask to speak to someone who can address your questions, some of which may include: What information does the firm have to substantiate the claims made for the product? Be aware that sometimes firms supply so-called proof of their claims by citing undocumented reports from satisfied consumers, or "internal" graphs and charts that could be mistaken for evidence-based research. Does the firm have information to share about tests it has conducted on the safety or efficacy of the ingredients in the product? Does the firm have a quality control system in place to determine if the product actually contains what is stated on the label and is free of contaminants? Has the firm received any adverse event reports from consumers using their products?

NURSING IMPLICATIONS

When a nurse is caring for a patient who is involved with dietary supplements (using them, intending to use them, or asking questions about them), the major nursing implication is mainly patient education.

1. Be prepared to teach clients how to do the following:
   a. Detect fraudulent products and deceptive advertising.
   b. Purchase quality products if they intend to use supplements.
   c. Read product labels.
   d. File a report if side effects are experienced.
   e. Recognize that dietary supplements can cause harm, the reasons they can be harmful, and the types of reactions that may occur.
   f. Reduce the chances of suffering adverse effects from supplement use.
2. Counsel patients to seek expert advice from their physicians before beginning any supplement regime.

The following information will assist you in preparing a teaching plan.

Fraudulent Products

Consumers need to be on the lookout for fraudulent products. These are products that don't do what they say they can or don't contain what they say they contain. At the very least, they waste consumers' money, and they may cause physical harm.

Fraudulent products often can be identified by the types of claims made in their labeling, advertising, and promotional literature. Some possible indicators of fraud, according to the National Council Against Health Fraud, are the following:

1. Claims that the product is a secret cure and use of such terms as *breakthrough*, *magical*, *miracle cure*, and *new discovery*. If the product were a cure for a serious disease, it would be widely reported in the media and used by healthcare professionals.
2. "Pseudomedical" jargon, such as *detoxify*, *purify*, and *energize* to describe a product's effects. These claims are vague and hard to measure, and so they make it easier for success to be claimed.
3. Claims that the product can cure a wide range of unrelated diseases. No product can do that.
4. Claims that a product is backed by scientific studies but with no list of references or references that are inadequate. For instance, if a list of references is provided, the citations cannot be traced, or if they are traceable, the studies are out-of-date, irrelevant, or poorly designed.
5. Claims that the supplement has only benefits-and no side effects. A product "potent enough to help people will be potent enough to cause side effects."
6. Accusations that the medical profession, drug companies, and the government are suppressing information about a particular treatment. It would be illogical for large numbers of people to withhold information

about potential medical therapies when they or their families and friends might one day benefit from them.

Though often more difficult to do, consumers also can protect themselves from economic fraud, a practice in which the manufacturer substitutes part or all of a product with an inferior, cheaper ingredient and then passes off the fake product as the real thing but at a lower cost. Avoid products sold for considerably less money than competing brands.

Quality Products

Poor manufacturing practices are not unique to dietary supplements, but the growing market for supplements in a less restrictive regulatory environment creates the potential for supplements to be prone to quality-control problems. For example, the FDA has identified several problems where some manufacturers were buying herbs, plants, and other ingredients without first adequately testing them to determine whether the product they ordered was actually what they received or whether the ingredients were free from contaminants.

To help protect themselves, consumers should do the following:

1. Look for ingredients in products with the U.S.P. notation, which indicates the manufacturer followed standards established by the U.S. Pharmacopoeia.
2. Realize that the label term *natural* doesn't guarantee that a product is safe. Think of poisonous mushrooms—they are natural.
3. Consider the name of the manufacturer or distributor. Supplements made by a nationally known food and drug manufacturer, for example, have likely been made under tight controls because these companies already have in place manufacturing standards for their other products.
4. Write to the supplement manufacturer for more information. Ask the company about the conditions under which its products were made.

Reading and Reporting

Consumers who use dietary supplements should always read product labels, follow directions, and heed all warnings.

Supplement users who suffer a serious harmful effect or illness that they think is related to supplement use should call a doctor or other healthcare provider. He or she in turn can report it to the FDA. To file a report, consumers will be asked to provide:

1. Name, address, and telephone number of the person who became ill
2. Name and address of the doctor or hospital providing medical treatment
3. Description of the problem
4. Name of the product and store where it was bought

Consumers also should report the problem to the manufacturer or distributor listed on the product's label and to the store where the product was bought.

Expert Advice

Before starting a dietary supplement, it is always wise to check with a medical doctor. It is especially important for people who have the following characteristics:

1. Pregnant or breastfeeding
2. Chronically ill
3. Elderly
4. Under 18
5. Taking prescription or over-the-counter medicines. Certain supplements can boost blood levels of certain drugs to dangerous levels.

Harm

Can dietary supplements be harmful? Under some circumstances, anything we ingest can be harmful, even ordinary food, and the same applies to dietary supplements. A dietary supplement (DS), especially one with multiple ingredients, can be harmful under one of the following circumstances (REASONS), assuming it is not a poison and it has been used by at least some individuals without adverse effects. Each circumstance has been substantiated by actual events of poisoning from dietary supplements in some individuals:

R   Raw impurities: The DS is not pure. It is mixed with some known or unknown ingredient or ingredients that are harmful at least to some individuals.

E   Excess levels of ingredients used: Intentionally or unintentionally the manufacturer has included an excess level of some of the ingredients. The excess substances have proved harmful to some consumers.

A   Allergic reactions to some ingredients in the dietary supplement for some individuals: The occurrence of this type of adverse effects is probably one of the most common observations among the consumers.

S   Systemic poisoning: This means the ingredients in the dietary supplement are distributed via the blood stream to various parts of the body and produce general poisonous effects in the body of some users. Most of the time, the cause of such poisoning is difficult to assess. One possibility is the interaction of ingredients in the body to a harmful by-product. Or, the ingredients interact with body organs or fluid to produce general by-products that interact among themselves to produce another by-product that is harmful.

O   Overdosing oneself: This is another common situation when adverse effects occur. Many users do not comply with the written instructions on the label. Instead of one tablet a day, three may be taken. Instead of swallowing a capsule, some open it and chew on the powder.

N   Negative reactions in some individuals because of a specific sensitivity: The substance is harmless for the average adult but may be harmful to infants, small children, and some elderly. The substance is not harmless under normal circumstances but may be harmful to individuals with certain clinical conditions, such as pregnancy, high blood pressure, and kidney diseases.

S   Safety of the product has not been carefully evaluated: In spite of legal requirements, many manufacturers have failed to conduct safety testing of their products.

Any consumer who enjoys using dietary supplements for whatever reasons, for example, nutritional benefits, clinical therapy, reversal of aging, is advised to perform a minimum amount of "homework" so that the chances of suffering adverse effects can be reduced. The following HOPES criteria serve as a good start:

H   *Health* status is an important clue. Are you sick? Do you have a terminal illness? Are you pregnant? You must be careful with the potential effect of any dietary supplement. The precaution applies even if you are taking the dietary supplement with an intention that it may cure your illness.

O   *Overacting* is a human weakness. When it comes to a dietary supplement, avoid it if you can. Even if it works and makes you feel better, there is no need to be excited. It may be a chance occurrence. Most important of all, do not overdose immediately because it "works." That is, if the label recommends 2 tablets a day, do not take 4 or 5.

P   *Product* description is your major weapon for self-protection. Read the label several times. Ask yourself the following questions: Is there a name for the product? Are the ingredients listed? Is there a recommended daily dosage? Are there precaution statements? Is there a name and address for the manufacturer? It is not a good idea to put something in your mouth if there is no name and address for the manufacturer. Why? Because, if there is something wrong, no one can trace it to the manufacturer. The store where you buy it may have obtained it from a distributor. Without the manufacturer, no one knows what is inside, and your doctor cannot treat you if you show harmful effects.

E   *Education* is invariably a part of any health program. If you are serious about taking dietary supplements and willing to spend money on one or more such products, then you have the responsibility of educating yourself about dietary supplements. Talk to your friends with similar interest. Read up on products, claims, and effects. Use the toll-free numbers for the FDA, FTC, and state consumer protection agencies to find out about any dietary supplement you are taking.

S *Symptoms* from taking a dietary supplement are of course valuable indications that there is something wrong with the product. If you detect a slight sign of unwelcome symptoms in your body, stop the supplement immediately and seek medical attention.

Your HOPES of a minimum protection from adverse effects of any dietary supplement is to implement these five simple steps.

FDA ENFORCEMENT

The FDA uses many tools to enforcement laws and regulations and some are described below:

1. Warning letters: The FDA sends a warning letter to inform a manufacture that one or more of its products is illegal or needs correction. Responses are then processed between the FDA and the manufacturers.
2. Recalls: Recalls are actions taken by a firm to remove a product from the market. Recalls may be conducted on a firm's own initiative, by FDA request, or by FDA order under statutory authority. There are three classes of recalls:
   - Class I recall—A situation in which there is a reasonable probability that the use of or exposure to a violative product will cause serious adverse health consequences or death
   - Class II recall—A situation in which use of or exposure to a violative product may cause temporary or medically reversible adverse health consequences or where the probability of serious adverse health consequences is remote
   - Class III recall—A situation in which use of or exposure to a violative product is not likely to cause adverse health consequences
3. Seizures: When the FDA decides that a product may pose danger to the public and recall is not implemented, it will work with the appropriate law enforcement agency to seize the product and remove it from the market.

Each of the above enforcement approach has been applied to manufacturers whose dietary supplements have raised the issues of safety or illegal claims. Some examples follow.

Warning Letters

In April 2007, the FDA sent a warning letter to the manufacturer of a dietary supplement affecting public safety and illegal claims. The company sells a dietary supple-

mented called "Cocaine." Its Web site use the following descriptions or claims:

- "The Legal Alternative"
- The product name is "Cocaine," and the letters in the product name appear to be spelled out in a white granular substance that resembles cocaine powder.
- "Speed in a Can"
- "Liquid Cocaine"
- "Cocaine - Instant Rush"
- "The question you have to ask yourself is: 'Can I handle the rush?'"
- "This beverage should be consumed by responsible adults. Failure to adhere to this warning may result in excess excitement, stamina, . . . and possible feeling of euphoria."
- Certain ingredients intended "to prevent, treat, or cure disease conditions." "Inositol . . . reduces cholesterol in the blood; it helps prevent hardening of the arteries, and may protect nerve fibers from excess glucose damage. Inositol has a natural calming effect and may be used in the treatment of anxiety, depression, and obsessive-compulsive disorder without the side effects of prescription medications."

According to the FDA, dietary supplements are products that are intended to supplement the diet. Street drug alternatives, meaning products that claim to mimic the effects of recreational drugs, are not intended to supplement the diet and, as a result, cannot lawfully be marketed as dietary supplements. Also, a dietary supplement may not bear claims that it prevents or treats a disease, except for authorized health claims about reducing the risk of a disease.

Since the outcome of each varies with conditions such as responses, remedies, legal actions, and so on, an interested party may access the FDA Web site to find more details about accessing the FDA's archive of warning letters.

Recalls

Some examples of class I recalls are listed in Table 11-1.

Seizures

On October 12, 2007, the FDA distributed this news release:

> At the request of the FDA, U.S. Marshals seized ~$71,000 of products from FulLife Natural Options, Inc., of Boca Raton, Florida, which marketed and distributed Charantea Ampalaya Capsules and Charantea Ampalaya Tea.
>
> Although these products are labeled as dietary supplements, they are being promoted by FulLife for use in treating serious conditions, such as diabetes, anemia, and hypertension, both in printed

TABLE 11-1   Recalled Dietary Supplements

Dietary Supplements Recalled	Reason	Recall Company	Manufacturer
LIVIRO3 Natural Energy Enhancer Nutritional Supplement Recall: May 2007	Containing the legal prescription drug ingredient Tadalafil (treating erectile dysfunction)	Ebek, Inc, Los Angeles, CA	West Coast Laboratories Inc, Gardena, CA
Avian-Rx tablets labeled to contain herbal ingredients to bulletproof your immune system. The primary ingredients on the label: star anise extract, shikimic acid, and *Hypericum perforatum*. Recall: July 2007	Unapproved drug claim that it can prevent "Bird Flu"	Hi-Tech Pharmaceuticals, Inc., Norcross, GA	Hi-Tech Pharmaceuticals, Inc., Norcross, GA
Metaboslim All Natural Fat Eater Apple Cider Vinegar Recall: October 2007	Containing undeclared sibutramine, an active legal pharmaceutical ingredient used for weight loss in treatment of obesity	Confidence Inc., Port Washington, NY	Island Vitamins Inc., Farmingdale, NY
V.MAX Herbal Stamina Enhancer for Men Dietary Supplement, Cordyceps Militaries, L-Arginine, Psyllium Husk Powder, Licorice Root, Astragalus Membranaceus, Steamed Panax Ginseng Recall: November 2007	Containing aminotadalafil, an analogue of tadalafil, a legal drug used to treat erectile dysfunction	Barodon S.F., Inc., Los Angeles, CA	MegaCare Inc., Las Vegas, NV
True Man Sexual Energy Nutriment, Men's formula, Natural Herbs Energy Max Energy Supplement Men's formula Natural Herbs Recall: December 2007	Containing various analogues of legal drug ingredients approved for treating erectile dysfunction (ED)	America True Man Health, Inc., West Covina, CA	H & L Industries, Inc., dba Natural Source Int'l, Inc., LaVerne, CA
Gripe Water All Natural Apple Flavor. An herbal supplement used to ease the gas and stomach discomfort often associated with colic, hiccups, and teething Recall: January 2008	Containing cryptosporidium, confirmed after investigating the illness of a 6-week-old infant in Minnesota who consumed the product. Cryptosporidium is a parasite that can cause intestinal infections.	MOM Enterprises, Inc., San Rafael, CA	Botanical Laboratories Inc., Ferndale, WA

and electronic (Web site) media distributed by the company.

FDA considers these products to be unapproved new drugs because they make claims related to the prevention or treatment of diseases in the products' labeling. Such seizures protect consumers who may rely on unapproved products and unsubstantiated claims associated with these products when making important decisions about their health.

Following an investigation of the firm's marketing practices, FDA officials advised FulLife that the claims related to prevention or treatment of diseases made these products subject to regulation as

drugs. Despite FDA's warnings, the firm failed to bring its marketing into compliance with the law. During subsequent inspections, FDA inspectors found that the offending claims were still being made.

On August 23, 2007, at the request of FDA, U.S. Marshals in the Northern District of Florida seized an estimated $41,000 worth of inventory of Glucobetic, Neuro-betic, Ocu-Comp, Atri-Oxi, Super-Flex, MSM-1000, and Atri-E-400 capsules being promoted and distributed by Charron Nutrition of Tallahassee, Florida, for use in treating diabetes, arthritis, and other serious health conditions.

PROGRESS CHECK ON ACTIVITY 4

TRUE/FALSE

Circle T for True and F for False.

1. T F I do not need to think about my total diet if I am taking dietary supplements.
2. T F Essential nutrients are safe, even when they are consumed in large doses.
3. T F I don't need to check with my doctor or health-care provider before using supplements if I have read the labels on these supplements.
4. T F All dietary supplements are risk free because they are sold over the counter.
5. T F Because vitamin and mineral supplements are widely used and generally considered safe, you may safely give them to your children.
6. T F If one plans to use a dietary supplement in place of drugs or in combination with any drug, one should tell one's healthcare provider first.
7. T F Dietary supplements, generally considered as safe, should not interact with prescription and over-the-counter (OTC) medicines.
8. T F When taking medication(s) or dietary supplement(s), advisories about these products should not be taken too seriously.
9. T F It is important to fully inform your doctor about the vitamins, minerals, herbals, or any other supplements you are taking before elective surgery.
10. T F Under the law, manufacturers of dietary supplements are not responsible for making sure their products are safe before they go to market.
11. T F Manufacturers of dietary supplements are responsible for determining that the claims on their labels are accurate and truthful.
12. T F If the FDA can prove that claims on marketed dietary supplement products are false and misleading, the agency may take action against products with such claims.
13. T F When searching on the Web, the directory sites of organizations included in all search engines are reliable.
14. T F Most nonprofit and government sites contain no advertising, and access to the site and materials offered are usually free.
15. T F While the Web can be a valuable source of accurate, reliable information, it also has a wealth of misinformation that may not be obvious.
16. T F Information from trained people is usually more much more reliable than that from lay people.
17. T F Even if a product may not help me, at least it won't hurt me.
18. T F When I see the term *natural*, it means that a product is healthful and safe.
19. T F A recall of a harmful product guarantees that all such harmful products will be immediately and completely removed from the marketplace.
20. T F It is appropriate to contact the manufacturer for more information about the specific product that one is purchasing.
21. T F When a nurse is caring for a patient who is involved with dietary supplements (using them, intending to use them, or asking questions about them), he or she should assist the patient in making appropriate choices through educating the patient and family regarding their use.
22. T F Fraudulent products often can be identified by the types of claims made in their labeling, advertising, and promotional literature.
23. T F According to the National Council Against Health Fraud, a product may be fraudulent if it contains claims such as *breakthrough, magical, miracle cure, new discovery, detoxify, purify, energize, cure a wide range of unrelated diseases*, and *only benefits but no side effects*.
24. T F Quality dietary supplements have no reason to carry the U.S.P. notation for their ingredients.
25. T F Nationally known food and drug manufacturers usually have tighter controls in their manufacturing methods for their products.
26. T F When a consumer starts to take a dietary supplement, he or she must check with a medical doctor.
27. T F Dietary supplements often contain plant products that may also be used in prescription medicine.

FILL-IN

28. Before starting a dietary supplement, it is always wise to check with a medical doctor. It is especially important for people who have the following characteristics:

    a. _____

    b. _____

    c. _____

    d. _____

    e. _____

29. The following minimal criteria should be followed when a person starts to take dietary supplements:

    H. _____

    O. _____

P. _____

E. _____

S. _____

REFERENCES

American Dietetic Association. (2000). *A Healthcare Professional's Guide to Evaluating Dietary Supplements.* Chicago: Author.

Bendich, A., & Deckelbaum, R. J. (Eds.). (2005). *Preventive Nutrition: The Comprehensive Guide for Health Professionals* (3rd ed.). Totowa, NJ: Humana Press.

Caballero, B., Allen, L., & Prentice, A. (Eds.). (2005). *Encyclopedia of Human Nutrition* (2nd ed.). Boston: Elsevier/Academic Press.

Davis, W. M. (2006). *Consumer's Guide to Dietary Supplements and Alternate Medicines: Servings of Hope.* New York: Pharmaceutical Products Press.

Di Pasquale, M. G. (2008). *Amino Acid and Proteins for the Athlete: The Anabolic Edge.* Boca Raton, FL: CRC Press.

Fairfield, K. (2007). Vitamin and mineral supplements for cancer prevention: Issues and evidence. *American Journal of Clinical Nutrition, 85*: 289s–292s.

Goodlad, R. A. (2007). Fiber can make your gut grow. *Nutrition, 23*: 434–435.

Higdon, J. (2007). *An Evidence-Based Approach to Dietary Phytochemicals.* New York: Thieme Medical.

Higdon, J. V. (2003). Tea catechins and polyphenols: Health effects, metabolism, and antioxidant functions. *Critical Reviews in Food Science and Nutrition, 43*: 89–143.

Huang, H. Y. (2007). Multivitamin/multimineral supplements and prevention of chronic disease: Executive summary. *American Journal of Clinical Nutrition, 85*: 265s–268s.

Jakubowski, H. (2003). On the health benefits of Allium sp. *Nutrition, 19*: 167–168.

Lagua, R. T., & Qaudio, V. S. (2004). *Nutrition and Diet Therapy: Reference Dictionary* (5th ed.). Ames, IA: Blackwell.

Marian, M. J., Williams-Muller, P., & Bower, J. (2007). *Integrating Therapeutic and Complementary Nutrition.* Boca Raton, FL: CRC Press.

Navarra, T. (2004). *The Encyclopedia of Vitamins, Minerals, and Supplements.* New York: Facts on File.

Ostlund, R. E. (2002). Phytosterols in human nutrition. *Annual Review of Nutrition, 22*: 533–549.

Rosenburg, I. H. (2007). Challenges and opportunities in the translation of the science of vitamins. *American Journal of Clinical Nutrition, 85*: 325s–327s.

Shils, M. E., & Shike, M. (Eds.). (2006). *Modern Nutrition in Health and Disease* (10th ed.). Philadelphia: Lippincott, Williams and Wilkins.

Smith, A. D. (2007). Folic acid fortification: The good, the bad, and the puzzle of vitamin B-1. *American Journal of Clinical Nutrition, 85*: 3–5 [Erratum: 86, 1256].

Stanner, S. A. (2004). A review of epidemiological evidence for the 'antioxidant hypothesis'. *Public Health Nutrition, 7*: 407–422.

Steyer, T. E. (2003). Use of nutritional supplements for the prevention and treatment of hypercholesterolemia. *Nutrition, 19*: 415–418.

Temple, N. J., Wilson, T., & Jacobs, D. R. (2006). *Nutrition Health: Strategies for Disease Prevention* (2nd ed.). Totowa, NJ: Humana Press.

Theobal, H. E. (2007). Low-dose docosahexanoic acid lowers diastolic blood pressure in middle-aged men and women. *Journal of Nutrition, 137*: 973–978.

Vaysse-Boue, C. (2007). Moderate dietary intake of myristic acid and alpha-linolenic acids increases lecithin-cholesterol acyltransferase activity in humans. *Lipids, 42*: 717–722.

CHAPTER 12

Alternative Medicine

Time for Completion
Activities: 1½ hours
Optional examination: ½ hour

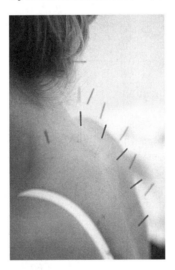

OBJECTIVES

Upon completion of this chapter the student should be able to do the following:

1. Identify five healing philosophies, approaches, and therapies not taught in medical schools.
2. Define complementary and alternative medicine (CAM):
   a. Describe the five domains or categories of CAM.
   b. List at least two examples in each domain and state the principal methods used in each.
3. Name at least five products or devices related to alternative medicine.
4. Describe the principle involved in using acupuncture as a complementary therapy in Western medicine.
5. Discuss ways to evaluate and provide reliable information to clients regarding the use of alternative medical treatment and practices.

GLOSSARY

Acupuncture: the use of very fine, thin wire needles inserted into the skin at specific sites in the body. A complementary therapy widely employed by licensed physicians. The needles used have received FDA approval.

Alternative: therapy used alone to treat an illness.

Biological-based: therapies employing herbs, special foods, and treatment with megadose vitamins and minerals and other ingested substances, such as laetrile or bee pollen.

Complementary: therapy used in addition to conventional therapy.

Complementary and alternative medicine (CAM): those therapies and medical practices not currently part of conventional medicine.

Conventional: therapies widely accepted and practiced by the mainstream medical community.

Energy therapy: a system that employs energy fields originating within the body or from electromagnetic fields outside the body.

Holistic: therapy that includes treatment of the whole person.

Homeopathic: a complete alternative medical system whose basic principle is "like cures like."

Laetrile: an unapproved compound used as an anticancer treatment. Contains cyanide. Drug is not available in the United States. Side effects are severe and can cause death.

Manipulative or body-based: methods based on manipulation and/or movement of the body, for example, chiropractic or massage therapy.

Mind-body therapy: techniques employed to facilitate the mind's capacity to affect body function and systems. Only two are considered mainstream: cognitive-behavioral approaches and patient education.

Naturopathic: a complete alternative medical system that emphasizes natural healing.

Preventive: therapy that seeks to prevent health problems from arising.

St.-John's-wort: an herb used as an alternative treatment for depression.

BACKGROUND INFORMATION

For more than a decade alternative medicine has played an increasing role in the health of Americans. In view of the extensive claims about its effectiveness, the information in this chapter is based on the following premises:

1. The purpose is to inform and not to recommend diagnosis, treatment, or cure.
2. Although nutrition and diet therapy are the subject matters of this book, their role in alternative medicine is only one consideration. To provide a meaningful picture of alternative medicine, this chapter discusses its entire spectrum, which includes diet and nutrition or human metabolism.
3. To ensure its accuracy and the absence of bias, all information in this chapter has been derived from educational materials distributed by the National Center for Complementary and Alternative Medicine, a unit within the U.S. National Institutes of Health.

Complementary and alternative medicine (CAM) covers a broad range of healing philosophies, approaches, and therapies. Generally, it is defined as those treatments and healthcare practices not taught widely in medical schools, not generally used in hospitals, and not usually reimbursed by medical insurance companies.

Many therapies are termed *holistic*, which means that the healthcare practitioner considers the whole person, including physical, mental, emotional, and spiritual aspects. Many therapies are also known as *preventive*, which means that the practitioner educates and treats the person to prevent health problems from arising, rather than treating symptoms after problems have occurred.

People use these treatments and therapies in a variety of ways. Therapies are used alone, in combination with other alternative therapies, or in addition to conventional therapies. Some approaches are consistent with physiological principles of Western medicine, while others constitute healing systems with a different origin. While some therapies are far outside the realm of accepted Western medical theory and practice, others are becoming established in mainstream medicine.

Complementary and alternative health care and medical practices are those health care and medical practices that are not currently an integral part of conventional medicine. The list of practices that are considered CAM changes continually as CAM practices and therapies that are proven safe and effective become accepted as "mainstream" healthcare practices.

A therapy is generally called *complementary* when it is used in addition to conventional treatments; it is often called *alternative* when it is used instead of conventional treatment. (Conventional treatments are those that are widely accepted and practiced by the mainstream medical community.) Depending on how they are used, some therapies can be considered either complementary or alternative. Complementary and alternative therapies are used in an effort to prevent illness, reduce stress, prevent or reduce side effects and symptoms, or control or cure disease.

Unlike conventional treatments for diseases, complementary and alternative therapies are often not covered by insurance companies. Patients should check with their insurance provider to find out about coverage for complementary and alternative therapies.

Patients considering complementary and alternative therapies should discuss this decision with their doctor or nurse, as they would any therapeutic approach, because some complementary and alternative therapies may interfere with their standard treatment or may be harmful when used with conventional treatment.

PROGRESS CHECK ON BACKGROUND INFORMATION

FILL-IN

1. Complementary and alternative medicine (CAM) are treatments and healthcare practices generally not:

   a. _____

   b. _____

   c. _____

2. Holistic treatment generally means that the healthcare practitioner considers the whole person, including aspects that are:

   a. _____

   b. _____

   c. _____

   d. _____

3. Name six products or devices related to alternate medicine:

   a. _____

   b. _____

   c. _____

   d. _____

   e. _____

   f. _____

TRUE/FALSE

Circle T for True and F for False.

4. T F Preventive therapy that seeks to prevent health problems from arising is generally taught in medical schools.

5. T F Biologically based therapies that employ herbs, special foods, and treatment with megadose vitamins and minerals and other ingested substances are completely ineffective in the eyes of most of the conventional medical practitioners in the United States.

6. T F Cognitive-behavior approach is a mind-body therapy not widely accepted by the conventional medical practitioner.

7. T F Patient education is critical in the employment of complementary and alternative medicine.

8. T F Acupuncture therapy uses very fine, thin needles inserted into the skin at specific sites in the body to achieve certain healing effect. It is widely accepted by conventional medical practitioners in the United States.

ACTIVITY 1:

Categories or Domains of Complementary and Alternative Medicine

Today, CAM practices may be grouped within five major domains: (1) alternative medical systems, (2) mind-body interventions, (3) biologically based treatments, (4) manipulative and body-based methods, and (5) energy therapies. The individual systems and treatments making up these categories are too numerous to list in this document. Thus, only limited examples are provided within each.

ALTERNATIVE MEDICAL SYSTEMS

Alternative medical systems involve complete systems of theory and practice that have evolved independent of and often prior to the conventional biomedical approach. Many are traditional systems of medicine that are practiced by individual cultures throughout the world, including a number of venerable Asian approaches.

Traditional Chinese medicine emphasizes the proper balance or disturbances of qi (pronounced chi or chee), or vital energy, in health and disease, respectively. Traditional Chinese medicine consists of a group of techniques and methods, including acupuncture, herbal medicine, oriental massage, and qi gong (a form of energy therapy described more fully later). Acupuncture involves stimulating specific anatomic points in the body for therapeutic purposes, usually by puncturing the skin with a needle.

Ayurveda is India's traditional system of medicine. Ayurvedic medicine (meaning "science of life") is a comprehensive system of medicine that places equal emphasis on body, mind, and spirit, and strives to restore the innate harmony of the individual. Some of the primary Ayurvedic treatments include diet, exercise, meditation, herbs, massage, exposure to sunlight, and controlled breathing.

Other traditional medical systems have been developed by Native American, Aboriginal, African, Middle Eastern, Tibetan, and Central and South American cultures.

Homeopathic and naturopathic medicine are also examples of complete alternative medical systems. Homeopathic medicine is an unconventional Western system that is based on the principle that "like cures like," namely, that the same substance that in large doses produces the symptoms of an illness, in very minute doses cures it. Homeopathic physicians believe that the more dilute the remedy, the greater its potency. Therefore, they use small doses of specially prepared plant extracts and minerals to stimulate the body's defense mechanisms and healing processes to treat illness.

Naturopathic medicine views disease as a manifestation of alterations in the processes by which the body naturally heals itself and emphasizes health restoration rather than disease treatment. Naturopathic physicians employ an array of healing practices, including diet and clinical nutrition; homeopathy; acupuncture; herbal medicine; hydrotherapy (the use of water in a range of temperatures and methods of applications); spinal and soft-tissue manipulation; physical therapies involving electric currents, ultrasound and light therapy; therapeutic counseling; and pharmacology.

MIND-BODY INTERVENTIONS

Mind-body interventions employ a variety of techniques designed to facilitate the mind's capacity to affect bodily function and symptoms. Only a subset of mind-body interventions are considered CAM. Many interventions that have a well-documented theoretical basis, for example, patient education and cognitive-behavioral approaches, are now considered "mainstream." Meditation; certain uses of hypnosis; dance, music, and art therapy; and prayer and mental healing still are categorized as complementary and alternative.

BIOLOGICAL-BASED THERAPIES

This category of CAM includes natural and biological-based practices, interventions, and products, many of which overlap with conventional medicine's use of dietary supplements. Included in this category are herbal, special dietary, orthomolecular, and individual biological therapies.

Herbal therapies employ individual or mixtures of herbs for therapeutic value. An herb is a plant or plant part that produces and contains chemical substances that act upon the body. Special diet therapies, such as those proposed by Drs. Atkins, Ornish, Pritikin, and Weil, are believed to prevent and or control illness as well as promote health. Orthomolecular therapies aim to treat disease with varying concentrations of chemicals, such as magnesium, melatonin, and megadoses of vitamins. Biological therapies include, for example, the use of laetrile and shark cartilage to treat cancer and bee pollen to treat autoimmune and inflammatory diseases.

MANIPULATIVE AND BODY-BASED METHODS

This category includes methods that are based on manipulation and/or movement of the body. For example, chiropractors focus on the relationship between structure (primarily the spine) and function, and how that relationship affects the preservation and restoration of health, using manipulative therapy as an integral treatment tool. Some osteopaths, who place particular emphasis on the musculoskeletal system, believing that all of the body's systems work together and that disturbances in one system may affect function elsewhere in the body, practice osteopathic manipulation. Massage therapists manipulate the soft tissues of the body to normalize those tissues.

ENERGY THERAPIES

Energy therapies focus either on energy fields originating within the body (biofields) or those from other sources (electromagnetic fields). Biofield therapies are intended to affect the energy fields, whose existence is not yet experimentally proven, that surround and penetrate the human body. Some forms of energy therapy manipulate biofields by applying pressure and/or manipulating the body by placing the hands in, or through, these fields. Examples include Qi gong, Reiki, and Therapeutic Touch. Qi gong is a component of traditional Chinese medicine that combines movement, meditation, and regulation of breathing to enhance the flow of vital energy (qi) in the body, to improve blood circulation, and to enhance immune function. Reiki, the Japanese word representing *Universal Life Energy*, is based on the belief that by channeling spiritual energy through the practitioner the spirit is healed, and it in turn heals the physical body. Therapeutic Touch is derived from the ancient technique of "laying-on of hands" and is based on the premise that it is the healing force of the therapist that affects the patient's recovery and that healing is promoted when the body's energies are in balance. By passing their hands over the patient, these healers identify energy imbalances.

Bioelectromagnetic-based therapies involve the unconventional use of electromagnetic fields—such as pulsed fields, magnetic fields, or alternating current or direct current fields—to, for example, treat asthma or cancer, or manage pain and migraine headaches.

PROGRESS CHECK ON ACTIVITY 1

FILL-IN

1. The five major domains of CAM practices are:

   a. _____

   b. _____

   c. _____

   d. _____

   e. _____

2. Traditional Asian medicine consists of mainly the following techniques and methods:

   a. _____

   b. _____

   c. _____

   d. _____

3. Name five of the primary Ayurvedic treatments:

   a. _____

   b. _____

   c. _____

   d. _____

   e. _____

4. Name five of the practices that naturopathic physicians will employ in healing:

   a. _____

   b. _____

   c. _____

   d. _____

   e. _____

5. Examples of energy therapy that manipulate biofields by applying pressure and/or manipulating the body by placing the hands in, or through, these fields are:

   a. _____

   b. _____

   c. _____

TRUE/FALSE

Circle T for True and F for False.

6. T F Alternative medical systems involve complete systems of theory and practice that have evolved independent of and often prior to the conventional biomedical approach.

7. T F Traditional Asian medicine emphasizes the proper balance or disturbances of qi (pronounced chi), or vital energy, in health and disease, respectively.

8. T F The basic principles of traditional Asian medicine principles and Ayurvedic medicine are completely different.

9. T F Homeopathic physicians use small doses of specially prepared plant extracts and minerals to stimulate the body's defense mechanisms and healing processes in order to treat illness.

10. T F Naturopathic medicine views disease as a manifestation of alterations in the processes by which the body naturally heals itself and emphasizes health restoration rather than disease treatment.

11. T F Meditation; certain uses of hypnosis; dance, music, and art therapy; and prayer and mental healing are ineffective therapies in the minds of conventional medical practitioners.

12. T F Herbal therapies that employ individual or mixtures of herbs for therapeutic value are not effective means of treating any diseases.

13. T F Use of laetrile and shark cartilage to treat cancer has been proven to be effective.

14. T F Bee pollen to treat autoimmune and inflammatory diseases has not been proven to be effective.

15. T F Chiropractors focus on the relationship between structure (primarily the spine) and function, and how that relationship affects the preservation and restoration of health by using manipulative therapy.

16. T F Energy therapies focus either on energy fields originating within the body (biofields) or those from other sources (electromagnetic fields).

17. T F Qi gong is a component of traditional Asian medicine that combines movement, meditation, and regulation of breathing to enhance the flow of vital energy (qi) in the body, to improve blood circulation, and to enhance immune function.

18. T F Therapeutic Touch is very similar to the form of qi gong treatment that applies energy to the patient through an external source.

ACTIVITY 2:

Products, Devices, and Services Related to Complementary and Alternative Medicine

According to Amazon.com, there are more than 500 books on various products, devices, and services related to alternative medicine. The following are some that have attracted much attention from the government and consumers:

1. Acupuncture
2. Cancell/Entelev
3. Gerson therapy
4. Gonzalez protocol
5. Immuno-augmentative therapy
6. Coenzyme Q10
7. Laetrile
8. St.-John's-wort
9. Cartilage (bovine and shark)
10. Hydrazine sulfate
11. Mistletoe

This chapter is not the proper forum to explore all of them. Instead, three specific examples are provided-acupuncture, laetrile, and St.-John's-wort. Acupuncture has no dietary significance. It is included here as an illustration of nondietary alternative medicine. Laetrile and St.-John's-wort have direct relationships to our diet because they are ingested for desired effects.

ACUPUNCTURE

Introduction

Acupuncture is one of the oldest, most commonly used medical procedures in the world. Originating in China more than 2000 years ago, acupuncture began to become better known in the United States in 1971, when *New York Times* reporter James Reston wrote about how doctors in China used needles to ease his abdominal pain after surgery. Research shows that acupuncture is beneficial in treating a variety of health conditions. In the past two decades, acupuncture has grown in popularity in the United States. A Harvard University study published in 1998 estimated that Americans made more than five million visits per year to acupuncture practitioners. The report from a Consensus Development Conference on Acupuncture held at the National Institutes of Health (NIH) in 1997 stated that acupuncture is being "widely" practiced-by thousands of physicians, dentists, acupuncturists, and other practitioners-for relief or prevention of pain and for various other health conditions. NIH has funded a variety of research projects on acupuncture. These grants have been awarded by the National Center for Complementary and Alternative Medicine (NCCAM), the Office of Alternative Medicine (OAM, NCCAM's predecessor), and other NIH institutes and centers. Traditional Chinese medicine theorizes that there are more than 2000 acupuncture points on the human body, and that these connect with 12 main and 8 secondary pathways called meridians. Chinese medicine practitioners believe these meridians conduct energy, or qi (pronounced chee or chi), throughout the body. Qi is believed to regulate spiritual, emotional, mental, and physical balance and to be influenced by the opposing forces of yin and yang.

According to traditional Chinese medicine, when yin and yang are balanced, they work together with the natural flow of qi to help the body achieve and maintain health. Acupuncture is believed to balance yin and yang, keep the normal flow of energy unblocked, and maintain or restore health to the body and mind.

Traditional Chinese medicine practices (including acupuncture, herbs, diet, massage, and meditative physical exercise) all are intended to improve the flow of qi. Western scientists have found meridians hard to identify because meridians do not directly correspond to nerve or blood circulation pathways. Some researchers believe that meridians are located throughout the body's connective tissue; others do not believe that qi exists at all.

Such differences of opinion have made acupuncture an area of scientific controversy. Several processes have been proposed to explain acupuncture's effects, primarily those on pain. Acupuncture points are believed to stimulate the central nervous system (the brain and spinal cord) to release chemicals into the muscles, spinal cord, and brain. These chemicals either change the experience of pain or release other chemicals, such as hormones, that influence the body's self-regulating systems. The biochemical changes may stimulate the body's natural healing abilities and promote physical and emotional well-being.

There are three main mechanisms under consideration:

- Conduction of electromagnetic signals: Western scientists have found evidence that acupuncture points are strategic conductors of electromagnetic signals. Stimulating points along these pathways through acupuncture enables electromagnetic signals to be relayed at a greater rate than under normal conditions. These signals may start the flow of pain-killing biochemicals, such as endorphins, and of immune system cells to specific sites in the body that are injured or vulnerable to disease.
- Activation of opioid systems: Research has found that several types of opioids may be released into the central nervous system during acupuncture treatment, thereby reducing pain.
- Changes in brain chemistry, sensation, and involuntary body functions: Studies have shown that acupuncture may alter brain chemistry by changing the release of neurotransmitters and neurohormones in a positive way.

Acupuncture also has been documented to affect the parts of the central nervous system related to sensation and involuntary body functions, such as immune reactions and processes whereby a person's blood pressure, blood flow, and body temperature are regulated.

Preclinical studies have documented acupuncture's effects, but they have not been able to fully explain how acupuncture works within the framework of the Western system of medicine.

Clinical Studies

According to the NIH Consensus Statement on Acupuncture:

Acupuncture as a therapeutic intervention is widely practiced in the United States. While there have been many studies of its potential usefulness, many of these studies provide equivocal results because of design, sample size, and other factors. The issue is further complicated by inherent difficulties in the use of appropriate controls, such as placebos and sham acupuncture groups. However, promising results have emerged, for example, showing efficacy of acupuncture in adult postoperative and chemotherapy nausea and vomiting and in postoperative dental pain. There are other situations such as addiction, stroke rehabilitation, headache, menstrual cramps, tennis elbow, fibromyalgia, myofascial pain, osteoarthritis, low back pain, carpal tunnel syndrome, and asthma, in which acupuncture may be useful as an adjunct treatment or an acceptable alternative or may be included in a comprehensive management program. Further research is likely to uncover additional areas where acupuncture interventions will be useful.

Increasingly, acupuncture is complementing conventional therapies. For example, doctors may combine acupuncture and drugs to control surgery-related pain in their patients. By providing both acupuncture and certain conventional anesthetic drugs, some doctors have found it possible to achieve a state of complete pain relief for some patients. They also have found that using acupuncture lowers the need for conventional painkilling drugs and thus reduces the risk of side effects for patients who take the drugs.

Currently, one of the main reasons Americans seek acupuncture treatment is to relieve chronic pain, especially from conditions such as arthritis or lower back disorders. Some clinical studies show that acupuncture is effective in relieving both chronic (long-lasting) and acute or sudden pain, but other research indicates that it provides no relief from chronic pain. Additional research is needed to provide definitive answers.

FDA's Role

The U.S. Food and Drug Administration (FDA) approved acupuncture needles for use by licensed practitioners in 1996. The FDA requires manufacturers of acupuncture needles to label them for single use only.

Relatively few complications from the use of acupuncture have been reported to the FDA when one considers the millions of people treated each year and the number of acupuncture needles used. Still, complications have resulted from inadequate sterilization of needles and from improper delivery of treatments. When not delivered properly, acupuncture can cause serious adverse effects, including infections and punctured organs.

LAETRILE

Laetrile is a compound that has been used as an anticancer treatment in humans worldwide. It is not approved by the Food and Drug Administration for use in the United States. The term *laetrile* is an acronym (laevorotatory and mandelonitrile) used to describe a purified form of the chemical amygdalin. Amygdalin is a plant compound that contains sugar and produces cyanide. Amygdalin is found in the pits of many fruits and raw nuts. It is also found in other plants, such as lima beans, clover, and sorghum. Cyanide is believed to be the active cancer-killing ingredient in laetrile.

Although the names laetrile, Laetrile, and amygdalin are often used interchangeably, they are not the same product. The chemical make-up of Laetrile patented in the United States is different from the laetrile/amygdalin produced in Mexico. The patented Laetrile is a semisynthetic form of amygdalin, while the laetrile/amygdalin manufactured in Mexico is made from crushed apricot pits.

Amygdalin was first isolated in 1830 and was used as an anticancer agent in Russia as early as 1845. Its first recorded use in the United States as a treatment for cancer was in the 1920s. The early pill form of amygdalin was considered too toxic, and work with the compound was discontinued. In the 1950s, a reportedly nontoxic, semisynthetic form of amygdalin was developed and patented in the United States as Laetrile. Laetrile gained popularity in the 1970s as a single anticancer agent and as part of a metabolic therapy program consisting of a special diet, high-dose vitamin supplements, and pancreatic enzyme proteins that aid in the digestion of food. By 1978, more than 70,000 people in the United States had reportedly been treated with Laetrile.

Laetrile is administered by mouth (orally) as a pill. It can also be given by injection into a vein (intravenously) or muscle. Laetrile is commonly given intravenously over a period of time and then orally as maintenance therapy (treatment given to help extend the benefit of previous therapy).

The side effects associated with laetrile treatment are like the symptoms of cyanide poisoning. The symptoms include nausea and vomiting, headache, dizziness, bluish discoloration of the skin due to a lack of oxygen in the blood, liver damage, abnormally low blood pressure, droopy upper eyelid, difficulty walking due to damaged nerves, fever, mental confusion, coma, and death. The side effects can be increased by eating raw almonds or crushed fruit pits; eating certain types of fruits and vegetables including celery, peaches, bean sprouts, and carrots; or taking high doses of vitamin C. The side effects of laetrile appear to depend on the method of administration. More severe side effects are experienced when laetrile is given by mouth than when it is given by injection.

In nearly half a century, laetrile in the United States has gone through some "stormy weathers" scientifically, medically, legally, and commercially:

1. Scientifically, it is the position of the federal government that there is no sound scientific evidence to support the therapeutic claims for laetrile.
2. Medically, not all licensed physicians consider laetrile as a form of treatment for cancer. Physicians who use this substance as a curative agent on cancer patients are subject to prosecution.
3. Legally, there are several fronts:
   a. Several lawsuits have been filed on the constitutional rights of cancer patients to obtain laetrile to treat their conditions without interference from the government or the medical community.

b. The FDA has declared it is illegal to sell interstate laetrile or products claimed to contain laetrile as an ingredient. The products from several companies have been seized and some companies have been prosecuted.

c. States and federal governments have prosecuted licensed physicians who use laetrile to treat cancer patients.

The availability of laetrile in Mexico is a well known fact. Many cancer patients and/or their relatives and friends have visited Mexico to buy the substance. This is the action of a private citizen, and it is difficult for the United States government to intervene unless the person with the substance crosses the border between the two countries. It is illegal to bring laetrile into this country.

ST.-JOHN'S-WORT

St.-John's-wort (*Hypericum perforatum*) is a long-living plant with yellow flowers. It contains many chemical compounds. Some are believed to be the active ingredients that produce the herb's effects, including the compounds hypericin and hyperforin.

How these compounds actually work in the body is not yet known, but several theories have been suggested. Preliminary studies suggest that St.-John's-wort might work by preventing nerve cells in the brain from reabsorbing the chemical messenger serotonin, or by reducing levels of a protein involved in the body's immune system functioning.

St.-John's-wort has been used for centuries to treat mental disorders as well as nerve pain. In ancient times, doctors and herbalists (specialists in herbs) wrote about its use as a sedative and treatment for malaria as well as a balm for wounds, burns, and insect bites. Today, St.-John's-wort is used by some people to treat mild to moderate depression, anxiety, or sleep disorders.

Depressive illness comes in different forms. The three major forms are described here. Each can vary from person to person in terms of symptoms experienced and the severity of depression.

In major depression, people experience a sad mood or loss of interest or pleasure in activities for at least 2 weeks. In addition, they have at least four other symptoms of depression. Major depression can be mild, moderate, or severe. If it is not treated, it can last for 6 months or more.

In dysthymia, a milder, but more chronic form of depression, people experience a depressed mood for at least 2 years (1 year for children) accompanied by at least two other symptoms of depression.

In bipolar disorder, also called manic depression, a person has periods of depressive symptoms that alternate with periods of mania. Symptoms of mania include an abnormally high level of excitement and energy, racing thoughts, and behavior that is impulsive and inappropriate.

Some people still hold outdated beliefs about depression, for example, that the emotional symptoms caused by depression are "not real." However, depression is a real medical condition. It can be treated effectively with conventional medicine, including antidepressant drugs and certain types of psychotherapy.

St.-John's-wort has been used as an alternative therapy for depression. Some patients who take antidepressant drugs do not experience relief from their depression. Other patients have reported unpleasant side effects from their prescription medication, such as a dry mouth, nausea, headache, or effects on sexual function or sleep. Sometimes people turn to herbal preparations like St.-John's-wort because they believe "natural" products are better for them than prescription medications, or that natural products are always safe. Neither of these statements is true (discussed further later). Finally, cost can be a reason. St.-John's-wort costs less than many antidepressant medications, and it is sold without a prescription (over the counter).

In Europe, St.-John's-wort is widely prescribed for depression. In the United States, St.-John's-wort is not a prescription medication, but there is considerable public interest in it. St.-John's-wort remains among the top-selling herbal products in the United States.

St.-John's-wort products are sold in the following forms:

- Capsules
- Teas—the dried herb is added to boiling water and steeped for a period of time
- Extracts—specific types of chemicals are removed from the herb, leaving the desired chemicals in a concentrated form

Does St.-John's-wort work as a treatment for depression? There has been scientific research to try to answer this question. The general observation is as follows. In Europe, results from a number of scientific studies have supported the effectiveness of certain extracts of St.-John's-wort for depression. In the United States several clinical studies have concluded that this herb is not effective in treating depression. Irrespective of scientific evidence, many consumers in this country take a supplement of St.-John's-wort regularly to treat depression.

Are there any risks to taking St.-John's-wort for depression? Yes, many so—called natural substances can have harmful effects—especially if they are taken in too large a quantity or if they interact with something else the person is taking.

Research from the NIH has shown that St.-John's-wort interacts with some drugs—including certain drugs used to control HIV infection (such as indinavir). It may also interact with drugs that help prevent the body from rejecting transplanted organs (such as cyclosporine). Using St.-John's-wort limits these drugs' effectiveness. Also, St.-John's-wort is not a proven therapy for depression.

If depression is not adequately treated, it can become severe and, in some cases, may be associated with suicide. Consult a healthcare practitioner if you or someone you care about may be experiencing depression. People can experience side effects from taking St.-John's-wort. The most common side effects include dry mouth, dizziness, gastrointestinal symptoms, increased sensitivity to sunlight, and fatigue.

Herbal products such as St.-John's-wort are classified as dietary supplements by the U.S. Food and Drug Administration (FDA), a regulatory agency of the federal government. The FDA's requirements for testing and obtaining approval to sell dietary supplements are less strict than its requirements for drugs (see Chapter 11). Unlike drugs, herbal products can be sold without requiring studies on dosage, safety, or effectiveness.

The strength and quality of herbal products are often unpredictable. Products can differ in content not only from brand to brand, but from batch to batch. Information on labels may be misleading or inaccurate.

Consult Chapter 11 on dietary supplements.

NURSING IMPLICATIONS

Regarding alternative medicine, the nurse's role is educational:

1. Be prepared to answer client questions.
2. Evaluate all information before providing it to a client.
3. Chart any alternative or complementary therapies the client is using; some may be contraindicated to traditional medicine.

Questions and answers for the nurse and the client are discussed in the following sections

How Can I Find More Information About Complementary and Alternative Medical Practices?

Ask your healthcare provider about complementary and alternative medical treatments and practices in general, and about those particular practices used for your specific health problems.

Increasingly, healthcare providers are becoming familiar with alternative treatments or are able to refer you to someone who is. For scientific information about the safety and effectiveness of a particular treatment, ask your healthcare provider to obtain valid information for you.

If your healthcare provider cannot provide information, medical libraries, public libraries, and popular bookstores are good places to find information about particular complementary and alternative medical practices.

Also, you may want to ask practitioners of complementary and alternative health care about their practices. Many practitioners belong to a growing number of professional associations, educational organizations, and research institutions that provide information about complementary and alternative medical practices. Many organizations are developing Web sites.

Remember that these organizations may advocate a specific therapy or treatment and may be unable to provide complete and objective health information.

How Can I Find a Practitioner in My Area?

To find a qualified complementary and alternative medical healthcare practitioner, you may want to contact medical regulatory and licensing agencies in your state. These agencies may be able to provide information about a specific practitioner's credentials and background. Many states license practitioners who provide alternative therapies such as acupuncture, chiropractic services, naturopathy, herbal medicine, homeopathy, and massage therapy.

You may also locate practitioners by asking your healthcare provider or by contacting a professional association or organization. These organizations can provide names of local practitioners and provide information about how to determine the quality of a specific practitioner's services.

When Considering Complementary and Alternative Therapies, What Questions Should Patients Ask Their Healthcare Provider?

The following are basic questions many patients ask:

- What benefits can be expected from this therapy?
- What are the risks associated with this therapy?
- Do the known benefits outweigh the risks?
- What side effects can be expected?
- Will the therapy interfere with conventional treatment?
- Is this therapy part of a clinical trial? If so, who is sponsoring the trial?
- Will the therapy be covered by health insurance?

How Do I Evaluate Medical Resources on the Web?

The number of Web sites offering health-related resources grows every day. Many sites provide valuable information, while others may have information that is unreliable or misleading. This short guide contains important questions you should consider as you look for health information online. Answering these questions when you visit a new site will help you evaluate the information you find. There are 10 things you should know:

1. Who runs this site? Any good health-related Web site should make it easy for you to learn who is responsible for the site and its information.

2. Who pays for the site? It costs money to run a Web site. The source of a Web site's funding should be clearly stated or readily apparent. For example, Web addresses ending in ".gov" denote a federal government-sponsored site. You should know how the site pays for its existence. Does it sell advertising? Is it sponsored by a drug company? The source of funding can affect what content is presented, how the content is presented, and what the site owners want to accomplish on the site.

3. What is the purpose of the site? This question is related to who runs and pays for the site. An "About This Site" link appears on many sites; if it is there, use it. The purpose of the site should be clearly stated and should help you evaluate the trustworthiness of the information.

4. Where does the information come from? Many health and medical sites post information collected from other Web sites or sources. If the person or organization in charge of the site did not create the information, the original source should be clearly labeled.

5. What is the basis of the information? In addition to identifying who wrote the material you are reading, the site should describe the evidence that the material is based on. Medical facts and figures should have references (such as to articles in medical journals). Also, opinions or advice should be clearly set apart from information that is "evidence based" (that is, based on research results).

6. How is the information selected? Is there an editorial board? Do people with excellent medical qualifications review the material before it is posted?

7. How current is the information? Web sites should be reviewed and updated on a regular basis. It is particularly important that medical information be current. The most recent update or review date should be clearly posted. Even if the information has not changed, you want to know whether the site owners have reviewed it recently to ensure that it is still valid.

8. How does the site choose links to other sites? Web sites usually have a policy about how they establish links to other sites. Some medical sites take a conservative approach and don't link to any other sites. Some link to any site that asks, or pays, for a link. Others only link to sites that have met certain criteria.

9. What information about you does the site collect, and why? Web sites routinely track the paths visitors take through their sites to determine what pages are being used. However, many health Web sites ask for you to "subscribe" or "become a member." In some cases, this may be so that they can collect a user fee or select information for you that is relevant to your concerns. In all cases, this will give the site personal information about you.

Any credible health site asking for this kind of information should tell you exactly what they will and will not do with it. Many commercial sites sell "aggregate" (collected) data about their users to other companies, information such as what percentage of their users are women with breast cancer, for example. In some cases, they may collect and reuse information that is "personally identifiable," such as your ZIP code, gender, and birth date. Be certain that you read and understand any privacy policy or similar language on the site, and don't sign up for anything that you are not sure you fully understand.

10. How does the site manage interactions with visitors? There should always be a way for you to contact the site owner if you run across problems or have questions or feedback. If the site hosts chat rooms or other online discussion areas, it should tell visitors what the terms of using this service are. Is it moderated? If so, by whom, and why? It is always a good idea to spend time reading the discussion without joining in, so that you feel comfortable with the environment before becoming a participant.

PROGRESS CHECK ON ACTIVITY 2

FILL-IN

1. The three main proposed mechanisms for acupuncture are:

    a. _____

    b. _____

    c. _____

2. Name five side effects of laetrile treatment:

    a. _____

    b. _____

    c. _____

    d. _____

    e. _____

3. Name three places where information about complementary and alternative medicine (CAM) practices can be obtained:

    a. _____

    b. _____

    c. _____

4. Important questions one should consider as one looks for health information online are:

    a. _____

    b. _____

c. _____

d. _____

e. _____

f. _____

g. _____

h. _____

i. _____

j. _____

TRUE/FALSE

Circle T for True and F for False.

5. T F Traditional Chinese medicine is based on the presence of qi and its travel in the body through the meridians, and the balance of yin and yang that works with natural qi in the body.

6. T F Qi is believed to regulate spiritual, emotional, mental, and physical balance and to be influenced by the opposing forces of yin and yang.

7. T F Traditional Chinese medicine practices (including acupuncture, herbs, diet, massage, and meditative physical exercise) all are intended to improve the flow of qi.

8. T F Meridians exist in a form that can be identified by Western scientists.

9. T F One of the main reasons Americans seek acupuncture treatment is to relieve chronic pain, especially from conditions such as arthritis or lower back disorders.

10. T F Laetrile is an effective compound that has been used as an anticancer treatment in humans worldwide.

11. T F The term *laetrile* is an acronym used to describe a purified form of the chemical amygdalin.

12. T F The names laetrile, Laetrile, and amygdalin mean the same product.

13. T F The laetrile/amygdalin manufactured in Mexico is made from crushed apricot pits.

14. T F Laetrile is commonly given intravenously over a period of time and then orally as maintenance therapy (treatment given to help extend the benefit of previous therapy). The side effects of laetrile treatment are usually fairly mild.

15. T F The side effects of laetrile are similar regardless of the method of administration.

16. T F St.-John's-wort is classified as a dietary supplement by the U.S. Food and Drug Administration (FDA).

17. T F The composition of St.-John's-wort and how it might work are well understood.

18. T F Scientific evidence shows that St.-John's-wort is useful for treating mild to moderate depression but is of no benefit in treating major depression of moderate severity.

19. T F Since St.-John's-wort is classified by FDA as a dietary supplement, it is safe and has no side effects.

20. T F Regarding CAM, a nurse must be able to answer patient's questions and evaluate information before providing advice.

21. T F Healthcare practitioners are obligated to provide complementary and alternative medical treatments and practices in general, and those particular practices used for your specific health problems.

22. T F CAM practitioners do not have to be certified in the United States.

REFERENCES

Allison, D. B. (2001). Alternate treatments for weight loss: A review. *Critical Reviews in Food Science and Nutrition, 41*: 1–28.

Baser, K. H. C. (2005). New trends in the utilization of medical and aromatic plants. *Acta Horticulturae, 676*: 11–23.

Bendich, A., Deckelbaum, R. J. (Eds.). (2005). *Preventive Nutrition: The Comprehensive Guide for Health Professionals* (3rd ed.). Totowa, NJ: Humana Press.

Coulston, A. M., Rock, C. L., & Monsen, E. L. (Eds.). (2001). *Nutrition in the Prevention and Treatment of Disease.* San Diego, CA: Academic Press.

Das, U. (2007). Functional food products and phytotherapy for chronic diseases. *HerbGram, 75*: 65–66.

Davis, W. M. (2006). *Consumer's Guide to Dietary Supplements and Alternate Medicines: Servings of Hope.* New York: Pharmaceutical Products Press.

Eastwood, M. (2003). *Principles of Human Nutrition* (2nd ed.). Malden, MA: Blackwell Science.

Etkin, N. L. (2006). *Edible Medicines: An Ethnopharmacology of Food.* Tuscon, AZ: University of Arizona Press.

Evans, M. (2001). Ripe for study: Complementary and alternative treatments for obesity. *Critical Reviews in Food Science and Nutrition, 41*: 35–37.

Garrow, D. (2006). Association between complementary and alternative medicine use, preventive care practices, and use of conventional medical services. *Diabetes Care, 29*: 15–19.

Harrison, R. A. (2004). Who and how many people are taking herbal supplements? A survey of 21,923 adults. *International Journal for Vitamin and Nutrition Research, 74*: 183–186.

Hollander, J. M. (2008). Complementary and alternate medicine and the management of the metabolic syndrome. *Journal of American Dietetic Association, 108*: 495–509.

Higdon, J. (2007). An Evidence-Based Approach to Dietary Phytochemicals. New York: Thieme Medical.

Mahan, L. K., Escott-Stump, S. (Eds.) (2008). *Krause's Food and Nutrition Therapy* (12th ed.). Philadelphia: Elsevier Saunders.

Marian, M. J., Williams-Muller, P., & Bower, J. (2007). *Integrating Therapeutic and Complementary Nutrition.* Boca Raton, FL: CRC Press.

Mathieu, J. (2005). Herbs and cancer treatment. *Journal of American Dietetic Association: 105,* 22, 24.

Mueller, M. S. (2005). Medical Plants in Tropical Use Experience Facts. Stuttgart, NY: Thieme.

Palmer, S. (2007). Can diet or supplements relieve your arthritis aches and inflammation? *Environmental Nutrition, 30*(8): 1, 4.

Pittler, M. H. (2005). Complementary therapies for reducing body weight: A systematic review. *International Journal of Obesity and Related Metabolic Disorders, 29*: 1030–1038.

Purcell, K. (2005). Survey shows 36% of U.S. adults use CAM. *HerbGram, 65*: 66.

Rivin, R. S. (2006). Is garlic alternate medicine? *Journal of Nutrition, 136*: 713s–715s.

Sarkar, S. (2007). Functional foods as self-care and complementary medicine. *Nutrition and Food Science, 37*: 160–167.

Shapiro, A. C. (2001). Guidelines for responsible nutrition counseling on complementary and alternate medicine. *Nutrition Today, 36*: 291–297.

Shils, M. E., & Shike, M. (Eds.). (2006). *Modern Nutrition in Health and Disease* (10th ed.). Philadelphia: Lippincott, Williams and Wilkins.

Temple, N. J., Wilson, T. & Jacobs, D. R. (2006). *Nutrition Health: Strategies for Disease Prevention* (2nd ed.). Totowa, NJ: Humana Press.

Touger-Decker, R. (2003). Complementary and alternate medicine: Competencies for dietetics professionals. *Journal of American Dietetic Association, 103*: 1465–1469.

Vangsness, S. (2005). Education and knowledge of dietetic interns regarding herbs and dietary supplements: Preparing for practice. *Topics in Clinical Nutrition, 20*: 269–276.

Vickery, C. E. (2006). Complementary and alternate medicine education in dietetics programs: Existent but not consistent. *Journal of American Dietetic Association, 106*: 860–866.

Walker, A. F. (2006). Herbal medicine: The science of the art. *Proceedings of Nutrition Society, 65*: 145–152.

CHAPTER **13**

Food Ecology

Time for completion
Activities: 1 hour
Optional examination: ½ hour

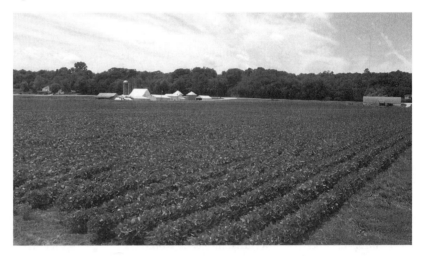

OBJECTIVES

Upon completion of this chapter, the student should be able to do the following:

1. Describe the appropriate methods for the safe handling, storage, and preparation of food to prevent illness by:
   a. recognizing agents that cause food-borne illness.
   b. knowing ways to minimize contamination.
   c. becoming familiar with regulations regarding the protection of food.
2. Describe the appropriate methods for handling, storing, and preparing food to conserve nutrients by becoming knowledgeable about:
   a. nutrition labeling.
   b. pasteurization, enrichment, and fortification of foods.

GLOSSARY

Bacteria: small unicellular microorganisms. They are spherical (cocci), rod shaped (bacilli), comma shaped (vibrios), or spiral (spirochetes). The symptoms produced by the bacteria depend on the type of bacteria ingested.

Enrichment: the addition of thiamin, niacin, riboflavin, and iron to bread and cereal products. The amount added to foods is set by the federal government.

Fortification: the addition of one or more nutrients not originally present in the food.

GRAS: generally recognized as safe. These are additives that have been used for a long time without known ill effects. Substances and additives sanctioned by the FDA prior to 1958.

Pasteurization: the practice of heating milk to 140°F for 30 seconds to kill disease-producing bacteria, or to 161°F for 15 seconds.

Restoration: replacing food nutrients that were present before processing but were destroyed by the processing.

URI: upper respiratory infection.

Virus: a minute microorganism much smaller than a bacterium. It has no independent cell activity. Viruses reproduce inside a host cell. More than 200 disease-producing viruses have been identified.

BACKGROUND INFORMATION

No matter how thorough an individual's knowledge is regarding the nutritional value of foods, unless the food is safe, there can be no optimal diets. No matter how carefully selected, food can only provide nourishment and health if it has been handled in such a way that it is neither contaminated nor a source of food-borne illness. Certain organisms that are transmitted to humans through food cause illness and sometimes death.

Modern food technology and sanitation practices have greatly reduced the threat of commercial food contamination. Food labelings have enabled consumers to be aware of the contents of food purchased. However, unsafe food-handling practices and nutrient losses from food preparation persist and continue to create problems even in modern societies. This is especially true in any group-eating environments, including healthcare facilities, shelter and retirement centers, schools, and restaurants.

Information on food safety has been derived from the following Web sites of U.S. government agencies:

1. U.S. Department of Agriculture (USDA): www.usda.gov
2. Food Safety Inspection Service of the USDA: www.fsis.gov
3. Food and Drug Administration: www.fda.gov
4. Centers for Disease Controls: www.cdc.gov
5. A combined government Web site: www.foodsafety.gov

Once you reach a Web site, you can search for such relevant words or phrases as:

- Salmonella
- Food poisoning
- Recalls
- Meat contamination

As for nutrient status in foods, the two most common government Web sites are:

1. U.S. Department of Agriculture: www.usda.gov
2. Food and Drug Administration: www.fda.gov

Once you reach a Web site, you can search for relevant words or phrases such as:

- Enrichment
- Cooking and nutrients
- Food labels

ACTIVITY 1:

Food Safety

CAUSES OF FOOD-BORNE ILLNESS

The three most common biological agents of illness that are transmitted to people from the food supply are bacteria, parasites, and viruses. The two most common factors causing transmission are human carelessness and lack of knowledge of food handling. Examples of causative factors include:

1. Contamination of the water supply
2. Sewage seeping into livestock food
3. Poor personal hygiene—for example, from the oral-fecal route, not washing hands after using the toilet
4. Improper storage of raw foods, especially eggs, meats, fish, poultry, and dairy products
5. Improper storage of cooked foods—for example, using deep pans for storage of hot food, which slows the cooling of food
6. Improper preparation of foods—for example, under-cooking food, especially pork and pork products
7. Improper holding temperatures—that is, above 40°F and below 140°F; improper thawing of frozen food, such as at room temperature
8. Poor health practices, especially in group settings; examples include sneezing and coughing onto food, blowing nose over food, not washing hands before handling food, and handling food with hands that have open sores or boils
9. Contamination by organisms transmitted from food handler to food or equipment and cross-contamination between foods
10. Lack of knowledge by food handlers of the potential hazards of the organisms they carry

For reference purposes, Table 13-1 describes the characteristics of some common food-borne diseases.

BACTERIA AND FOOD TEMPERATURE

To minimize the risk of food-borne illnesses, all individuals should take care to keep food clean to prevent bacteria from multiplying, and to adequately cook fresh and frozen meat, fish, poultry, and eggs.

The majority of cases of food poisoning are from bacteria or toxin from the bacteria. If we know what causes bacteria to multiply, we can take preventive measures. Given a few pathogens and favorable conditions, a harmless food can quickly become a source of illness.

TABLE 13-1   Characteristics of Different Food-Borne Diseases

Disease and Organism That Causes It	Source of Illness	Symptoms	Prevention Methods
Salmonellosis *Salmonella* (bacteria; more than 1,700 kinds)	May be found in raw meats, poultry, eggs, fish, milk, and products made with them. Multiplies rapidly at room temperature.	Onset: 12–48 hours after eating. Nausea, fever, headache abdominal cramps, diarrhea, and sometimes vomiting. Can be fatal in infants, the elderly, and the infirm.	Handling food in a sanitary manner. Thorough cooking of foods. Prompt and proper refrigeration of foods.
Staphylococcal food poisoning Staphylococcal enterotoxin (produced by *Staphylococcus aureus* bacteria)	The toxin is produced when food contaminated with the bacteria is left too long at room temperature. Meats, poultry, egg products, tuna, potato and macaroni salads, and cream-filled pastries are good environments for these bacteria to produce toxin.	Onset: 1–8 hours after eating. Diarrhea, vomiting, nausea, abdominal cramps, and prostration. Mimics flu. Lasts 24–48 hours. Rarely fatal.	Sanitary food handling practices. Prompt and proper refrigeration of foods.
Botulism Botulinum toxin (produced by *Clostridium botulinum* bacteria)	Bacteria are widespread in the environment. However, bacteria produce toxin only in an anaerobic (oxygenless) environment of little acidity. Types A, B, and F may result from inadequate processing of low-acid canned foods, such as green beans, mushrooms, spinach, olives, and beef. Type E normally occurs in fish.	Onset: 8–36 hours after eating. Neurotoxic symptoms, including double vision, inability to swallow, speech difficulty, and progressive paralysis of the respiratory system. Obtain medical help immediately. Botulism can be fatal.	Using proper methods for canning low-acid foods. Avoidance of commercially canned low-acid foods with leaky seals or with bent, bulging, or broken cans. Toxin can be destroyed after a can is opened by boiling contents hard for 10 minutes—not recommended.
Perfringens food poisoning *Clostridium perfringens* (rod-shaped bacteria)	Bacteria are widespread in environment. Generally found in meat and poultry and dishes made with them. Multiply rapidly when foods are left at room temperature too long. Destroyed by cooking.	Onset: 8–22 hours after eating (usually 12). Abdominal pain and diarrhea. Sometimes nausea and vomiting. Symptoms last a day or less and are usually mild. Can be more serious in older or debilitated people.	Sanitary handling of foods, especially meat and meat dishes and gravies. Thorough cooking of foods. Prompt and proper refrigeration.
Shigellosis (bacillary dysentery) *Shigella* (bacteria)	Food becomes contaminated when a human carrier with poor sanitary habits handles liquid or moist food that is then not cooked thoroughly. Organisms multiply in food stored above room temperature. Found in milk and dairy products, poultry, and potato salad.	Onset: 1–7 days after eating. Abdominal pain, cramps, diarrhea, fever, sometimes vomiting, and blood, pus, or mucus in stools. Can be serious in infants, the elderly, or debilitated people.	Handling food in a sanitary manner. Proper sewage disposal. Proper refrigeration of foods.

continues

TABLE 13-1   (continued)

Disease and Organism That Causes It	Source of Illness	Symptoms	Prevention Methods
Campylobacterosis *Campylobacter jejuni* (rod-shaped bacteria)	Bacteria found on poultry, cattle, and sheep and can contaminate the meat and milk of these animals. Chief food sources: raw poultry and meat and unpasteurized milk.	Onset: 2–5 days after eating. Diarrhea, abdominal cramping, fever, and sometimes bloody stools. Lasts 2–7 days.	Thorough cooking of foods. Handling food in a sanitary manner. Avoiding unpasteurized milk.
Gastroenteritis *Yersinia enterocolitica* (non-spore-forming bacteria)	Ubiquitous in nature, carried in food and water. Bacteria multiply rapidly at room temperature, as well as at refrigerator temperatures (4° to 9°C). Generally found in raw vegetables, meats, water, and unpasteurized milk.	Onset: 2–5 days after eating. Fever, headache, nausea, diarrhea, and general malaise. Mimics flu. An important cause of gastroenteritis in children. Can also infect other age groups and, if not treated, can lead to other more serious diseases (such as lymphadenitis, arthritis, and Reiter's syndrome).	Thorough cooking of foods. Sanitizing cutting instruments and cutting boards before preparing foods that are eaten raw. Avoidance of unpasteurized milk and unchlorinated water.
Cereus food poisoning *Bacillius cereus* (bacteria and possibly their toxin)	Illness may be caused by the bacteria, which are widespread in the environment, or by an enterotoxin created by the bacteria. Found in raw foods. Bacteria multiply rapidly in foods stored at room temperature.	Onset: 1–18 hours after eating. Two types of illness: (1) abdominal pain and diarrhea, and (2) nausea and vomiting. Lasts less than a day.	Sanitary handling of foods. Thorough cooking of foods. Prompt and adequate refrigeration.
Cholera *Vibrio cholera* (bacteria)	Found in fish and shellfish harvested from waters contaminated by human sewage. (Bacteria may also occur naturally in Gulf Coast waters.) Chief food sources: seafood, especially types eaten raw (such as oysters).	Onset: 1–3 days. Can range from "subclinical" (a mild uncomplicated bout with diarrhea) to fatal (intense diarrhea with dehydration). Severe cases require hospitalization.	Sanitary handling of foods. Thorough cooking of seafood.
Hemorrhagic colitis (gastroenteritis, intestinal disorders) Escherichia coli O157:H7 (entero- hemorrhagic E. coli or EHEC)	Undercooked or raw hamburger (ground beef) has been implicated in many of the documented outbreaks; however, E. coli O157:H7 outbreaks have implicated alfalfa sprouts, unpasteurized fruit juices, dry-cured salami, lettuce, game meat, and cheese curds. Raw milk was the vehicle in a school outbreak in Canada.	The illness is characterized by severe cramping (abdominal pain) and diarrhea, which is initially watery but becomes grossly bloody. Occasionally vomiting occurs. Fever is either low-grade or absent. The illness is usually self-limited and lasts for an average of 8 days. Some individuals exhibit watery diarrhea only.	Handling food in a sanitary manner. Thorough cooking of foods. Prompt and proper refrigeration of foods.
Parahaemolyticu food poisoning *Vibrio parahaemolyticus* (bacteria)	Organism lives in salt water and can contaminate fish and shellfish. Thrives in warm weather.	Onset: 15–24 hours after eating. Abdominal pain, nausea, vomiting, and diarrhea. Sometimes fever, headache, chills, and mucus and blood in the stools. Lasts 1–2 days. Rarely fatal.	Sanitary handling of foods. Thorough cooking of seafood.

continues

TABLE 13-1   (continued)

Disease and Organism That Causes It	Source of Illness	Symptoms	Prevention Methods
Gastrointestinal disease Enteroviruses rotaviruses parvoviruses	Viruses exist in the intestinal tract of humans and are expelled in feces. Contamination of foods can occur in three ways: (1) when sewage is used to enrich garden/farm soil; (2) by direct hand-to-food contact during the preparation of meals; and (3) when shellfish-growing waters are contaminated by sewage.	Onset: After 24 hours. Severe diarrhea, nausea, and vomiting. Respiratory symptoms. Usually lasts 4–5 days but may last for weeks.	Sanitary handling of foods. Use of pure drinking water. Adequate sewage disposal. Adequate cooking of foods.
Hepatitis Hepatitus A virus	Chief food sources: shellfish harvested from contaminated areas, and foods that are handled a lot during preparation and then eaten raw (such as vegetables).	Jaundice, fatigue. May cause liver damage and death.	Sanitary handling of foods. Use of pure drinking water. Adequate sewage disposal. Adequate cooking of foods.
Listeriosis *L. Monocytogenes.*	Associated with such foods as raw milk, supposedly pasteurized fluid milk, cheeses (particularly soft-ripened varieties), ice cream, raw vegetables, fermented raw-meat sausages, raw and cooked poultry, raw meats (all types), and raw and smoked fish. Its ability to grow at temperatures as low as 3°C permits multiplication in refrigerated foods.	The onset time to serious forms of listeriosis is unknown but may range from a few days to 3 weeks. The onset time to gastrointestinal ymptoms is unknown but is probably greater than 12 hours. The manifestations of listeriosis include septicemia, meningitis (or meningoencephalitis), encephalitis, and intrauterine or cervical infections in pregnant women, which may result in spontaneous abortion (2nd/3rd trimester) or stillbirth. The onset of the aforementioned disorders is usually preceded by influenza-like symptoms including persistent fever. It was reported that gastrointestinal symptoms such as nausea, vomiting, and diarrhea may precede more serious forms of listeriosis or may be the only symptoms expressed.	Handling food in a sanitary manner. Thorough cooking of foods. Prompt and proper refrigeration of foods.
Mycotoxicosis Mycotoxins (from molds)	Produced in foods that are relatively high in moisture. Chief food sources: beans and grains that have been stored in a moist place.	May cause liver and/or kidney disease.	Checking foods for visible mold and discarding those that are contaminated. Proper storage of susceptible foods.

continues

TABLE 13-1 (continued)

Disease and Organism That Causes It	Source of Illness	Symptoms	Prevention Methods
Giardiasis *Giardia lamblia* (flagellated protozoa)	Protozoa exist in the intestinal tract of humans and are expelled in feces. Contamination of foods can occur in two ways: (1) when sewage is used to enrich garden/farm soil; and (2) by direct hand-to-food contact during the preparation of meals. Chief food sources: foods that are handled a lot during preparation.	Diarrhea, abdominal pain, flatulence, abdominal distention, nutritional disturbances, "nervous" symptoms, anorexia, nausea, and vomiting.	Sanitary handling of foods. Avoidance of raw fruits and vegetables in areas where the protozoa is endemic. Proper sewage disposal.
Amebiasis *Entamoeba histolytica* (amoebic protozoa)		Tenderness over the colon or liver, loose morning stools, recurrent diarrhea, change in bowel habits, "nervous" symptoms, loss of weight, and fatigue. Anemia may be present.	Sanitary handling of foods. Avoidance of raw fruits and vegetables in areas where the protozoa is endemic. Proper sewage disposal.

Source: C. L. Ballentine and M. L. Herndon, FDA Consumer, July–August 1982, pp. 25–28.

Bacteria thrive in foods that are moist, warm, good sources of protein, and low in acid. A few thrive in the absence of oxygen supply (anaerobic). These bacteria are usually in home-canned low-acid foods where they produce the deadly botulism toxin.

The time-temperature factor is critical in preventing bacteria from multiplying. After purchasing food, it is essential to minimize the opportunity for bacteria incubation by properly storing, preparing, and handling food. Figure 13-1 depicts the effects of temperature on potential disease-producing organisms.

Observation of safe food preparation practices is an effective way to prevent food-borne illness. These practices, which all family members should observe, are listed below.

SAFE FOOD-PREPARATION PRACTICES

Observe personal hygiene:

1. Hands should always be clean whenever food is handled. Hot water and soap should be used to wash hands after going to the bathroom, before handling cooked foods, and after handling raw food.
2. A person who is ill should not prepare food.
3. During food preparation, contact between hands and the mouth, nose, or hair should be avoided, as should coughing and sneezing over foods. Tissues or handkerchiefs should be used to prevent contamination.
4. Tasting food with fingers and utensils used during preparation is not advised, even if the cooking temperature is very hot.

The following guidelines apply to the food environment:

1. All kitchen equipment and utensils should be thoroughly cleaned before being used with any foods.
2. Cooked foods should not be allowed to stand at room temperature for more than two to three hours whenever feasible. Exposure of food to temperatures between 5°C and 60°C (40°F and 140°F) should be kept to a minimum. The practice of preparing foods a day or several hours before eating should be done with care and avoided if possible.
3. Hot foods should never be allowed to cool slowly to room temperature before refrigerating. The slow cooling period provides an ideal growth temperature for bacteria. Foods should be refrigerated immediately after removing from a steam table or warming oven. A shallow pan, cold running water, or ice bath can be used to cool foods rapidly for storage. A large amount of food in a big container requires additional cooling time before all the contents are below 7°C (45°F), potentially creating an environment for bacteria to grow.
4. When leftovers are served, the food should be heated until all parts reach a temperature of 74°C (165°F). This destroys all vegetative cells of bacteria. Whenever applicable, food should be chopped into small pieces and boiled to destroy any susceptible vegetative cells of the bacteria. No cooling should be permitted after preparation—the food should be served hot.
5. Certain popular foods—stuffed turkey, gravies, cream pies and puddings, sandwiches, and salads—are

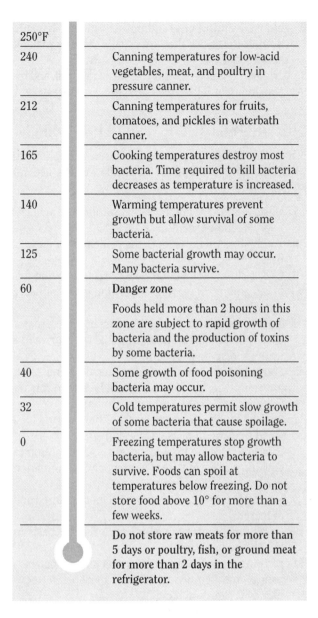

250°F	
240	Canning temperatures for low-acid vegetables, meat, and poultry in pressure canner.
212	Canning temperatures for fruits, tomatoes, and pickles in waterbath canner.
165	Cooking temperatures destroy most bacteria. Time required to kill bacteria decreases as temperature is increased.
140	Warming temperatures prevent growth but allow survival of some bacteria.
125	Some bacterial growth may occur. Many bacteria survive.
60	**Danger zone** Foods held more than 2 hours in this zone are subject to rapid growth of bacteria and the production of toxins by some bacteria.
40	Some growth of food poisoning bacteria may occur.
32	Cold temperatures permit slow growth of some bacteria that cause spoilage.
0	Freezing temperatures stop growth bacteria, but may allow bacteria to survive. Foods can spoil at temperatures below freezing. Do not store food above 10° for more than a few weeks.
	Do not store raw meats for more than 5 days or poultry, fish, or ground meat for more than 2 days in the refrigerator.

FIGURE 13-1   Temperature Guide to Food Safety
Source: Distributed by the U.S. Department of Agriculture.

frequent culprits in food poisoning. When preparing roast turkey, do not stuff the bird but cook the stuffing separately. If turkey is stuffed with raw fillers, avoid stuffing it the night before. If stuffing is cooked separately, it should be cooked immediately after mixing, especially if in a large quantity. Stuffing is an excellent place for bacteria to grow, and if a large amount of lukewarm stuffing is permitted to stand at room temperature, the organisms will surely multiply.

6. Gravies and broths are quite susceptible to bacterial contamination, especially as leftovers. These foods should be placed in the refrigerator as soon as possi-

ble. Gravy or broth should not be held in the refrigerator more than one or two days, and it should be reheated or boiled for several minutes before serving. A reheated dressing should not be permitted to stay at room temperature.

7. Cream pies and puddings are also often involved in food poisoning. People dislike keeping these items in the refrigerator, because they can become soggy. However, leaving them at room temperature can allow bacteria to multiply rapidly. Ideally, such pastries should be prepared as close to serving time as possible.

8. Items such as ham sandwiches, turkey and chicken salads, and deviled eggs require special attention. One good practice is to freeze the sandwiches immediately after preparation and thaw them whenever they are needed. Chicken salads may be prepared by using frozen chicken cubes, which will thaw as the salad stands. The entire salad dish should be kept cool.

CASE HISTORIES OF FOOD POISONING IN THE UNITED STATES

Salmonella

On April 12, 2008, the Food and Drug Administration (FDA) announced that at least 21 people in 13 states have been diagnosed with salmonellosis that was caused by the same strain of *Salmonella* that was found in the recently recalled unsweetened Puffed Rice and unsweetened Puffed Wheat Cereals produced by Malt-O-Meal.

The recalled products were distributed nationally under the Malt-O-Meal brand name as well as under private label brands including Acme, America's Choice, Food Club, Giant, Hannaford, Jewel, Laura Lynn, Pathmark, Shaw's, ShopRite, Tops, and Weis Quality.

Salmonella is a type of bacteria that can cause serious and sometimes fatal infections in young children, frail or elderly people, and others with weakened immune systems. Symptoms of food-borne *Salmonella* infection include nausea, vomiting, fever, diarrhea, and abdominal cramps. In persons with poor health or weakened immune systems, *Salmonella* can invade the bloodstream and cause life-threatening infections.

Listeriosis

On November 13, 2000, healthcare providers at a hospital in Winston-Salem, North Carolina, contacted the local health department about three cases of listeriosis within a 2-week period in recent Mexican immigrants.

The FDA together with the local authorities investigated this outbreak of *Listeria monocytogenes* infections, implicating noncommercial, homemade, Mexican-style fresh soft cheese produced from contaminated raw milk sold by a local dairy farm as the causative agent.

Culturally appropriate education efforts are important to reduce the risk for *L. monocytogenes* transmission through Mexican-style fresh soft cheese.

All patients were Hispanic and 10 were pregnant women. Infection with *L. monocytogenes* resulted in five stillbirths, three premature deliveries, and two infected newborns. On hospital admission, the women reported symptoms that included fever, chills, headache, abdominal cramps, stiff neck, vomiting, and photophobia. Patients had eaten the following food items purchased from door-to-door vendors: Queso fresco, a Mexican-style fresh soft cheese; and hotdogs. Illness was not associated with purchases at specific markets or supermarkets, eating raw fruits or vegetables, deli products, other cheeses (e.g., American, cheddar, mozzarella, and blue/Gorgonzola), or other dairy products.

Various members of the Hispanic immigrant community made the Mexican-style fresh soft cheese from raw milk in their homes. Inspectors found unlabeled homemade cheese in all three of the small local Latino grocery stores they visited in Winston-Salem. In addition, many persons regularly sold the cheese in parking lots and by going door to door. Owners of two local dairies reported selling raw milk. Milk samples were obtained from these two Forsyth County dairies and from three dairies in neighboring counties. *L. monocytogenes* isolates were obtained from nine patients, three cheese samples from two stores, one cheese sample from the home of a patient, and one raw milk sample from a manufacturing grade dairy.

As a result of this outbreak, North Carolina health authorities stopped the sale of raw milk by the dairy farm to noncommercial processors and educated store owners that it is illegal to sell unregulated dairy products. Officials cited the outbreak as sufficient reason to strengthen laws prohibiting the sale of raw milk except to regulated processors.

Despite laws prohibiting the sale and consumption of raw milk and raw milk products, such practices persist in some communities as a result of consumers' taste preferences and for cultural reasons. The popularity of queso fresco has resulted in several outbreaks in Hispanic communities since the 1980s. In 1985, an outbreak of septic abortions attributed to *L. monocytogenes* occurred among Hispanics in Los Angeles and Orange counties, California. In 1997, three outbreaks occurred in Hispanic communities in northern California and Washington.

Because queso fresco in these communities is produced in private homes, food safety regulations are difficult to enforce. However, the following approaches have some success:

1. Massive education programs using Spanish-speaking health providers with background on cultural practices. The targets are Hispanic consumers, especially pregnant women.

2. Intense training of grandmothers in the Hispanic communities since they are usually the ones making the soft cheeses.
3. Stringent regulatory action on use of raw milk and responsibility of sellers (vendors, grocery stores).

RESPONSIBILITIES OF HEALTH PERSONNEL

A health practitioner should emphasize the following when educating a client, an institution, or the general public:

1. Observe sanitary practices that minimize the likelihood of food-borne illness.
2. Teach all family members the principles of cleanliness.
3. Check closely for sanitary, safe practices being followed among all personnel working in a healthcare setting.
4. Make your clients aware that bacteria are a major cause of food-borne illness, and that they thrive in a warm, moist environment.
5. Foods kept at a temperature between 60°F and 125°F for more than two hours may not be safe to eat.
6. Observe good hand-washing technique.
7. Advise individuals not to work with or around food when they are ill or have any skin lesions.
8. If insecticides are used, counsel extreme caution in cooking and eating areas to prevent contamination of food.
9. Regularly inspect all areas where food is stored and prepared.
10. Perform laboratory cultures on a regular basis in healthcare facilities.
11. Encourage mandatory regular teaching of food personnel and demonstrations of appropriate techniques of safe food handling.
12. Check the source of supply of food items (supplier).
13. Purchase only those food items that meet government regulations for safety, such as pasteurized milk and dairy products, USDA inspected meats, and fish.

PROGRESS CHECK ON ACTIVITY 1

FILL-IN

1. Describe five ways in which a food may be contaminated by a food handler.

    a. _____

    b. _____

    c. _____

    d. _____

    e. _____

2. The storage temperature of perishable foods must be below _____°F or above _____°F in order to retard the growth of bacteria.

   a. 32, 200
   b. 40, 140
   c. 60, 170
   d. 80, 190

3. What is the major causative agent in food-borne illness? _____

   _____

4. Describe how temperature and moisture affect the growth of organisms. _____

   _____

5. List five prevention methods for contamination of foods.

   a. _____
   b. _____
   c. _____
   d. _____
   e. _____

6. List the most common gastrointestinal symptoms of food-borne illness. _____

   _____

TRUE/FALSE

Circle T for True and F for False.

7. T F Leftover food should be cooled completely before it is refrigerated.
8. T F Cooking reduces the number of pathogenic bacteria but does not destroy all of them.
9. T F Cooking may not provide protection against food contaminated with staphylococcus.
10. T F Cooking destroys most parasites and viruses.

Case Study

You are invited to the residence of a friend who runs a day care center for the elderly. She has six residents plus her own family, and has hired a person to cook who has had no previous training. While you are visiting, you observe the following procedures (comment on the food-handling practices in each instance given):

11. A pot of homemade beef vegetable soup was made the night before and left on the counter overnight because there was not room to refrigerate it. The cook is not concerned because she has plans to reheat it before serving.

   _____

   _____

12. The cook takes several cans of green beans from a cupboard to heat and two of them are rusty at the seams. One has a little leakage, but none of the cans is bulging. Should you warn her not to use them? Explain.

   _____

   _____

13. The cook assembles the ingredients for potato salad before she begins preparation. She then takes a break and runs a few errands before she prepares the potato salad.

   _____

   _____

14. The cook takes the cutting board from under the sink near the water pipes and cuts and finely chops all the vegetables, fruits, and meats she plans to use for the next two meals. She then puts them in a deep, open pan and refrigerates them.

   _____

   _____

ACTIVITY 2:

Nutrient Conservation

Nutrients may also be lost during processing or preservation of foods. At home, nutrients can also be lost during storage, preparation, and cooking of foods.

Using good food-preparation methods to maximize nutrient retention is especially important when the diet is limited or low in certain nutrients. The following measures are recommended to minimize loss during storage, preparation, and cooking.

STORAGE

1. Avoid bruising soft, fresh produce such as berries and peaches.
2. Store perishable items at the recommended temperature, usually in the refrigerator or freezer.
3. Store foods, except fresh meats, in containers that allow little room for air to circulate, or wrap the foods in moisture- and vapor-proof material.

4. Package green vegetables in such a way that they stay crisp. Keep them slightly moist, not wet. (Washed lettuce keeps well if wrapped loosely in a clean towel and enclosed in a plastic bag.)
5. Store less perishable items (such as canned foods, dry cereals, cooking oils) in a cool, dry place.
6. If foods are not stored in opaque or colored glass containers, store away from the light.
7. Use fresh foods as quickly after harvesting as possible.
8. Store food in glass jars in a dark place.
9. Plan for fast turnover of food on the shelf or in the refrigerator to avoid long storage times. Use leftovers as soon as possible.

PREPARATION

1. Prepare fresh produce as close to time of use as is practical.
2. Use a very sharp knife for cutting fresh produce.
3. Avoid soaking cut fruits and vegetables, especially if they are your major source of any water-soluble nutrients.
4. When appropriate, scrub vegetables instead of paring them and leave them whole instead of cutting them.
5. If paring is desired, pare as thinly as possible. If practical (as for beets and potatoes), peel after cooking.
6. Use clean fresh vegetable parings for making stock for soup.
7. Use the liquid from canned fruit as an ingredient in homemade fruit punch.
8. Save time, fuel, and nutrients by eating raw fruits and vegetables often.
9. Avoid reheating leftover cooked vegetables by using them in cold salads.
10. Discard bruised or dried outside leaves of vegetables.

COOKING

1. Cook vegetables for the shortest time possible, just until tender.
2. If cooking any type of vegetable in water, make sure it is boiling rapidly before vegetable is added.
3. Cook vegetables in the smallest amount of water practical for the type of pan, but take care not to scorch them. A small volume of water is especially helpful to reduce nutrient loss when cooking vegetables that are cut into small pieces. Cover the pan tightly to minimize the amount of water needed.
4. Steam, microwave, or pressure cook clean, whole, unpeeled vegetables.
5. Stir-fry vegetables the Asian way.
6. Plan meals so that vegetables can be served as soon as they are cooked.
7. Heat canned vegetables in the liquid in which they are packed.
8. Use cooking liquid from vegetables and drippings from meat for gravy, sauces, soup stock, or for cook-

ing grains such as rice. Small amounts of cooking liquid can be saved and stored in the freezer.
9. Do not add baking soda when cooking vegetables, even though it makes green vegetables stay brightly colored.

FOOD ADDITIVES AS NUTRIENTS

To process food and preserve nutrients, chemical substances are added to foods. While these procedures are necessary, they have confused the consumer and changed the nutrient content of many foods. In addition, new foods are being introduced to the consumer daily for which the nutrient content is unknown. Some measures to protect and enlighten the consumer have been established by the government.

The FDA enforces laws and regulations to ensure that food is safe, wholesome, and properly labeled. Outside substances are present, intentionally and accidentally, in food as a result of processing, storage, or packaging. Some substances are intentionally added to food to enhance its nutritional value. This takes two forms:

1. Enrichment: The addition of thiamin, niacin, riboflavin, and iron to bread, flour, and cereal products in amounts set by the government. The word *restoration* is sometimes used when the addition of nutrients to a food is to restore it to its original quality. These are nutrients that have been lost through manufacturing or processing.
2. Fortification: Addition to food of one or more nutrients not originally present or occurring only in minute amounts. Some examples are: adding vitamin D to milk, adding vitamins A and D to skim milk and nonfat dry milk; adding iodine to salt; and adding fluoride to water.

Nonnutritive additives do not improve quality. They preserve food and prevent unwanted changes (for example, antioxidants).

All additives to food must be approved by the FDA. There is a category of additives generally recognized as safe (known as GRAS). These substances are sanctioned by the FDA and have been in widespread use over a long period of time without known ill effects. All others must undergo rigid testing before being added to foods.

To protect consumers and educate them about their nutrient intakes, the FDA has established regulations for food labeling.

Nutritional labeling is mandatory on FDA-regulated products as of January 1993 (see Chapter 1). There is a standardized format for presenting the information.

SUMMARY

The government's role and the individual's role in conserving nutrients are important considerations for health personnel.

Safeguarding the food supply, appropriate selection and purchase of foods, label reading, and knowledge of nutrition principles can prevent illness and improve health.

RESPONSIBILITIES OF HEALTH PERSONNEL

When counseling a client, an institution, or the general public, a health practitioner should do the following:

1. Teach clients that many foods lose nutrients, especially vitamins, during storage.
2. Teach clients that food storage at warm temperatures increases nutrient loss as well as bacterial and insect growth.
3. Make clients aware that nutrients are lost by unnecessary trimming, dissolving, soaking, or cooking foods in water.
4. Teach clients that nutrients are lost by overcooking.
5. Teach clients and families that proper food storage, preparation, and cooking techniques can improve their nutritional status.
6. Educate consumers about the advantages of properly reading nutrition labels.
7. Encourage clients to learn the general principles of nutrition.
8. Encourage food producers to maintain high-quality products.

PROGRESS CHECK ON ACTIVITY 2

FILL-IN

1. Nutrition labeling is not mandatory in which two circumstances?

    a. _____

    b. _____

2. List three advantages to nutrition labeling.

    a. _____

    b. _____

    c. _____

3. Identify three practices to preserve nutrient content of foods during storage.

    a. _____

    b. _____

    c. _____

4. Identify at least six food preparation and cooking practices that keep nutrient loss at a minimum.

    a. _____

    b. _____

    c. _____

    d. _____

    e. _____

    f. _____

Define the following terms:

5. Enrichment _____

6. Fortification _____

7. Restoration _____

8. Name two types of food additives and give one example of each.

    a. _____

    b. _____

REFERENCES

Balkin, K. F. (2004). *Food-Borne Illnesses.* San Diego, CA: Greenhaven Press.

Brennfleck, J. (2006). *Diet and Nutrition Sourcebook.* Detroit, MI: Omnigraphics.

Curtis, P. A. (2005). *Guide to Food Laws and Regulations.* Ames, IA: Blackwell.

D'Mello,. P. F. (Ed.). (2003). *Food Safety: Contaminants and Toxins.* Cambridge, MA: CABI.

De Leon, S. Y., Meacham, S. L., & Claudio, V. S. (2003). *Global Handbook on Food and Water Safety: For the Education of Food Management, Food Handlers, and Consumers.* Springfield, IL: Charles C. Thomas.

Entis, P. (2007). *Food Safety: Old Habits, New Perspectives.* Washington, DC: ASM Press.

Food and Agriculture Organization. 2006. *Food Safety Risk Analysis: A Guide for National Food Safety Authorities.* Rome, Italy: Author.

Friedman, M., Mottram, D. S. (Eds.). (2005). *Chemistry and Safety of Acrylamide.* New York: Springer.

Griffin, C. (Ed.). (2005). *Consumer Food Safety.* Bradford, England: Emerald Group.

Griffiths, M. (Ed.). (2005). *Understanding Pathogen Behaviour Virulence, Stress Response and Resistance.* Cambridge, MA: Woodhead.

Grover, J. (Ed.). (2008). *Food.* Detroit, MI: Greenhaven Press.

Harris, N. (Ed.). (2004). *Genetically Engineered Foods.* San Diego, CA: Greenhaven Press.

Hoffmann, S. A., & Taylor, M. R. (Eds.). (2005). *Toward Safer Food.* Washington, DC: Resources for the Future.

Jongen, W. (Ed.). (2005). *Improving the Safety of Fresh Fruit and Vegetables.* Boca Raton, FL: CRC Press.

Kallen, S. A. (2005). *Food Safety.* Detroit, MI: Greenhaven Press.

Lasky, T. (2007). *Epidemiological Principles and Food Safety.* Oxford, England: Oxford University Press.

Marrion, N. (2006). *What to Eat.* New York: North Point Press.

Matthews, K. R. (2006). *Microbiology of Fresh Produce.* Washington, DC: ASM Press.

McElhatton, A., & Marshall, R. J. (2007). *Food Safety: A Practical and Case Approach.* New York: Springer.

McSwane, D., Rue, N. R., & Linton, R. (2005). *Essentials of Food Safety and Sanitation.* Upper Saddle River, NJ: Pearson/Prentice Hall.

National Restaurant Association Educational Foundation. (2007). *Food Preparation: Competency Guide.* Upper Saddle River, NJ: Pearson-Prentice Hall.

Ortega, Y. R. (Ed.). (2006). *Foodborne Parasites.* New York: Springer.

Rasco, B. A., & Bledsoe, G. (2005). *Bioterrorism and Food Safety.* Boca Raton, FL: CRC Press.

Roberts, J. A. (2006). *The Economics of Infectious Disease.* Oxford, England: Oxford University Press.

Schmidt, R. H., & Rodrick, G. E. (Eds.). (2003). *Food Safety Handbook.* Hoboken, NJ: Wiley-Interscience.

United States government Web sites:

a. U.S. Department of Agriculture: www.usda.gov

b. Food Safety Inspection Service of the USDA: www.fsis.gov

c. Food and Drug Administration: www.fda.gov

d. Centers for Disease Controls: www.cdc.gov

e. A combined government Web site: www.foodsafety.gov

Nutrition and Diet Therapy for Adults

CHAPTER 14

Overview of Therapeutic Nutrition

Time for completion
Activities: 1 hour
Optional examination: ½ hour

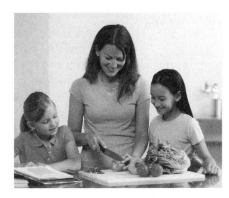

OBJECTIVES

Upon completion of this chapter, the student should be able to do the following:

1. Define the principles of diet therapy.
2. Explain the objectives of diet therapy.
3. Describe the methods used to adapt a normal diet to treat a specific clinical disorder.
4. Identify the most common therapeutic diets used in clinical care.

GLOSSARY

Acculturation: traditions, values, or religious beliefs that compose a way of life (see Chapter 2).

Ascites: an abnormal accumulation of fluid in the peritoneal cavity resulting in distention of the abdomen.

Diet therapy: The use of any diet for restoring or maintaining optimal nutritional status and body homeostasis.

Distention: stretching, enlarging.

Edema: abnormal accumulation of fluid in body tissues (intercellular space).

Gastritis: inflammation of the stomach.

Liquid diet: a modified diet consisting of foods that pour or become liquid at body temperature (see Activity 2).

Mechanically altered diet: a regular diet that has been modified in texture and/or seasoning, depending on the medical needs of the patient (see Activity 2).

Milieu: surroundings, environment.

Modified diet: a regular diet that has been altered to meet specific requirements of individuals with a disease or disorder.

Peritoneal: pertaining to the serous membrane lining the walls of the abdominal and pelvic cavities.

Satiety: feeling of fullness, satisfaction.

BACKGROUND INFORMATION

Basic Principles

Therapeutic nutrition is based on the modification of the nutrients or other aspects of a normal diet to meet a person's nutritional needs during an illness. An understanding of the basics of normal nutrition is a prerequisite to the study of the principles of diet therapy. A nurse's background in anatomy, physiology, and pathophysiology will facilitate the clinical application of these principles.

The purpose of diet therapy is to restore or maintain an acceptable nutritional status of a patient. This is accomplished by modifying one or more of the following aspects of the diet:

1. Basic nutrient(s)
2. Caloric contribution
3. Texture or consistency
4. Seasonings

In adapting a normal diet to treat a disease, one or more of these modifications may be needed to restore or maintain the good nutritional status of a given patient. In general, all therapeutic diets must consider physical factors, clinical disorders, and the patient's total acculturation.

In many cases the patient may require an alteration of feeding methods in order to accomplish the stated purpose of diet therapy. It may also become necessary to alter the feeding intervals. These changes will be discussed in Activity 2.

The nurse's role is critical in helping a patient adjust to a modified diet by acting as the coordinator, interpreter, and teacher of diet therapy. Meeting the patient's nutritional needs involves the coordination of the medical, dietary, and nursing staff. In larger hospitals, the nurse maintains liaisons among the patient, the physician, and the dietitian; assists the patient at meals; observes the patient's response to foods and beverages; charts pertinent information; and supports and supplements the primary instruction given by the dietitian. In small hospitals, nursing homes, and community nursing services, the nurse may be responsible for planning, supervising, and teaching the modified diet. In many cases, the nurse may need to interpret the diet and make food selections both for the patient and the kitchen personnel.

It is important to emphasize that in the practice of medical nutrition therapy one must consider the following:

1. The professional healthcare providers in each clinic, hospital, or other medical institution practice diet therapy according to their experience, available resources and cultural preferences of the patients in addition to the medical diagnosis and treatment. So, the details about any dietary regimen may differ from those presented in this book. Your instructor will explain the status where applicable.
2. The Internet is a valuable tool that helps both care providers and patients to learn more about the dietary care the patient is receiving. Therefore, it is important to access a specific Web site using a popular search engine where applicable.

Kinds and Uses of Exchange Lists

Exchange lists for calculating various modified diets are employed by nutritionists, dietitians, and other health professionals to accurately calculate the amounts and kinds of foods required. These include exchange lists for diabetes, weight reduction or gain, renal disorders, and phenylketonuria. The bases for all these lists are the food groups for selecting a balanced diet. Food lists are classified primarily on their key nutrients, all the foods in a particular group having approximately the same set of nutrients. When diets are calculated, for whatever reason, the recommended servings are intended to provide at least 80 percent of the RDAs/DRIs for all nutrients. When the health professional instructs a client, he or she does not use the figures from nutrients when instructing. Instead, figures are given in terms of foods that will meet the nutrient requirement. The Food Guide Pyramid, therefore, is very practical. The patient can use it to plan menus, order meals in restaurants, and make grocery lists. Checking the foods selected from each group can give the patient and counselor an estimate of how adequate the diet is. The food groups do not account for ethnic and mixed dishes, and will need to be interpreted according to variations acceptable to the client. Supplements to the food groups can be added whenever the diet is not adequate for a particular individual.

The Food Exchange System of Dietary Control

Created by the American Dietetic Association and the American Diabetes Association, this system is widely used in planning all kinds of diets. It is based on exchange lists, which group foods according to their carbohydrate, protein, and fat content. Caloric content of the diet can be calculated when these are known. Diets can therefore be designed to modify basic nutrients, energy value, texture, and/or seasonings (primarily sodium content) (see

Activity 3). The percentage of each of the energy nutrients (carbohydrate, protein, and fat) in the diet can be figured to meet the dietary guidelines for Americans. The exchange system is presented in Appendix F.

Renal Diet Exchange System

For patients with renal disease, the exchange lists become even more detailed. These individuals must be able to pick foods from each of the lists in a renal exchange diet that do not exceed their prescribed levels of sodium, potassium, calcium, and protein, as well as managing total calories and any fluid restrictions. Renal patients are usually counseled several times by the health team and closely followed to assess compliance and needed nutrient changes. Since these diets are very individualized, an exchange list for renal patients is not included in this book. See Chapter 20 for details on the treatment of renal disorders.

Exchange Lists for Phenylketonuria (PKU)

According to the nature of the metabolic error that causes the birth of an infant with PKU, the exchanges are created for two main purposes: to furnish adequate nutrition for rapid growth and a healthy child, while keeping the phenylalanine level low enough to prevent the mental retardation and other unacceptable changes that take place when rigid diet control is not imposed.

The exchange lists for PKU infants and children are not within the scope of this book, but the health professional should be aware that these lists are available and be proficient in providing caregivers of these children with instructions concerning them. See Chapter 28 for more details on PKU, the disease, and treatment. Also, Web sites are the best resources.

The use of the labeling laws as discussed in Chapter 1 will add to the ability of the professional to provide additional information to consumers when they are interpreting these lists. Consumers who learn to read the labels will find that they are more confident and better able to follow diet instructions when using any of the lists.

Health Team

Under the current system in a hospital, the nutrition and dietary care of a patient is managed by a health team of three core members: doctor, nurse, and dietitian. Other health professionals also participate in the care, including pharmacists, physical therapists, and so on.

The role of each of the three core members is as follows. The doctor orders the diet, the dietitian implements it, and the nurse coordinates meals and nutrition requirements with other clinical treatments for a patient.

To comply with legal requirements, a dietitian must be registered with the American Dietetic Association. This person carries the title of Registered Dietitian (R.D.) The word *dietitian* in this book refers to this health professional.

Medical Terms

For many years, terms such as *diet therapy, dietary management, nutrition therapy, therapeutic diets,* and *nutrition feedings* have been used interchangeably. The United States Congress, working with the American Dietetic Association, recently passed legislation that recognizes medical nutrition therapy (MNT) as a covered Medicare benefit. At present, only a few chronic disorders are covered by this act, but the number will grow.

PROGRESS CHECK ON BACKGROUND INFORMATION

FILL-IN

1. What is the major principle of therapeutic nutrition? _____

    _____

    _____

2. State the purpose of diet therapy. _____

    _____

    _____

3. Describe the methods used to adapt a normal diet to a disease condition. _____

    _____

    _____

4. What are the four most common therapeutic diet modifications?

    a. _____

    b. _____

    c. _____

    d. _____

5. Identify four illness factors that affect food consumption.

    a. _____

    b. _____

    c. _____

    d. _____

6. Explain the nurse's role in helping a patient adjust to a therapeutic diet modification.

    a. _____

    b. _____

    c. _____

    d. _____

ACTIVITY 1:

Principles and Objectives of Diet Therapy

Health professionals in care of the hospitalized patient must consider the physiological, psychological, cultural, social, and economic factors of the patient. Illness may alter any of these factors.

The stress of illness brings about many fears in the hospitalized patient and often causes personality changes. Immobilization can disrupt nutritional balance and interfere with patient care. In addition, drug therapy often reduces food intake and interferes with nutrient utilization. The disease process itself modifies food acceptance. Food preferences may revert to those of childhood favorites. Symbolic security foods may be desired. Some patients express their fear, frustration, and hostility by rejecting food and showing resentment toward everyone connected with it.

Another major source of stress is the frequent necessity to modify the diet. When confronted with this necessity, patients often respond irrationally and refuse to accept the change. The health team can help a hospitalized patient accept a therapeutic diet by recognizing the many factors that affect the patient and then helping with the adjustment. In this milieu, the nurse becomes the key to the success or failure of a modified diet.

The patient's nutritional needs are evaluated according to past nutrition practices and the clinical disorder. If nutritional status was poor before admission, the patient's needs will be greater than those of a well-nourished patient. Each analysis must be individualized.

The focus of diet therapy is on the patient's identified needs and problems. The diet plan should be relevant to the nature of the illness and its effects on the body. It should be based on sound, scientific rationale in line with current nutrition concepts. The nurse should question a prescribed diet that shows no apparent relationship to the disease. It is helpful to educate the patient by providing a rationale and expected effects of the modified diet.

PROGRESS CHECK ON ACTIVITY 1

FILL-IN

1. List five factors that affect the nutritional care of the hospitalized patient.

    a. _____

    b. _____

    c. _____

    d. _____

    e. _____

2. List four ways that the stress of illness affects food acceptance.

    a. _____

    b. _____

    c. _____

    d. _____

3. What is the focus of diet therapy?

    _____

    _____

4. Upon which principle is therapeutic nutrition based? _____

    _____

    _____

5. What is the purpose of diet therapy? _____

    _____

    _____

ACTIVITY 2:

Routine Hospital Diets

REGULAR DIETS

The "normal," "regular," or "house" diet is the most frequently used of all diets in hospitals. A normal diet, like a modified diet, is of great importance in a therapeutic sense. When a patient eats well, the body's damaged tissues (from the illness) are continuously repaired and maintained.

The normal diet in a hospital must meet the RDAs/DRIs. During illnesses, the additional stress is often accommodated by increasing these allowances. The daily food groups are often the basis for dietary planning. The normal hospital diet has no restrictions of food choice.

MECHANICALLY ALTERED OR FIBER-RESTRICTED DIETS

These diets are the second most common hospital diets. They differ from a normal diet in texture and seasonings, depending on the needs of the patient. The diet is a nutritionally adequate diet. The following differentiates these two types of diets.

Mechanically Altered Diet

The mechanically altered diet is limited to soft foods for those who have difficulty chewing food because of missing teeth or poorly fitting dentures. The seasonings and preparation of this diet are the same as those for a normal diet.

Table 14-1 describes foods permitted in a mechanically altered diet.

Fiber-Restricted Diet

The fiber-restricted diet differs from the normal diet in being reduced in fiber content and soft in consistency. It serves as a transition to a normal diet following surgery, in acute infections and fevers, and in gastrointestinal disturbances.

Table 14-2 describes foods permitted and prohibited in a soft, fiber-restricted diet. Table 14-3 provides a sample menu for a fiber-restricted diet.

LIQUID DIETS

A liquid diet consists of foods that will pour or are liquid at body temperature. The nutritive value of liquid diets is low and, consequently, such diets are used only for very limited periods of time. Liquid diets may be clear-liquid or full-liquid. They are standard hospital diets. The liquid diet is used for various reasons. One objective is to keep fecal matter in the colon at a minimum. The clear-liquid diet may be used after surgery. The diet can replace fluids lost from vomiting or diarrhea. The clear-liquid diet is composed mainly of water and carbohydrates. It is only a temporary diet, since it is nutritionally inadequate. Its use is typically limited to 24 to 36 hours.

Clear-Liquid Diet

This diet permits tea, coffee or coffee substitute, and fat-free broth. Ginger ale, fruit juices, flavored gelatin, fruit ices, and water gruels (strained and liquefied cooked cereals) are sometimes given. Small amounts of fluid are given to the patient every hour or two. For example, the diet is used for 24 to 48 hours following acute vomiting, diarrhea, or surgery.

TABLE 14-1 Foods Permitted in a Mechanically Altered Diet

Food Types	Foods Permitted
Milk	All forms
Cheeses	All forms
Eggs	Any cooked form
Breads	White, rye without seeds, refined whole wheat; corn bread; any cracker not made with whole grains; French toast made from permitted breads; spoon bread; pancakes, plain soft rolls
Cereals	All cooked, soft varieties; puffed flakes and noncoarse ready-to-eat varieties
Flour	All forms
Meats, fish, poultry	Small cubed and finely ground or minced forms; as ingredients in creamed dishes, soups, casseroles, and stews
Seafoods	Any variety of fish without bone (canned, fresh, or frozen; packaged prepared forms in cream sauces); minced, shredded, ground, and finely chopped shellfish
Legumes, nuts	Fine, smooth, creamy peanut butter; legumes (if tolerated) cooked tender, finely chopped, mashed, or minced
Potatoes	White potatoes: mashed, boiled, baked, creamed, scalloped, cakes, au gratin; sweet potatoes: boiled, baked, mashed
Soups	All varieties, preferably without hard solids such as nuts and seeds
Fruits	Raw: avocado, banana; cooked and canned: fruit cocktail, cherries, apples, apricots, peaches, pears, sections of mandarin oranges, grapefruits, or oranges without membranes; all juices and nectars
Vegetables	All juices; all vegetables cooked tender, chopped, mashed, canned, or pureed; canned, pureed, or paste forms of tomato
Sweets	Marshmallow and chocolate sauces; preserves, marmalade, jelly, jam; candy: hard, chocolate, caramels, jellybeans, marshmallows, candy corn, butterscotch, gumdrops, plain fudge, lollipops, fondant mints; syrup: sorghum, maple, corn; sugar: granulated, brown, maple, confectioner's; honey, molasses
Desserts	All plain or certain flavored varieties (permitted flavorings include liquids, such as juice; finely chopped or pureed fruits without solid pieces of fruit, seeds, nuts, etc.); gelatins, puddings; ice cream, ice milk, sherbet; water ices; cakes, cookies, cake icing; cobblers
Fats	Butter, margarine, cream (or substitutes), oils and vegetable shortenings, and bacon fat; salad dressings, tartar sauce, sour cream
Seasonings	Salt, pepper, soy sauce, vinegar, catsup; all other herbs, especially finely chopped or ground, that can be tolerated

TABLE 14-2   Foods Permitted and Prohibited in a Fiber-Restricted Diet

Food Types	Foods Permitted	Foods Prohibited
Milk	All milk and milk products without added ingredients; condensed and evaporated milk, chocolate milk and drink; cocoa and hot chocolate; yogurt and whey	Any milk product with prohibited ingredients
Cheese	Cottage cheese, cream cheese, mild cheese, and any cheese not prohibited	Any sharp, strongly flavored cheese; any cheese with prohibited ingredients
Eggs	Poached, scrambled, soft- and hard-cooked eggs; salmonella-free egg powder (pasteurized)	Raw or fried eggs
Breads and equivalents	Breads: white, Italian, Vienna, French, refined whole wheat, corn bread, spoon bread, French toast, seedless rye; muffins, English muffins, pancakes, rolls, waffles; melba toast, rusk, zwieback; biscuits, graham crackers, saltines, and other crackers not made with whole grains	Breads: any variety with seeds or nuts; Boston brown, pumpernickel, raisin, cracked wheat, buckwheat; crackers: all made with whole grain; rolls: any made with whole grain, nuts, coconut, raisins; tortillas
Cereals	Cooked and refined dry cereals	Dry, coarse cereals such as shredded wheat, all bran, and whole grain
Flours	All varieties except those prohibited	Any made with whole-grain wheat or bran
Beverages	All types	None
Meat, fish, poultry*	Meats: beef, liver, pork (lean and fresh), lamb, veal; poultry: turkey, chicken, duck, Cornish game hens, chicken livers; fish: all types of fresh varieties, canned tuna and salmon	Fried, cured, and highly seasoned products such as chitterlings, corned beef, cured and/or smoked products, most processed sausages, and cold cuts; meats with a lot of fat; geese and game birds; most shellfish; canned fish such as anchovies, herring, sardines, and any strongly flavored seafoods
Legumes, nuts	Fine, creamy, smooth peanut butter	Most legumes, nuts, and seeds
Fruits	Raw: avocado, banana; canned or cooked: apples, apricots, cherries, peaches, pears, plums, sections of oranges, grapefruits, mandarin oranges without membranes, stewed fruits (except raisins), fruit cocktail, seedless grapes; all juices and nectars	All raw fruits not specifically permitted; all dried fruits; fruits with seeds and skins
Vegetables	All juices; canned or cooked: asparagus, beets, carrots, celery, eggplant, green or wax beans, chopped kale, mushrooms, peas, spinach, squash, shredded lettuce, chopped parsley, green peas, pumpkin; tomato: stewed, pureed, juice, paste	All those not specifically permitted
Fats	Butter, margarine, cream (or substitute), oil, vegetable shortening, mayonnaise, French dressing, crisp bacon, plain gravies, sour cream	Other forms of fats and oils, salad dressings, highly seasoned gravy
Soups	Any made from permitted ingredients: bouillon (powder or cubes), consommé, cream soups; strained soups: gumbos, chowders, bisques	Soups made from prohibited ingredients; split pea and bean soups; highly seasoned soups such as onion
Potatoes	White potatoes: scalloped, boiled, baked, mashed, creamed, au gratin; sweet potatoes: mashed	White potatoes: fried, caked, browned, and in salad; yams
Rice and equivalents	Rice (white or brown), macaroni, spaghetti, noodles, Yorkshire pudding	Wild rice, bulgur, fritters, bread stuffing, barley
Sweets	Sugar: granulated, brown, maple, confectioner's; candy: mints, butterscotch, chocolate, caramels, fondant, plain fudge; syrups: maple, sorghum, corn; jelly, marmalade, preserves, jams; honey, molasses, apple butter; chocolate sauces	All candies containing nuts, coconut, and prohibited fruits Jelly beans, marshmallows, gumdrops, and candy corn

continues

TABLE 14-2   (continued)

Food Types	Foods Permitted	Foods Prohibited
Desserts	Cake, cookies, custard, pudding, gelatin, ice cream, cobblers, ice milk, sherbet, water ice, cream pie with graham cracker crust; all plain or flavored without large pieces of fruits	Any products containing nuts, coconut, or prohibited fruits
Miscellaneous	Sauces: cream, white, brown, cheese, tomato; vinegar, soy sauce, catsup; all finely ground or chopped spices and herbs served in amounts tolerated by the patient	Spices and sauces that the patient is unable to tolerate, such as red pepper, garlic, curry, mustard; pickles; olives; popcorn, potato chips, Tabasco and Worcestershire sauces

*Cooked tender—may be broiled, baked, creamed, stewed, or roasted.

TABLE 14-3   Sample Menu for a Fiber-Restricted Diet

Breakfast	Lunch	Dinner
Orange juice, ½ c	Tomato soup, ½ c	Soup, creamed, ½ c*
Farina, ½ c	Cod, broiled, 2–3 oz	Beef, stew meat, tender, 3–4 oz
Egg, soft-boiled, 1*	Potato, baked, medium, 1	White rice, ½ c
Bacon, crisp, 2 strips*	Toast, 1 slice	Asparagus, canned, ½ c
Toast, 1 slice	Butter or margarine, 1 tsp	Toast, 1 slice
Butter or margarine, 1 tsp	Pudding, plain, ½ c	Butter or margarine, 1 tsp
Jam, 1–3 tsp	Coffee or tea, 1–2 c	Gelatin, flavored, ½ c
Milk, 1 c	Sugar, 1–3 tsp	Coffee or tea, 1–2 c
Coffee or tea, 1–2 c	Cream, 1 tbsp*	Cream, 1 tbsp*
Sugar, 1–3 tsp	Salt, pepper	Sugar, 1–3 tsp
Cream, 1 tbs*		Salt, pepper
Salt, pepper		

*Egg, bacon, and cream may be omitted to lower the fat content of the diet.

The primary objective of the diet is to relieve thirst and to help maintain water balance. Broth provides some sodium, and fruit juices contribute potassium. The inclusion of carbonated beverages, sugar, and fruit juices furnishes a small amount of carbohydrate. This diet is deficient in nutrients and provides about 600 calories per day. Severe malnutrition results from an extended use of this diet. A sample menu for a clear-liquid diet is shown in Table 14-4.

DIET FOR DYSPHAGIA

The dysphagia diet changes the texture of foods. It is used for those clients who have difficulty swallowing, for example, those with partial paralysis of the throat following a CVA (stroke), or patients undergoing radiation treatment for neck and throat cancers. The diet reduces the risk of food going into the trachea and getting into the lungs. It also makes it easier to chew and move food around in the mouth. Liquids are particularly difficult to swallow. Any liquids are thickened to a semisolid consistency. Table 14-5 describes the types of foods suitable for a patient with dysphagia.

PROGRESS CHECK ON ACTIVITY 2

MULTIPLE CHOICE

Circle the letter of the correct answer.

1. The clear-liquid diet:

   a. replaces lost body fluids.
   b. provides a nutritionally adequate diet.
   c. includes any food that pours.
   d. is never used after surgery.

2. Which of the following groups of food would be allowed on a clear-liquid diet?

   a. strained cream of chicken soup, coffee, and tea
   b. tomato juice, sherbet, and strained cooked cereal
   c. raspberry ice, beef bouillon, and apple juice
   d. tea, coffee, and eggnog

TABLE 14-4   Sample Menu for a Clear-Liquid Diet

Breakfast	Lunch	Dinner
Clear juice, ⅔ c	Clear juice, ⅔ c	Clear juice, ⅔ c
Coffee or tea	Broth (chicken, beef, or vegetable), ⅔ c	Broth (chicken, beef, or vegetable), ⅔ c
Sugar	Flavored gelatin, ½ c	Fruit ice or flavored gelatin, ½ c
Snack	Coffee or tea	Coffee or tea
Juice, ⅔ c or broth, clear, ½ c	Sugar	Sugar
	Snack	Snack
	Flavored ice, ½ c	Carbonated beverage

TABLE 14-5   Dysphagia Diet Guidelines

1. The diet consists of small, frequent, high protein, high calorie meals supplemented with calorie-dense high protein snacks between meals.
2. The texture of foods that are served must be of pudding or pureed consistency.
3. Some foods that meet these criteria:
   a. Hot cereals and custards (nonfat dry milk powder or pureed cottage cheese may be added to increase food value).
   b. Custard style yogurt without fruit or nuts (egg yolk may be blended in to increase food value).
   c. Mashed potatoes (with added dry milk powder and egg yolks); can also be used to thicken liquids to a semisolid consistency.
   d. Gelatins, ice cream, and sherbets become liquid at room temperature, are considered liquids, and should be eaten only if approved by the physician or speech-language pathologist.
   e. Liquid nutrition supplements such as Ensure, Ensure HN, Sustacal, or Carnation Instant Breakfast can be used if thickened to the appropriate texture.
   f. Flavorings, salt, or finely ground herbs and spices may be added if tolerated by the patient.
   g. Avoid highly seasoned, irritating, and acidic foods.
   h. If the patient tolerates hot foods, be certain that they are served hot to avoid food contamination. Serve all cold foods cold.
4. Serve all foods attractively, and in an odor-free, clean environment.

3. The dysphagia diet:
   a. is of semisolid consistency.
   b. is followed by clear-liquid diet.
   c. does not include milk in any form.
   d. is given to patients with acute respiratory infections.

4. The dysphagia diet:
   a. may contain mild spices.
   b. includes no protein foods.
   c. includes no commercial supplements.
   d. is commonly given immediately after surgery.

5. The protein content of the dysphagia diet:
   a. can be increased by adding lactose to beverages.
   b. can be increased by adding dried milk to mashed potatoes.
   c. cannot be varied.
   d. is always adequate.

6. The clear-liquid diet:
   a. is given to all patients with chewing difficulties.
   b. may be used after surgery.
   c. includes milk foods.
   d. is nutritionally adequate.

7. The mechanically altered diet:
   a. is a standard diet in health facilities.
   b. is always served to children under 12 years old.
   c. is similar to a high-residue diet.
   d. does not nourish as well as a regular diet.

8. A major difference between the regular and the fiber-restricted diet is the:
   a. nutrient content.
   b. texture of the foods.
   c. energy values.
   d. satiety value of the food.

9. It is not unusual for the fiber-restricted diet to be:
   a. ordered to precede the clear-liquid diet.
   b. ordered for a patient with dysphagia.
   c. ordered to succeed the clear-liquid diet.
   d. used in place of the clear-liquid diet.

10. Which of the following foods would not be included in a fiber-restricted diet?
    a. ground beef
    b. leg of lamb
    c. roast chicken
    d. grilled pork chops

11. Cellulose is:
    a. a complete protein.
    b. an indigestible carbohydrate.

c. a saturated fat.

d. an essential mineral.

12. Texture of food refers to its:

    a. color.

    b. flavor.

    c. consistency.

    d. satiety value.

13. Which of the following groups of food would be allowed on the dysphagia diet?

    a. coffee, bananas, and sponge cake

    b. salt, sherbet, and scrambled eggs

    c. butter, angel food cake, and fried chicken

    d. ginger ale, chocolate ice cream, and cocoa with marshmallows

    e. none of the above

FILL-IN

14. Adapt the following menu to meet the needs of a patient on a fiber-restricted diet: fresh fruit cup, oatmeal with milk and sugar, bran muffin, and butter. _____

    _____

    _____

15. Indicate which of the following foods would be allowed on a fiber-restricted diet by writing Y (yes) and N (no):

    _____ a. banana nut bread

    _____ b. roast chicken breast

    _____ c. baked halibut

    _____ d. french fries

    _____ e. angel food cake

    _____ f. black coffee

    _____ g. celery sticks

    _____ h. tapioca pudding

    _____ i. coconut cookies

    _____ j. tossed salad

ACTIVITY 3:

Diet Modifications for Therapeutic Care

The underlying concept in planning a therapeutic diet is that it is based on a normal balanced diet. The regular or house diets used during acute care can be modified to meet specific conditions, since they are already balanced diets. In addition to meeting specific needs, the changes that may be required must take into account many specific factors affecting the patient.

The modifications most generally used deal with four aspects of foods: basic nutrients, energy value, texture or consistency, and seasonings.

MODIFYING BASIC NUTRIENTS

The quantity and quality of the protein, fat, carbohydrate, vitamins, water, and minerals in a diet may be modified. An increase is used to correct deficiencies or provide extra nutrients for repair of body tissue. The increase may involve one or more nutrients, but combinations are frequent, since all nutrients have interrelated functions. Examples are a high-protein, high-carbohydrate, and high-vitamin diet for postoperation and an iron-rich diet for iron-deficiency anemia. The diet for a malnourished patient upon admission to the hospital may require increases in all the nutrients. A nutrient-rich diet is not necessarily accepted by the patient. The patient with a chronic, debilitating illness may be anorexic and present quite a challenge to the health team.

Nutrients may be reduced in a diet because the patient can metabolize only a certain amount. For example, a person with high blood sugar requires a diet low in simple carbohydrate. High serum lipids require a low-fat diet. When a diseased kidney cannot excrete excess minerals, a reduced intake of minerals is prescribed, as well as a monitored fluid intake.

MODIFYING ENERGY VALUE

The calculated diet is used to adjust caloric intake to regulate body weight. Calculations are based on the caloric value of foods which is the number of calories per gram a food will furnish when metabolized by the body. Adjustments are made in the amounts of carbohydrate, protein, and fat contained in the diet. For example, an underweight patient may need a 3000-calorie diet while an overweight patient may need only 1500 calories. The diabetic diet is also a calculated diet. The nutrient values are calculated individually in order to ensure that daily requirements for each are met. A 1000-calorie diet containing only fat and carbohydrate can be developed, if there is no concern for nutrient adequacy. Patients with certain malabsorptive disorders may require diets with increased energy value along with adjustments in the amount of a specific nutrient.

MODIFYING TEXTURE OR CONSISTENCY

Modification of foods' texture or consistency is used to: provide ease of chewing, swallowing, or digestion; rest the whole body or an affected organ; and bring a patient back to a regular diet. It is widely used in combination with other modifications. Patients with gastrointestinal diseases or trauma to the mouth and throat frequently are given diets altered in texture. Postsurgery patients may progress from liquid to regular diets, as tolerated. Patients with heart disorders may be prescribed diets altered in texture to ease digestion to rest the damaged heart.

The dysphagia diet may be utilized to fill a variety of needs for patients requiring alterations in texture.

MODIFYING SEASONINGS

Seasonings are usually adjusted to individual tolerances, but a few are not advised in certain diseases. Salt restriction is prescribed for various conditions, including sodium retention in the body, edema, ascites, and others.

Whatever the modification, the goal of diet therapy remains the same: to restore and maintain good nutritional status. Nutrient supplements of vitamins, minerals, and high-protein formulas are needed for highly restricted diets, anorexia, and impaired absorption and metabolism.

A planned diet is successful only when it is eaten. The diet must be individualized to take into account the psychological and cultural factors that influence food acceptance. In addition, the food must be attractively presented, palatable, and safe. The patient's environment at mealtime is also an important factor, as is the attitude of the individuals serving the meals.

NURSING IMPLICATIONS

1. Recognize the unique position of the nurse in promoting dietary compliance to modified diets:
   a. Assess nutritional status.
   b. Observe and document nutritional intake.
   c. Evaluate response to diet therapy.
   d. Teach or support the diet teaching and diet therapy ordered for the client.
2. Be aware that diet therapy, alone or in conjunction with other treatment, may play an important role in the prevention and treatment of disease by:
   a. lessening severity of symptoms.
   b. decreasing need for medication.
   c. delaying onset of disease or delaying progression.
   d. increasing resistance to diseases or speeding recovery.
3. provide the client and caregivers with nutrition information, encouragement, education, and referrals as needed.
4. Recognize the social, cultural, and psychological aspects that influence nutritional status of hospitalized clients and intervene when needed.
5. Continue to update knowledge regarding diet therapy.

PROGRESS CHECK ON ACTIVITY 3

FILL-IN

1. What are the four basic modifications made in a diet?

   a. _____

   b. _____

   c. _____

   d. _____

2. Give an example and the rationale for decreasing a nutrient in the diet. _____

   _____

   _____

3. Name three situations where diet supplementation would be needed:

   a. _____

   b. _____

   c. _____

4. Explain how a diet can be individualized and still provide the correct modifications. _____

   _____

   _____

ACTIVITY 4:

Alterations in Feeding Methods

It is estimated that protein energy malnutrition (PEM) is present in 25%–50% of all medical surgical patients. The most common reason is exhausted nutrient reserves when entering a facility. In addition, hospitalized patients who were previously stable can experience malnutrition in as little as two weeks.

Of particular significance are those patients at high risk for whom oral feedings are inadequate, such as being on five days or more of clear liquids. Other high-risk patients who may require alternate feeding methods are those with eating disorders, malabsorption syndromes, cancer, or a hypermetabolic condition such as burns. Whenever a patient cannot or will not eat, for any one of myriad reasons, an alternate method of feeding should be employed.

There are two parenteral or intravenous feeding methods. One method injects nutrients into the blood via a peripheral vein (for example, a vein in the arm, near the surface). The other method injects nutrients into the blood via a central vein (those deeper into the central portion of the system; for example, the subclavian located under the collarbone).

SPECIAL ENTERAL FEEDINGS (TUBE FEEDINGS)

Enteral (tube) feedings are used only for patients who have enough functioning of the GI tract to digest and absorb their food. They are also used when the patient cannot eat enough regular food to promote healing, even though the GI tract is functional. Frequently, an oral supplement has been added to the diet (such as Ensure from Ross Laboratories) before tube feedings are considered, but it has been insufficient. After careful assessment of nutritional status, tube feedings are added as an additional supplement. Tube feedings must be provided that meet the individual patient's needs. Many new commercial modular formulas are available.

A tube feeding is a nutritionally adequate diet of liquified foods administered through a tube into the stomach or duodenum. These foods are commercially available. From the standpoint of accuracy in measuring, sanitation, and convenience, most hospitals prefer commercial mixtures. These mixtures can be milk-based formulas, lactose-free formulas, meat-based formulas, and residue-free formulas. Tube feedings usually furnish one calorie per milliliter. A 24-hour intake of three liters would furnish 3000 calories.

Enteral feedings have several advantages, including the following:

1. It is more economical to feed enterally than intravenously, considering equipment, time, and foods used.
2. It is safer to feed enterally than intravenously. The risk of fluid and electrolyte imbalances and infection is less than for intravenous feedings.

Some disadvantages of enteral feedings include the following:

1. Nutritional inadequacy for certain patients (not enough protein and calories)
2. Overnutrition for certain patients (excess calories and formula)
3. Diarrhea or constipation
4. Vomiting
5. Problems of preparation and safety. Bacterial contamination can be a factor if preparation is not carefully controlled.
6. Home-prepared tube feedings are not recommended. Prepared formulas are preferred over the use of home-blenderized diets, which can clog tubes, are not sterile, and in which nutrient composition is not well defined.

Depending on the patient and the circumstances, some or all of the above problems can be avoided or remedied.

There is an increasing movement back toward use of more enteral feedings. Recent studies indicate that the intestinal bacteria will translocate to other areas, become pathogenic, and create sepsis when they are not fed.

Enteral feedings depend on enteral formulas. There are three categories of commercial enteral formulas:

1. Standard, intact, or routine enteral formulas
2. Elemental or defined enteral formulas
3. Disease-specific enteral formulas

Standard enteral formulas have existed for many years with a few commercial products coming to the market 30 years ago. Now, there are more than 35 products in the market. They are used for routine feedings for patients who need them as prescribed by physicians. Each product is made of regular foods and individual nutrients.

Defined enteral formulas contain specific nutrients or modified nutrients, including simple and complex carbohydrates, amino acids, peptides, fatty acids, triglycerides, and so on. There are about 15 or so in the market.

Disease-specific enteral formulas are available for five or more clinical disorders such as those of the kidney, liver, pancreas (diabetes), lung, and the immune system.

There are four companies that manufacture most of the products although some smaller companies manufacture one or two of these formulas. Table 14-6 describes the type of enteral formulas and the companies manufacturing them.

PARENTERAL FEEDINGS VIA PERIPHERAL VEIN

Nutrient fluids entering a peripheral vein can be saline with 5%–10% dextrose (clinically represented by D5W or D10W); amino acids; electrolytes; vitamins; and medications. Intravenous fluids may be either isotonic, hypotonic, or hypertonic. Both hypotonic and hypertonic solutions create a shift in body fluids. Hypotonic solutions draw fluid from the blood vessels into the interstitial spaces and cells. Hypertonic solutions create the opposite effect; they draw fluids out of interstitial spaces into the blood.

When enteral feedings are contraindicated, feeding by a peripheral vein is often used. This type of feeding is safer than feeding by a central vein, but it fails to provide adequate calories and other nutrients for repair and replacement of losses. The dangers of overloading with fluid in order to meet caloric needs are inherent in using solutions via the peripheral vein. Some examples of nutrient quantities in these solutions will illustrate the clinical problem. For example, 2500 cc of D5W provides 425 calories and 0 g protein; 200 cc of 3.5% amino acid solution provides 70 g protein, 280 calories, but 0 g carbohydrate to spare protein. A 10% fat emulsion (intralipids may be used via the peripheral vein) furnishes 1 calorie per 1 cc emulsion, contains no amino acids, and is not compatible with any other added nutrients. It elevates serum cholesterol levels and is questionable in its ability to promote nitrogen balance by sparing protein.

PARENTERAL FEEDING VIA CENTRAL VEIN (TOTAL PARENTERAL NUTRITION [TPN])

When a patient is severely depleted nutritionally or if the GI tract cannot be used, parenteral feeding via a catheter inserted into a central vein (usually the subclavian to the superior vena cava) can provide adequate nutrition. The solution for TPN is a sterile mixture of glucose, amino acids, and micronutrients. The intralipids are not given

TABLE 14-6   Manufacturers and Enteral Formulas

Manu-facturers	Standard formulas	Elemental formulas	Formulas for kidney disorder	Formulas for liver disorder	Formulas for Diabetes	Formulas for lung disorders: [COPD Formulas]	Formulas for lung disorders: [ARDS Formulas]	Immune system disorder
Nestle	Probalance® Nutren® 1.0 Nutren® 1.0 with fiber Nutren® 1.5 Nutren® 1.5 fiber Replete® Replete® with fiber	F.A.A.® Peptamen® Peptamen® with FOS Peptamen® 1.5 Peptamen® VHP	Nutren® Renal Renalcal®	Nutren® Hepatic	Glytrol®	Nutren® Pulmonary		Crucial®
Norvatis	Compleat® Fibersource® Fibersource® HN Isocal® Isocal® HN Isosource® Isosource® HN Isosource® VHN Novasource® 2.0 Traumacal® Ultracal®	Peptinox® Peptinox® DT Subdue® Subdue® plus Tolerex® Vivonex® plus Vivonex® RTF Vivonex® TEN	NovaSource® Renal		Diabetisource® AC Rosource® Diabetic	NovaSource® Pulmonary		Impact® Impact® 1.5 Impact® Gtutamine Impact® with Fiber
Ross Products	Jevity® Jevity® 1.2 Jevity® 1.5 Osmolite® Osmolite® 1 cal Osmolite® 1.2 cal Osmolite® 1.5 cal Promote® Promote® with fiber Twocal® HN	Optimental® Vital® HN	Nepro® Suplena®		Glucema® Select	Pulmocare®	Oxepa®	Perative® Pivot® 1.5
Hormol Healthlabs			Hepatic-Aid® II					

in this solution and may be administered via a peripheral vein. The amounts of micronutrients added are based on the individual's blood chemistry. Multivitamin preparations can be added to the TPN solutions, except for B_{12}, K, or folic acid, which are given separately.

TPN has many advantages. It can be used for long periods of time to meet the individual body's total nutritional needs. The solutions can be adjusted according to individual needs by increasing or decreasing any or all of the nutrients.

TPN also has many disadvantages. The solutions are very expensive, and they support rapid growth of bacteria and fungi. The rate of infusion must be adhered to rigidly, around the clock. Dressing changes are done using sterile technique. Careful monitoring of the patient's response and corrective measures when needed are mandatory for safe administration of these solutions.

NURSING IMPLICATIONS

The responsibilities or implications for nutritional support by the nursing staff are varied and many. A brief summary of some of these implications follows:

1. Discard all unused, cloudy, or sedimented fluids.
2. Do not add drugs and other mixtures to a solution containing protein.
3. Refrigerate solutions until they are used.
4. Be aware that dates should be on tube feedings, and that they should not be given past 24 hours of date.
5. Be alert for signs of gas, regurgitation, cramping, and diarrhea, and be prepared to intervene.
6. Take necessary precautions when using nutrient solutions because they are excellent sources for bacterial growth.
7. Be especially alert for signs of hypo- or hyperglycemia when TPN is used and intervene if necessary.
8. Assist the patient in adjusting to an alternate feeding method. Many patients experience stress due to fear and concern of unfamiliar feeding methods.
9. Encourage and practice good oral hygiene measures with the patient, even though he or she is not eating by mouth.
10. Encourage early ambulation, which makes use of the muscles and increases the use of calcium and protein. Physical activity also raises morale.

PROGRESS CHECK ON ACTIVITY 4

MULTIPLE CHOICE

Circle the letter of the correct answer.

1. Which of the following is an important concern for the nurse who is providing nutrition by peripheral vein?

   a. calorie overload
   b. contamination of the injection site
   c. fluid overload
   d. all of the above

2. The solution used for TPN consists of:

   a. glucose, amino acids, and micronutrients.
   b. glucose, amino acids, and fatty acids.
   c. 10% dextrose in saline and vitamins.
   d. commercial hydrolyzed mixtures.

3. Which of the following vitamins would need to be given separately instead of added to a formula?

   a. thiamin, niacin, and riboflavin
   b. the fat-soluble vitamins
   c. B_{12}, K, and folic acid
   d. none of the above

TRUE/FALSE

Circle T for True and F for False.

4. T F Nutrient fluids via peripheral vein are as adequate for long-term feedings as those via central vein.
5. T F Tube feedings are always commercial preparations.
6. T F Parenteral feedings will sustain the fluid and electrolyte balance of a postoperative patient.
7. T F TPN can be used for long periods of time and still maintain cell integrity.
8. T F Enteral feedings are more likely to become contaminated than parenteral ones.

MATCHING

Match the statement to the appropriate fluid.

9. Draws fluid from interstitial spaces into the blood.
10. Does not create a fluid shift.
11. Draws fluid from blood into interstitial spaces.

a. isotonic fluid
b. hypotonic fluid
c. hypertonic fluid

FILL-IN

12. Define tube feedings. _____

    _____

    _____

13. List two advantages and two disadvantages of enteral feeding.

    a. _____

    _____

    b. _____

    _____

14. List two conditions requiring TPN.

    a. _____

    b. _____

15. List three important nursing measures for a patient receiving TPN.

    a. _____

    _____

    b. _____

    _____

    c. _____

    _____

16. List three types of formulas used in tube feedings and describe the major difference of each from the other.

    a. _____

    _____

    b. _____

    _____

    c. _____

    _____

REFERENCES

Abrams, S. A. (2005). Calcium supplementation during childhood: Long-term effects on bone mineralization. *Nutrition Reviews, 63*: 251–255.

Block, A., Maillet, J. O., Winkler, M. F., & Howell, W. H. (2006). *Issues and Choices in Clinical Nutrition and Practice.* Philadelphia: Lippincott, Williams and Wilkins.

Bogden, J. D., & Klevay, L. M. (Eds.). (2000). *Clinical Nutrition of the Essential Trace Elements and Minerals: The Guide for Health Professionals.* Totowa, NJ: Humana Press.

Brazin, L. R. (2006). *Internet Guide to Medicinal Diets and Nutrition.* New York: Haworth Information Press.

Caballero, B., Allen, L., & Prentice, A. (Eds.). (2005). *Encyclopedia of Human Nutrition* (2nd ed.). Boston: Elsevier/Academic Press.

CRC. *Handbook of Chemistry and Physics* (85th ed.). (2004). Boca Raton, FL: CRC Press.

Deen, D., & Hark, L. (2007). *The Complete Guide to Nutrition in Primary Care.* Malden, MA: Blackwell.

Droke, E. A. (2008). Dietary fatty acids and minerals. In Chow, C. K. (Ed.). *Fatty Acids in Foods and Their Health Implications.* Boca Raton, FL: CRC Press.

Eckhert, C.D. (2006). Other trace elements. In Shils, M. E. (Ed.). *Modern Nutrition in Health and Disease* (10th ed., pp. 338–350). Philadelphia: Lippincott, Williams and Wilkins.

Escott-Stump, S. (2002). *Nutrition and Diagnosis-Rrelated Care* (5th ed.). Philadelphia: Lippincott, Williams and Wilkins.

Food and Agriculture Organization. (2002). *Human Vitamin and Mineral Requirements: Report of a Joint FAO/WHO Expert Consultation.* Rome, Italy: World Health Organization.

Gupta, V. B., Anitha, S., Hegde, M. L., Zecca, L., Garruto, R. M., & Ravid, R., et al. (2005). Aluminium in Alzheimer's disease: Are we still at a crossroad? *Cellular and Molecular Life Sciences, 62*(2):143–58.

Higdon, J. (2003). *An Evidence-Based Approach to Vitamins and Minerals: Health Implications and Intake Recommendations.* New York: Thieme.

Iannotti, L. L. (2006). Iron supplementation in childhood: Health benefits and risks. *American Journal of Clinical Nutrition, 84*: 1261–1276.

Kaplan, R. J. (2006). Beverage guidance system is not evidence-based. *American Journal of Clinical Nutrition, 84*: 1248–1249.

Lane, H. W. (2002). Water and energy dietary requirements and endocrinology of human space flight. *Nutrition, 18*: 820–828.

Lopez, M. A., & Martos, F. C. (2004). Iron availability: An updated review. *International Journal of Food Sciences and Nutrition, 55*(8): 597–606.

Mahan, L. K., & Escott-Stump, S. (Eds.). (2008). *Krause's Food and Nutrition Therapy* (12th ed.). Philadelphia: Elsevier Saunders.

Mann, J., & Truswell, S. (Eds.). (2007). *Essentials of Human Nutrition* (3rd ed.). New York: Oxford University Press.

Moore, M. C. (2005). *Pocket Guide to Nutritional Assessment and Care* (5th ed.). St. Louis, MO: Elvesier Mosby.

Mosby's Medical, Nursing and Allied Health Dictionary. (2002). (6th ed.). St. Louis, MO: Elsevier Health Sciences.

Navarra, T. (Ed.). (2004). *The Encyclopedia of Vitamins, Minerals, and Supplements* (2nd ed.). New York: Facts on File.

Neilsen, F. H. (2001). Other trace elements. In Bnowman, B. A. & Russell, R. M. (Eds.). *Present Knowledge in Nutrition* (8th ed., pp. 384–400). Washington, DC: ILSI Press.

Otten, J. J., Pitzi Hellwig, J., & Meyers, L. D. (Eds.). (2006). *Dietary Reference Intakes: The Essential Guide to Nutrient Requirements.* Washington, DC: National Academy Press.

Papanikolaou, G., & Pantopoulos, K. (2005). Iron metabolism and toxicity. *Toxicology and Applied Pharmacology, 202*(2): 199–211.

Sardesai, V. M. (2003). *Introduction to Clinical Nutrition* (2nd ed.). New York: Marcel Dekker.

Shils, M. E., & Shike, M. (Eds.). (2006). *Modern Nutrition in Health and Disease* (10th ed.). Philadelphia: Lippincott, Williams and Wilkins.

Water, Sanitation, and Health Protection and Human Environment (WHO). (2005). *Nutrients in Drinking Water.* Geneva, Switzerland: World Health Organization.

Webster-Gandy, J., Madden, A., & Holdworth, M. (Eds.). (2006). *Oxford Handbook of Nutrition and Dietetics.* Oxford, England: Oxford University Press.

Yves, R., Mazue, A., & Durlach, J. (2001). *Advances in Magnesium Research: Nutrition and Health.* Eastleigh, England: John Libby.

CHAPTER

15

Diet Therapy for Surgical Conditions

Time for completion
Activities: 1 hour
Optional examination: ½ hour

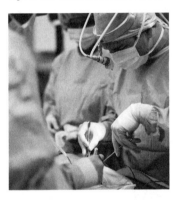

OBJECTIVES

Upon completion of this chapter, the student should be able to do the following:

1. Identify the physiological and psychological effects of body trauma or stress.
2. Contrast the outcomes of surgery in a patient with poor nutritional status and in a patient with good nutritional status.
3. Explain the rationale for the importance of the nutrients most needed during the surgical experience.
4. List the major nutritional problems encountered in preoperative patients and possible solutions to these problems.
5. Describe the diet therapy regime for the postoperative patient and rationale for its use.
6. Identify common foods and fluids suitable for replacing losses and promoting healing in the surgical patient.
7. Relate nursing interventions to the nutritional care of the surgery patient.

GLOSSARY

Acidosis: an accumulation of excess acid or depleted alkaline reserve (bicarbonate content) in the blood and body tissues. It almost always occurs as part of a disease process.

Ambulatory: able to walk; not confined to bed.

Calcification: process in which organic tissue becomes hardened by deposition of lime salts in the tissues.

Capillary walls: the sides of the minute blood vessels (capillaries). Capillaries connect the smallest arteries with the smallest veins.

Coenzymes: enzyme activators, such as vitamins, that enter into a variety of body processes.

Collagen: the protein in connective tissue and bone matrix.

Colloidal osmotic pressure: the pressure that develops on either side of a membrane. The colloid does not pass through the membrane, so therefore keeps the concentration of the solution approximately equal to that of circulating blood. The colloidal substance is a protein; therefore, when protein in the diet is depleted, edema develops because the solution can then pass from inside the membrane into the tissues.

Connective tissue: fibrous insoluble protein that holds cells together; collagen represents approximately 30% of body protein.

Decubitis ulcers: inflammation, sore, or ulcer over a bony prominence (exercise, movement, good skin care, and a high-protein, high-vitamin diet are needed for prevention).

Dehiscence: splitting open; separation of all the layers of a surgical wound.

Dehydration: the loss or deprivation of water from the body or tissues.

Diuresis: increased excretion of urine.

Duodenum: the first portion of the small intestine extending from the pylorus to the jejunum. It is about 10 inches long and both the common bile duct and pancreatic duct empty into it.

Edema: swelling; the body tissues contain an excess amount of tissue fluid.

Enteral nutrition: fed by way of the small intestine.

Evisceration: extrusion of the internal organs; disembowelment.

Exudate: fluid with a high content of protein and debris that has escaped from blood vessels and deposited on tissues.

Hyperglycemia: glucose in the blood elevated above the normal limit.

Hypoglycemia: blood sugar below the normal limit.

Interstitial: pertaining to or situated between parts or in the interspaces of a tissue.
 a. **fluid:** the extracellular fluid bathing most tissues, excluding fluid in the lymph and blood vessels.
 b. **tissue:** connective tissue between cells.

Intravenous: within the veins.

Parenteral nutrition: not fed through the alimentary canal but rather by subcutaneous, intramuscular, intrasternal, or intravenous injection.
 a. **via central vein:** in the central portion of the system.
 b. **via peripheral vein:** near the surface.

Peripheral veins: veins away from the central portion of the system; near the surface.

Peristalsis: the wormlike movement by which the alimentary canal propels its contents, consisting of a wave of contractions passing along the tube.

Plasma protein: the liquid part of the blood and lymph is the plasma. Plasma contains numerous chemicals and protein, glucose, and fats. Protein in plasma prevents undue leakage of fluids out of the capillaries.

Prothrombin: a chemical substance in the blood that interacts with calcium salts to produce thrombin, which clots blood.

Subclavian vein: a large vein located under the collarbone that unites with the interior jugular and forms the innominate vein.

Superior vena cava: the principal vein draining the upper portion of the body. Formed by the junction of right and left innominate veins, it empties into the right atrium of the heart.

BACKGROUND INFORMATION

The nutritional status of the patient before, during, and after surgery is important to a rapid and successful recovery. Factors affecting pre- and postoperative conditions are introduced below.

Effects of Stress

All kinds of stress or trauma deplete body stores and interfere with ingestion, digestion, and metabolism. Injury, accidents, trauma, burns, cancer, illness, fever, infections, loss of blood and other fluids, loss of body tissues, and other conditions requiring surgery can significantly deplete body substances in a patient. Such injuries or stress require an increased amount of nutrients for repair. These problems are usually compounded by psychological stress such as anxiety, fear, and pain, which greatly interfere with the desire or ability to eat.

During periods of stress there may be reduced function of the gastrointestinal (GI) tract. Muscular activity is lowered in the digestive tract. This may cause abdominal distention, gas pains, and constipation. In some cases, the nervous system may be stimulated by these conditions, resulting in nausea, vomiting, and diarrhea. Prolonged stress results in depleted liver glycogen and the wasting of muscle tissue.

Effects of Nutrition

Good nutrition prior to surgery leads to effective wound healing, increases resistance to infection, shortens convalescence, and lowers the mortality rate.

Poor nutrition prior to surgery leads to poor wound healing, dehydration, edema, excessive weight loss, decubitis ulcers, increased infections, potential liver damage, and a high mortality rate.

Most patients are not at optimum nutritional status when they are admitted to a healthcare facility. If surgery is to be performed, the patient's nutritional status must be improved by an appropriate dietary regimen prior to surgery. This minimizes surgical risk. Unfortunately, this is not always possible due to the acute need for surgery. Some also believe that such consideration is given low priority because of poor hospital practice, limited staffing, lack of communication, relatively low urgency, and so on.

Nutrients for the Surgical Experience

The following are nutrients considered important for persons undergoing surgery:

1. Protein is needed to build and repair damaged tissue.
2. Carbohydrate and fat are needed to spare protein and furnish energy.
3. Glucose is necessary to prevent acidosis and vomiting.
4. Vitamins:
   a. Vitamin C is required to hasten wound healing and collagen formation.
   b. Vitamin B complex is needed to form the coenzymes for metabolism, especially of carbohydrates.
   c. Vitamin K is needed to promote blood clotting.
5. Minerals:
   a. Zinc is needed to aid wound healing.
   b. Iron is needed to permit hemoglobin synthesis to replace blood loss.

Surgery Outcome

There is strong evidence that nutrition plays an important role in the outcomes of surgical cases. Some recent clinical findings are listed below.

1. In a National Veterans Affairs Surgical Risk Study of 87,000 noncardiac surgical cases, nutrition played an important role in surgical success. The preoperative serum albumin levels, an indicator of nutritional status, were the strongest predictors of patients who would show complications or die within 30 days.
2. A Veterans Affairs study found that malnourished patients who received postsurgical total parenteral nutrition support had fewer noninfectious complications than controls.
3. One study found that the number of days in the ICU and days on a ventilator were highest among those patients that did not receive postoperative enteral feeding. Length of hospital stay, infectious complications, hospital costs, and antibiotic usage were highest in the study's "unfed" group.
4. In a study of 300 patients undergoing major surgical procedures, malnutrition was associated with increased rates of morbidity and mortality.
5. A report by the National Institutes of Health, the American Society for Parenteral and Enteral Nutrition, and the American Society for Clinical Nutrition advocates the nutrition assessment of surgical patients via laboratory and physical data in combination with a subjective global assessment (SGA). The SGA encompasses food intake, maldigestion, and malabsorption and is useful in determining the effects of malnutrition on organ function and body composition.

PROGRESS CHECK ON BACKGROUND INFORMATION

MULTIPLE CHOICE

Circle the letter of the correct answer.

1. Effects of stress on the body include all except:
   a. stimulation of the desire to eat.
   b. depletion of body tissues.
   c. depressed GI functioning.
   d. decreased liver glycogen.

2. Poor nutrition prior to surgery may result in all of the following except:
   a. increased resistance to infection.
   b. dehydration.
   c. edema.
   d. liver damage.

FILL-IN

List four effects of good nutritional status on the outcome of surgery.

3. _____
4. _____
5. _____
6. _____

MATCHING

Some nutrients have been identified as being very important in the surgical experience. Match the nutrient at the left with the letter of its major function at the right.

7. Glucose
8. Vitamin C
9. Protein
10. B complex
11. Iron

a. builds and repairs tissue
b. blood clotting
c. synthesis of hemoglobin
d. aids in wound healing and collagen formation
e. prevents acidosis and vomiting
f. provides coenzymes for metabolism

Match the word with its definition.

12. Dehiscence
13. Evisceration
14. Collagen
15. Interstitial
16. Diuresis

a. excessive urine
b. connective tissue
c. between the cells
d. splitting open
e. disembowelment

TRUE/FALSE

Circle T for True and F for False.

17. T F Physical stress reduces functioning of all body organs.
18. T F Psychological stress depletes body stores.
19. T F If the patient is not fed orally he or she won't get edema and ascites.
20. T F Most patients have adequate nutritional status prior to surgery.
21. T F The postoperative serum albumin level is the strongest predictor of patients who show complications or die within 30 days.
22. T F The number of days in ICU and days on a ventilator probably is the highest among patients that did not receive postoperative enteral feeding.
23. T F Malnutrition is not related to increased rate of morbidity and mortality.
24. T F Subjective global assessment (SGA) encompasses food intake, maldigestion, and malabsorption and is useful in determining the effects of malnutrition on organ function and body composition.

ACTIVITY 1:

Pre- and Postoperative Nutrition

PREOPERATIVE NUTRITION

The major nutritional problems in the preoperative period are undernutrition and overnutrition. Both the undernourished and obese patients present special needs.

The undernourished patient, because of a lack of the major nutrients necessary for recovery, is at higher risk in surgery than a patient of normal weight. Protein deficiency is most common among these patients. Low protein storage will predispose the patient to shock, less detoxification of the anesthetic agent by the liver, increased edema at the incision site, and decreased antibody formation. The last factor increases the risk of infection. Intravenous feeding of solutions that are more concentrated in nutrients prior to surgery is one way to replenish nutrient storage. This assumes that surgery can be postponed for a time. Aggressive oral nutrition, although more time consuming, can accomplish the same goals.

Obese patients are at higher health risk in surgery than those of normal weight. Excess fat complicates surgery, puts a strain on the heart, increases the risk of infection and respiratory problems, and delays healing. The risks of dehiscence and evisceration are greater in the obese patient. Preexisting conditions such as hypertension and diabetes, which are prevalent in obese persons, also increase risks. There is no quick way for an obese person to safely lose weight prior to surgery. If time permits, a low-calorie diet, high in the essential nutrients, should be attempted. Starvation or fad diets are obvi-

ously not recommended preoperatively. Conversely, a reduction diet after surgery is not in the patient's best interest when the need for all nutrients is high. If weight loss is needed, a low-calorie diet should not be instituted until healing is complete.

Dietary considerations for an adequately nourished patient prior to surgery are also important. The special nutritional needs of surgical interventions should be met. The preoperative diet for these persons should be rich in carbohydrate, protein, minerals, vitamins, and fluids. This diet will assist in a rapid recovery as it promotes wound healing and decreases the risk of infections and other complications.

If a patient has preexisting conditions—for example, diabetes—the blood sugar should be stabilized before surgery. Other problems such as anemia, dehydration, acidosis, or electrolyte imbalances should be corrected before the surgical procedure.

POSTOPERATIVE NUTRITION

The goal of postoperative diet therapy is to replace body losses as soon as possible. Energy, protein, and ascorbic acid are major factors in achieving rapid wound healing. Fluid replacement is another major concern. Minerals and other vitamins also play a vital role in recovery.

The postoperative diet may be liquid, soft, or of regular consistency, but it must be high in calories, protein, vitamins, minerals, and fluids.

RATIONALE FOR DIET THERAPY
Protein

100–200 grams of high-quality protein per day are needed:

1. Up to 1 pound of tissue protein per day may be lost through bleeding, high metabolic rate (using protein for energy), from exudate, and catabolism of muscle tissue as well as from surgery itself.
2. Plasma protein loss from hemorrhage or wound bleeding may occur. Loss of plasma protein and blood volume increases the risk of shock. Extra protein is required to replace these losses.
3. Fever and inflammation that may accompany surgery can be reduced by an increased supply of protein.
4. When antibody production decreases, infections increase. A high protein intake can reduce the risk of infection.
5. Edema may develop due to an imbalance of colloidal osmotic pressure. Serum protein levels must be increased to reduce edema. Edema at the incision site may also develop, slowing healing. This is another reason for protein intake.
6. Bone healing is delayed if the protein intake is not high. The bone marrow is considered a special protein that anchors minerals and favors calcification.

7. Hormones and enzymes are protein substances. A lack of protein can lower production of these vital substances.

8. In the liver, protein combines with fat for removal. This prevents fatty infiltration. Thus, increased protein can protect the body against liver damage. When a protein combines with a fat, the product is a lipoprotein.

Fluids

There must be sufficient fluids to replace potential losses from vomiting, fever, diuresis, drainage, and exudates. Preventing dehydration is of great importance. Up to seven liters of fluid per day may be needed. Because the body tends to retain sodium and fluid postoperatively, total fluid intake and output must be measured and recorded to assure proper fluid balance.

Calories

If the caloric intake in the postoperative patient is inadequate, protein will be used for energy rather than for tissue rebuilding and wound healing. More than half of ingested proteins will be used to provide energy in the absence of sufficient carbohydrates and fats. A minimum of 2800 calories per day from carbohydrates and fat must be available to spare protein for its primary purpose. Review the protein-sparing action of carbohydrates in Chapters 4 and 5. An example of protein-sparing action is if a patient has had extensive surgery that requires 250 grams of protein for tissue building and repair, the total caloric content of the diet should range from 4000 to 6000 calories.

Vitamins

Vitamin C availability is imperative. The role of vitamin C, as you will recall, is to supply the cementing material of connective tissue, capillary walls, and new tissue. Depending on the nature and extent of the surgery, the patient may need 6 to 20 times the RDAs/DRIs.

Vitamin K is also of special concern because of its function in blood clotting. Intestinal bacteria synthesis of this vitamin is decreased because of the use of antibiotics. Any liver damage reduces prothrombin formation, which can be corrected by the presence of more vitamin K.

The need for B complex vitamins increases with rising caloric requirements. These vitamins function as coenzymes in carbohydrate and protein metabolism, the formation of hemoglobin, and the prevention of anemia.

Minerals

Minerals are of great importance in the replacement of electrolytes simultaneously lost with fluid from the body. The amount and kinds of minerals to be replaced are determined by the type of surgery and extent of loss in the patient. Certainly, sodium, chloride, phosphorus, potas-sium, and iron will need replacing and an increase in calcium supply is mandatory if bone surgery or loss is involved. Table 15-1 lists food sources of some of the most essential nutrients needed by surgical patients.

PROGRESS CHECK ON ACTIVITY 1

MULTIPLE CHOICE

Circle the letter of the correct answer.

1. The major nutritional problems that the health team encounters among patients scheduled for surgery are _____ and _____.

   a. anxiety
   b. undernutrition
   c. pain
   d. overnutrition

2. Low protein reserves can cause all except which of the following conditions?

   a. shock and edema
   b. muscle wasting
   c. anxiety
   d. liver damage

3. Sufficient fluids are supplied in the diet to replace losses from all except:

   a. edema.
   b. diuresis.
   c. vomiting.
   d. drainage.

TRUE/FALSE

Circle T for True and F for False.

4. T F A minimum of 1200 calories per day from carbohydrate and fat is required for protein-sparing of the postoperative patient.

5. T F The major problem in preoperative patients is under- or overnutrition.

6. T F Decreased protein increases antibody formation.

7. T F It is more important to increase total calories than carbohydrate in the preoperative diet.

FILL-IN

8. Using the following menu, indicate the major nutrients supplied by each food listed by placing an X in the appropriate column.

	Pro	CHo	Thia	Nia	Ribo	Fe	Vit C
Oyster stew	—	—	—	—	—	—	—
Whole wheat garlic toast	—	—	—	—	—	—	—
Green pepper and cabbage slaw	—	—	—	—	—	—	—
Raisin rice pudding with orange sauce	—	—	—	—	—	—	—

TABLE 15-1   Some Food Sources of the Nutrients Identified as Essential to a Successful Surgery

Protein		Vitamin C	Vitamin B Complex*	Vitamin K	Iron	Zinc
Complete:	Milk Eggs Meat Fish Poultry	Citrus fruits Sweet and hot peppers Greens Strawberries	1. Thiamin: pork, oysters, organ meats, enriched bread and cereals	Green leafy vegetables† Fruits Cereals Meats	Liver Heart Eggs Raisins Prunes Whole wheat and enriched cereals and breads Apricots, dried Red meats Oysters Pork Almonds	Shellfish (especially oysters) Dairy products Eggs Whole grain cereals
Incomplete:	Vegetables Grains Nuts and seeds	Broccoli Tomatoes Cantaloupe Cabbage	2. Riboflavin: milk, milk products, organ meats muscle meats, oysters, enriched bread and cereals			
			3. Niacin: liver, tuna, peanuts and peanut butter, peas, pork, enriched bread and cereals			

*Others not listed of this group will be supplied if these three B vitamins in the diet are adequate.
†Best source

ACTIVITY 2:

The Postoperative Diet Regime

GOALS OF DIETARY MANAGEMENT

The main goal of postoperative nutritional and dietary care is for the patient to regain a normal body weight. This is brought about by a positive nitrogen balance and subsequent muscle formation and fat deposition. This goal can be achieved by first correcting all fluid and electrolyte imbalances and giving appropriate transfusions. The second step is to provide carefully planned dietary and nutritional support for the patient, with special emphasis on those nutrients discussed at the beginning of this chapter. The third step is to monitor food intake by maintaining a detailed record of what is consumed.

A postoperative dietary regimen also requires aggressive nutritional support that is needed to maintain normal body functions and tissues. Tissue maintenance is especially important since additional losses may result from postoperative bed confinement and ensuing muscle atrophy. Nutritional supports should also attempt to replace tissue (such as muscle, bone, blood, exudate, and skin) that may have been lost during the trauma of surgery. Any malnourishment should be remedied if it has not already been treated. Plasma protein should be supplied to control or prevent edema and shock. Plasma protein also provides vital components for the synthesis of albumin, antibodies, enzymes, and other necessary substances, which may have been lost through bleeding or the escape of fluids. Finally, plasma protein also accelerates the healing of wounds.

Inadequate nutritional supports increase morbidity and mortality, delay the return of normal body functions, and retard the process of tissue rebuilding. Inadequate nutrition prevents wounds from healing at a normal pace and causes edema and muscular weakness. Most importantly, all of these consequences prolong convalescence and discomfort for the patient.

FEEDING THE PATIENT IMMEDIATELY AFTER THE OPERATION

Since a patient usually cannot tolerate solid food immediately after an operation, it is withheld anywhere from a few hours to two or three days. A feeding that is too early may nauseate the patient and cause vomiting and possible aspiration. This results in further fluid and electrolyte losses, discomfort, and potential pneumonia. The following outline lists the various types of dietary support that can be used during this short part of the postoperative period.

1. No food by mouth (NPO)
2. Intravenous feeding: blood transfusion, fluids and electrolytes, 5% dextrose, vitamin and mineral supplements, protein-sparing solutions (with or without Intralipid), combinations of above
3. Oral feeding: routine hospital progressive liquid diets with or without supplements, liquid-protein supplements with or without nonprotein calories, combinations of above
4. A combination of oral and intravenous feedings

Many clinicians feel that it is not worthwhile to provide aggressive nutritional support during such a short period of food deprivation. This decision is justified in a well-nourished individual who can afford temporary catabolic losses and would not be able to efficiently use the supplied protein or calories. As described in Activity 1, the majority of patients do not fit this category. The attending physician must decide if the patient is well nourished and if enteral or parenteral feedings can be tolerated. If the feedings can be tolerated, a subsequent decision must be made on benefits of these exogenous nutrients. The health professional may, after his or her assessment of the patient's status, request the physician to evaluate the patient and prescribe additional feedings.

Blood transfusions and fluid and electrolyte compensation are administered to those patients needing them. Some doctors prescribe 5% dextrose solution in saline or water, but the amount given is limited by the patient's tolerance. Another problem is that a concentrated dextrose solution may cause thrombosis in the peripheral veins. Because of the relatively low nutrient density of dextrose solution, it should not be used as a long-term means of feeding. It has been claimed generally that the infusion of dextrose spares some body protein from breakdown to provide needed calories. Recently various medical centers have experimented with the infusion of protein-sparing solutions made up mainly of essential amino acids. The preliminary trials have been very encouraging. However, if such means are used every day, it may not only be expensive, but further deteriorate fragile peripheral veins. Some hospitals use vitamin and mineral supplements as well as protein-sparing solutions.

Although solid foods are withheld from patients immediately after an operation, most hospitals provide patients with oral feedings after their intestinal functions return to normal (as early as 24 hours after the operation). The feedings consist of routine hospital progressive diets (see Chapter 14). This stepwise postoperative feeding may cover one to three days, depending on the patient's tolerance, strength, and type of operation or trauma.

Some patients may be able to start with a soft diet, while others must begin with a clear liquid diet. Progressive feedings occasionally may be supplemented with commercial formulas. Some patients are given liquid-protein supplements with or without nonprotein calories if they can tolerate the feedings. Again, depending on the patient and his or her condition, a combination of feeding methods, including total parenteral nutrition (see Chapter 14), may be used. For patients requiring tube feeding, consult the detailed procedures described in Chapter 14.

At this early stage of postoperative recovery, physicians, nurses, and dietitians should work closely to determine whether dextrose solution or oral liquid diets should be continued. This is important, since both types of feeding may not be nutritionally sound without concentrated supplements. Nutritional supports, including fluids, electrolytes, protein, calories, and other nutrients, should be carefully reviewed. Finally, a long-term aggressive postoperative dietary treatment should be planned and executed to combat the catabolic consequences of trauma and to bring about a speedy recovery.

DIETARY MANAGEMENT FOR RECOVERY

When a patient can tolerate regular hospital foods, the health team should plan and prescribe an appropriate diet. Experts in clinical nutrition have tried for a number of years to develop a postoperative diet that will provide patients with an optimal amount of nutrients. In general, the following diet prescription should satisfy most clinical conditions that involve trauma:

1. 40–50 kcal/kg body weight/d
2. 12%–15% of total calories as protein
3. Well-balanced intakes of the established RDAs/DRIs
4. Carefully monitored intakes of vitamins A, K, C, B_{12}; folic acid; and the minerals, iron and zinc

To illustrate the protein and calorie composition of such a diet, Table 15-2 includes two examples (40 kcal and 50 kcal/d) for a man weighing 70 kg.

TABLE 15-2	Approximate Protein and Calorie Content of a Postoperative Diet for a Male Patient Weighing 70 kg		
kcal/kg Body Weight	Total Daily Kilocalories	Approximate Dietary Protein (g)	Total Calories from Protein (%)
40	2800	84	12
50	3500	131	15

If the patient has a minimal amount of tissue and blood loss, a sound preoperative nutritional status, a moderate to good appetite, and no sign of surgical complications, a diet of 35 to 40 kcal/kg is probably sufficient. However, the diet for a postoperative patient should be individualized, especially the serving sizes and the frequency of feeding. Patients usually tolerate solids better if the feedings are small and frequent.

Both carbohydrates and fats are important sources of calories, and they should be provided in about equal quantities to constitute 85%–88% of the total calories. (If this reduces the patient's appetite, less fat should be consumed.) The calories from carbohydrates and fats used to correct hypermetabolism supply energy for all processes of rebuilding and repairing, and spare protein for anabolic purposes.

If the patient is given solid food, a good quantity of fruits and vegetables should be included in meals in addition to protein, fat, and carbohydrate. Refer to Chapter 14 for planning a high-protein, high-calorie, balanced diet. The need for vitamins A, K, C, B_{12}, and folic acid in a postoperative regimen requires special attention. Vitamins A and C have been proven experimentally and clinically to assist in wound healing as well as tissue repair. Vitamin A is well known for its role in maintaining epithelial structures, and vitamin C is important for collagen synthesis. In addition, vitamin A acid (retinoic acid) has recently been shown to assist in wound healing and is currently suspected to be a possible curative agent for certain types of human cancer.

The body's ability to clot blood postoperatively depends on an adequate supply of vitamin K. Folic acid and vitamin B_{12} are necessary for the synthesis and turnover of all body cells, especially red blood cells, and should be amply provided. The postoperative use of antibiotics may inhibit the formation of these three important vitamins by the intestinal flora, thus partially reducing the body's supply. Therefore, patients must be monitored for deficiencies of these nutrients and given adequate supplementation.

The importance of iron and zinc cannot be underestimated. Iron is vital for hemoglobin synthesis and is used to compensate for blood loss and possible anemia.

Zinc has a definitive role in wound healing and clinical supplementation with zinc postoperatively is now common. Zinc sulphate is the preferred form, given in dosage amounts of 18–22.5 mg/day. (See Table 15-1 for food sources of these essential nutrients.)

There are differences with the dietary care of patients undergoing different types of surgery, such as digestive tract, gynecological organs, or pancreas. Space limitation does not permit discussions of details for each surgical condition. However, the next section presents a discussion of important considerations in the nutritional and dietary care of a patient with part of the intestine surgically removed.

GASTROINTESTINAL SURGERY: AN ILLUSTRATION

According to some professionals, early removal of the nasogastric tube, early oral feeding, and a reasonable transition to a regular diet is safe and tolerated in most patients after gastrointestinal (GI) surgery. The patients who may not benefit from or tolerate this more progressive postoperative care are those who have had emergency GI surgery. In terms of the first postoperative meals, the ideal approach may be to allow patients to select their foods and beverages. Those patients who are nauseated or not hungry are more likely to choose clear liquids, and those who are hungry and feeling well will choose from a regular diet.

As an illustration, we will study the dietary care of a patient undergoing partial removal of the GI tract.

The normal small intestine is 300–800 cm (10–25 ft) in length (⅓ jejunum and ⅔ ileum). The normal colon (large intestine) is about 150 cm (10 ft). Most nutrients are absorbed in the jejunum. Nine liters of fluid per day enters the small bowel. Normally, all but 1 liter is absorbed proximal to the colon. The colon absorbs more than 80% of the remaining fluid, and can absorb up to 3–4 liters daily. The colon also has the capability to salvage energy by the fermentation of complex carbohydrate and soluble fiber to short chain fatty acids.

Short-bowel syndrome refers to a surgical loss of significant distal ileum, ileocecal valve, and/or colon. The result is a faster overall transit and the potential for greater loss of fluid and nutrient. Following a resection, the ileum has a greater ability to adapt than the jejunum. The adaptation depends on the size of section of ileum or colon removed or nonfunctional. The function of the remaining bowel may further be handicapped by:

- Mucosal disease
- Bacterial overgrowth
- Rapid gastric emptying
- Excessive gastric acid with inactivation of pancreatic lipase and deconjugation of bile salts, or pancreatic insufficiency

If 100 cm or more of terminal ileum is removed, there is impairment of the absorption of vitamin B_{12} and bile salts, which means the absorption of fat and fat soluble vitamins will also be affected. If there is less than 100 cm of remaining jejunum or ileum (without a colon or ileocecal valve) or less than 50 cm of small bowel attached to the colon, central parenteral nutrition may be required until clinical conditions indicate otherwise.

The process of intestinal adaptation is facilitated by complex foods and continues for one or more years in adults. Stool output with diarrhea may depend on the type of carbohydrate consumed, simple or complex. Excessive eating is an important adaptive response to maldigestion and malabsorption.

Thus, approaches to diet therapy for a patient with short-bowel syndrome are as follows:

During the initial postoperative period, recommended management includes no food by mouth, with intravenous feeding of electrolytes and central parenteral feeding if indicated. Increase oral intake gradually, which will be determined by patient response and clinical status, starting with 6 small feedings per day, avoiding hyperosmolar liquids.

Advance to regular diet, mostly unrestricted with high calories and protein intake. In most patients, lactose is well tolerated except those with a significant amount of jejunum removed.

Some patients require supplements of vitamins and some trace elements and minerals. Some patients require supplemental calcium, magnesium, and zinc. If the distal ileum is removed, the patient may need Vitamin B_{12} injection via vein or musculature.

The attending physician will prescribe a constant monitoring of blood chemistry especially levels of vitamins and minerals, organ integrity, bone density, and urinary analysis for components and volumes.

If patient has no ileum or colon, dehydration is the greatest concern. Sipping an oral rehydration solution containing a calculated amount of sodium can reduce the need for intravenous fluid. There are several acceptable commercial preparations, though it is important to consider palatability and patient rejection.

If a patient's colon is intact and functioning, encourage the consumption of soluble fiber which is fermented to short-chain fatty acids in the large intestine. Supplemental medium chain triglycerides can increase total calories when absorbed in the small bowel and the colon. Restrict the following:

- Oxalate because it can bind calcium especially in a supplement
- Sugars to avoid diarrhea
- Fat if steatorrhea is present and more than 100 cm of distal ileum is removed

Consider the use of enteral feeding. Several acceptable commercial preparations are available.

NURSING IMPLICATIONS

Recognizing that inadequate nutritional support may increase morbidity and mortality during the early postoperational period, the nurse should do the following:

1. Recognize that malnutrition even in the short period of 1–3 days postoperatively may retard the healing process.
2. Monitor the patient closely and provide nourishment as soon as bowel sounds are present.
3. Check for other feeding methods that will furnish adequate nutrients, if oral feedings are contraindicated.
4. Assess total fluid intake carefully and compare total fluid losses to avoid circulating overload.
5. Be aware that any weight gain during this period may be indicative of excess fluids.
6. Recognize the need for extra nutrients and fluids if the patient has elevated temperature.
7. Request specific written orders for change of diet and/or feeding method as the condition indicates.
8. Provide aggressive nutritional support during the early postoperative period as well as in subsequent convalescence.
9. Refer to the nutritional support team for assistance if the facility has one. Otherwise, work within the health team of which you are part.
10. Document all changes, requests, and rationales carefully.

PROGRESS CHECK ON ACTIVITY 2

FILL-IN

1. State the main goal of dietary management in the postoperative period. _____

   _____

   _____

2. List three ways this goal can be achieved.

   a. _____

   b. _____

   c. _____

3. Describe the three major functions of plasma protein.

   a. _____

   b. _____

   c. _____

4. Identify five intravenous feedings that may be used in the immediate postoperative period.

   a. _____

b. _____

c. _____

d. _____

e. _____

5. Describe the normal progression of routine hospital diets and approximate time periods of use for each (consult Chapter 12 if in doubt about the time periods). _____

_____

_____

Situation

Johnny B, 5'6", 150 lb, wrecked his motorcycle. He was wearing a helmet, but sustained a mild concussion. In addition, he received a compound fracture of the left femur and multiple lacerations of the arms, face, and upper body. He was in surgery for three hours. The diet prescription is for a soft diet in six feedings with the following specifications: 45 kcal/kg body weight/day, 15% of total calories as protein, 55% as carbohydrate, and the remainder as fat. Answer the following questions about this situation.

6. What is the total kcal content of Johnny's diet? Round to nearest whole number. _____

_____

7. How many grams of protein per day will he receive? _____

_____

8. How many grams of fat are in his diet order?

_____

9. How many grams of carbohydrate will Johnny get? _____

_____

10. Write a 1-day menu, including the three snacks, that will satisfy the diet requirements.

Breakfast

_____

_____

_____

Mid-AM

_____

_____

Lunch

_____

_____

_____

Mid-PM

_____

_____

Dinner

_____

_____

H.S. (Hour of Sleep)

_____

_____

REFERENCES

American Dietetic Association. (2006). *Nutrition Diagnosis: A Critical Step in Nutrition Care Process.* Chicago: Author.

Babor, S. (2005). Early feeding compared with parenteral nutrition after oesophageal or oesophagastric resection and reconstruction. *British Journal of Nutrition, 93*: 509–513.

Beham, E. (2006). *Therapeutic Nutrition: A Guide to Patient Education.* Philadelphia: Lippincott, Williams and Wilkins.

Buchman, A. (2004). *Practical Nutritional Support Technique* (2nd ed.). Thorofeue, NJ: SLACK.

Deen, D., & Hark, L. (2007). *The Complete Guide to Nutrition in Primary Care.* Malden, MA: Blackwell.

Escott-Stump, S. (2002). *Nutrition and Diagnosis-Related Care* (5th ed.). Philadelphia: Lippincott, Williams and Wilkins.

Garrow, J. S. (2000). *Human Nutrition and Dietetics* (10th ed.). New York: Churchill Livingston.

Haas, E. M., & Levin, B. (2006). *Staying Healthy with Nutrition: The Complete Guide to Diet and Nutrition Medicine* (21st ed.). Berkeley, CA: Celestial Arts.

Hark, L., & Morrison, G. (Eds.). (2003). *Medical Nutrition and Disease* (3rd ed.). Malden, MA: Blackwell.

Kang, I. (2007). Mineral deficiency in patients who have undergone gastrectomy. *Nutrition, 23*: 318–322.

Ljungqvist, O. (2005). To fast or not to fast before surgical stress. *Nutrition, 21*: 885–886.

Lopez Hellin, J. (2008). Nutritional modulation of protein metabolism after gastrointestinal surgery. *European Journal of Clinical Nutrition, 62*: 254–262.

Luis, D. A. (2007). Clinical and biochemical outcomes after a randomized trial with a high dose of enteral arginine formula in postsurgical head and neck cancer patients. *European Journal of Clinical Nutrition, 61*: 200–204.

Luo, M. H. (2008). Depletion of plasma antioxidants in surgical intensive care unit patients requiring paenteral feeding: Effects of parental nutrition with or without alanyl-glutamine dipeptide supplementation. *Nutrition, 24*: 37–44.

Mahan, L. K., & Escott-Stump, S. (Eds.) (2008). *Krause's Food and Nutrition Therapy* (12th ed.). Philadelphia: Elsevier Saunders.

Mann, J., & Truswell, S. (Eds.). (2007). *Essentials of Human Nutrition* (3rd ed.). New York: Oxford University Press.

Marian, M. J., Williams-Muller, P., & Bower, J. (2007). *Integrating Therapeutic and Complementary Nutrition.* Boca Raton, FL: CRC Press.

Mertes, N. (2006). Safety and efficacy of a new parental lipid emulsion (SMOFlipid) in surgical patients: A randomized, double-blind multicenter study. *Annals of Nutrition & Metabolism, 50*: 253–259.

Moore, M. C. (2005). *Pocket Guide to Nutritional Assessment and Care* (5th ed.). St. Louis, MO: Elvesier Mosby.

Payne-James, J., & Wicks, C. (2003). *Key Facts in Clinical Nutrition* (2nd ed.). London: Greenwich Medical Media.

Sardesai, V. M. (2003). *Introduction to Clinical Nutrition* (2nd ed.). New York: Marcel Dekker.

Shils, M. E., & Shike, M. (Eds.). (2006). *Modern Nutrition in Health and Disease* (10th ed.). Philadelphia: Lippincott, Williams and Wilkins.

Sungurtekin, H. (2004). The influence of nutritional status on complications after major intraabdomnal surgery. *Journal of American College of Nutrition, 23*: 227–232.

Thomas, B., & Bishop, J. (Eds.). (2007). *Manual of Dietetic Practice* (4th ed.). Ames, IA: Blackwell.

Webster-Gandy, J., Madden, A., & Holdworth, M. (Eds.) (2006). *Oxford Handbook of Nutrition and Dietetics.* Oxford, England: Oxford University Press.

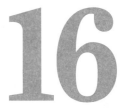

CHAPTER **16**

Diet Therapy for Cardiovascular Disorders

Time for completion
Activities: 1½ hours
Optional examination: ½ hour

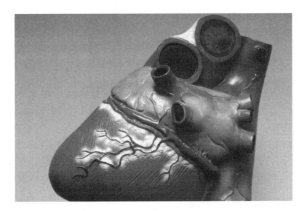

OBJECTIVES

Upon completion of this chapter, the student should be able to do the following:

1. Discuss the recommendations regarding the role of diet in preventing heart disease.
2. Describe and state the rationale of diet therapies used for the different heart disorders.
3. List the foods allowed, limited, and forbidden on selected therapeutic diets for heart disorders.
4. Identify resources available for patient education.
5. Identify nursing implications involved in the use of modified diets in cardiovascular disease.

GLOSSARY

Atherosclerosis: thickening of the inside walls of arteries by deposits of fat or cholesterol substances (plaques).
Cardiovascular: of or relating to the heart and blood vessels.
Cerebrovascular accident (CVA): when the blood vessels in the cerebrum (brain) are deprived of oxygen by an obstruction (occluded). This may be due to plaque formation, thrombus (blood clot), or aneurism (rupture of

the blood vessel). Absence of oxygen to brain tissue for more than 5 to 6 minutes leads to irreversible cerebral changes and tissue death. Commonly called a "stroke."

Cholesterol: a fatlike substance manufactured in the liver from saturated fats, including body fat. It is widely distributed in the body tissues and serves many important functions.

Coronary: encircling (like a crown).

Coronary arteries: two large arteries that branch from the ascending aorta and supply the heart muscle with blood.

Coronary heart disease (CHD): the coronary arteries supply all of the blood to the heart muscle. Occlusion, most often caused by narrowing of the vessels by plaque (atherosclerosis), deprives it of its nutrients and causes death to the part of the heart muscle that is occluded. When the occlusion is complete, myocardial infarction results (*see* coronary occlusion).

Coronary occlusion: closing off of a coronary artery-most often caused by the plaques of atherosclerosis. When the occlusion is complete, myocardial infarction (MI) results.

Hyperlipoproteinemia: the presence of abnormally high levels of lipoproteins in the serum.

Hypertension: blood pressure elevated above the normal range for age and sex.

Lipoproteins: the form in which lipids are transported in the blood. There are four main classes of lipoproteins: chylomicrons, very-low-density lipoproteins, low-density lipoproteins, and high-density lipoproteins.

   a. **Low-density lipoproteins (LDLs)** transport 60%–75% of the serum cholesterol. They carry from the liver to the body cells (including blood vessels). High serum levels of LDLs, therefore, increase the risk of CHD (see above).

   b. **High-density lipoproteins (HDLs)** transport 20%–25% of plasma cholesterol. They are believed to collect excess cholesterol from body cells and carry it back to the liver to be excreted or used for making bile.

Myocardial infarction (MI): death of tissue of an area of the heart muscle as a result of oxygen deprivation, which in turn was caused by an obstruction of the blood supply (*see* coronary heart disease). Commonly referred to as a "heart attack."

Triglycerides: the principal form of fat in foods and in the body, consisting of three fatty acids and glycerol.

BACKGROUND INFORMATION

More than half the people who die in this country each year die of heart and blood vessel disease. About 75% of all adult hospitalized patients show symptoms of heart problems even though they are admitted for other causes. The high occurrence of these health problems means

that the nurse should have accurate information about available dietary treatments for heart problems and the rationale for their use.

There is no known single cause of heart disease. However, the presence of a combination of certain factors predisposes a person to high risk of the disease. Some personal characteristics, such as a family history of heart disease, sex, and age cannot be changed, but dietary factors and stressful lifestyles can be modified. Therefore, the diets discussed in this chapter serve two goals: to reduce or prevent further damage to the cardiovascular system, and to prevent development of the disorder in yet unaffected individuals.

Current Consensus

The National Cholesterol Education Program (NCEP) is one of three principal programs administered by the Office of Prevention, Education, and Control of the National Heart, Lung, and Blood Institute (NHLBI) of the National Institutes of Health (NIH). It came about after years of trials and scientific evidence that linked blood cholesterol levels to coronary heart disease. These trials showed that levels could be lowered safely by both diet and drugs (see Table 16-1).

The First Report of the Expert Panel on Detection, Evaluation, and Treatment of High Blood Cholesterol in Adults was produced in 1988. An additional report was published in 1991 that presented recommendations for high blood cholesterol in children and adolescents. The Second Report by the Expert Panel, in 1993, included evidence that had emerged since 1991 and updated recommendations for the management of high blood cholesterol in adults. This edition includes assessments for cholesterol lowering in women, the elderly, and young adults as well as physical activity and weight loss as components of diet therapy.

TABLE 16-1   Criteria for Treatment Intervention in Adults

Classification based on total cholesterol

< 200 mg/dl—desirable level
200–239 mg/dl—borderline high blood cholesterol
≥ 240 mg/dl—high blood cholesterol

Classification based on LDL cholesterol

< 130 mg/dl—desirable LDL cholesterol
130–159 mg/dl—borderline high risk
≥ 160 mg/dl—high risk

Source: Second Report of the Expert Panel on Detection, Evaluation and Treatment of High Blood Cholesterol in Adults, September 1993, and Report of the Expert Panel on Blood Cholesterol Levels in Children and Adolescents, September 1991.

The third report (ATP 3), May 2001, updates clinical guidelines for cholesterol testing and management. It reports and expands indications for intensive cholesterol-lowering therapy in clinical practice. Many persons have high risk for CHD and will benefit from more intensive treatment than was recommended in ATP 1 and 2.

ATP 3 continues to use LDL cholesterol as the primary target of cholesterol-lowering therapy; therefore, the primary goals are stated in terms of LDL. There have been some modifications in lipid and lipoprotein classifications. Compare Tables 16-1 and 16-2. This report is available at the Web site, www.nih.gov. ATP 4, the fourth report, is in the planning and preparation stage.

The reports outline "heart-healthy" eating for the general population, as well as treatment for persons with high cholesterol levels, or those at high risk for developing CHD.

Guidelines have been established for health professionals, patients, and the public. Among these important guidelines are two of particular interest to students of nutrition:

1. To increase the knowledge of health professionals regarding the major role that diet plays in reducing blood cholesterol.
2. To improve the knowledge, skills, and attitudes of students in the health professions regarding high blood cholesterol and its management.

See Table 16-2.

You are encouraged to add these publications to your database for clinical practice, as the reports present guidelines that are the responsibility of not only physicians but also nurses, dietitians, pharmacists, and all other members of the health team. The patient is, of necessity, the center of this team and must be educated to make the dietary and lifestyle changes necessary to reduce CHD risk.

Implementing dietary guidance with the use of nutrition labeling and standards of identity is one example of steps being taken to help Americans implement the guidelines. (Refer to Table 16-3.) The major objective for this sweeping revision is to increase the availability of health-promoting foods.

Nutritional Risk Factors in Heart Disease

The risk factors of heart disease include the following:

1. Elevated serum cholesterol
2. Elevated serum triglycerides
3. Obesity
4. Hypertension
5. Generally poor eating habits and a sedentary lifestyle

All of these factors can be altered by diet and exercise.

ACTIVITY 1:

The Lipid Disorders

DEFINITIONS

The term used most frequently in describing the lipid disorders is *hyperlipoproteinemia* (hyper = excess, lipoprotein = fat and protein, emia = in blood, which translates as excess level of fat/protein complex in blood). It refers to higher than normal levels of certain lipids in the blood.

Cholesterol and triglycerides are water-insoluble lipids, carried in the blood by lipoproteins. Diet, genetics, and acquired factors affect the circulating levels of one or more lipoproteins.

Lipoproteins are lipids combined with proteins. They are called apolipoproteins. Three main classes of lipoproteins are very-low-density lipoproteins (VLDL), low-density lipoproteins (LDL), and high-density lipoproteins (HDL). LDL and HDL mainly transport cholesterol, and VLDL transports triglycerides.

The liver makes cholesterol from saturated fat. The amount of cholesterol synthesized is directly related to the quantity of saturated fat consumed. LDLs carry cholesterol to the artery plaques. Plaque formation is directly related to the amount of LDLs present. The connection is cholesterol, LDLs, plaques, and coronary heart disease. HDLs carry cholesterol away from the plaques to the liver, to the gallbladder, and into the intestines, where it is excreted. HDLs, therefore, lower the risk of CHD. It appears that a person with a high HDL level is less likely to develop the disease than a person with a low HDL level. On the other hand, the reverse

TABLE 16-2	ATP III Classification of LDL, Total, and HDL Cholesterol (mg/dl)	
LDL Cholesterol		
< 100	Optimal	
100–129	Near optimal/above optimal	
130–159	Borderline high	
160–189	High	
≥ 190	Very high	
Total Cholesterol		
< 200	Desirable	
200–239	Borderline high	
≥ 240	High	
HDL Cholesterol		
< 40	Low	
≥ 60	High	

Source: Third Report of the Expert Panel on Evaluation and Treatment of High Blood Cholesterol in Adults, May 2001.

TABLE 16-3   Descriptive Labeling Terms Approved by the FDA: A Translation to Components Important in a Cholesterol-Lowering Diet*

Nutrient	Free	Low	Reduced/Less/Fewer	Other
All	Synonyms for "Free": "Free of," "No," "Zero," "Without," "Trivial Source of," "Negligible Source of," "Dietary Insignificant Source of"	Synonyms for "Low": "Contains a Small Amount of, "Low Source of," "Low in"	Synonyms for "Reduced/Less/Fewer": "Reduced in," "Lower," "Low"	
Total calories	Less than 5 calories/reference serving	Less than 40 calories/reference serving	Reduced by at least 25%	
Total fat	Less than 0.5 g/reference serving	3 g or less/reference serving Meal and main dish products: 3 g or less per 100 g product and 30% or less calories from fat	Reduced by at least 25%	"__% Fat Free" "__% Lean," must meet requirements for "Low Fat"
Saturated fat	Less than 0.5 g/reference serving, levels of trans-fatty acids must be 1% or less of total fat	1 g or less/reference serving and 15% or less of calories from saturated fatty acids Meal and main dishes products: 1 g or less per 100 g, and less than 10% of calories from saturated fat	Reduced by at least 25%	
Cholesterol	Less than 2 mg/reference serving; saturated fat content must be 2 g or less	20 mg or less/reference serving; saturated fat content must be 2 g or less per serving Meal and main dish products: 20 mg or less per 100 g, with saturated fat content less than 2 g/100 g	Reduced by at least 25% Contains 2 g or less saturated fat per reference serving	
Sodium	Less than 5 mg/reference serving	140 mg or less/reference serving Meal and main dish products: 140 mg or less/100 g of food	Reduced by at least 25%	"Very Low Sodium," "Very Low in Sodium": 35 mg or less/reference serving

*The new FDA labeling requirements make it possible for patients to determine how many grams of total fat and saturated fat are contributed by a serving of a particular food. In addition, the new nutrition label will indicate in a "Percent Daily Value" column the percent the food contributes to the maximum amount of fat allowed in a 2,000-calorie diet that meets recommendations for less than 30% of calories from fat, and less than 10% of calories from saturated fat (see Module 1). Patients will also be able to use the fat and cholesterol descriptors that are now defined by the FDA.

Source: Second Report of the Expert Panel on Detection, Evaluation and Treatment of High Blood Cholesterol in Adults, September 1993.

applies to blood LDL levels; that is, a high LDL level increases the risk of heart disease.

CHOLESTEROL AND LIPID DISORDERS

When we talk about blood cholesterol, we now refer to three forms: total, LDL, and HDL. Some health-screening procedures measure the LDL cholesterol since it reflects the actual risk of atherosclerosis. To calculate LDL cho-

lesterol, one may use the following formula (quantities are in mg/dl):

$$\text{LDL cholesterol} = \text{total cholesterol} - \text{HDL cholesterol} - \frac{\text{triglycerides}}{5}$$

Normally, the plasma levels of different forms of lipid exist within certain limits. However, particular individuals may deviate from such norms and develop hyperlipidemia, or an elevated level of serum lipid. Three main types of lipid are involved in this condition: cholesterol (an excess of which is called hypercholesterolemia), triglyceride (hypertriglyceridemia), and certain forms of lipoprotein (hyperlipoproteinemia). Hyperlipoproteinemia is usually associated with hypercholesterolemia or hypertriglyceridemia, or both, although the reverse is not necessarily true. Any of the hyperlipidemias is undesirable because it may potentiate atherosclerosis or cause its associated clinical symptoms.

DIETARY MANAGEMENT

To treat a patient with a lipid disorder, the attending physician uses laboratory data and clinical examination to type the patient. The typing uses many data: sex, age, symptoms, blood and laboratory tests, family history, and so forth. After the physician has typed the patient, the dietitian implements the appropriate dietary treatment according to the diagnosis. This is not the proper forum to discuss details for treating individual patients.

The second approach involves the public and is applicable to all individuals. It has one goal: to lower blood cholesterol while maintaining adequate diet. At present, the dietary management of a person with high blood (total or LDL) cholesterol is being promoted by three major groups: the American Heart Association (AHA), the National Cholesterol Education Program (NCEP), and other private health groups. All three groups target the amount and type of fats we eat.

NCEP RECOMMENDATIONS

Dietary intervention is the first priority in lowering blood cholesterol. The NCEP has also issued a guide for foods low in saturated fat and cholesterol. (See Tables 16-3 through 16-6.)

The NCEP has other recommendations that are of importance in patient care and public health programs:

1. The use of blood cholesterol as a means of classifying the risk of atherosclerosis for the population: The two classifications are based on plasma total cholesterol or LDL cholesterol (Table 16-1). These classifications can be applied if a person's blood cholesterol is known through screening or other means.
2. Using the LDL cholesterol recommendations, one can make a careful study of a person's blood lipid and set goals.

THIRD EDITION OF NCEP (ATP 3)

ATP 3 recommends a multifaceted approach to reduce the risk for CHD. This approach is designated therapeutic lifestyle changes or TLC. The major features of TLC are reduction in saturated fat and cholesterol intakes, weight reduction, and physical activity. If the patient cannot achieve LDL of < 100mg/dl by diet alone, LDL-lowering drugs can be started simultaneously. Table 16-4 lists the nutrient composition of the TLC diet. Notice the increase in the amount of fiber in this diet. Fiber, especially soluble forms, helps to lower cholesterol by removing it via excretion in feces. The TLC diet generally follows the *Dietary Guidelines for Americans 2000*. One exception is that total fat is allowed to range from 25% to 35% of total calories, provided saturated fats and trans-fatty acids are kept low. A higher intake of total fat, mostly in the form of unsaturated fat, can help to reduce triglycerides and raise HDL cholesterol in persons with metabolic syndrome. Examples of daily food choices that meet the dietary guidelines are found in Table 16-5. Table 16-6 delineates the types of fat, cholesterol, and omega-3 content of meat, fish, and poultry, which is a helpful tool in planning diet therapy.

METABOLIC SYNDROME

A constellation of major risk factors, life-habit risk factors, and emerging risk factors constitute a condition called metabolic syndrome. Factors characteristic of metabolic syndrome are abdominal obesity, elevated triglycerides, small LDL particles, low HDL, hypertension, insulin resistance, and prothrombotic and proinflammatory states (see Table 16-8).

Metabolic syndrome is a secondary target of risk-reduction therapy after the primary target LDL cholesterol.

TABLE 16-4 Nutrient Composition of the TLC Diet

Nutrient	Recommended Intake
Saturated fat*	Less than 7% of total calories
Polyunsaturated fat*	Up to 10% of total calories
Monounsaturated fat	Up to 20% of total calories
Total fat	25%–35% of total calories
Carbohydrate†	50%–60% of total calories
Fiber	20%–30 g/day
Protein (approximately)	15% of total calories
Cholesterol	Less than 200 mg/day
Total calories (energy)‡	Balance energy intake and expenditure to maintain desirable body weight/ prevent weight gain

*Trans-fatty acids are another LDL-raising fat that should be kept at a low intake.
†Carbohydrate should be derived predominantly from foods rich in complex carbohydrates including grains, especially whole grains, fruits, and vegetables.
‡Daily energy expenditure should include at least moderate physical activity (contributing approximately 200 kcal per day).

TABLE 16-5   Examples of Daily Food Choices That Meet the Dietary Guidelines

Food Group	No. of Servings	Serving Size	Some Suggested Foods
Vegetables	3–5	1 c leafy/raw	Leafy greens, lettuce
		½ c other	Corn, peas, green beans, broccoli, carrots, cabbage, celery, tomato, spinach, squash, bok choy, mushrooms, eggplant, collard and mustard greens
		¾ c juice	Tomato juice, vegetable juice
Fruits	2–4	1 piece fruit	Orange, apple, applesauce, pear, banana, grapes,
		½ c diced fruit	grapefruit, tangerine, plum, peach, strawberries and other berries, melons, kiwi, papaya, mango, lychee
		¾ c fruit juice	Orange juice, apple juice, grapefruit juice, grape juice, prune juice
Breads, cereals, pasta, grains, dry beans, peas, potatoes, and rice	6–11	1 slice	Wheat, rye or enriched breads/rolls, corn and flour tortillas
		½ bun, bagel, muffin	English muffin, bagel, muffin, cornbread
		1 oz dry cereal	Wheat, corn, oat, rice, bran cereal, or mixed-grain cereal
		½ c cooked cereal	Oatmeal, cream of wheat, grits
		½ c dry beans or peas	Kidney beans, lentils, split peas, black-eyed peas
		½ c potatoes	Potato, sweet potato
		½ c rice, noodles, barley, or other grains	Pasta, rice, macaroni, barley, tabbouli
		½ c bean curd	Tofu
Skim/low-fat dairy products	2–3	1 c skim, 1% milk	Low/nonfat yogurt, skim milk, 1% milk, buttermilk
		1 oz low-fat, fat-free cheese	Low-fat cheeses
Lean meat, poultry, and fish		≤6 oz/day—Step I Diet	Lean and extra-lean cuts of meat, fish, and skinless poultry, such as sirloin, round steak, skinless chicken, haddock, cod
		≤5 oz/day—Step II Diet	
Fats and oils	≤6–8*	1 tbsp soft margarine	Soft or liquid margarine, vegetable oils
		1 tbsp salad dressing	
		1 oz nuts	Walnuts, peanuts, almonds, pecans
Eggs		≤4 yolks/week—Step I Diet	Used in preparation of baked products
		≤2 yolks/week—Step II Diet	
Sweets and snack foods		In moderation	Cookies, fortune cookies, pudding, bread pudding, rice pudding, angel food cake, frozen yogurt, candy, punch, carbonated beverages
			Low-fat crackers and popcorn, pretzels, fat-free chips, rice cakes

*Includes fats and oil used in food preparation, also salad dressings and nuts.

The risk factors can be reduced by weight reduction and physical activity. The risk factors of the metabolic syndrome correlate to enhanced risk for CHD at any given LDL level. Abdominal obesity is more highly correlated than is an elevated body mass index (BMI).

SPECIAL CONSIDERATIONS FOR DIFFERENT POPULATION GROUPS

Men, aged 35 to 65 years have a higher risk of CHD than do women. Middle-aged men in particular have a high prevalence of risk factors, and are predisposed to abdom-

inal obesity and the metabolic syndrome. A large fraction of all CHD occurs in men of middle age. For those who carry relatively high risks, intensive LDL-lowering therapy is needed.

For women, aged 45 to 75 years, onset of CHD is generally delayed by 10–15 years compared with that of men; most CHD in women occurs after age 65. CHD in women younger than 65 occurs in those with multiple risk factors and the metabolic syndrome. Previous belief that the protective effect of estrogen in women accounted for the gender difference in risk for CHD has been cast in doubt in clinical trials of the use of hormone

TABLE 16-6   Saturated Fat, Total Fat, Cholesterol, and Omega-3 Content of Meat, Fish, and Poultry in 3-Ounce Portions Cooked Without Added Fat

Source	Saturated Fat g/3 oz	Total Fat g/3 oz	Cholesterol mg/3 oz	Omega-3 g/3 oz
Lean Red Meats				
Beef (rump roast, shank, bottom round, sirloin)	1.4	4.2	71	—
Lamb (shank roast, sirloin roast, shoulder roast, loin chops, sirloin chops, center leg chop)	2.8	7.8	78	—
Pork (sirloin cutlet, loin roast, sirloin roast, center roast, butterfly chops, loin chops)	3.0	8.6	71	—
Veal (blade roast, sirloin chops, shoulder roast, loin chops, rump roast, shank)	2.0	4.9	93	—
Organ Meats				
Liver				
Beef	1.6	4.2	331	—
Calf	2.2	5.9	477	—
Chicken	1.6	4.6	537	—
Sweetbread	7.3	21.3	250	—
Kidney	0.9	2.9	329	—
Brains	2.5	10.7	1,747	—
Heart	1.4	4.8	164	—
Poultry				
Chicken (without skin)				
Light (roasted)	1.1	3.8	72	—
Dark (roasted)	2.3	8.3	71	—
Turkey (without skin)				
Light (roasted)	0.9	2.7	59	—
Dark (roasted)	2.0	6.1	72	—
Fish				
Haddock	0.1	0.8	63	0.22
Flounder	0.3	1.3	58	0.47
Salmon	1.7	7.0	54	1.88
Tuna, light, canned in water	0.2	0.7	25	0.24
Shellfish				
Crustaceans				
Lobster	0.1	0.5	61	0.07
Crab meat				
Alaskan King Crab	0.1	1.3	45	0.38
Blue Crab	0.2	1.5	85	0.45
Shrimp	0.2	0.9	166	0.28
Mollusks				
Abalone	0.3	1.3	144	0.15
Clams	0.2	1.7	57	0.33
Mussels	0.7	3.8	48	0.70
Oysters	1.3	4.2	93	1.06
Scallops	0.1	1.2	56	0.36
Squid	0.6	2.4	400	0.84

Source: Dietary Guidelines for Americans. 2000. Washington, DC: USDA.

replacement therapy (HRT) to reduce risk of CHD in postmenopausal women. Cholesterol-lowering drug therapy is preferred to HRT.

With older adults (men > 65 years and women > 75 years), most new CHD events and coronary deaths occur in this age group. A high level of LDL cholesterol and a low level of HDL still are predictive of the development of CHD in older persons, but TLC is the primary therapy for older people, followed by drug therapy if they are at higher risk because of multiple risk factors or advanced atherosclerosis.

Young adults (men 20 to 35 years, women 20 to 45 years): CHD is rare in this group except in those with severe risk factors such as family history, diabetes, heavy smoking, and so on. Life-habit changes and early detection and intervention of elevated LDL cholesterol can delay or prevent onset of CHD later in life.

RACIAL AND ETHNIC GROUPS

African-Americans have the highest overall CHD mortality rate of any ethnic group in the United States, particularly at younger ages. It is accounted for by the high prevalence of coronary risk factors. Hypertension, diabetes mellitus, cigarette smoking, obesity, physical inactivity, and multiple CHD risk factors occur more frequently in this population than in white populations.

Other ethnic groups and minority populations in the United States vary somewhat in baseline CHD risk, but the evidence is not sufficient to modify general recommendations for cholesterol management in these populations.

Sample menus based on the TLC diet for men and women aged 25 to 49 years, as well as sample menus for several ethnic and regional groups, are found in Appendix B.

THE ROLE OF FISH OILS

In population and clinical studies omega-3 fatty acids, eicosapentaennic acid (EPA), and decosahezaenoic acid (DHA) found in fatty fish such as albacore tuna, herring, lake trout, mackerel, salmon, and sardines, have been shown to reduce sudden cardiac death, reduce serum triglyceride levels, and retard the accumulation of plaques in blood vessels. Omega-3 fatty acids can also reduce metabolic processes that increase the risk of heart diseases. The matter of safety must consider:

1. Intake of more than 3 grams/day of omega-3 fatty acid from capsules can cause bleeding in some patients, so this should be done only on a physician's advice.
2. Mercury contamination of fish is an established risk. Federal agencies have issued guides about eating fish with a potential presence of mercury. Chapter 9 discusses a detailed list of mercury content of commercial fish and shellfish and should be consulted for details.

Also, alpha linolenic acid (ALA) found in tofu, soybeans, canola oil, walnuts, flaxseeds, and their oils, can convert into omega-3 fatty acids in the body.

The American Heart Association provides the following guide in the consumption of omega-3 fatty acids for reducing cardiovascular risk:

1. For the general population:
   - Eat a variety of fish (fatty fish) at least twice a week.
   - Include oils and food rich in ALA (flaxseed, canola, and soybean oils; flaxseed and walnuts).
2. For patients with cardiovascular diseases: Consume 1 gm/day of EPA+DHA, preferably from fatty fish. Use of capsule supplements must be under a physician's guide.
3. For patients with high triglyceride levels: 2 to 4 grains of EPA+DI IA per day, provided in capsules under a physician's supervision.

DRUG MANAGEMENT

As we have discussed, dietary management has two approaches: patient specific or the population as a whole.

Initiation of drug therapy depends upon whether it is used for primary prevention (no evidence of CHD) or secondary prevention (evidence of atherosclerotic disease). The physician makes the decision after careful assessment of all factors.

In primary prevention, at least six months of intensive diet therapy and counseling are usually prescribed before considering drug therapy. Even one year of diet therapy may be considered if the patient is not at immediate risk. If, at this time, the LDL cholesterol still remains above the target level, drug therapy may be added to diet therapy.

For those individuals with severely elevated LDL cholesterol at the beginning, diet therapy alone will not be adequate. Drug therapy is started simultaneously.

All nondrug treatments should be tried: diet modification (the TLC diet), weight control, exercise, and smoking cessation, before drugs are initiated. The drugs have many side effects, are expensive, and are usually used for the rest of the patient's life. For these reasons diet therapy and exercise are the safest and best treatment and should certainly be used as long as possible before drugs are prescribed.

Both prescription and over-the-counter (OTC) drugs are available. The OTC drugs are nicotinic acid or their derivatives.

Table 16-7 lists drugs used at present.

NURSING IMPLICATIONS

Physicians usually refer patients to registered dietitians or other qualified nutritionists for medical nutrition therapy, which is the term for nutritional intervention and guidance provided by a nutritional professional. However,

TABLE 16-7   Drugs Affecting Lipoprotein Metabolism

Drug Class, Agents and Daily Doses	Lipid/Lipoprotein Effects	Side Effects	Contraindications	Clinical Trial Results
HMB CoA reductase inhibitors (statins)*	LDL ↓18–55% HDL ↑5–15% TG ↓7–30%	Myopathy Increased liver enzymes	Absolute: • Active or chronic liver disease Relative: • Concomitant use of certain drugs	Reduced major coronary events, CHD deaths, need for coronary procedures, stroke, and total mortality
Bile acid Sequestrants‡	LDL ↓15–30% HDL ↑3–5% TG No change or increase	Gastrointestinal distress Constipation Decreased absorption of other drugs	Absolute: • dysbeta-lipoproteinemia • TG > 400 mg/dL Relative: • TG > 200 mg/dL	Reduced major coronary events and CHD deaths
Nicotinic acid¶	LDL ↓5–25% HDL ↑15–35% TG ↓20–50%	Flushing Hyperglycemia Hyperuricemia (or gout) Upper GI distress Hepatotoxicity	Absolute: • Chronic liver disease • Severe gout Relative: • Diabetes • Hyperuricemia • Peptic ulcer disease	Reduced major coronary events, and possibly total mortality
Fibric acids§	LDL ↓5–20% (may be increased in patients with high TG) HDL ↑10–20% TG ↓20–50%	Dyspepsia Gallstones Myopathy Unexplained non-CHD deaths in WHO study	Absolute: • Severe renal disease • Severe hepatic disease	Reduced major coronary events

*Lovastatin (20–80 mg), pravastatin (20–40 mg), simvastatin (20–80 mg), fluvastatin (20–80 mg), atorvastatin (10–80 mg), cerivastatin (0.4–0.8 mg).
‡Cholestyramine (4–16 g), colestipol (5–20 g), colesevelam (2.6–3.8 g).
¶Immediate release (crystalline) nicotinic acid (1.5–3 g), extended release nicotonic acid (Niaspan[R]) (1–2 g), sustained release nicotinic acid (1–2 g).
§Gemfibrozil (600 mg BID), fenofibrate (200 mg), clofibrate (1000 mg BID).
Source: Third Report of the Expert Panel on Evaluation and Treatment of High Blood Cholesterol in Adults, May 2001.

the nurse has the closest contact with the patient and in many instances may be the primary teacher.

If you are the primary teacher:

1. Work with the health team to implement all treatment goals: careful assessment, diet counseling, monitoring, and follow-up.
2. Provide explicit patient instruction and use good counseling techniques to teach the patient how to follow the prescribed diet. Use an approved, up-to-date diet manual, or other acceptable sources of material.
3. Provide the patient with a list of foods to be used, limited, or omitted from the diet.
4. Provide an explanation of the reasons these foods are controlled.
5. Encourage the use of prompts to help patients remember.
6. Make arrangements for diet consultation with the dietitian or nutritionist to reinforce teaching.
7. Provide the patient with a list of possible side effects, if drug therapy is used.
8. Be able to check the diet tray and recognize any errors in the food served.
9. Lend assistance to the patient in selecting an adequate menu within the limitations of the diet.
10. Remind the patient to check labels when shopping and describe what to look for. Meet with any others who are directly concerned in shopping and food preparation.
11. Discuss appropriate cooking methods.
12. Recommend reliable resources, either persons or materials, when necessary.
13. Encourage the support of family and friends.
14. Involve patients in their care through self-monitoring.
15. Utilize case management and collaborative care of pharmacists, dietitians, and all other members of the health team.

TABLE 16-8	Clinical Identification of the Metabolic Syndrome	
Risk Factor	**Defining Level**	
Abdominal Obesity*	Waist Circumference†	
Men	> 102 cm (> 40 in)	
Women	> 88 cm (> 35 in)	
Triglycerides	≥ 150 mg/dl	
HDL cholesterol		
Men	< 40 mg/dl	
Women	< 50 mg/dl	
Blood pressure	≥ 130/≥ 85 mmHg	
Fasting glucose	≥110 mg/dl	

*Overweight and obesity are associated with insulin resistance and metabolic syndrome. However, the presence of abdominal obesity is more highly correlated with the metabolic risk factors than is an elevated body mass index (BMI). Therefore, the simple measure of waist circumference is recommended to identify the body weight component of the metabolic syndrome.
†Some male patients can develop multiple metabolic risk factors when the waist circumference is only marginally increased, e.g., 94–102 cm (37–39 in). Such patients may have a strong genetic contribution to insulin resistance. They should benefit from changes in life habits, similarly to men with categorical increases in waist circumference.
Source: Third Report of the Expert Panel on Evaluation and Treatment of High Blood Cholesterol in Adults, May 2001.

PROGRESS CHECK ON ACTIVITY 1

FILL-IN

1. List the five nutritional risk factors for heart disease.

    a. _____

    b. _____

    c. _____

    d. _____

    e. _____

2. Define TLC. _____

3. Name the three major features of the TLC diet.

    a. _____

    b. _____

    c. _____

4. A combination of major risk factors, life habit factors, and emerging risk factors identify a condition known as _____.

5. The total fat allowed in a LDL-lowering diet is _____ % of total calories.

6. The most characteristic feature in the identification of metabolic syndrome is _____
_____ .

7. Statins are the most commonly prescribed drugs for _____ .

8. Which drug is currently available OTC?

    _____ .

MULTIPLE CHOICE

Circle the letter of the correct answer.

9. Amount of fiber per day recommended in the TLC diet is:

    a. 10–15 g
    b. 15–20 g
    c. 20–30 g
    d. 30–40 g

10. Most deaths from coronary heart disease occur in which of these age groups?

    a. men age 35–45 years, women age 45–65 years
    b. men over age 65 years, women over age 75 years
    c. minority groups of all ages
    d. a and b
    e. a, b, and c

11. Which of the following groups of foods would be most suitable for a patient on a TLC diet?

    a. beef rounds, lamb, coconut, pasta
    b. tofu, chicken, catfish, peanut butter
    c. duck, avocado, shrimp, almonds
    d. liver, bologna, sherbert, olives

LIST

12. List at least eight techniques a nurse should use when teaching a patient about cholesterol-lowering diet therapy.

    _____

    _____

    _____

    _____

    _____

    _____

    _____

    _____

PRACTICE QUESTION

Write a 1-day menu for a 45-year-old Mexican-American woman on the TLC diet. Write your menu first, then check Appendix B and grade yourself on how well you did.

ACTIVITY 2:

Heart Disease and Sodium Restriction

Dietary sodium restriction is an important part of the medical treatment for hypertension and congestive heart failure. Although hypertension is a symptom, not a disease, it is one leading contributor to heart attack and stroke and is also associated with kidney diseases. For these reasons, controlling hypertension is one way to prevent the development of these conditions. Congestive heart failure occurs when the heart fails to pump out the returning blood fast enough, allowing blood to accumulate in the right side of the heart. This raises venous pressure (pressure in the vein from the accumulation of blood), causing fluid retention (edema) in the heart and its associated parts.

DIET AND HYPERTENSION

Secondary hypertension is caused by some known factor, such as a kidney disorder. The cause of essential or primary hypertension is unknown. Dietary factors that may cause high blood pressure include obesity and excessive use of salt. Some believe that caffeine in coffee and alcoholic beverages can potentiate the condition. New research indicates that calcium deficiency may be a factor in hypertension.

A low-sodium diet is usually supplemented with drug therapy (antihypertensives). Most antihypertensives contain diuretics. While most diuretics remove water and sodium from the body, some also remove potassium. Since the patient frequently is overweight, a low-calorie diet is also prescribed. Weight loss by itself will often reduce blood pressure, especially in males. The diet should be individually prescribed and tailored to the patient's need for sodium and calorie reduction. Since there are different levels of sodium restriction and many levels of calorie restriction, the diet order must be specific to be effective. A diet order that reads "salt poor, low cal" is unacceptable. Sodium is ordered in milligrams or grams, and calories by a specific number designed to help the patient lose weight. An adequate diet under 1200 calories daily is difficult to plan; it results in low patient compliance, especially with long-term usage. A normal level of protein of high biological value is recommended. Fats in the diet are moderately low and the types of fat flexible. Unsaturated fats used within the caloric allowance are more acceptable than saturated fats. Carbohydrates provide up to 50% of the total caloric intake, but concentrated sweets are not recommended. High-potassium foods should be encouraged if drug therapy causes loss of this mineral in the urine. Some physicians prescribe special potassium supplements.

DIET AND CONGESTIVE HEART FAILURE

The treatment for congestive heart failure consists of rest to reduce the demands on the heart; drug therapy to strengthen the heartbeat and slow it down; and diet therapy to reduce edema and decrease the workload on the heart. The dietary regimen is as follows:

1. Reduce edema. A low-sodium diet is used, usually in the moderate to low range. It is difficult to severely reduce the sodium intake of a patient because such a diet is most unpalatable.
2. Decrease workload. The diet may be of soft consistency and divided into five or six small meals per day. If the patient is overweight, the diet may also be restricted in calories. Fluids are not usually restricted, but excess fluid intake is not allowed. Although individual need varies, 2000 to 3000 ml of fluid per day is acceptable.

Some patients with hypertension and/or congestive heart failure may also require a modification of fat or cholesterol intake.

When a patient with this clinical disorder loses 6% or more of body weight (fat and muscle, not water) in half a year, the condition is known as cardiac cachexia (CC).

CC signals poor prognosis with increased mortality. When this patient undergoes nutritional therapy before an operation, he or she may have a better survival rate after an operation. Therefore identifying the susceptible patient is a priority, meaning that an appropriate nutritional intervention can be implemented before the patient develops CC.

A patient with CC suffers wasting of muscle mass, bone atrophy, lower bone density, and severe loss of fat storage. Some potential candidates and causes for CC may include the following:

1. Senior patients suffering from anorexia, difficulty in chewing and swallowing, nausea from medications, depression, and isolation.
2. Patients undergoing diuretic treatment, where micronutrient and antioxidant deficiencies created by the therapy can also precipitate malnutrition or muscle wasting. Micronutrients involved include selenium, copper, zinc, and magnesium. The diuretic therapy may also precipitate calcium losses. These nutrient deficiencies increase the rate of oxidative stress, one major cause of muscle wasting.
3. Other potential problems that may lead to CC include abnormal clinical conditions such as higher requirement for resting energy expenditure, lower capacity to exercise, and edema.

CC can lead to serious problems for the patient. When diagnosed early it can be treated. Therapy includes but is not limited to nutritional intervention, drug management, scheduled physical activity, use of medical devices, and heart transport.

THE SODIUM-RESTRICTED DIET

The average intake of sodium in the American diet ranges from 3 to 8 grams per day. Although some sodium is essential for body functioning, the amount needed is approximately ½ to 1 gram daily. The main source of sodium in our diets is table salt (sodium chloride). Salt is about 40% sodium by weight. It is used extensively in food processing for items such as processed meats (lunch meat, ham, bacon, canned meats, and fish), dried foods, sauerkraut, olives, and pickles. It is used in baking and cooking, and then used again at the dining table. In addition, most foods contain some sodium before any processing or cooking takes place. Some unprocessed foods are higher in naturally occurring sodium than others. For example, meats, milk, and eggs are high in natural sodium, whereas most plant foods are low. There are exceptions. Beets, spinach, chard, and kale are fairly high in sodium. Fruits, oils, sugars, and cereal grains contain only a trace of sodium or none at all, if no sodium chloride is added in processing. If a diet is based on the basic food groups, unsalted bread/butter and unprocessed grains and meats are used, and no salt is used during cooking or at the table, then the diet contains approximately 500 mg sodium. It is not difficult to see how we can "overdose" our foods with sodium.

The Diet Guidelines for Americans recommends the use of salt and sodium in moderation (see Chapter 1.) Four levels of sodium restriction are recommended by the American Heart Association to control a patient's sodium intake. The levels vary from 250 mg up to 3 to 5 grams of sodium daily.

The DASH diet (Dietary Approach to Stop Hypertension) from the NIH is more commonly recommended to prevent or control hypertension than is the AHA diet. The eating plan is rich in various nutrients believed to benefit blood pressure and in other factors involved in maintaining good health. The sodium content is ~2400 mg/day. Access DASH from the following Web site: www.nhlbi.nih.gov/health/public/heart/hbp_low/recap.htm.

Mild Sodium Restriction (3 to 5 Grams Daily)

This is a regular diet that omits only salty foods and the use of salt at the table. Salt may be used lightly in cooking; for example, use half the amount stated in the recipe. This diet is used frequently after discharge from the hospital, when edema is under control. A wide variety of foods from the basic food groups is recommended. Table 16-9 illustrates the foods to avoid within each food group.

TABLE 16-9   Foods Excluded in a 3- to 5-Gram Sodium Diet

Meat Group
1. Cured, canned, or smoked meats and fish
2. Canned dried beans, meat stews, soups
3. Meat analogs, e.g., imitation bacon bits
4. Cheeses: regular, processed
5. Frozen TV dinners
6. Ready-prepared meats in gravy or sauces
7. Kosher meats

Grain Group
1. Salty crackers
2. Rolls with salted tops
3. Seasoned mixes (e.g., stuffing, pasta, rice)

Milk Group
1. Cheese spreads
2. Processed cheese (cheese spreads)
3. Cheese: Roquefort, blue, camembert
4. Salted buttermilk

Fruit and Vegetable Group
1. Any vegetable prepared in brine
2. Sauerkraut
3. Canned tomatoes; tomato juice
4. Tomato sauce or paste
5. V-8 juice

Other
1. Salted sauces and seasonings: barbecue sauce, chili sauce, meat sauce, Worcestershire sauce, etc.; any type of salt, including tenderizers and flavor enhancers
2. Salted snacks: chips, pretzels, popcorn, nuts, pickles, olives, seeds
3. Miscellaneous: mustard, relishes, bacon drippings, bouillon cubes, catsup, etc.

Moderate Sodium Restriction (1000 Milligrams Daily)

This diet is used both in the hospital and at home. In addition to avoiding the foods indicated for the 3- to 5-gram sodium diet, the diet has the following restrictions:

1. No more than 2 c milk per day.
2. No more than 5 oz meat per day. One egg may be substituted for 1 oz meat.
3. No salt in cooking.
4. Bread and butter beyond three servings daily should be unsalted.
5. No commercial mixes or regular canned vegetables.

Strict Sodium Restriction (500 Milligrams Daily)

This diet is used primarily for hospitalized patients, though it may be followed at home. The restrictions, however, result in low patient compliance except in a hospital setting. In addition to the restrictions indicated for 3- to 5-gram and 1000-mg sodium diets, two other restrictions are required to lower the dietary sodium to 500 mg:

1. No bread and butter that has salt added
2. No vegetables that are naturally high in sodium content

Severe Sodium Restriction (250 Milligrams Daily)

The substitution of low-sodium milk for regular milk in the 500-mg sodium diet will lower the dietary sodium content to 250 mg.

The *Exchange Lists for Meal Planning*, issued by the American Dietetic Association and the American Diabetic Association (see Appendix F), may be modified for the various levels of sodium restriction. This booklet is a helpful tool for diet planning, particularly when a caloric or fat modification is also necessary.

Some drinking water is high in sodium, especially if water softeners are used. Patients on low-sodium diets should ascertain their drinking water's sodium content and, if necessary, use distilled water.

Many drugs, both prescription and over-the-counter, contain high levels of sodium. Patients need to be made aware of these.

NURSING IMPLICATIONS

The nurse should follow the following guidelines.

1. Be aware that sodium-restricted diets are unpalatable, especially at very restricted levels.
2. Be prepared to offer alternative seasonings to enhance flavor and encourage the patient to consume an adequate diet.
3. Caution patients to read the labels on foods and to avoid self-medication. Check medications received in the hospital, and, if they are too high in sodium, ask about alternates.
4. Check trays of all patients on sodium-restricted diets to make sure salt has not been included accidentally.
5. Recognize that patients with congestive heart failure tend to have poor appetites. Accurate intake and out-put records are necessary. Meal sizes and intervals may need adjusting.
6. Check for inadequate potassium intake when antihypertensives are used.
7. Be aware that iodine intake may be low when salt is restricted.
8. Do not suggest salt substitutes without asking the physician first: there may be impaired renal function or, if a potassium supplement is being used, a patient could develop hyperkalemia. Salt substitutes are high in potassium.

PROGRESS CHECK ON ACTIVITY 2

FILL-IN

1. Complete Exercise 16-1.
2. Write a day's menu for a person on a 500-mg sodium diet with no calorie restriction (use separate sheet).
3. List 10 appropriate seasonings that may be used in place of salt.

    a. _____
    b. _____
    c. _____
    d. _____
    e. _____
    f. _____
    g. _____
    h. _____
    i. _____
    j. _____

Exercise 16-1

Complete Each Column with the Appropriate Information

Diet	Disease or Condition	Foods Allowed	Foods Limited	Foods Forbidden	Nursing Implications
5000 mg sodium					
1000 mg sodium					
500 mg sodium					
250 mg sodium					

ACTIVITY 3:

Dietary Care After Heart Attack and Stroke

MYOCARDIAL INFARCTION (MI): HEART ATTACK

Priority is given to life-saving measures immediately following a myocardial infarction (MI). An intravenous line (IV) is prepared and inserted. If needed, the IV can be used to administer drugs and regulate fluid and electrolyte balance.

The goals of diet therapy are to reduce the workload of the heart, restore and maintain electrolyte balance and, after a brief period of undernutrition, to maintain an adequate nutritional intake. The diet therapy progresses as follows:

1. For the first 24 to 48 hours after oral feedings are ordered by the physician, the patient receives only clear liquids.
2. The liquid diet is followed by a low-residue diet, and then a soft diet. Foods are divided into five to six small meals. The diet also may be restricted in sodium, if necessary.
3. Beverages containing caffeine are omitted.
4. The physician may prescribe fluid restriction, if intake and output records warrant.
5. Constipation may accompany a restriction of fiber and/or fluids. Nursing measures to solve this complication are needed.
6. A gradual return to regular foods, with a restriction of sodium, fat, and/or cholesterol for certain patients.

CEREBROVASCULAR ACCIDENT (CVA): STROKE

As with a myocardial infarction, the first measures taken by health professionals after a cerebrovascular accident are life saving, not dietary. Ongoing therapy focuses on restoring and maintaining adequate nutrition. Diet therapy after a CVA progresses as follows:

1. An intravenous line is used for the first 24 to 48 hours. Careful monitoring is necessary. Fluids must be restricted if cerebral edema is present.
2. If the patient is comatose, tube feeding will be the diet of choice after IV therapy. Oral liquid feedings may begin when the patient is conscious. If the patient develops paralysis of one side of the throat, he or she will choke more easily on liquids than on semisolids. In the event of such paralysis, very thick liquids or very soft solids may be necessary.
3. Eventually, with training, the patient may return to a regular diet.

4. Depending on the patient, the diet may be low in calories, sodium, fat, and/or cholesterol.

After the initial emergency measures, the health team will implement many care procedures, and those affecting eating and diet will include the following:

1. An evaluation of the patient is made by a speech therapist and an occupational therapist.
2. The patient's food and beverage tolerance is observed, applying aspiration when necessary.
3. Initially, the patient is fed thickened liquids with a consistence of a nectar, honey, or pudding when indicated.
4. Commercial preparations such as roll thickeners (Thick It) or other prethickened products may be ordered from the food service department.
5. Standard procedures indicate the texture of the food be modified according to the dysphagia diet used routinely in hospitals. This diet progresses in 4 stages.
   Stage 1: Diet is pureed.
   Stage 2: Diet is mechanically changed to a semisolid and moist consistence that is cohesive with the following characteristics:
   a. Presence of some chewing ability
   b. Meats that are grounded or minced
   c. Fruits and vegetables fork-mashable
   d. No dry food such as bakery products (bread, crackers)
   Stage 3: Diet is advanced to soft solids with the following characteristics:
   a. More chewing ability
   b. Meats that can be cut easily
   c. Fruits and vegetables that are not hard and crunchy
   d. Sticky food
   e. Foods with little moisture
   Stage 4: Diet is a regular one with solid textures.

There are other considerations for a patient suffering from a stroke:

1. Visual impairment
2. Low appetite
3. Use of tube feedings
4. Food-drug interactions
5. Lifestyle modification if indicated

The health team is familiar with all the above issues and adjustments. Lifestyle modification is an important public concern. The issues cover exercise, lowering blood pressure, salt intake, and the quantity and quality of fat consumed. Government and private institutions have made recommendations, most of which have been presented in various chapters in this book. Use the index to find the appropriate chapter for more details.

NURSING IMPLICATIONS

The responsibilities of the nurse include the following:

1. Assess food deficits as soon as oral feedings are resumed, and take measures to restore sufficient intake.
2. Allow self-feeding for both MI and CVA patients as soon as possible.
3. Position the patient to allow maximum use of his or her remaining abilities and to give the patient some control.
4. Schedule nursing care and treatment far enough in advance of meals to let the patient rest before eating.
5. Relieve pain before meals are served.
6. Promote comfort, relieve anxiety, and be very patient.
7. Explain all restrictions in the patient's diet.
8. Teach diet restrictions when the patient is able to listen (when anxiety and fear have diminished).
9. Make arrangements for those involved in food purchasing and preparation to be involved in the teaching session with the dietitian.

PROGRESS CHECK ON NURSING IMPLICATIONS

FILL-IN

1. List four objectives of diet therapy for a patient who has had a myocardial infarction.

   a. _____

   b. _____

   c. _____

   d. _____

2. List as many nursing measures as you can think of to assist a stroke victim to ingest an adequate diet.

   a. _____

   b. _____

   c. _____

   d. _____

   e. _____

   f. _____

   g. _____

   h. _____

   i. _____

   j. _____

PROGRESS CHECK ON ACTIVITY 3

FILL-IN

1. List five hidden sources of sodium.

   a. _____

   b. _____

   c. _____

   d. _____

   e. _____

2. List 10 seasonings that may be used freely on a low-sodium diet.

   a. _____

   b. _____

   c. _____

   d. _____

   e. _____

   f. _____

   g. _____

   h. _____

   i. _____

   j. _____

3. State five nursing measures applicable to the feeding of a CVA patient with right-sided hemiplegia who is not comatose.

   a. _____

   b. _____

   c. _____

   d. _____

   e. _____

4. Explain the rationale for a diet therapy that specifies "soft 2 g sodium in 6 feedings" for a 5-day, post-MI patient. _____

   _____

   _____

   _____

   _____

MULTIPLE CHOICE

Circle the letter of the correct answer.

5. Which of the following menus would be the best choice for a person on a 1-g sodium, low-cholesterol diet?

   a. split pea soup, crackers, tuna salad, ice cream, and tea
   b. scrambled eggs, baked potato, fruit salad, baked apple, and skim milk
   c. broiled fresh trout with lemon, baked potato, sliced tomato salad, skim milk, and peach halves
   d. prime rib roast, broccoli, mashed potatoes, sliced pineapple, and tea

6. From the following list, which foods would be most suitable for a person on a 500-mg sodium diet?

   a. tuna fish salad with lettuce
   b. sliced turkey with cranberry sauce
   c. scalloped potatoes and ham
   d. honey and peanut butter sandwich

REFERENCES

American Dietetic Association. (2006). *Nutrition Diagnosis: A Critical Step in Nutrition Care Process.* Chicago: Author.

Beham, E. (2006). *Therapeutic Nutrition: A Guide to Patient Education.* Philadelphia: Lippincott, Williams and Wilkins.

Bendich, A., & Deckelbaum, R. J. (Eds.). (2005). *Preventive Nutrition: The Comprehensive Guide for Health Professionals* (3rd ed.). Totowa, NJ: Humana Press.

Burrowes, J. D. (2007). Preventing heart disease in women: What is new in diet and lifestyle recommendations. *Nutrition Today, 42*: 242–247.

Chow, C. K. (2006). Does potassium-enriched salt or sodium reduction reduce cardiovascular mortality and medical expenses? *American Journal of Clinical Nutrition, 84*: 1552–1553.

Coulston, A. M., Rock, C. L., & Monsen, E. L. (Eds.). (2001). *Nutrition in the Prevention and Treatment of Disease.* San Diego, CA: Academic Press.

Deen, D., & Hark, L. (2007). *The Complete Guide to Nutrition in Primary Care.* Malden, MA: Blackwell.

Dietary guidelines for Americans (6th ed.). (2005). Washington, DC: United States Department of Agriculture (USDA) and United States Department of Health and Human Services (U.S.-DHHS). www.healthierus.gov.

Haas, E. M., & Levin, B. (2006). *Staying Healthy with Nutrition: The Complete Guide to Diet and Nutrition Medicine* (21st ed.). Berkeley, CA: Celestial Arts.

Hill, A. M. (2007). Combining fish-oil supplements with regular aerobic exercise improves body composition and cardiovascular disease risk factors. *American Journal of Clinical Nutrition, 85*: 1267–1274.

Klein, S. (2007). Waist circumference and cardiometabolic risk: A consensus statement from Shaping America's Health: Association for Weight Management and Obesity Prevention: NAASO, The Obesity Society: The American Society for Nutrition; and The American Diabetes Association. *American Journal for Nutrition, 85*: 1197–1202.

Lichtenstein, A. H. (2008). Cardiovascular disease. In Thompson, L. U., & Ward, W. E., (Eds.). *Optimizing Women's Health Through Nutrition.* Boca Raton, FL: CRC Press.

Lopez-Miranda, J. (2006). Monounsaturated fat and cardiovascular risk. *Nutrition Reviews, 64,* (10, part 2): s2–s12.

Mahan, L. K., & Escott-Stump, S. (Eds.). (2008). *Krause's Food and Nutrition Therapy* (12th ed.). Philadelphia: Elsevier Sauders.

Mann, J. (2007). Dietary carbohydrate: Relationship to cardiovascular disease and disorders of carbohydrate metabolism. *European Journal of Clinical Nutrition, 61*: s100–s111.

Mann, J., & Truswell, S. (Eds.). (2007). *Essentials of Human Nutrition* (3rd ed.). New York: Oxford University Press.

Mead, A. (2006). Dietary guidelines on food and nutrition in the secondary prevention of cardiovascular disease-evidence from systemic reviews of randomized controlled trials (2nd update). *Journal of Human Nutrition and Dietetics, 19*: 401–419.

Merchant, A. T. (2008). Interrelation of saturated fat, trans fat, alcohol intake, and subclinical atherosclerosis. *American Journal of Clinical Nutrition, 87*: 168–174.

NHLBI. (2001). Third Report of the Expert Panel on Detection, Evaluation, and Treatment of High Blood Cholesterol in Adults (Adult Treatment Panel III) Executive Summary. Washington, DC: National Cholesterol Education Program (NCEP), National Heart, Lung, and Blood Institute.

Ordovas, J. M. (2007). Nutrition in the genomics era: Cardiovascular disease risk and the Mediterranean diet. *Molecular Nutrition and Food Research, 51*: 1293–1299.

Rudolph, T. K. (2007). Acute effects of various fast-food meals on vascular functions and cardiovascular disease risk markers: The Hamburg Burger Trial. *American Journal of Clinical Nutrition, 86*: 334–340.

Ryan, D. (2007). Bioactivity of oats as it relates to cardiovascular disease. *Nutrition Research Reviews, 20*: 147–162.

Shils, M. E., & Shike, M. (Eds.). (2006). *Modern Nutrition in Health and Disease* (10th ed.). Philadelphia: Lippincott, Williams and Wilkins.

Stipanuk, M. H. (Ed.). (2006). *Biochemical, Physiological and Molecular Aspects of Human Nutrition* (2nd ed.). St. Louis, MO: Elsevier Saunders.

Temple, N. J., Wilson, T., & Jacobs, D. R. (2006). *Nutrition Health: Strategies for Disease Prevention* (2nd ed.). Totowa, NJ: Humana Press.

CHAPTER

17

Diet and Disorders of Ingestion, Digestion, and Absorption

Time for completion
Activities: 1–½ hours
Optional examination: ½ hour

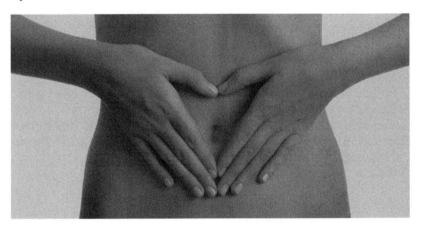

OBJECTIVES

Upon completion of this chapter, the student should be able to do the following:

1. List the diet modifications used in certain gastrointestinal disorders.
2. Explain the rationale for the use of diet modifications.
3. Describe the diet modification sequence and progression.
4. List foods that meet the diet requirements.
5. State nursing implications for dietary care.

GLOSSARY

Antiemetics: an agent (drug) that relieves vomiting.

Aspiration: the act of inhaling. Pathological aspiration of vomitus or mucus into the respiratory tract (lungs) may occur when a patient is unconscious or under the effect of anesthesia.

Cachexia: general wasting of the body, especially during chronic disease.

Cholinergic: an agent (drug) that stimulates the action of the sympathetic nerves.

Colostomy: creation of an opening between the colon and surface of the body. A surgical procedure.

Defecate: to eliminate waste and undigested food from the rectum.

Esophageal varices: varicose veins in the esophagus.

Flatulence: excessive formation of gas in intestinal tract.

Gallstones: precipitation of cholesterol crystals in the gallbladder to form stones.

Gastrectomy: removal of part of the stomach.

Helicobacter pylori (H. pylori): common rod-shaped bacteria that live in the gastrointestinal tract around the pyloric valve, lower gastric antrum, and upper duodenal bulb. They are well known for their role in chronic gastritis and, more recently, in the gastric ulcer process.

Hemorrhoidectomy: surgical removal of varicose veins in the mucosa either outside or just inside the rectum.

Ileostomy: creating an opening between the ileum and the surface of the body by establishing a stoma (*see* Stoma) on the abdominal wall.

Ileum: distal portion of the small intestine extending from jejunum to cecum.

Immunotherapy: passive immunization of an individual with preformed antibodies. It activates the entire immune system to fight off disease. Most recently used in terminology relating to treatment of cancer.

Intraluminal: within the lumen (wall) of a tubular structure.

Jejunum: part of the small intestine extending from the duodenum to the ileum.

Mucosa (mucous membrane): the membrane that lines the tubular organs of the body.

NSAIDS: nonsteroidal anti-inflammatory drugs.

Osteomate: one who has had an ostomy (colostomy or ileostomy). These are surgical procedures for creating an opening to the outside of the body for the elimination of waste.

Pectin: a carbohydrate that forms a gel when mixed with a sweetened liquid.

Pylorus: a distal part of the stomach opening into the duodenum. Contains many glands that secrete hydrochloric acid.

Stoma: a mouthlike opening. A surgical opening kept open for drainage and other purposes.

Varices: plural for varix; an enlarged, tortuous vein, artery, or lymph vessel.

BACKGROUND INFORMATION

The gastrointestinal (GI) tract extends from the mouth to the anus. All disturbances related to food intake, digestion, absorption, and elimination affect the GI tract and usually require special diets. Such diets were among the very first ever used in the treatment of diseases. Unfortunately, many have not changed much since they were first used, even though recent research has shown that some of the diets used to treat diseases are ineffective and incompatible with the clinical conditions of patients. Two notable examples include the diets for diverticular diseases and peptic ulcer.

Psychological factors play a role when we consider many disorders of the GI tract. The digestive system is said to "mirror the human condition." If this is true, then specific foods do not cause the problem in all cases; rather, the psychological state of the body that receives them can be responsible. Stress factors such as anxiety, fear, work pressure, grief, emotional makeup, and coping patterns have a great deal to do with how or if foods are tolerated. If a person has specific food allergies or a physiological basis for food intolerance (such as an enzyme deficiency), then the offending foods obviously should not be eaten. Otherwise, as in the case of an ulcer patient, there is no sound basis for the traditional diet therapy that permits only soft, white, or mildly flavored foods.

Frequently, patients who have experienced traditional diet therapy will challenge a prescription of modern diet therapy. Nurses must understand and be prepared to explain the newer concepts of dietary management.

ACTIVITY 1:

Disorders of the Mouth, Esophagus, and Stomach

MOUTH

Cleft Lip and/or Palate

A congenital defect of newborns, cleft lip and/or palate is corrected by a series of surgeries after the infant reaches a weight safe enough to withstand a surgical procedure. These infants have a high nutritional requirement to prepare for surgery and rapid growth. The care provider must practice care in the positioning and feeding of these children to prevent aspiration. Certain types of nipples and/or tubing may be required for infant feeding. Families need counseling in the feeding and care of these infants. Nurses should receive additional training when caring for and teaching others to care for such patients.

Dental Caries

Almost all children in the United States are afflicted with decayed teeth, and about 30% of Americans past the age of 25 wear full dentures. While poor dental hygiene (improper brushing, not flossing, and failing to get checkups) may account for part of the problem, much is dietary in nature. Lack of essential nutrients such as calcium, phosphorus, fluorine, and vitamins D, A, and C affect tooth and gum formation and development. Because both deciduous ("baby") and permanent teeth are formed in utero (before birth), the diet of the mother affects the offspring's teeth. Fetuses are not parasites and cannot necessarily derive adequate amounts of each nutrient needed for development from the mother. Some children are born without all of their permanent teeth buds, and, in this case, it is prudent to maintain deciduous teeth as long as possible.

A youngster's diet affects the strength and function of his or her teeth. Milk, juice, or sweetened drinks left in the bottle against an infant's gums during sleep can cause decay of newly erupted teeth. This is known as the "baby bottle syndrome." Children learn to like sweets if they receive them early in their diet. It is believed that the high use of concentrated sweets, especially the sticky type, is the main culprit in the formation of cavities (dental caries).

Health promotion measures that will benefit oral tissues throughout life include a well-balanced diet with adequate amounts of essential nutrients, limitation or omission of sweets, and proper oral hygiene and dental care.

Dentures

The wearing of dentures can be a mixed blessing. If properly fitted, they provide the ability to ingest a variety of foods not possible otherwise. Dentures are cosmetically attractive and improve self-esteem, but there are disadvantages associated with them. As bone recedes after teeth have been extracted, frequent realignments are mandatory for proper fit. Loose dentures may collect particles underneath them, causing pain. Rubbing between dentures and the gum tissue creates sore spots that can lead to inflammation or even tumors. The health of the gums on which dentures rest determines the success of wearing dentures. An adequate supply of vitamins A and C, along with other nutrients, is essential to gum tissue integrity.

Many older people have ill-fitting dentures or no dentures at all, even though they may have no teeth. This can cause great difficulty in chewing food, and therefore, in the digestion of food. This leads to a decreased intake of fiber and other essential nutrients, since unchewed and undigested foods are not absorbed. The effect of this condition on health is obvious.

Whenever dental problems exist or dentures are absent, the mechanical soft diet is preferred, since it provides adequate nutrition and ease of chewing. Chapter 12 provides additional information on the mechanical soft diet.

Fractured Jaw

The nutritional needs for a person following the trauma of a fractured jaw are high, as in other types of fractures.

The treatment of choice is to wire the jaws together, which poses obvious problems with eating. A diet high in protein, calories, minerals, and vitamins is necessary for proper healing. Liquid food must pass through a straw without moving the jaw. Care must be taken to prevent choking, and a wire cutter must be close at hand to cut the wire if choking occurs. As the person is usually home for a considerable length of time before the wires are removed, the caretaker must be taught how to use the wire cutter. Since the practice of oral hygiene is difficult, the oral tissues must be cleaned by a special and thorough procedure to prevent bacterial growth. Lack of adequate cleaning can cause cavities and produce odors that decrease the appetite. Table 17-1 lists examples of foods suitable for the person with a fractured jaw.

ESOPHAGUS: HIATAL HERNIA

The esophagus is separated from the stomach by the diaphragm. When the stomach partially protrudes above the diaphragm because of the weakening of the diaphragm opening, hiatal hernia results. Hiatal hernia is usually treated with antacids and a low-fat diet. Six small feedings per day are recommended, and fluids are taken between meals. Foods that irritate esophageal mucosa are eliminated—for example, orange, tomato, or grapefruit juices. Alcoholic beverages should be avoided. Patients should not eat within two hours of bedtime. Extra fluids and laxative foods help to prevent constipation that can put pressure on the esophagus. Patients should not lie down or bend over after eating. Extra height in the form of pillows or an elevated bed-head for sleeping is recommended. If the patient is obese, weight loss will improve the clinical condition. Fats are usually avoided, since they tend to lower esophageal pressure and add calories.

STOMACH: PEPTIC ULCER
Dietary Management

Peptic ulcer is the most common of the problems affecting the upper GI tract. An ulcer is an erosion of the stomach, pylorus, or duodenum. Ulcers occur only in areas affected by excess hydrochloric acid and pepsin (an enzyme). The most common location is the duodenal bulb, because the gastric contents emptying through the pyloric valve are most concentrated in acid at this point. The following are the major causative factors of peptic ulcer:

1. Increased acidity and secretion of gastric juices
2. Decreased secretion of mucous lining and buffers
3. Prolonged use of nonsteroidal anti-inflammatory drugs (NSAIDs) such as aspirin, ibuprofen, and others
4. *Helicobacter pylori* (*H. pylori*) infection—Infection by this bacteria, along with hydrochloric (HCl) acid and pepsin secretion, is now believed to be a major cause of ulcers.

TABLE 17-1   Foods for a Patient with a Fractured Jaw

Composition of feedings	These are oral feedings composed of approximately 250 g carbohydrate 115 g protein 110 g fat 2400 calories
General instructions	1. Follow the family menu as closely as possible, if the meal pattern is adequate. 2. Plan for the increase in protein by using meats of all kinds (beef, pork, poultry, lamb, veal, fish, organ meats) and meat substitutes such as eggs, cottage cheese, other soft cheeses, and yogurt. 3. All meats should be lean and, with the exception of beef, should be well cooked; beef may be used raw or rare if desired. Use sufficient broth when blending. 4. All meats, vegetables, breads should be cubed before being added to blender. Eggs should be added last when blending. 5. If butter or margarine is used, it should be very soft or melted before adding to mixture. 6. It may be necessary to strain the mixture after it has been blended to prevent clogging. 7. Variety can be obtained by using soups, vegetable juices, or broths for blending instead of milk, but be aware that this lowers total caloric intake. 8. The patient should participate in the selection of the various meats, vegetables, and pastas that go into the blender.

Meal plan for oral liquid feedings

Breakfast	Lunch	Dinner
Strained juice	Fruit drink	Fruit eggnog
Hot blended drink	Hot blended drink	Hot blended drink
Coffee/cream/sugar if desired	Coffee/cream/sugar if desired	Beverage of choice
or Beverage of choice	or Beverage of choice	

Supplemental Feedings

To increase caloric intake over 2400 add any of these: fruit drink, fruit eggnog, a thick milkshake, liquid gelatin, chocolate milk, malted milk, or regular eggnog. Dry milk powder or vitamin supplements may be added to increase nutrients upon recommendations of the physician.

Recipes: follow for those items marked

Recipes for oral feedings:

Hot Blended Drink #1

½ c cooked refined cereal such as farina, grits, cream of wheat, etc.

1 c hot milk*

2 soft-cooked eggs

1 tsp melted butter or margarine

½ tsp salt (optional)

Mix all ingredients except fat. Blend to desired consistency and strain. Add the melted fat and salt. Reheat to desired temperature.

Hot Blended Drink #2

½ c cubed poultry, veal, pork, lamb, or cheese

½ c cooked rice or pasta

½ c cooked vegetable of choice

1–2 slices whole wheat bread, cubed

1½ c milk*

1 tsp melted butter or margarine

½ tsp salt (optional)

Blend the meat or substitute separately with ½ c of the milk for approximately 2 minutes. Add rice or pasta, vegetable, and bread. Add remaining milk and salt. Blend to desired consistency. Strain the mixture. Add the melted fat and reheat to desired temperature before serving.

(continues)

TABLE 17-1   (continued)

Hot Blended Drink #3

½ c chopped raw or rare beef or ground beef patty

1 c broth*

½ c cooked or canned vegetable of choice

½ c cooked potato (without skins)

1 c milk, tomato juice, or cream soup*

1 tsp melted butter or margarine

½ tsp salt (optional)

Blend beef and broth together for approximately 2 minutes. Add other ingredients except fat. Blend together to desired consistency. Strain. Add fat and salt. Heat to desired temperature before serving.

Fruit Drink

1 banana or ½ c any canned or cooked fruit

⅔ c fruit juice, preferably a vitamin C source (orange, grapefruit)*

Blend. Strain. Chill before serving.

Fruit Eggnog

To the above recipe for fruit drink, add 2 tsp lemon juice, 1 tbsp sugar, and 1 egg. Blend. Strain. Serve cold.

*All liquids used may be increased to thin the mixture to the consistency that will not clog a straw.

Treatment goals for the peptic ulcer are to relieve pain, heal erosion, prevent complications, and prevent recurrences. Therapy usually includes rest, antacids, and anticholinergics. Physicians recommend reduction of ulcer-predisposing factors such as stress, hurried or skipped meals, and excess coffee, colas, smoking, and aspirin.

Current drug therapy for ulcers now includes the use of histamine receptor blockers (H2 blockers) such as Tagamet, Zantac, Axid, and Pepsid. Some newer, more potent drugs approved for use help ulcers to heal more rapidly. Antacids are still used as standard therapy, the preferred ones being those with a magnesium or aluminum base, such as Maalox or Mylanta. Calcium-based antacids (e.g., Tums) are thought to stimulate acid secretions and are not generally recommended. Antibiotics, including Flagyl, Achromycin, and Amoxil, are used to counter the *H. pylori* bacteria. (The drugs mentioned are brand names. Consult the *Physician's Desk Reference* for more information.)

These drugs are used in tandem with the general measures of adequate rest, sleep, and stress-reduction measures that have always been standards.

Principles of Diet Therapy for Peptic Ulcer Disease

1. A highly restrictive diet is no longer ordered for peptic ulcer. The diet is a regular one that follows dietary guidelines, with enough increases for tissue healing and promotion of optimal nutritional status. The condition of the individual, determined after a complete nutritional assessment, will determine the amount of calories and nutrients needed.

2. Another change that has occurred in the dietary management of peptic ulcer is that of the meal pattern: Patients are advised to eat three meals a day without snacks, especially at bedtime. This change from former meal plans is to avoid the production of excess acid.

3. Meal size should be moderate; large meals cause distention and pain.

4. There is no need to eliminate a particular food unless it causes repeated discomfort.

5. Dietary fiber, especially soluble dietary fiber, is not restricted. In fact, it is encouraged according to patient tolerance.

6. Individualized tolerances include:
   a. Seasonings: Hot chilies and black pepper are common irritants; other than these, the individual may have any seasonings that do not cause a problem.
   b. Alcohol: High-proof alcohols (80 proof) and beer are potent gastric juice stimulants and should be avoided. Some patients tolerate small amounts of wine when taken with a meal.
   c. Coffee (regular and decaffeinated), tea, and colas are to be avoided as they are gastric stimulants. If small amounts of coffee are used, the coffee should be drunk with or after a meal to minimize its effects.

7. General recommendations:
   a. Avoid aspirin and other NSAIDS. If pain medication is needed, use the acetaminophen types (e.g., Tylenol).

b. Eliminate smoking.

c. Eat slowly in a calm environment.

d. Antidepressant therapy may be prescribed for some patients as a sedative and for relaxation.

e. If a patient is in acute pain when admitted, the diet will require modification to lessen symptoms. The regular diet will be reordered when the pain is gone. Most diet manuals in facilities contain some form of modified diet therapy suitable for these conditions.

Patients and physicians accustomed to the traditional diets have been slow to accept the liberal diet. Most hospitals generally offer the minimum fiber diet initially to ulcer patients (see Chapter 14). Individual changes are made toward a regular diet as the patients and their conditions indicate acceptance and improvement.

Nursing responsibilities in treating ulcer patients are as follows:

1. Explain the rationale for use of the newer diet therapy (some patients are very fearful and skeptical of the less restrictive diet).
2. Evaluate the diet for nutritional adequacy after individual changes have been made.
3. Encourage the consumption of laxative foods, especially if the patient is prescribed antacids, which cause constipation.
4. Explain the adoption of a less stressful lifestyle to help prevent a recurrence.
5. Intervene on the patient's behalf if the prescribed diet is not tolerated.

GASTRIC SURGERY FOR ULCER DISEASES

Perforation and hemorrhage are two major complications of ulcer disease for which surgery is indicated. The types of surgical procedures can be found in all nursing and medical texts, but space prohibits discussion here. After the initial period of NPO and fluid and electrolyte replacement, and when peristalsis has returned, oral feedings may be resumed. The necessity for optimum nutrition following gastric surgery is the same as in any other operation, but postgastrectomy diet therapy (which must be ordered by the physician) differs in some respects. In general the health practitioner should follow these basic principles:

1. Implement a progressive diet for a 2-week course.
2. Keep meals small (1 to 2 oz each) and frequent (hourly). Low carbohydrate clear liquids with ½ slice toast or two crackers are appropriate for first feedings.
3. Increase the size of feedings by 1 oz daily.
4. Use a six-meal, low-carbohydrate, high-protein, moderate-fat, diet by approximately day 10 to day 16, if conditions permit.
5. Introduce simple, mild, low-fiber, and easily digested foods, such as cream of wheat or rice, sugar-free gelatin, soft-cooked (poached) eggs, mashed potatoes, and tender beef or chicken. Milk and regular carbonated beverages are not included, and liquids are given separately from solid foods. These precautions are to prevent development of the "dumping syndrome."
6. Resume a regular diet gradually.

The "dumping syndrome" is a complication of gastric surgery that may occur a short time after recovery from the operation, after eating is resumed. It may also be the delayed type, occurring from one to five years after a gastrectomy. It is more likely to occur in the patient who has had two-thirds or more of the stomach removed.

The process is as follows: Food reaches the jejunum 10 to 15 minutes after eating. With part of the stomach removed, the food is not digested properly and, instead of being delivered slowly, it is "dumped" quickly into the small intestine. The patient then experiences nausea, cramping, weakness, dizziness, cold sweating, a rapid pulse, and possibly vomiting. These symptoms of shock occur as the concentrated foodstuff draws water from the body tissues into the intestine. The symptoms are especially severe when the meal is high in simple carbohydrate, which can exert high osmotic pressure. Two to three hours after the meal, hypoglycemic symptoms may occur, because the absorbed monosaccharides, especially glucose, cause a rapid rise in blood glucose. This, in turn, stimulates the body to produce more insulin that quickly removes the excess glucose from the blood, resulting in hypoglycemia.

The aim of diet therapy is to provide the patient with optimum nutrition that will control these symptoms:

1. Small, frequent meals (that will not overload the jejunum) eaten slowly.
2. No liquid during meals and the following hour; the absence of liquid slows absorption.
3. High-protein foods for tissue repair and moderately high-fat foods to add calories and delay the time food is emptied from the stomach.
4. Moderate to low amounts of complex carbohydrate foods (which are digested more slowly).
5. No milk, sugar, sweets, desserts, alcohol, or sweetened beverages. All of these pass rapidly into the jejunum and pull fluid there. Also, simple sugars stimulate insulin release and so should be avoided.
6. Raw foods as tolerated (low-fiber types are usually given).

Table 17-2 presents an antidumping diet, and Table 17-3 provides a sample menu.

NURSING IMPLICATIONS

1. Encourage a supine position after meals to decrease the force of gravity.
2. Advise mouth rinsing before meals as cholinergic blocking agents can cause dryness of mouth.

TABLE 17-2   Permitted and Prohibited Foods in an Antidumping Diet

Food Group	Foods Permitted	Foods Prohibited
Breads	All breads and crackers except those noted	Breads with nuts, jams, or dried fruits or made with bran
Fats	Margarine, butter, oil, bacon, cream, mayonnaise, French dressing	None
Cereals and equivalents	All grains, rice, spaghetti, noodles, and macaroni except those noted	Presweetened cereals
Eggs	All egg dishes	None
Meats	All tender meats, fish, poultry	Highly seasoned or smoked meats
Beverages	Tea, coffee, broth, liquid unsweetened gelatin, artificially sweetened soda (½–1 hour before and after meals)*	No milk or alcohol; carbonated beverages if not tolerated; beverages with meal unless symptoms begin to subside†
	The following foods are to be added as patient tolerance and condition progress.	
Vegetables	Mashed potato, all tender vegetables (peas, carrots, spinach, etc.)	Creamed; gas-forming varieties if not tolerated (cabbage, broccoli, dried beans and peas, etc.)
Fruits	Fresh or canned (unsweetened or artificially sweetened); one serving citrus fruit or juice	Canned with sugar syrup; avoid sweetened dried fruits; e.g., prunes, figs, dates
Dairy products	Milk, cheese, cottage cheese, yogurt, etc.	Introduce small amounts of dairy to determine tolerance
Miscellaneous	Salt, catsup, mild spices, smooth peanut butter	Pickles, peppers, chili powder, nuts, olives, candy, milk gravies

*Some practitioners prefer 1 to 2 hours before and after meals.
†Some practitioners permit 4 oz of fluid with a meal.

TABLE 17-3   Sample Menu Plans for Antidumping Diets

	Soon after Surgery		Later after Surgery	
	Sample 1	Sample 2	Sample 1	Sample 2
Breakfast	Egg, poached, 1 Toast, 1 slice Butter, 1 tsp Banana, ½	Egg, scrambled, 1 Toast, 1 slice Butter, 1 tsp Peaches, ½ c	Cream of wheat, ½ c Butter, 1 tsp Egg, soft-cooked, 1	Juice, tomato, 4 oz Oatmeal, ½ c Bacon, crisp, 2 slices Toast, 1 slice Butter, 1 tsp
Snack	Gelatin, fruit-flavored, unsweetened, 1 c	Smooth peanut butter, 2 oz Crackers, 2	Gelatin, fruit-flavored Crackers, 4	Diet soda Crackers, 4
Lunch	Chicken breast, stewed, 3 oz Potato, mashed, ½ c Butter, 2 tsp	Fish, 3 oz Rice, ½ c Spinach, ½ c Butter, 2 tsp	Roast beef, 3 oz Rice, ½ c Peas, buttered, ½ c	Beef patty, 3 oz Potato, ½ c Asparagus, ½ c Butter, 2 tsp
Snack	Soft-cooked egg Crackers, 4	Gelatin, fruit-flavored, unsweetened, 1 c	Juice, orange, ½ c Crackers, 2	Apple juice Crackers, 4
Dinner	Meat, 3 oz Rice with grated cheese, ½ c Asparagus, tips, ½ c Margarine, 1 tsp	Turkey, sliced, 3 oz Potato, baked, 1 Butter, 2 tsp Tomato, 2 slices	Beef, 3 oz Potatoes, mashed, 1 c Carrots, ½ c Tomato, sliced, ½ Butter, 2 tsp	Chicken, 3 oz Noodles, 3 oz Spinach, ½ c Margarine, 1 tsp
Snack	Bread, 1 slice Meat, 2 oz Margarine, 1 tsp	Peach, halves canned, unsweetened	Smooth peanut butter Crackers (2)	Sandwich: Bread, 2 slices Mayonnaise, 2 tsp Meat, 2 oz

3. Emphasize eating slowly in a relaxed, pleasant environment.
4. Explain the reasons for diet restrictions to the patient and family or care provider.
5. Be aware that vitamin B$_{12}$ by injection may be necessary following total gastrectomy, because the intrinsic factor necessary for its absorption will be lost. Make sure that the patient understands the need for this treatment.
6. Check weight and caloric intake frequently.

PROGRESS CHECK ON ACTIVITY 1

FILL-IN

1. Fill out the section in Exercise 17-1 for the low-residue diet, listing all diseases or conditions for which this diet is applicable.

2. a. Fill out the section in Exercise 17-1 for foods suitable for a patient with a gastric ulcer.

   b. Repeat Exercise 17-1, using foods suitable for dumping syndrome.

3. Explain the rationale for the important changes in diet therapy for peptic ulcers. _____

   _____

   _____

4. Make a 1-day meal plan for a patient who is four days postgastrectomy.

ACTIVITY 2:

Disorders of the Intestines

DIETARY FIBER INTAKE

The structural parts of brans, husks of whole grain products, hulls, skins, and seeds are important sources of fiber. A low-fiber and a low-residue diet are not the same. Residue is the portion of the diet that contributes to the content of the feces. Dietary fiber is the portion of food that cannot be digested by the human body.

We can provide the patient with a low-fiber diet or a diet in which the amount of fiber is regulated. This is used for preoperative and postoperative states of lower gastrointestinal surgery or a condition in which decreased fecal bulk is desired such as diverticulitis, ulcerative colitis, Crohn's disease, or any time stenosis of the esophageal or intestinal lumen occurs. Simply put, we can provide a nutritionally adequate diet that leaves a minimum of residue in the colon by limiting the amount of fiber.

The fiber content of a diet can be reduced with the following practices:

1. Use young, very tender, cooked vegetables.
2. Omit foods with seeds, skin, and structural fiber, such as berries, celery, cabbage, corn, and peas.
3. Peel fruits and vegetables and cook to soften fiber.
4. Puree or strain foods.
5. Use only refined white breads and cereals.
6. Omit fruits and vegetables and use only strained juices.

Exercise 17-1   A practice on the dietary management of selected disorders and nursing implications

Complete the chart by filling in the information for each column.

Diet	Disease or Condition	Foods Allowed	Foods Limited	Foods Forbidden	Nursing Implications
Low-Residue					
Diet					
Gastric Ulcer					
Dumping Syndrome					

Table 17-4 shows the foods permitted in a low- to moderate-fiber or residue-restricted diet. Table 17-5 shows a sample menu for a low- to moderate-fiber or residue-restricted diet.

The most common of the intestinal disorders that occasionally affect people are constipation and diarrhea. Both disorders are usually managed with simple changes in diet and lifestyle. Other, more severe intestinal conditions are diverticular disease, inflammatory bowel disease (IBD), and cancer.

CONSTIPATION

Because constipation is a symptom, many variables have been implicated in its treatment. One cause is related to the stress and strain of modern life. Poor personal habits may be responsible, including irregular routine and meals, inadequate rest and exercise, tension, and ignoring the body's need to defecate. Some medications that contain iron, aluminum, or calcium can cause constipation. Regular use of laxatives also is a contributing

TABLE 17-4 Foods Permitted in Low- to Moderate-Fiber or Residue-Restricted Diets	
Foods and Daily Servings Permitted	
Meat, equivalents	Beef, veal, ham, liver, and poultry (broiled, baked, or stewed to tender); fish, fresh or salt (broiled, baked); canned tuna or salmon; shellfish, tender meat only
Milk, milk products	Whole, skim, chocolate; buttermilk, yogurt (2 c daily including amount in food preparation)
Cheese	Cottage, cream, American, Muenster, and Swiss 1 c milk = 1 oz cheese
Eggs	All varieties except fried
Grain, grain products	Bread (Italian, Vienna, or French); toast (French or melba); crackers (saltines or soda); rolls (plain, soft, or hard); others: biscuits, zwieback, rusk All above prepared with refined whole wheat or rye Cereals (ready-to-eat, cooked, all prepared from refined grains); oatmeal Flours from refined grains other than graham or bran White rice Plain spaghetti, noodles, and macaroni
Potatoes	Potatoes without skin (creamed, mashed, scalloped, boiled, baked); sweet potatoes without skin
Fruits	Daily allowance: 2 servings All juices and nectars; fruit, ripe and fresh (peeled, without seeds), frozen, or canned; grapes, bananas, apricots, plums, peaches, pears, cherries, avocados, citrus fruits (segments only; e.g., oranges, grapefruit, tangerine, honeydew, cantaloupe, pineapple, and nectarines)
Vegetables	Daily allowance: 1 serving for vegetables, with no limitation on juices Vegetables, well-cooked or canned: green and waxed beans, carrots, asparagus, beets, eggplant, mushrooms, onions, cauliflower, peas, winter squash, pumpkin, cabbage Vegetables, cooked, chopped: turnip greens, broccoli, spinach, kale, collards Vegetables, raw, chopped: lettuce
Beverages	Coffee (regular, decaffeinated), tea; others: soft drinks, cereal beverages All drinks may be flavored with permitted fruits. Broth and cream-based soups made from other permitted ingredients
Candies, sweets	Plain candies, jelly, honey, syrup, sugar, jelly beans, mints
Fats	Cream: regular, dried substitutes, sour; dressings: mayonnaise and mayonnaise-type, all must be plain; regular smooth salad oil; butter, margarine, oils; others: crisp bacon, shortenings
Desserts	All must be plain and made from permitted ingredients: pie, cakes, cookies, pudding, gelatin, sherbet, ice cream
Miscellaneous	Spices and herbs (ground or finely chopped); flavorings: soy sauce, vinegar, salt, monosodium glutamate, chocolate, catsup, and all commercial flavoring extracts; sauces and gravies: mild and made from permitted ingredients

TABLE 17-5   Sample Menu for Low- to Moderate-Fiber or Residue-Restricted Diet

Breakfast	Lunch	Dinner
Tomato juice, ½ c	Melted cheese sandwich:	Roast beef, tender, 3 oz
Egg, poached, 1	White bread, 2 slices	Potato, mashed, 1 c
Toast, white bread, 1 slice	Cheese, mild, 2 oz	Carrots, cooked, ½ c
Bacon, 2 slices	Green beans, ½ c	Orange juice, strained, ½ c
Margarine	Apple juice, ⅓ c	White bread, 1 slice
Jelly	Gelatin, 1 c	Margarine
Coffee or tea	Vanilla wafers, 2	Ice cream, ½ c
	Coffee or tea	Coffee or tea
	Snacks	
	Milk, 1 c	
	Cookies, plain, 2	

factor. Ideal treatment requires adopting good health habits to restore regularity and break the laxative cycle.

A regular balanced diet high in fiber and fluids is recommended to avoid constipation. Eight to ten glasses of fluids daily should be consumed. Foods high in fiber include whole grains and raw fruits and vegetables. If the patient cannot tolerate the latter, cooked ones may be used. Prune juice, apple juice, figs, and raisins are especially helpful. Bran with a high fiber content is an effective agent.

Nursing Implications

1. Explain the benefits of a high-fiber diet. In addition to increasing bulk, the foods that provide fiber are high in vitamins and minerals.
2. Discourage regular and excessive use of laxatives.
3. Reassure patients that a daily bowel movement is not an absolute necessity. It may not be normal for them.
4. Advise gradual inclusion of high-fiber foods in the diet. Excess dietary fiber at the beginning may cause cramping and gas. This can discourage patients from continuing the diet.
5. Encourage a high fluid intake, especially of water.

DIARRHEA

Diarrhea in infants, small children, and the elderly can be serious if prolonged, especially if an infection is present. Common mild diarrhea of short duration usually responds well to simple treatment. Diarrhea is functional when related to stress, irritation of the bowel, or a change in the regular routine, such as traveling. It is organic if it is caused by a GI lesion. Treatment includes eliminating the underlying cause, using antidiarrheal drugs as needed, and using appropriate diet therapy.

Diet therapy during severe diarrhea is characterized by the following:

1. No oral feeding for first 24 to 48 hours. Intravenous (IV) fluids are used to replace electrolytes and water.

If the need for IV fluids continues beyond 72 hours, amino acids and vitamins may be added. If diarrhea is prolonged, total parenteral nutrition (TPN) is necessary.

2. Resumption of oral feedings: First day include clear liquids with a minimum of sugar. Second day progressively introduce a minimum-residue diet (see Tables 17-4 and 17-5), high in protein. Calcium supplements are provided. Applesauce and raw apples may be used for their pectin content, which can thicken the stools. Implement gradual progression of a low-fiber, low-residue, soft, solid-to-regular diet as the situation improves.

Mild diarrhea usually responds to the following: reducing the total food intake, especially carbohydrate and fat; limiting residue; and replacing fluids. A bland low-residue diet may ease the discomfort.

Nursing implications for individuals or patients with diarrhea:

1. Note daily weight changes.
2. Keep accurate daily records of intake and output.
3. Do not permit carbonated beverages. Use flat soda or ginger ale if carbonated beverages are desired.
4. Relieve any pain before serving meals.
5. Employ diversionary tactics during meals.
6. Offer replacements later, if patient does not finish food when it is first offered.

DIVERTICULAR DISEASE

Diverticuli are herniations (pockets or sacs) of intestinal mucosa through the muscles of the bowel wall. The process is referred to as diverticulosis. If accompanied by inflammation, the disorder is called diverticulitis. It is important to distinguish between the two, as the diet therapy used is different for each.

One cause of diverticulosis appears to be related to a lack of fecal bulk, which increases intraluminal pressure.

The treatment of diverticulosis is aimed at preventing inflammation. A high-fiber diet is prescribed. Fiber sources include bran, whole grains, and fruits and vegetables. Pepper and chili powder, sometimes nuts and corn, may be eliminated.

Diverticulitis requires special attention. During acute periods when the diverticuli are inflamed and there is pain, tenderness, nausea, vomiting, and distention, fecal residue may add to the discomfort. Diet therapy during this period may be limited to clear liquids progressing to full liquids, then to low-residue and to regular high-fiber diet as the inflammation subsides. Severe diverticulitis is usually treated by surgical methods (colostomy, bowel resection).

Nursing implications are as follows:

1. Patient education is most important here, as all diverticular disease was formerly treated with a low-residue diet.
2. The older patient should be especially reassured, as most diverticulosis occurs in the elderly, and they become most anxious on a high-fiber diet.
3. A symptomatic patient should be encouraged to rest and to take medicines as prescribed.
4. Patients who are malnourished on admission should be replenished nutritionally to facilitate healing and recovery.

INFLAMMATORY BOWEL DISEASE

Inflammatory bowel disease is a term used for ulcerative colitis and Crohn's disease. Both may have the related condition of short bowel syndrome if there have been repeated surgeries that removed sections of the bowel as the disease progressed.

Both ulcerative colitis (UC) and Crohn's disease have increased in incidence in the United States. They have similar pathophysiology and clinical symptoms, but are prevalent in different groups. They both have severe nutritional consequences, but are separate diseases. Crohn's can occur anywhere in the GI tract, but UC is confined to the colon and rectum. The pattern of disease in Crohn's is that of a chronic disorder, often involving the entire intestinal wall. This may cause complications, such as partial or complete obstruction and the formation of fistulas. The inflammatory processes in UC, on the other hand, are usually acute and are limited to the mucosa and submucosa of the intestine. The patient may have periods of remission.

Diet therapy for inflammatory bowel disease is based upon the common clinical symptoms of bloody diarrhea and the various associated nutritional problems.

Ulcerative Colitis (UC)

Primarily a disease of young adults, especially women, ulcerative colitis is a life-threatening disorder. While the cause is unknown, one major culprit is related to psychological factors. The disorder is characterized by widespread ulceration and inflammation of the colon, fever, chronic bloody diarrhea, edema, and anemia. The patient is severely malnourished, suffering from avitaminosis, negative nitrogen balance, dehydration, electrolyte imbalances, and skin lesions. Patients are nervous, anorexic, and in pain. The obvious need for maximum nutrition for a patient who cannot eat is a challenge to the health team.

The treatment of UC includes rest, sedation, antibiotics, antidiarrheal drugs, and rigorous diet therapy. Surgical removal of the diseased portion of the bowel is the treatment of choice, if other medical procedures fail. Diet therapy includes the following:

1. A regular, high-fiber diet supplemented with formula feeding, as tolerated
2. High protein: 125 to 150 g
3. High calorie: 3000+ calories
4. High vitamins/minerals, especially vitamins C, B complex, and K
5. Moderate fat or as tolerated
6. Dairy products usually eliminated to avoid secondary lactose intolerance, or lactose-free products used
7. IV fluids used in addition to oral feedings to correct fluid and electrolyte losses due to diarrhea
8. TPN is most effective when the bowel has been shortened or the disease is extensive

Crohn's Disease

Crohn's disease is another manifestation of inflammatory bowel disease. It is particularly prevalent in industrial areas and among the 55 to 60 age group. It has an insidious onset and is characterized by tenderness, pain, diarrhea, and cramping in the right lower quadrant of the bowel. There is less blood in the stool than in ulcerative colitis, but increased secretion of mucus by the bowel. The patient runs a low-grade fever.

Widespread involvement of the small bowel results in malabsorption of fat, protein, carbohydrates, vitamins, and minerals, and subsequent weight loss. Vitamin B_{12} deficiency may occur, leading to macrocytic anemia and neurologic damage. Bile salt losses lead to cholelithiasis, diarrhea, and steatorrhea. There may also be anemia due to loss of blood in the stool. Children with Crohn's disease show retarded growth patterns.

As with UC, the effects of malabsorption are widespread. Malabsorption of vitamins C and K leads to capillary fragility, hemorrhagic tendencies, and petechiae. Malabsorption of calcium and vitamin D puts the patient at risk for osteomalacia and osteoporosis. The bone pain that is a frequent symptom of both UC and Crohn's is due to this impairment. Tetany and paresthesia are also related to calcium and magnesium malabsorption. The whole vitamin B complex is destroyed, giving rise to glossitis, cheilosis, skin changes, and peripheral neuritis.

The rational for diet therapy for both diseases is to restore nutrient deficits, prevent further losses, promote healing, and repair and maintain body tissue.

NURSING IMPLICATIONS

Nursing responsibilities for patients with ulcerative colitis or Crohn's disease include the following:

1. Be aware that the patient's need for high levels of food and fluids parallels that of a burn patient.
2. Interpret the diet to the patient and family member or care provider. A young person on a bland low-residue diet for long periods of time becomes discouraged.
3. Be aware that, if steroid-type medication is used, sodium restriction may also become necessary.
4. Do not confuse fluid retention with nutritional improvement (body weight gain).
5. Keep careful daily records: fluid intake and output, weight changes, nutrient intake, and calorie counts.
6. Seek outside resources for the patient (counselor, therapist) as needed. Work closely with dietitian and other health team members.
7. Provide the patient with the rationale for strict medical management and the side effects of same.
8. Provide education for continuing diet therapy for UC and Crohn's. It is based on:
   a. Restoring adequate nutrition intake
   b. Correcting deficits, usually with supplements
   c. Preventing further losses
   d. Controlling substances that do not absorb well, such as fats
   e. Promoting the healing and repairing and maintaining of tissue
9. Any number of commercial preparations to add additional calories in easily digestible form may be obtained from the local pharmacy, (MCT, Portagen, etc.).
10. The diet for both UC and Crohn's remains:
    a. High protein: 120%–150% of the RDA. Assuming 60 g/day as recommended for healthy adults, the diet would contain from 72–90 g/day of HBV protein.
    b. High vitamin, especially those found to be most deficient.
    c. High minerals as needed by the individual (especially iron, which may be administered by transfusion; calcium, zinc, and potassium if diarrhea persists).
    d. Low residue to regular. Recent research indicates that the low-residue diet as diet of choice for IBD may become obsolete, as the bland low-residue diet did for diverticulosis and ulcers. Five-year trials of patients with IBD showed that a regular diet with appropriate increases in protein, vitamins, minerals, and calories for healing leads to more improvement and fewer hospitalizations than traditional diet therapy. While more research will be necessary to confirm this study, the nurse should stay abreast of the changing nature of diet therapy.
    e. High calorie to spare the protein for tissue healing and rebuilding.
    f. Supplemental defined formula as needed.

GASTRIC SURGERY FOR SEVERE OBESITY

According to the National Institutes of Diabetes, Digestive, and Kidney Diseases, stomach surgery is one option for severe obesity. Severe obesity is a chronic condition that is difficult to treat through diet and exercise alone. Gastrointestinal surgery is the best option for people who are severely obese and cannot lose weight by traditional means or who suffer from serious obesity-related health problems. The surgery promotes weight loss by restricting food intake and, in some operations, interrupting the digestive process. As in other treatments for obesity, the best results are achieved with healthy eating behaviors and regular physical activity.

People who may consider gastrointestinal surgery include those with a body mass index (BMI) above 40, about 100 pounds of overweight for men and 80 pounds for women (see Appendix B for a BMI conversion chart). People with a BMI between 35 and 40 who suffer from type 2 diabetes or life-threatening cardiopulmonary problems such as severe sleep apnea or obesity-related heart disease may also be candidates for surgery.

Gastrointestinal surgery for obesity, also called bariatric surgery, alters the digestive process. The operations promote weight loss by closing off parts of the stomach to make it smaller. Operations that only reduce stomach size are known as restrictive operations, because they restrict the amount of food the stomach can hold. Some operations combine stomach restriction with a partial bypass of the small intestine. These procedures create a direct connection from the stomach to the lower segment of the small intestine, literally bypassing portions of the digestive tract that absorb calories and nutrients. These are known as malabsorptive operations.

Restrictive Operations

As a result of this surgery, most people lose the ability to eat large amounts of food at one time. After an operation, the person usually can eat only ¾ to 1 cup of food without discomfort or nausea. Also, food has to be well chewed. Although restrictive operations lead to weight loss in almost all patients, they are less successful than malabsorptive operations in achieving substantial, long-term weight loss. About 30% of those who undergo this surgery achieve normal weight, and about 80% achieve some degree of weight loss. Some patients regain weight. Others are unable to adjust their eating habits and fail to lose the desired weight. Successful results depend on the patient's willingness to adopt a long-term plan of healthy eating and regular physical activity.

A common risk of restrictive operations is vomiting, which is caused when the small stomach is overly stretched by food particles that have not been chewed well. In a small number of cases, stomach juices may leak into the abdomen, requiring an emergency operation. In less than 1% of all cases, infection or death from complications may occur.

Malabsorptive Operations

In addition to the risks of restrictive surgeries, malabsorptive operations also carry greater risk for nutritional deficiencies. This is because the procedure causes food to bypass the duodenum and jejunum, where most iron and calcium are absorbed. Menstruating women may develop anemia because not enough vitamin B_{12} and iron are absorbed. Decreased absorption of calcium may also bring on osteoporosis and metabolic bone disease. Patients are required to take nutritional supplements that usually prevent these deficiencies. Depending on the particular method of bypass, some patients must also take water-soluble vitamins A, D, E, and K supplements.

These operations may also cause dumping syndrome. This means that stomach contents move too rapidly through the small intestine. Symptoms include nausea, weakness, sweating, faintness, and sometimes diarrhea after eating.

The more extensive the bypass, the greater the risk for complications and nutritional deficiencies. Patients with extensive bypasses of the normal digestive process require close monitoring and life-long use of special foods, supplements, and medications.

Surgery to produce weight loss is a serious undertaking. Anyone thinking about surgery should understand what the operation involves. Patients and physicians should carefully consider the benefits and risks.

COLOSTOMY AND ILEOSTOMY

Many intestinal diseases not responsive to medical and dietary measures must be treated surgically. Depending on the location of the obstruction or disease, a colostomy or an ileostomy may be performed.

Colostomy

In a colostomy, the rectum and anus are removed. The remaining intestine is led to the outside through a hole in the abdomen. Because this surgical procedure diverts fecal material from the distal colon and rectum, where fluids are normally absorbed, patients with colostomies have stools with high water content.

Diet therapy is characterized by the following:

1. A well-balanced diet that is appropriate for the preoperative patient is indicated. See Chapter 15 for diet planning.
2. The initial postoperative diet is clear liquid, followed by a high-soluble fiber diet as tolerated. Progress as rapidly as possible to a regular diet. Nutrient supplements are provided as needed.
3. General goals are to promote healing and prevent odor, constipation, and diarrhea.
4. Each patient must experiment with the diet. The patient can identify those foods to be limited or avoided.

The nursing implications in caring for this group of patients include the following:

1. Colostomy patients have real concerns about odors and flatulence. Help them with corrective measures. For example, spinach and parsley have deodorizing action and a commercial deodorant may be used in the bag.
2. A diet must be evaluated for adequacy, if certain food items are prohibited.
3. Eating slowly and thorough chewing can prevent swallowing air.
4. Patients with colostomy usually progress rapidly as they gain control over the elimination process and adapt well to changes in lifestyle.
5. Emotional support for the patient and family is mandatory.
6. Compile information regarding outside resources that will help patients.

Ileostomy

This surgery is indicated for intractable ulcerative colitis, Crohn's disease, and cancer of the colon. An ileostomy bypasses the colon and rectum, and the distal ileum is led to the outside of the body through an opening in the abdomen. Since the surgery is performed higher in the intestine, the waste material is mainly in fluid form. There are great losses of fluid, sodium, vitamin K, and other essential nutrients. Fat absorption is poor and vitamin B_{12} absorption is reduced or absent. Body-weight loss is high.

Diet therapy after the operation is as follows:

1. The diet progresses from clear liquids to a high-soluble fiber diet as tolerated. New foods are given one at a time to test the patient's tolerance.
2. Nutritional supplements and/or TPN may be needed in the early stages.
3. Vitamin B_{12} injections are given at scheduled times to prevent pernicious anemia.
4. Extra fluid is required. Orange juice and bananas are high in potassium, while extra salt with food increases sodium intake.

5. The progression to a regular diet is longer for the patient with an ileostomy than a patient with a colostomy.

NURSING IMPLICATIONS

Nursing implications for caring for this group of patients include the following:

1. Provide emotional support and encouragement to eating adequately.
2. Work closely with the dietary department, and plan for the family of the patient to participate.
3. Be aware that the same nursing measures are applicable to colostomy and ileostomy patients.
4. Become familiar with obesity and the role of surgery. The nurse's role is extremely important before, during, and after the operation. Apart from clinical nursing considerations, the significant role of nutrition in patient care during these three phases should be acknowledged. The implementation of proper enteral and parenteral nutrition revolves around the close working relationships among the doctor, the nurse, and the dietitian.

PROGRESS CHECK ON ACTIVITY 2

MATCHING

1. Indicate which of the following foods would be allowed on a minimum-residue diet by writing Y (yes) or N (no) in the blanks:

   _____ a. broccoli with hollandaise sauce
   _____ b. bouillon
   _____ c. applesauce
   _____ d. fresh pears
   _____ e. sherbet
   _____ f. fruitcake
   _____ g. poached egg
   _____ h. macaroni
   _____ i. pecan waffles
   _____ j. broiled chicken

MULTIPLE CHOICE

Circle the letter of the correct answer.

2. Residue is that part of food that:

   a. remains longest in the GI tract.
   b. is indigestible.
   c. is left uneaten after the meal.
   d. is inedible.

3. IBD is the result of which of these factors?

   a. short bowel syndrome
   b. infectious processes
   c. inadequate diets
   d. malabsorption

4. An appropriate diet for the patient with IBD would allow the basic principles of optimum nutrition and would:

   a. be increased in fiber.
   b. contain extra fats for energy.
   c. be decreased in fiber.
   d. be decreased in sodium.

5. Patients with colostomies usually gain control of evacuation faster than patients with ileostomies because:

   a. they have better preoperative nutritional status.
   b. they have better neuromuscular functions.
   c. the surgery site is lower in the gut.
   d. the surgical site heals more quickly.

6. General goals of diet therapy following a colostomy are to promote healing and prevent:

   a. constipation.
   b. diarrhea.
   c. odors.
   d. all of the above.

7. The restricted-residue diet:

   a. is always very high in calories.
   b. is very similar to the full-liquid diet.
   c. may be inadequate in vitamins and minerals.
   d. is nutritionally adequate.

8. The minimum-residue diet:

   a. is always very high in calories.
   b. is very similar to the full-liquid diet.
   c. may be inadequate in vitamins and minerals.
   d. is nutritionally adequate.

9. Which of the following foods are allowed on a minimum-residue diet?

   a. milkshake, hamburger, and french fries
   b. tomato wedge, scrambled egg, and broiled bacon
   c. chicken sandwich on white bread with butter
   d. all of the above

10. Which of these foods would be included in a high-fiber diet?

    a. whole wheat bread, prunes, celery
    b. carrot sticks, bran cereal, apples
    c. coconut bars, pecan rolls, oatmeal
    d. all of the above

11. If the minimum-residue diet must be used for a period of time, the physician should:

    a. alternate it weekly with the high-iron diet.
    b. substitute the full-liquid diet.

c. add fresh fruit juices before each meal.

d. prescribe a vitamin and mineral supplement.

FILL-IN

12. Name 10 foods high in fiber content.

a. _____

b. _____

c. _____

d. _____

e. _____

f. _____

g. _____

h. _____

i. _____

j. _____

13. List five goals for feeding a patient with an inflammatory bowel disease.

a. _____

b. _____

c. _____

d. _____

e. _____

14. List five nursing implications for nutritional care of the osteomate.

a. _____

b. _____

c. _____

d. _____

e. _____

TRUE/FALSE

Circle T for True and F for False.

15. T F Severe obesity is a chronic condition that does not respond to treatment through diet and exercise alone.

16. T F Bypass surgery should be considered for a female who is 30 pounds overweight.

17. T F Following bypass surgery, a patient should be able to resume original eating habits to control body weight.

18. T F Restrictive surgeries for chronic obesity promote weight loss by decreasing the size of the stomach.

19. T F Malabsorptive operations may cause nutritional deficiencies because the diet therapy is too restrictive.

20. T F The nurse's role in the nutritional care of a patient with bypass surgery is extremely important before, during, and after the operation.

REFERENCES

Alanis, A. D. (2005). Antibacterial properties of some plants used in Mexican traditional medicine for the treatment of gastrointestinal disorders. *Journal of Enthnopharrmacology, 22*: 153–157.

American Dietetic Association. (2006). *Nutrition Diagnosis: A Critical Step in Nutrition Care Process.* Chicago: American Dietetic Association.

Beham, E. (2006). *Therapeutic Nutrition: A Guide to Patient Education.* Philadelphia: Lippincott, Williams and Wilkins.

Bendich, A., & Deckelbaum, R. J. (Eds.). (2005). *Preventive Nutrition: The Comprehensive Guide for Health Professionals* (3rd ed.). Totowa, NJ: Humana Press.

Buchman, A. (2004). *Practical Nutritional Support Technique* (2nd ed.). Thorofeue, NJ: SLACK.

Coulston, A. M., Rock, C. L., & Monsen, E. L. (Eds.). (2001). *Nutrition in the Prevention and Treatment of Disease.* San Diego, CA: Academic Press.

Deen, D., & Hark, L. (2007). *The Complete Guide to Nutrition in Primary Care.* Malden, MA: Blackwell.

Eastwood, M. (2003). *Principles of Human Nutrition.* (2nd ed.). Malden, MA: Blackwell Science.

Escott-Stump, S. (2002). *Nutrition and Diagnosis-Related Care.* (5th ed.). Philadelphia: Lippincott, Williams and Wilkins.

Fauci, A. S., Braunwald, E., Kapser, D. L., Hauser, S. L., Longo, D. L., Jameson, J. L. et al. (Eds.). (2008). *Harrison's Principles of Internal Medicine* (17th ed.). New York: McGraw-Hill.

Garrow, J. S. (2000). *Human Nutrition and Dietetics.* (10th ed.). New York: Churchill Livingston.

Haas, E. M., & Levin, B. (2006). *Staying Healthy with Nutrition: The Complete Guide to Diet and Nutrition Medicine* (21st ed.). Berkeley, CA: Celestial Arts.

Hark, L., & Morrison, G. (Eds.). (2003). *Medical Nutrition and Disease.* (3rd ed.). Malden, MA: Blackwell.

Hay, D. W. (2001). *Blackwell's Primary Care Essentials: Gastrointestinal Diseases.* Ames, IA: Blackwell.

Lagua, R. T., & Qaudio, V. S. (2004). *Nutrition and Diet Therapy: Reference Dictionary* (5th ed.). Ames, IA: Blackwell.

Mahan, L. K., & Escott-Stump, S. (Eds.). (2008). *Krause's Food and Nutrition Therapy* (12th ed.). Philadelphia: Elsevier Saunders.

Mann, J., & Truswell, S. (Eds.). (2007). *Essentials of Human Nutrition* (3rd ed.). New York: Oxford University Press.

Minocha, A., & Adamec, C. (2004). *The Encyclopedia of the Digestive System and Digestive Disorders.* New York: Facts On File.

Mistkovitz, P., & Betancourt, M. (2005). *The Doctor's Guide to Gastrointestinal Health Preventing and Treating Acid Reflux, Ulcers, Irritable Bowel Syndrome, Diverticulitis, Celiac Disease, Colon Cancer, Pancreatitis, Cirrhosis, Hernias and More.* Hoboken, NJ: Wiley.

Paajanen, L. (2005). Cow milk is not responsible for most gastrointestinal immune-like syndromes—evidence from a population-based study. *American Journal of Clinical Nutrition 82*: 1327–1335.

Payne-James, J., & Wicks, C. (2003). *Key Facts in Clinical Nutrition* (2nd ed.). London: Greenwich Medical Media.

Sardesai, V. M. (2003). *Introduction to Clinical Nutrition* (2nd ed.). New York: Marcel Dekker.

Shils, M. E., & Shike, M. (Eds.). (2006). *Modern Nutrition in Health and Disease* (10th ed.). Philadelphia: Lippincott, Williams and Wilkins.

Temple, N. J., Wilson, T., & Jacobs, D. R. (2006). *Nutrition Health: Strategies for Disease Prevention* (2nd ed.). Totowa, NJ: Humana Press.

Thomas, B., & Bishop, J. (Eds.). (2007). *Manual of Dietetic Practice* (4th ed.). Ames, IA: Blackwell.

Webster-Gandy, J., Madden, A., & Holdworth, M. (Eds.). (2006). *Oxford Handbook of Nutrition and Dietetics.* Oxford, England: Oxford University Press.

Yamada, T., Hasler, W. L., Inadomi, J. M., Anderson, M. A., & Brown, R. S., Jr. (2005). *Handbook of Gastroenterology* (2nd ed.). Lippincott, Williams and Wilkins.

CHAPTER 18

Diet Therapy for Diabetes Mellitus

Time for completion
Activities: 1½ hours
Optional examination: ½ hour

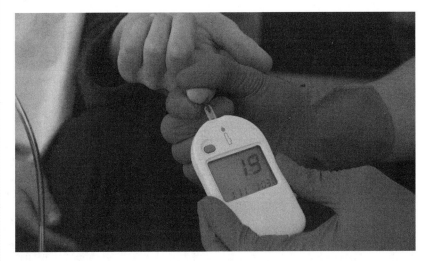

OBJECTIVES

Upon completion of this chapter, the student should be able to do the following:

1. Explain the use of the exchange system in dietary control.
2. Identify the exchange groups and their subcategories.
3. List the carbohydrate, protein, fat, and energy values of each list of foods in the exchange groups.
4. Plan an appropriate menu for a person with a clinical condition that requires a calculated diet.
5. Describe the use of the calculated diet in controlling diabetes mellitus.
6. Describe the use of the calculated diet in controlling weight.
7. Describe the nursing implications appropriate to the disorders.

GLOSSARY

Atherosclerosis: formation of plaques containing cholesterol and other liquid material within the lumina of the arteries.
Endogenous: produced within the body.

Gestational diabetes: A high blood glucose level that develops during pregnancy. Usually there is a return to normal following childbirth, but these women may develop NIDDM later in life.

Glycemic index: A measurement of how fast starches and sugars metabolize in the blood stream. It indicates how quickly specific foods affect blood sugar levels based on a scale of 1 to 100. Glycemic control refers to the use of these specific foods to help control blood sugar levels. The application of this concept is still being debated and, therefore, will not be included in this chapter.

High biological value: refers to complete proteins that supply abundant amounts of essential amino acids for synthesis of new tissues.

Hyperglycemia: condition that occurs when the glucose in the blood exceeds the normal range (the normal range for blood sugar levels is 70 to 120 mg/ml).

Hypoglycemia: condition that occurs when the glucose in the blood falls below normal range.

Hypoglycemic agent: a drug sometimes used by diabetics not receiving insulin to assist in lowering blood sugar levels. It is not a hormone.

IDDM: insulin-dependent diabetes mellitus.

Insulin: hormone produced in the beta cells of the pancreas that controls blood glucose levels. It is the only hormone that lowers blood sugar.

Ketoacidosis: formation and accumulation of ketone bodies in body tissues and fluids.

NIDDM: Non-insulin-dependent diabetes mellitus.

Polydipsia: excessive thirst.

Polyphagia: excessive hunger.

Polyunsaturated: a fat that has two or more double bonds into which hydrogen can be added.

Polyuria: excessive urination.

Triglycerides: the type of fat that is the body's main form of stored energy.

BACKGROUND INFORMATION

In 2007, the American Dietetic and Diabetes Associations updated its 2003 food exchange lists for diabetic patients. However, the principles and basic guidelines remain the same in the new revision with the following differences:

1. There is a large increase in the number of entries for food items.
2. The nutritional contributions of each food are provided for: gm/serving, protein, fat, carbohydrate, saturated fatty acids, trans fats, polyunsaturated fats, cholesterol, sodium, fiber, and sugars.
3. The source of data for each food is identified when available, e.g., U.S. Department of Agriculture, food labels, and so on.

The new list contains a large number of foods and is impractical to reproduce completely in Appendix F.

However, we will provide examples of foods selected from the 2007 edition. Also for ease of use, we exclude the complete listing of nutrient data for each selected food in Appendix F. The instructors will provide an explanation for the extent of coverage of the food exchange lists in this chapter. Also, the Web sites of the two professional organizations are making available the complete 2007 food exchange lists.

As explained in Chapter 1, the exchange lists remain the definitive tool used to plan diet therapy for persons with diabetes, and may be modified to meet specific needs.

The caloric value of a diet can be regulated by the number of servings allowed per day from each group. Obviously, the number of servings will depend on how many calories are prescribed in the diet plan, which depends on age, gender, and activity level, and if that individual needs to lose or gain weight.

Consistent with the 3rd edition (2001) of the NCEP guidelines as discussed in Chapter 1, the diet should contain not more than 25%–35% of total calories from fat. Of this amount, not more than 7% should come from saturated fat. Review Chapter 16 for particulars on the NCEP guidelines.

Product labels provide valuable information regarding the types of fats in products, although the percent of trans fats does not appear on labels at present.

Because of the incidence of atherosclerosis in patients with non-insulin-dependent diabetes mellitus (NIDDM), the kind of fats used is an important factor in diet management.

Control of the diet is still depending on the monitoring of the total amount of carbohydrate and the type of fats used. For clients who need to limit their sodium intake, foods in each list that contain 400 mg or more of sodium are marked with a symbol (a salt shaker).

The use of food exchange groups will not be new to the student who has studied the information on normal nutrition in Part I. Only a brief review of the principles is provided here. As explained above, Appendix F lists selected foods from the 2007 edition of the food exchange lists. These food groups are useful because they do the following:

1. Permit nutrients to be counted in foods.
2. Facilitate meal planning by balancing the meal with choices from each group.
3. Enable a patient to comply with diet instructions with minimal effort because of their easy application.
4. Allow a certain flexibility and variety, and reduce diet monotony.
5. Emphasize foods containing more fiber and foods low in sodium.
6. Ensure a reduced intake of saturated fats and cholesterol by a systematic procedure.
7. Enable a patient to raise or lower caloric content as needed.

8. Teach food selection in a practical way.
9. Regulate the intake of carbohydrate, protein, and fat, and permit the calculation of a diet for the overweight, underweight, or diabetic patient.

The exchange groups and their assigned values are listed in Table 18-1.

The student should remember the caloric values for the three major nutrients: carbohydrate: 1 g = 4 calories; protein: 1 g = 4 calories; fat: 1 g = 9 calories. While alcohol is not a nutrient, it does furnish 7 calories per gram and is a factor to be considered in weight control. Because body fat contains some water, a pound of body fat equals 3500 calories. Diet calculations are based on calories per kilogram (kg) of body weight. The conversion 1 kg = 2.2 lb is important.

ACTIVITY 1:

Diet Therapy and Diabetes Mellitus

Diabetes mellitus is characterized by an inability to metabolize carbohydrate due to a deficiency of insulin or a deficiency of receptor sites. The metabolism of protein and fat is also affected.

Glucose is the form of carbohydrate that is carried in the blood; all carbohydrate breaks down to glucose. Without glucose, the cells have no energy source and have to use muscle protein and tissue fat as an alternate. Without insulin, glucose cannot go from the blood into the cells. This glucose accumulates in the blood, producing hyperglycemia. The sources of blood glucose are:

1. Carbohydrate (CHO): 100% of digestible CHO converted to glucose.
2. Protein: 58% converted to glucose.
3. Fat: 10% converted to glucose.
4. Glycogen (the liver's emergency supply of carbohydrate): converted to glucose when other sources are used up. Muscle tissue also contains glycogen that may be used in emergencies.

Blood glucose is controlled by two hormones from the beta cells of the pancreas: insulin, which lowers blood sugar, and glucagon, which raises it. A third hormone, somatostatin, regulates the secretions of these two hormones.

TREATMENT AND DIET THERAPY

Although the cornerstone of treatment for diabetes mellitus is diet therapy, there are some differences in the way that the therapy is applied, depending upon the type of diabetes present.

The general classification of diabetes is based upon two major types: type I, insulin-dependent diabetes mellitus (IDDM); and type II, non-insulin-dependent diabetes mellitus (NIDDM). Eighty-five to ninety percent of the diabetic population is non-insulin dependent; the other 10 to 15 percent is insulin-dependent. The following discussion illustrates some of the similarities and differences between these types of diabetes.

TABLE 18-1   Outline of the American Diabetes Association Food Exchange Lists

Food Group						
Number	Nutrient	Food Lists	CHO (g)	Protein (g)	Fat (g)	Kcal
1.	Carbohydrates	Starch	15	3	–	80
		Fruit	15	–	–	60
		Milk:				
		Skim	12	8	0–1	90
		Low fat	12	8	5	120
		Whole	12	8	8	150
		Other CHO				
		Vegetable	15*			
			5	2	–	25
2.	Meat and meat substitutes	Very lean	–	7	0–1	35
		Lean	–	7	3	55
		Medium fat	–	7	5	75
		High fat	–	7	8	100
3.	Fat	Monounsaturated	–	–	5	45
		Polyunsaturated	–	–	5	45
		Saturated	–	–	5	45

*Or 1 starch, or 1 fruit, or 1 milk. Some will also count as 1 or more fat(s).

Type I—IDDM

This is the most severe form of diabetes, occurring most often in childhood or young adulthood. It may, or may not, be an inherited trait. Recent research indicates that the islet cells of the pancreas may have been damaged, either by a disease (such as rubella) or by certain chemicals that were toxic, which led to the onset of the disease. The classic symptoms of IDDM are polydipsia, polyphagia, and polyuria, accompanied by rapid weight loss and often ketoacidosis.

IDDM has a rapid onset, is very unstable, and causes metabolic imbalances that are difficult to control. For these reasons the diet is very carefully planned and coordinated with the insulin and exercise regime. Failure to time and regulate the meals with these factors will result in great fluctuations in blood glucose, ranging from acute hypoglycemia to extreme hyperglycemia. Diet therapy is discussed at length later in this chapter.

Type II—NIDDM

NIDDM has a much stronger genetic link than does IDDM. The majority of these clients are older adults because the onset is slow, and they are usually obese. Some endogenous insulin is still produced, making it unnecessary for them to take insulin, except in unusual situations (such as surgery or other stressors).

Obesity, physical inactivity, and hypertension are strong risk factors for the onset of NIDDM. The symptoms are similar to those of IDDM, except there is no weight loss and very rarely ketoacidosis. NIDDM is a milder form of diabetes and is most often controlled with weight loss and an exercise program. Occasionally an oral hypoglycemic drug will be necessary.

Persons with NIDDM have a high incidence of atherosclerosis, making it advisable to counsel them on the need for reduced fat intake as well as reduced calories.

As we have advanced in our knowledge of treatments for diabetes, diabetic persons are living longer. They have increased risks of developing major complications such as kidney disease, vascular disease, nerve impairment, and diseases of the retina of the eye. In fact, as much as 20% of the diabetic population becomes blind. Fluctuations of blood glucose from uncontrolled diabetes are thought to be one important factor in the onset of these conditions, making it even more imperative to manage and monitor the diet carefully.

BASIC NUTRITION REQUIREMENTS

Basic nutrition requirements will be determined by several factors. Some of the guidelines used are physical assessment, health and diet histories, and laboratory reports. These factors, combined with the psychological aspects of the client, will help the physician or healthcare specialist determine the diet prescription.

Nutrient Balance

In the most widely used diabetic diet plans, daily carbohydrate intake provides 50%–55% of the daily caloric requirement. Protein of high biological value is emphasized for diabetic diets, especially for children and adolescents. Protein provides 15%–20% of the daily caloric intake. Emphasis is placed on using polyunsaturated fats and limiting cholesterol in the remaining 30% of calories permitted for dietary fat.

An example will serve to illustrate the concept of nutrient balance: Mr. X is placed on a 1500 calorie per day diabetic diet. The nutrient balance is 50% carbohydrate, 20% protein, and 30% fat. What is the number of grams of each nutrient used in the daily diet plan?

1. Carbohydrate
   1500 calories $\times$ .50 = 750 calories
   750 calories/(4 calories/g) = 187 g carbohydrate, rounded to 190 g
2. Protein
   1500 calories $\times$ .20 = 300 calories
   300 calories/(4 calories/g) = 75 g protein
3. Fat
   1500 calories $\times$ .30 = 450 calories
   450 calories/(9 calories/g) = 50 g fat

The diet prescription will be 190 g carbohydrate, 75 g protein, and 50 g fat. The amount of food from each of the exchange lists will be chosen to satisfy these nutrient requirements.

Alcohol usage is determined by the attending physician. Because alcohol contains 7 calories per gram and no nutrients, it is usually substituted for fats in the diet. A chart showing the caloric content of individual servings of alcohol (one glass of wine or one glass of beer, for example) helps those diabetics who drink.

CALORIC REQUIREMENTS

Daily caloric need includes basal metabolism, activity rate, and physiological stress (such as a growth spurt or pregnancy). If the patient is overweight, the caloric range is usually 1200 to 1500 calories per day. If the patient is thin, young (growing), and male, it may be as high as 4000 calories per day.

Tables 18-2A and 18-2B contain food plans at four caloric levels, using the exchange system. They also meet the nutrient balance concept, as previously discussed, of approximately 50% carbohydrate, 20% protein, and 30% fat. Complex carbohydrates containing good amounts of fiber are emphasized when menu planning is done, as well as the use of lean protein foods and very little animal fat. There are many ways to calculate daily caloric need for an adult diabetic patient. The methods include the three categories discussed in the following sections.

TABLE 18-2A Meal Plans at Four Caloric Levels Using the Exchange System

Food Group	Daily Food Distribution			
(total/day)	1000 kcal	1200 kcal	1500 kcal	1800 kcal
Carbohydrates group*				
Starch/bread list	4	5	6	9
Vegetable list	3	3	4	4
Fruit list	3	3	4	4
Milk list (skim)	2	2	2	2
Meat and meat substitute group				
Meat (lean)	3	4	5	6
Fat				
Polyunsaturated	1	1	2	2
Monounsaturated	1	1	2	2
Saturated	0	1	1	1

*Foods from the "Other Carbohydrates" list may be substituted for any foods in the carbohydrate group, as long as they do not exceed the total carbohydrate for the day and/or result in a diet that does not meet the criteria for nutritional adequacy (balance).

TABLE 18-2B Meal Plans for Four Caloric Levels Using the Exchange System

Food Group	Menu Pattern (Number of Exchanges Each Meal)			
(total/day)	1000 kcal	1200 kcal	1500 kcal	1800 kcal
Breakfast				
Carbohydrates:				
Starch/bread	1	1	2	2
Fruit	1	1	1	1
Milk	½	½	½	½
Meat or meat substitute	0	0	1	1
Fat	1	1	1	1
Lunch				
Carbohydrates:				
Starch/bread	1	2	2	3
Vegetable	1	1	2	2
Fruit	1	1	1	1
Milk	½	½	½	½
Meat	1	2	2	2
Fat	1	1	2	2
Dinner				
Carbohydrates:				
Starch/bread	1	1	1	3
Vegetable	2	2	2	2
Fruit	1	1	1	1
Milk	½	½	½	½
Meat	2	1	2	2
Fat	0	1	2	2
Snacks*				
Carbohydrate				
Starch/bread	1	1	1	1
Milk	½	½	½	½
Fruit	0	0	1	1
Meat	0	0	0	1

*Can be used afternoon or evening (HS).

Tables or Charts Method

Most healthcare providers such as medical clinics, weight loss centers, diabetic centers, and others use standard tables or charts that provide your daily caloric needs according to the standard variables such as race, age, sex, height, and physical activity.

Ideal Weights and Basal Energy Needs Method

For nearly four decades, health professionals have been using three fundamental assumptions based on available medical observation as a base of calculating daily caloric needs:

1. A table or chart has been developed to show the "ideal" or "desirable" weight of a man or a woman.
2. A person's basal energy needs are generally figured at 1 kcal/kg body weight/hr.
3. Three levels of caloric expenditure have been developed for three levels of physical activity.

An example is described below for calculating the daily caloric need of an adult patient:

Patient's desirable weight (DW)	= DW kg
Caloric need for sedentary patient	= DW kg × 20–25 kcal/kg
Caloric need for patient with light activity	= DW kg × 30 kcal/kg
Caloric need for patient with strenuous activity	= DW kg × 35 kcal/kg

Special considerations are made for other groups: childhood, adolescence, elderly, with adjustment made if the person is overweight or underweight. As a result of new scientific studies, this method is not as popular as it once was.

Individualized Method

Scientifically, the most sophisticated method of calculating daily caloric needs uses many equations that cover several variables: race, age, sex, height, body mass index, and physical activity. This method is used mainly by large medical and research centers and applies to all age groups.

However, for children and adolescents, the following individualized method is applicable and used frequently (for children, common estimates are based on age and sex):

Up to 1 year: 120 kcal/kg of body weight
1–10 years: 100–80 kcal/kg (declines as age increases)
Adolescence:
  Male
    11–15 years: average, 65 kcal/kg body weight
    6–20 years: average, 50 kcal/kg (high activity)
            40 kcal/kg (light activity)
            30 kcal/kg (sedentary)

Female
  11–15 years: average, 35 kcal/kg body weight
  16–up years: average, 30 kcal/kg body weight

However, of all methods mentioned previously, tables and charts are used by most clinics and healthcare providers.

After the patient's daily caloric need is determined, the physician (or dietitian) will prescribe the percentage of these calories from carbohydrate, protein, and fat, respectively. Then the permitted grams of these three nutrients can be calculated.

NUTRIENT DISTRIBUTION

When the daily amounts of protein, carbohydrate, and fat have been determined, they are converted into food servings and spread throughout the day into three meals and from one to three snacks, depending on the need for insulin injection, oral drugs, activity, or a combination of these. Large amounts of food, especially carbohydrates, should be avoided at any one time. A balance of meals throughout the day provides better control. The diabetic person should have regular meal hours to avoid fluctuations in blood glucose.

FOOD EXCHANGE LISTS

The exchange system of dietary control is widely used to manage the diet of a diabetic patient. This system permits flexibility in planning and preparation and allows measuring instead of weighing. It also offers a variety of food choices. However, the student will recognize, after studying the exchange lists, that it is not a suitable guide for planning meals for some ethnic groups or in all clinical situations. People from diverse cultural backgrounds may need nutrition counseling. Many times the illiterate or confused client will not understand the exchanges as written. Some clients have vision and/or hearing impairments. At such a time, students may wish to research the particular foods needed in order to individualize the diet or to simplify it. The dietitian in a nearby healthcare facility can be an excellent source for additional information, and can assist in designing appropriate diet instructions.

The exchange system provides equivalent food value for each food within a list; for example:

Starch list: B vitamins, iron, protein, and carbohydrate

Meat list: iron, zinc, B_{12}, protein, and varying fat contents

Milk list: carbohydrate, protein, varying fat contents, folacin and other vitamins from the B complex, vitamins A and D, and minerals

Vegetable list: vitamins A, E, C, and K; B complex; fiber; protein; and carbohydrate

Fruit list: vitamins, minerals, carbohydrate, and fiber

(Refer to Appendix F for the exchange lists.)

CARING FOR A DIABETIC CHILD

Caring for a diabetic child requires many special considerations, some of which are listed below:

1. Disease characteristics:
   a. The patient may be normal or underweight.
   b. Disease onset is abrupt and increases in severity during growth periods.
   c. Pancreatic cells cannot make insulin, and a diabetic child is insulin dependent.
   d. As the patient grows older, the requirement for insulin increases.
2. Dietary treatment goals:
   a. To permit normal growth and activity
   b. To control the disease
   c. To permit a normal school and social life with minimal restriction in freedom of movement and food choices
   d. To correspond with the action of insulin treatment. To achieve the above goals, the diet must recognize the child's food preferences and differ little from that of the patient's peers. Also, the child must be provided adequate food to permit normal development and activities.
3. Diet prescription and meal planning
   a. 75–90 kcal/kg of the child's ideal weight.
   b. 3.3 to 2.2 g of protein per kg body weight, with decreasing amount for increasing age.
   c. 50% of total calories from complex carbohydrate, 20% from protein, and 30% from fat.
   d. Three meals and three snacks daily usually, with other meal patterns determined by patient's clinical condition, amount of insulin needed, daily activities, and other factors.
   e. Meal plan coordinated with activities—sweets and extra fluids for strenuous and prolonged activities, eating a prescribed snack just before an exercise.
4. Patient compliance and education
   a. A young diabetic will accept a diet if it is not too different from that of his or her peers, and if it permits the child freedom in school and play.
   b. The patient should learn how to use the exchange lists for fast foods, which is included in the patient's booklets for meal planning. This permits the child to eat fast foods with his or her friends without deviating from the dietary prescription.

INSULIN PREPARATIONS, ORAL HYPOGLYCEMIC AGENTS (OHAS OR DIABETES PILLS), AND NEW DRUG THERAPY

Diet therapy must be coordinated with the patient's use of insulin or oral agent as prescribed by the attending physician. A pharmacist can help to interpret Tables 18-3 and 18-4 for the patient, and the specific medica-

tion that the patient has been prescribed should be emphasized.

The RN should:

1. Reinforce the pharmacist's teaching and help patients to understand the medication used to help control their diabetes. Interpret and explain these tables to the patient if no pharmacist is available.
2. Teach patients to use insulin or diabetic pills properly according to their prescription.
3. Coordinate meal and snack times with the prescribed medication.

Insulin Preparations

There are more than 20 types of insulin products available in four basic forms, each with a different time of onset and duration of action. The decision as to which insulin to choose is based on an individual's lifestyle, a physician's preference and experience, and the person's blood sugar level. Among the criteria considered in choosing insulin are:

- How soon it starts working (onset)
- When it works the hardest (peak time)
- How long it lasts in the body (duration)

Since 1982, most of the newly approved insulin preparations have been produced by inserting portions of DNA ("recombinant DNA") into special lab-cultivated bacteria or yeast. This process allows the bacteria or yeast cells to produce complete human insulin. Recombinant human insulin has, for the most part, replaced animal-derived insulin, such as pork and beef insulin. More recently, insulin products called "insulin analogs" have been produced so that the structure differs slightly from human insulin (by one or two amino acids) to change onset and peak of action. Table 18-3 lists some of the more common insulin preparations available today. Onset, peak, and duration of action are approximate for each insulin product, as there may be variability depending on each individual, the injection site, and the individual's exercise program.

Insulin Delivery Devices

All insulin delivery devices inject insulin through the skin and into the fatty tissue below. Most people inject the insulin with a syringe that delivers insulin just under the skin. Others use insulin pens, jet injectors, or insulin pumps. Several new approaches for taking insulin are under development.

Syringes

Syringes are hypodermic needles attached to hollow barrels that people with diabetes use to inject insulin. Insulin syringes are small with very sharp points. Most have a special coating to help the needles enter the skin as pain-

Table 18-3   Insulin Preparations

Type of Insulin	Examples	Onset of Action	Peak of Action	Duration of Action
Rapid-acting	Humalog (lispro) Eli Lilly	15 minutes	30–90 minutes	3–5 hours
	NovoLog (aspart) Novo Nordisk	15 minutes	40–50 minutes	3–5 hours
Short-acting (Regular)	Humulin R Eli Lilly Novolin R Novo Nordisk	30–60 minutes	50–120 minutes	5–8 hours
Intermediate-acting (NPH)	Humulin N Eli Lilly	1–3 hours	8 hours	20 hours
	Humulin L Eli Lilly	1–2.5 hours	7–15 hours	18–24 hours
Intermediate- and short-acting mixtures	Humulin 50/50 Humulin 70/30 Humalog Mix 75/25 Humalog Mix 50/50 Eli Lilly Novolin 70/30 Novolog Mix 70/30 Novo Nordisk	The onset, peak, and duration of action of these mixtures would reflect a composit of the intermediate and short- or rapid-acting components, with one peak of action.		
Long-acting	Ultralente Eli Lilly	4–8 hours	8–12 hours	36 hours
	Lantus (glargine) Aventis	1 hour	none	24 hours

Source: U.S. Food and Drug Administration

lessly as possible. Insulin syringes come in several different sizes to match insulin strength and dosage.

Insulin Pens

Insulin pens look like pens with cartridges, but the cartridges are filled with insulin rather than ink. They can be used instead of needles for giving insulin injections. Some pens use replaceable cartridges of insulin; other models are totally disposable after the prefilled cartridge is empty. A fine, short needle, like the needle on an insulin syringe, is on the tip of the pen. Users turn a dial to select the desired dose of insulin and press a plunger on the end to deliver the insulin just under the skin.

Jet Injectors

Insulin jet injectors may be an option for people who do not want to use needles. These devices use high-pressure air to send a find spray of insulin through the skin. Jet injectors have no needles.

Insulin Pumps

Insulin pumps are small pumping devices worn outside of your body. They connect by flexible tubing to a catheter that is located under the skin of your abdomen. The following recommendations are for a diabetic who likes to use this device:

- Program the pump to dispense the necessary amount of insulin.
- Usually, set the pump to give a steady small dose of insulin, but you can give an additional amount in a short time if needed, such as after a meal.
- If adjusted properly, these pumps allow close control of your insulin levels without multiple injections.
- Do not use this type of pump during physical activities that may damage the pump or disrupt the pump's connection to the body.
- You still need to monitor your blood glucose levels regularly if you use this type of device.

Oral Hypoglycemic Agents (OHAs or Diabetic Pills)

Insulin is produced by the beta cells in the islets of Langerhans in the pancreas. When glucose enters the blood, the pancreas should automatically produce the right amount of insulin to move glucose into the cells. People with type 2 diabetes either produce too little insulin, produce it too late to match the rise in blood glucose, or do not respond correctly to the insulin that is produced. Then glucose builds up in the blood, overflows into the urine, and passes out of the body. This means that the body loses its main source of energy even though the blood contains large amounts of glucose.

Diabetes pills work in one of three ways. They either stimulate the pancreas to release more insulin, increase the body's sensitivity to the insulin that is already present, or slow the breakdown of foods (especially starches) into glucose.

There are six categories of diabetes pills: sulfonylureas, meglitinides, nateglinides, biguanide thiazolidinediones, and alpha-glucose inhibitors. These are shown in Table 18-4.

New Drug Therapy

In 2006, the FDA approved the first ever inhaled insulin, Exubera, an inhaled powder form of recombinant human insulin for the treatment of adult patients with type 1 and type 2 diabetes. It is the first new insulin delivery option introduced since the discovery of insulin in the 1920s. This is a new, potential alternative for many of the more than 5 million Americans who take insulin injections.

NURSING IMPLICATIONS

Since diabetes is a lifelong disease, the client needs to learn to take responsibility for self-care. To promote this outcome requires extensive education.

Congress passed legislation allowing medical nutrition therapy (MNT) services to be compensated by insurance companies after the cost-effectiveness of such therapy was demonstrated. The registered dietitian (RD) is designated to be the primary teacher, but the nurse has a major role in the teaching process. In fact, diabetes education centers employ many RNs as well as RDs for teaching classes that help patients understand and control their disease (Certified Diabetes Educators). Nurses are part of a teaching team; therefore, they must be able to teach as well as reinforce the information that all diabetic clients need. The topics covered should include the following:

1. Explanation of the disease and why the diet will help the client control it
2. Principles of managing the diet:

Table 18-4 Oral Antidiabetes Medications

Category	Action	Generic Name	Brand Name	Manufacturer
Sulfonylurea	Stimulates beta cells to release more insulin	Chlorpropamide	Diabinese	Pfizer
		Glipizide	Glucotrol	Pfizer
		Glyburide	DiaBeta/Micronase/ Glynase	Aventis, Pharmacia and Upjohn
		Glimepride	Amaryl	Aventis
Meglitinide	Works with similar action to sulfonylureas	Repaglinide	Prandin	Novo Nordisk
Nateglinide	Works with similar action to sulfonylureas	Nateglinide	Starlix	Novartis
Biguanide	Sensitizes the body to the insulin already present	Metformin	Glucophage	Bristol Myers Squibb
		Metformin (long lasting)	Glucophage XR	Bristol Myers Squibb
		Metformin with glyburide	Glucovance	Bristol Myers Squibb
Thiazolidinedione (Glitazone)	Helps insulin work better in muscle and fat; lowers insulin resistance	Rosiglitazone	Avandia	GlaxoSmithKline
		Pioglitazone	Actos	Takeda Pharmaceuticals
Alpha-Glucose Inhibitor	Slows or blocks the breakdown of starches and certain sugars; action slows the rise in blood sugar levels following a meal	Acarbose	Precose	Bayer
		Miglitol	Glyset	Pharmacia and Upjohn

Source: U.S. Food and Drug Administration

a. Basic nutrition needs

b. Meal planning following the individual prescription

c. Menu planning that allows variety in the diet

d. Purchase and preparation practices appropriate to the diet therapy

e. Adjustments for illness or unusual activity, especially strenuous exercise

f. Diabetic foods

- Diabetic foods are different from dietetic foods. The first group is either sugar-free or reduced in sugar content. The second refers to foods reduced in sugar, sodium, protein, or some other nutrients.
- Diabetic foods are recommended for some but not all patients. Regular foods suitable for everyone are usually recommended, with only a few exceptions.

g. A relative or caretaker who can assist with meal planning should be present during patient education.

h. The patient should be provided with as much information as possible. Some examples include:

- Food exchange lists
- Diet plans, written or in picture form
- Scheduled meal times and frequency
- List of recommended cookbooks
- Audio cassettes (if client is vision impaired)

The patient's level of reading and comprehension must be considered, as well as any physical limitations. Diabetic patients required to restrict sodium intake must be taught basic knowledge of the sodium content of foods.

i. Some over-the-counter, prescription, or illicit drugs interfere with glucose test results. For example, experience has confirmed that prolonged excess vitamin C intake can lead to a false urinary glucose test.

3. How to monitor blood and urine, why it is needed, and how to keep good records

4. How to inject insulin: dosage, type, site rotation, and why timing of meals to insulin schedule is important

5. How to recognize symptoms of hypoglycemia or hyperglycemia and what to do about them

6. Why an exercise program is adjunct to diet therapy

7. Complications of uncontrolled diabetes, especially atherosclerosis, which is 25% higher in the diabetic population than in the nondiabetic population

8. Special dietary measures to prevent or delay onset of atherosclerosis: reduced fat intake, increased fiber intake

9. Dietary teaching begins with diagnosis or hospital admission, and not after discharge.

Since any comprehensive and successful diabetes management program must always include patient education, some special guidelines to assist in teaching follow.

Patient Education

A diabetic person may become ill from causes such as infection, trauma, and so on. Patients with a short-term illness should follow the guidelines indicated in Exhibit 18-1.

The patient is the most important member of the healthcare team. His or her participation and cooperation must be gained.

Who to Teach and How

1. Teaching one patient instead of a group of patients is more useful to the patient, although it is more costly in time and money.

2. If group education is used, patients should be sorted by their type of diabetes (e.g., young and insulin-dependent diabetics, obese patients using OHAs, and patients who are maintaining by diet alone). This sorting reduces confusion in the teaching process. If feasible, the use of both individualized and group education is ideal.

3. The benefits and limitations of using paraprofessionals to teach the patient should be considered.

4. The patient's history should be studied, especially the type of diet instructions he or she has previously received. This ensures that the patient will not receive contradictory information during an education session. Any information presented that seems to conflict with previous instructions should be explained to a patient's satisfaction.

5. At least one close relative or the patient's caretaker should be familiar with the information presented to the patient and should be present for the teaching sessions.

Some teaching aids and counseling services for diabetic persons include:

Local, city, and county diabetic programs and support groups

Private and public diabetic (clinical) centers

Professional sources of materials include drug companies, American Dietetic Association, American Diabetes Association, state health agencies, diabetes educators

Food models, films, and slides

Ethnic teaching materials

Demonstration kitchens and demonstration food portion sizes

Recipes and cookbooks

Evaluation and follow-up teaching by the nurse or a clinical nutrition specialist should be scheduled.

EXHIBIT 18-1   Sick Day Guidelines

1. Never omit the daily dosage of insulin, even if you feel too ill to eat your normal diet. You must consume some nourishment.
   a. If feasible, take fluids hourly. Keep a record. Use small amounts. Clear soups and broths will replace fluids lost in vomiting and in diarrhea.
   b. Liquids and carbohydrates are more easily tolerated during illness than proteins and fats. Determine the amount of carbohydrate you are allowed per meal and try to consume items listed below until you reach your carbohydrate allowance.
2. Check your diet plan. Food containing carbohydrates are fruits, milk, breads, and vegetables. Table 18-1 shows the amount of carbohydrate per exchange (serving) in each list. Multiply the carbohydrate amount by the number of exchanges allowed in each food group. An example for breakfast is

1 fruit	=	15 g carbohydrate
1 milk	=	12 g carbohydrate
2 bread	=	30 g carbohydrate
1 meat	=	0 g carbohydrate
1 fat	=	0 g carbohydrate
TOTAL	=	57 g carbohydrate

3. Fluids easily tolerated are listed below along with their carbohydrate equivalents:

15 g carbohydrate: ¾ c ginger ale; ⅓ c grape juice; ½ c orange juice; ½ c apple or pineapple juice

12 g carbohydrate: 1 c milk; 1 c chocolate milk; 1 c tomato soup; 1 c buttermilk; 1 c soy milk

15 g carbohydrate: 1 frozen juice bar; ½ c plain ice cream; ½ c regular gelatin (any flavor)

4. If you are still unable to eat after four or five liquid meals, call your physician for advice and take the following precautions:
   a. Stay warm in bed. If possible, have a relative or friend nearby in case of an insulin reaction.
   b. Test your urine for glucose (sugar) and acetone (ketone) every six hours or so. If blood glucose is over 250 mg/dl a test for ketones should be done every 4 hours. Have the results available when you call your physician. Even though you are now eating less (as a result of nausea and vomiting) than you usually do, your urine will show sugar and possible acetone. You will always need your normal insulin dose. Again, do not omit your daily insulin dose. Sometimes you may even need extra insulin. This may be in the form of regular insulin.
5. Call your physician if you are ill for more than 48 to 72 hours or if vomiting or diarrhea persists for more than a few hours. It is better to call sooner than to put yourself in jeopardy.
6. Be prepared. Keep the following or similar items on hand: paregoric, Maalox, Tylenol, milk of magnesia, glucagon, usual insulin, and refrigerated regular insulin. Take prescribed item(s) with physician's consent.

PROGRESS CHECK ON ACTIVITY 1

With the use of the exchange lists in Appendix F, complete the following:

1. Fill out Exercise 18-1 for a calculated diet for diabetes mellitus.

MULTIPLE CHOICE

Circle the letter of the correct answer.

2. Which of the following foods is not a member of any of the meat exchange groups?
   a. ½ c pinto beans
   b. soy milk, 1 c

Exercise 18-1

Complete the chart by filling in the information for each column.

Diet	Disease or Condition	Foods Allowed	Foods Limited	Foods Forbidden	Nursing Implications
Calculated	Diabetes Mellitus				

c. peanut butter, 1 tbsp
d. 1 hot dog

3. Which of the following statements correctly describes the action of insulin?

   a. Insulin controls the entry of glucose into the cell.
   b. Insulin regulates the conversion of glucose to glycogen.
   c. Insulin decreases the conversion of glucose to fat for storage as adipose fat tissue.
   d. Insulin allows fat to be converted to glucose as needed to return the blood glucose levels to normal.

4. The caloric value of a diabetic diet should be:

   a. increased above normal requirements to meet the increased metabolic demand.
   b. decreased below normal requirements to prevent glucose formation.
   c. the individual's normal energy requirement to maintain ideal weight.
   d. contributed mainly by fat to spare carbohydrate.

5. In the exchange system of diet control, an ounce of canned tuna may be exchanged for all except:

   a. the same amount of lean meat.
   b. ¼ c 4% cottage cheese.
   c. ½ c tofu, light.
   d. one egg.

6. The exchange system of diet control is based on principles of:

   a. equivalent food values.
   b. flexible food choices.
   c. nutritional balance.
   d. all of the above.

7. How much orange juice would substitute for the CHO in an uneaten slice of bread?

   a. ½ c
   b. ¾ c
   c. 1 c
   d. 1–½ c

8. The diabetic diet is designed for long-term use and contains a balance of:

   a. energy.
   b. nutrients.
   c. distribution.
   d. all of the above.

9. Sources of blood glucose include:

   a. carbohydrates.
   b. proteins.

c. fats.
d. all of the above.

10. If 50% of the total calories in a 1500 calorie diabetic diet is from carbohydrates, how many grams of carbohydrate will the diet contain? (Round to nearest whole number.)

    a. 50
    b. 150
    c. 190
    d. 210

11. Emphasis is placed on using polyunsaturated fats and limiting foods high in cholesterol in the diet of the diabetic. The reason for this is:

    a. to aid in the prevention of cardiovascular diseases.
    b. to aid in the digestive process.
    c. to prevent skin breakdown.
    d. to control blood sugar.

12. The daily intake of foods for the diabetic is spaced at regular intervals throughout the day. The reason for this is:

    a. to prevent hunger pangs.
    b. to avoid symptoms of hypoglycemia or hyperglycemia.
    c. to modify eating habits.
    d. to prevent obesity.

13. Sally, an 8-year-old diabetic, is ready to go home from the hospital. Sally's mother should know that:

    a. all of her food must be measured.
    b. she needs a snack before she exercises.
    c. she should always carry hard candy with her.
    d. all of the above.

TRUE/FALSE

Circle T for True and F for False.

14. T F The majority of adult-onset diabetics are underweight at the time the disease is discovered.

15. T F A diabetic diet is a combination of specific special foods that cannot be changed.

16. T F Diabetics should follow a low carbohydrate diet of about 50 g a day.

17. T F A medium-size fresh peach contains 10 g carbohydrate and 40 calories.

18. T F Insulin preparations now available are produced by recombinant DNA.

19. T F Insulin analogs differ from regular insulin in their onset and peak action.

20. T F Insulin is used to metabolize sugar in the body.

A diabetic patient in the hospital received insulin in the morning and ate breakfast, but was nauseated at lunch and could not eat. Circle T for the appropriate nursing interventions for this situation and F for the inappropriate ones.

21. T F Remove the lunch tray and tell the patient to let you know when he feels like eating.
22. T F Relieve the nausea by appropriate means.
23. T F Remove the lunch tray, asking the meal preparers to substitute liquids of equal value for the carbohydrate foods on the tray.
24. T F After you observe that the patient is better, offer him or her the liquids you ordered.

MATCHING

Match the foods in the left column with their nutrient values in the right column.

25. 1 slice bacon
26. 2 tbsp peanut butter
27. ½ c oatmeal
28. ½ c beets
29. ½ c tofu

   a. 12 g carbohydrate, 8 g protein, 5 g fat
   b. 15 g carbohydrate, 3 g protein
   c. 5 g carbohydrate, 2 g protein
   d. 7 g protein, 5 g fat
   e. 5 g fat

LISTING AND DESCRIPTION

30. List five nursing implications for dietary care of a diabetic patient.

   a. _____
   b. _____
   c. _____
   d. _____
   e. _____

31. Describe 5 of the 10 essential factors that a diabetic patient must know to control his or her disease.

   a. _____
   b. _____
   c. _____
   d. _____
   e. _____

FILL-IN

32. Calculate the carbohydrate, protein, and fat value of the following day's allowance:

	Carbohydrate (grams)	Protein (grams)	Fat (grams)
Milk (2%), 2 exchanges	_____	_____	_____
Vegetables, 3 exchanges	_____	_____	_____
Fruit, 3 exchanges	_____	_____	_____
Lean meat, 6 exchanges	_____	_____	_____
Medium fat meat, 2 exchanges	_____	_____	_____
Fat, 5 exchanges	_____	_____	_____
Bread, 6 exchanges	_____	_____	_____

33. Arrange the allowances in Question 32 into a day's menu:

   Breakfast   Lunch   Dinner   Snack

MULTIPLE CHOICE

Circle the letter of the correct answer.

34. The caloric value of the diet in Question 32 is approximately:

   a. 1250 calories.
   b. 1500 calories
   c. 1600 calories.
   d. 1850 calories.

35. An intake reduction of 1000 calories daily would enable an obese person to lose weight at which of the following rates:

   a. 1 lb per week
   b. 2 lb per week
   c. 3 lb per week
   d. 4 lb per week

36. Which two of the following food portions have the lowest caloric values:

   a. 4 oz lean meat
   b. 1 granola bar
   c. 1 slice raisin bread
   d. 1 8-oz glass of whole milk

SHORT ANSWERS

37. People with type II diabetes usually have one of the following conditions:

   a. _____
   b. _____
   c. _____

38. The three criteria that should be considered in choosing insulin are:

a. _____

b. _____

c. _____

39. The four basic types of insulin products are:

a. _____

b. _____

c. _____

d. _____

40. The three ways diabetes pills work in the body are:

a. _____

b. _____

c. _____

REFERENCES

American Diabetes Association. (2007). *Food Exchange Lists for Diabetes.* Alexandria, VA: Author.

American Dietetic Association. (2006). *Nutrition Diagnosis: A Critical Step in Nutrition Care Process.* Chicago: Author.

American Dietetic Association. (2007). *Food Exchange Lists for Diabetes.* Chicago: Author.

Beham, E. (2006). *Therapeutic Nutrition: A Guide to Patient Education.* Philadelphia: Lippincott, Williams and Wilkins.

Bendich, A., & Deckelbaum, R. J. (Eds.). (2005). *Preventive Nutrition: The Comprehensive Guide for Health Professionals* (3rd ed.). Totowa, NJ: Humana Press.

Buchman, A. (2004). *Practical Nutritional Support Technique* (2nd ed.). Thorofeue, NJ: SLACK.

Caballero, B., Allen, L., & Prentice, A. (Eds.). (2005). *Encyclopedia of Human Nutrition* (2nd ed.). Boston: Elsevier/Academic Press.

Coulston, A. M., Rock, C. L., & Monsen, E. L. (Eds.). (2001). *Nutrition in the Prevention and Treatment of Disease.* San Diego, CA: Academic Press.

D'Adamo, P. (2004). *Diabetes: Fight It with Blood Type Diet.* New York: Putman.

Deen, D., & Hark, L. (2007). *The Complete Guide to Nutrition in Primary Care.* Malden, MA: Blackwell.

Gibertson, H. R. (2003). Effect of low-glycemic-index dietary advice on dietary quality and food choice in children with type 1 diabetes. *American Journal of Clinical Nutrition, 77*: 83–90.

Green Pastor, J. (2003). How effective is medical nutrition therapy in diabetes care? *Journal of American Dietetic Association, 103*: 827–831.

Hark, L., & Morrison, G. (Eds.). (2003). *Medical Nutrition and Disease* (3rd ed.). Malden, MA: Blackwell.

Lewis, G., & Thomson, L. L. (2005). *Optimizing Glycemic Control with Diabetes Technology and Diabetes Medical Nutrition Therapy with Advanced Insulin Management.* Chicago: American Dietetic Association.

Mahan, L. K., & Escott-Stump, S. (Eds.). (2008). *Krause's Food and Nutrition Therapy* (12th ed.). Philadelphia: Elsevier Saunders.

Mann, J. I. (2006). Nutrition recommendations for the treatment and prevention of type 2 diabetes and the metabolic syndrome: An evidenced-based review. *Nutrition Reviews, 64*: 422–427.

Mann, J., & Truswell, S. (Eds.). (2007). *Essentials of human nutrition* (3rd ed.). New York: Oxford University Press.

Nasu, R. (2005). Effect of fruit, species and herbs on glucocidase activity and glycemic index. *Food Science and Technology Research, 11*: 77–81.

Nuttall, F. Q. (2007). Dietary management of type 2 diabetes: A personal odyssey. *Journal of American College of Nutrition, 26*(2): 83–94.

Physicians Committee for Responsible Medicine. (2002). *Healthy Eating for Life to Prevent and Treat Diabetes.* New York: John Wiley.

Powers, M. (2003). *American Dietetic Association Guide to Eating Right When You Have Diabetes.* New York: Wiley & Sons.

Reader, D. (2006). Impact of gestational diabetes mellitus nutrition practice guidelines implemented by registered dieticians. *Journal of American Dietetic Association, 106*: 1426–1433.

Ross, T., Boucher, J. L., & O'Connell, B. S. (Eds.). (2005). *American Dietetic Association Guide to Diabetes Medical Nutrition Therapy and Education.* Chicago: American Dietetic Association.

Shils, M. E., & Shike, M. (Eds.). (2006). *Modern Nutrition in Health and Disease* (10th ed.). Philadelphia: Lippincott, Williams and Wilkins.

Tahbaz, F. (2006). An audit of diabetes control, dietary management, and quality of life in adults with type 1 diabetes mellitus. *Journal of Human Nutrition and Dietetics, 19*(1): 1–3.

Thomas, A. M., & Gutierrez, Y. M. (2005). *American Dietetic Association Guide to Gestational Diabetes Mellitus.* Chicago: American Dietetic Association.

Thomas, B., & Bishop, J. (Eds.). (2007). *Manual of Dietetic Practice* (4th ed.). Ames, IA: Blackwell.

CHAPTER **19**

Diet and Disorders of the Liver, Gallbladder, and Pancreas

Time for completion
Activities: 1 hour
Optional examination: ½ hour

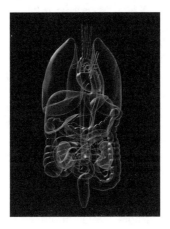

OBJECTIVES

Upon completion of this chapter, the student should be able to do the following:

1. Describe the major functions of the normal liver.
2. Identify the appropriate diet therapy for treating liver diseases and state the rationale for its use in treating hepatitis, cirrhosis, hepatic coma and liver failure, and cancer.
3. Describe the diet therapy used for liver transplantation.
4. Evaluate nursing interventions to promote optimal nutrition in a patient with liver disease.
5. Discuss the causes of gallbladder and pancreatic disorders, and describe how they affect food metabolism.
6. Identify the sequence of physiological events in which bile assists in the absorption and metabolism of foods.
7. Differentiate among cholecystitis, cholelithiasis, and cholecystectomy in relation to their effects on the digestion and metabolism of foods.
8. Describe and give examples of the diet therapy used for gallbladder disease.
9. Identify the major causes of pancreatitis.

10. Relate the association between pancreatitis and gallbladder disease.
11. Describe the diet therapy for pancreatitis and the reasons for its use.
12. Discuss appropriate nursing interventions for patients with gallbladder disease or pancreatitis.

GLOSSARY

Ascites: abnormal accumulation of serous fluid within the peritoneal cavity (the space between the abdominal walls and the pelvic cavity).

Calculi ("stones"): an abnormal concretion, usually of mineral salts, occurring in the body in hollow organs or passages.

Cholecystectomy: removal of the gallbladder by surgical procedure.

Cholecystitis: inflammation of the gallbladder, acute or chronic.

Cholecystokinin: a hormone secreted in the small intestine that stimulates gallbladder contraction and secretion of pancreatic enzymes.

Cholelithiasis: calculi in the common bile duct.

Cholesterol: a steroid alcohol found in animal fats, bile, blood, brain tissue, whole milk, egg yolk, liver, kidneys, adrenal gland, and the myelin sheath of nerve fibers.

Edema: abnormal accumulation of fluid in the intercellular spaces of the body.

Emulsify: to mix together two immiscible liquids. One is dispersed into the other in small drops.

Encephalopathy: any chronic degenerative disease of the brain.

Esophageal varices: varicose veins in the esophagus that occur most often as a result of obstruction of the portal circulation.

Fulminant: sudden, severe; occurring suddenly with great intensity.

Gallbladder (GB): the pear-shaped organ located below the liver which serves as a storage place for bile.

Hepatic: pertaining to the liver.

Hepatitis virus classification:

Hepatitis A virus (HAV), previously called infectious hepatitis, is spread by the oral-fecal route from an infected person through contaminated water and food. Although it is a very serious disease it does not cause chronic hepatitis or cirrhosis. A recent vaccine, better than gamma globulin, is now on the market.

Hepatitis B virus (HBV), formerly called serum hepatitis, is classified as a sexually transmitted disease (STD) because it is spread via body fluids, semen, saliva, tears, and by needle-sharing among drug users. It is a major factor in chronic liver disease and liver cancer. It can persist a lifetime in body fluids. Up to 75% of carriers are Asian.

Hepatitis C virus (HCV) is associated with chronic active hepatitis, liver cirrhosis, and liver cancer.

Hepatitis D virus (HDV), previously called non-A, non-B, is toxic to functional liver cells and may be related to the onset of HAV and HBV.

Hepatitis E virus (HEV), the newest of the discovered viral liver diseases, has a mortality rate of 80%–90%. It may be due to toxic liver injury such as with carbon tetrachloride or acetaminophen overdose. Pregnant women who contract HEV, usually in the third trimester, die of fulminant liver failure.

Jaundice: yellowness of the skin, mucous membranes, and excretions (jaundice is not a disease, but is a symptom of numerous disorders of the liver, gallbladder, and blood; it occurs when pigment in the blood is destroyed).

Marasmus: protein-calorie malnutrition, causing growth retardation and wasting of muscle.

Pancreas: a large elongated gland located transversely behind the stomach between the spleen and duodenum.

Portal (circulation): circulation of blood through layer vessels from the capillaries of one organ to those of another (applies here especially to passage of blood from the GI tract and spleen through the portal vein to the liver).

Psychotropic: capable of modifying mental activity; a drug that affects the mental state.

BACKGROUND INFORMATION

Liver

A normal liver regulates the proper digestion, metabolism, and absorption of food. The following is an outline of the liver's major functions:

1. Storage—The liver stores:
   a. Approximately 1 lb of glycogen, the body's emergency energy supply; this supply lasts 12 to 36 hours when used as the only energy source.
   b. More fat-soluble than water-soluble vitamins
   c. More iron than any other part of the body
2. Circulation—The liver regulates:
   a. Blood volume
   b. Blood transfer from the portal to systemic circulation
   c. Fluid transfers
3. Metabolism—The liver participates in:
   a. Carbohydrate metabolism by interconverting glucose and glycogen as needed; it also converts amino acids to glucose in the presence of excess protein or low carbohydrate level
   b. Fat metabolism by providing bile salts for emulsifying fat, cholesterol, and lipoproteins and by converting excess amino acid and carbohydrate to fats
   c. Protein metabolism by forming plasma proteins, prothrombin, and urea

4. Detoxification—The liver detoxifies all ingested:
   1. Drugs
   2. Poisons

From the functions of the liver listed, it should be obvious that a diseased liver adversely affects gastrointestinal function and the use of food.

Gallbladder and Pancreas

The gallbladder (GB) is an accessory organ to the gastrointestinal (GI) tract. The emulsification of fats by bile salts from the GB is an important contribution to the overall efficiency of GI functioning. Gallbladder disease is a common but potentially serious disorder. The most common disorder is cholelithiasis, or formation of gallstones. It develops in 10%–20% of the Western world's population. Nearly 80%–90% of gallstones are composed primarily of cholesterol.

Some population groups are more susceptible to GB disease, such as older men and women, and especially women who have borne children. Others include Native Americans and individuals using oral contraceptives and drugs that lower blood cholesterol levels. Heredity appears to have a major influence in the development of gallstones. Diet plays a role, but a minor one. For example, excess use of polyunsaturated fats can increase the incidence of GB disease.

Other contributing factors include obesity and intestinal diseases that involve the malabsorption of bile salts. Occasionally, the stress of pregnancy is responsible. Populations with a low intake of total fat appear to be less vulnerable to cholelithiasis.

Medical management of GB disease includes temporary use of drugs to dissolve the stones, and surgery if the patient is not undernourished or obese. An undernourished patient can be replenished, while an obese one can lose weight. The actual surgery (cholecystectomy) has less nutritional implication than believed previously. The procedure allows bile to enter the small intestine on a continuous basis. With time, the bile ducts may enlarge and store bile. Because of this adaptation, many clients resume a normal diet one to two months after surgery.

Because the pancreas is an important accessory organ of the GI tract and a major producer of digestive enzymes, any pancreatic disorder can seriously impair the body's ability to digest food. Reduced production of pancreatic enzymes may occur in cystic fibrosis, chronic pancreatitis, pancreatic cancer, or protein-calorie malnutrition. The pancreas may become inflamed and/or obstructed by chronic alcohol abuse or GB disease. Food eaten during these conditions becomes the source of excruciating pain, and the client will avoid eating. Consequently, the person's nutritional status is very poor. Determining the type of pancreatic disorder is of major importance when planning nutritional care for patients with pancreatitis.

ACTIVITY 1:

Diet Therapy for Diseases of the Liver

DIET THERAPY FOR HEPATITIS

Viral hepatitis, inflammation of the liver, is a major world health problem, causing the illness and death of millions of people. Currently scientists have discovered five types of hepatitis. They are described in the glossary. Even though they are unrelated in function, the goal of medical management and diet therapy for hepatitis of any type is to promote liver tissue healing.

Medical management for hepatitis includes (a) optimum nutrition for healing, (b) complete bed rest to reduce inflammation and metabolism, and (c) alcohol and all other drugs are prohibited to avoid further liver damage. Diet therapy appropriate for hepatitis includes the following considerations:

1. Protein: 1.2–1.5 g/kg body weight per day
2. Carbohydrate: no carbohydrate restriction; however, serum glucose should be monitored as hyper- and hypoglycemia can result from liver dysfunction.
3. Fat: 30% of calories, with restrictions only indicated with maldigestion due to reduced synthesis and secretions of bile acids
4. Energy (Calories): 25–35 kcal/kg body weight per day
5. A multivitamin mineral supplement at 100% of the RDAs/DRIs may be necessary.
6. Fluids and sodium restriction may be necessary if edema or ascites is present.
7. If adequate nutrition cannot be maintained by oral feedings, enteral feedings or TPN may be indicated.

Table 19-1 presents a sample menu for a high-carbohydrate, high-protein, high-vitamin, and moderate-fat diet. Food may need to be liquid at first; concentrated formulas can be used that contain a modified fat content, as tolerated by the patient.

DIET THERAPY FOR CIRRHOSIS

Cirrhosis is the final stage of certain liver injuries, including alcoholism, untreated hepatitis, biliary obstruction, and drug and poison ingestion. Malnutrition, chronic active hepatitis, and excessive intake of vitamin A for a prolonged time also induce cirrhosis. In fact, cited cases of vitamin A overdose that produced cirrhosis, and ultimately death, report doses ranging from 25,000 IU to 100,000 IU taken continuously for two to six years. The persons believed they were improving their health. The liver is unable to generate new cells, which are replaced with fibrous, nonfunctioning tissue.

Stages of Cirrhosis

Cirrhosis has early and late stages. The early stages affect the digestive system and cause such symptoms as nausea,

TABLE 19-1   Sample Menu for a Diet Containing Approximately 2500 kcal, 90 g of Protein, 300 g of Carbohydrate, and 100 g of Fat

Breakfast	Lunch	Dinner
Orange juice 1 c	Grape juice, ½ c	Lamb chop, 1
Eggs, scrambled	Tuna salad, ½ c	Carrots, cooked, 1 c
Muffin, whole wheat, 2	Lettuce leaves, 4	Cole slaw, with mustard and vinegar, 1 c
Margarine, 1 pat	Tomato, 2 slices	Potato, baked, 1 med
Coffee, tea	Bread, whole wheat, 2 slices	Margarine, 1 tbsp
Sugar	Milk, skim, 1 c	Milk, skim, 1 c
Salt, pepper	Coffee, tea	Fresh peach
Jelly	Sugar	Coffee, tea
Salt, pepper	Sugar	
	Salt, pepper	
Snack		
8 oz low-fat yogurt	Snack	
	4 sugar cookies	
	Apple juice, 1 c	

vomiting, distention, diarrhea, and anorexia. These symptoms are managed by a dietary plan similar to that for hepatitis. The rationale also is the same: to support residual liver function and prevent further cell destruction. Compliance with dietary and other medical recommendations will delay development of the late stages of the disease for years for some patients.

In the later stages of cirrhosis, the patient is severely malnourished. Edema, ascites, anemia, infections, intestinal bleeding, jaundice, and esophageal varices may be present. Renal failure also may occur. The patient is in critical condition. Primarily, a diet high in protein, carbohydrate, vitamins, and calories, and moderate in fat is preferred for advanced cirrhosis. However, other dietary changes are prescribed according to the patient's condition:

1. Protein—If hepatic coma is not indicated, protein remains at 75 to 100 g daily. If, however, the patient shows signs of impending coma, the physician should reduce protein intake to lessen the chance of coma.
2. Sodium—Edema and/or ascites is counteracted by a 500 to 1000 mg sodium (daily) diet. Fluid intake may be limited. Refer to Chapter 16 for sodium-restricted diets.
3. Texture—Esophageal varices, if present, are managed by semisolid or liquid diets to avoid potential rupture and hemorrhage. Tube feedings are not advised for patients with this complication. These patients should avoid coffee, tea, pepper, chili powder, and other irritating seasonings.

For a patient with poor appetite, other measures are used to provide adequate nutrients and calories. These include oral formulas high in nutrients and calories;

vitamin/mineral supplements; electrolyte replacements; hepatic aids; and parenteral feedings.

If the cirrhosis is alcohol induced, deficiency of magnesium and vitamin B complex is often present. Alcohol reduces vitamin absorption and increases mineral excretion.

HEPATIC ENCEPHALOPATHY (COMA)

Hepatic coma is caused by brain damage resulting from the inability of a damaged liver to metabolize ammonia compounds. Irritability, confusion, drowsiness, apathy, and irrational behavior precede the coma. Other signs are motor dysfunction and fecal breath odor. Ammonia is formed from protein in the intestines by bacterial action. The protein may be ingested or derived from blood (bleeding into the intestine). Treatment includes antibiotics, psychotropic drugs, enemas to remove blood and protein from the bowel, and diet therapy. Diet therapy in impending hepatic coma is as follows:

1. Protein intake is limited to 0 to 50 g daily, depending on the blood ammonia level. Note that dietary protein is derived chiefly from milk and meats and is of high biological value. It produces minimal ammonia because it is used optimally without waste; that is, it is not metabolized for energy.
   Supplemental branched chain amino acids (leucine, isoleucine, and valine) can be used as a source of protein for the heart, muscle, and brain, as well as for energy. They are not dependent on the liver but are metabolized by other body tissues.
2. The diet provides 1500 to 2000 calories per day, mainly derived from carbohydrates and fat. This reduces tissue breakdown and ammonia formation.

3. Vitamins are given intravenously; vitamin K is especially needed to reduce bleeding.
4. Fluid output is balanced by equal intake. Urine voided and other fluid lost are recorded.
5. TPN or enteral nutrition are also standard forms of diet therapy for liver failure.

CANCER OF THE LIVER

The diet for a patient with liver cancer is high in carbohydrate, protein, fluid, vitamins, and calories and moderate in fat. Alternate intervals of feeding (other than three meals a day) are indicated for all cancer patients, but especially when the liver is involved and the utilization of nutrients is compromised. The diet will be individualized to fit the patient's tolerance. For instance, when cancer patients develop an aversion to meat, meat substitutes are offered to satisfy the high protein need.

The type of protein-calorie malnutrition that develops during advanced liver disease and hepatic cancer is severe and is accompanied by the many complications common to marasmus. The malnourishment only adds to other clinical problems, making the restoration and maintenance of optimum nutrition difficult.

All liver disorders present a challenge to the nurse to provide adequate nutrition for the patient.

LIVER TRANSPLANTS

Liver transplantation for patients with end-stage liver disease is now a standard operation, and survival rate is acceptable within the current medical care system.

Persons considered candidates for transplantation include those with progressive, irreversible liver disease whose chances for survival are less than 10% without a transplant and for whom conventional treatment has failed. Diagnosis in adult candidates for transplantation include biliary cirrhosis, chronic active hepatitis, and fulminant liver failure with encephalopathy. Common diagnosis in child candidates are biliary atresia or inborn errors of metabolism. Patients with alcoholic cirrhosis, hepatic malignancies, or advanced lung and kidney disease are not considered candidates because their chances of survival are poor.

In general, nutrition therapy for a post liver transplant patient has the following objectives:

- Hasten wound healing.
- Reduce or prevent infection.
- Increase metabolism to preserve lean body mass.
- Normalize hydration.
- Supply adequate energy to permit physical therapy.

Major nutrition support after transplant includes the following:

1. Determine appropriate weight for diet calculation. The weight measure can be achieved with proper procedure.

2. 30–35 calories per kg weight, taking into consideration fever, infection, or other complications
3. Assuming renal function is normal, a diet offering 1.2–2 g of protein per kg per day is recommended. Protein requirements are increased due to:
   - Immunosuppressive medications can result in muscle or fat breakdown.
   - Wound healing status.
4. Food preferences and selections can pose a problem. Extensive assistance from caregivers is essential. Advises on food variety such as type, taste, texture are important. Small and frequent meals are encouraged.
5. Most patients cannot achieve the recommended nutrients intake without dietary supplements, though some do not welcome such products or procedures.
6. Enteral or tube feedings may be necessary to supply recommended intakes of calories, protein, and other nutrients in order to assist the patient to reach an acceptable improvement in the overall health and oral consumption.

At all times, the patient is monitored closely for clinical improvement in the following:

- Healing of wounds
- Infection
- Physical activity
- Adjustment to all aspects of nutrition intervention

One can determine when to start an oral diet by using the following guides:

- An intact digestive system is confirmed.
- All tubes are removed from the digestive system.
- Ability to chew and swallow.

Most liver recipients will be able to start oral intake within the first 1–2 days after transplantation. However, initial feedings should be in small amounts to observe patient response.

Initial feedings follow standard postsurgical hospital dietary management: clear fluids to a regular diet as rapidly as tolerated. Other considerations such as use of supplements, restriction of a nutrient (sodium, fats, or carbohydrate) should be individualized by the care team and the attending dietitian.

The issue of food safety, especially the occurrence of pathogens in the food, must be closely monitored. All standard hospital routine practices of excluding microbial contamination must be implemented. Any patient with a liver transplant is a good candidate for infection.

However, as time progresses, accumulated experience will allow hospital dietitians to implement more appropriate nutrition interventions for the patient after the transplant.

NURSING IMPLICATIONS

Responsibilities of the nurse in treating cirrhosis are as follows:

Dietary Plans

1. The dietary plan for each patient should be individualized according to clinical conditions, appetite, and so on. For example, a patient with advanced cirrhosis may be very hungry in the morning, and a large breakfast should be provided.
2. Many patients with ascites prefer frequent, small meals to large ones, which can cause discomfort by raising portal pressure.
3. Any meal planning must consider gastrointestinal disorders such as diarrhea, nausea, vomiting, and anorexia. Such conditions interfere, both physically and psychologically, with eating.
4. Low-sodium milk is more acceptable if flavoring such as honey or vanilla is added.
5. Patients do not like most oral nutrition formulas with medium-chain triglycerides (MCT) added. Experience confirms better acceptance by some patients when the beverage is served chilled.
6. Work with the dietitian to devise ways to encourage optimal intake.

Patient Monitoring

1. A careful record of food intake is useful.
2. Be alert to signs of impending coma.
3. Always balance fluid intake and output.

Teamwork

1. Teamwork is mandatory. The team includes the nurse, physician, dietitian, patient, and family members.
2. Conferences and strategy sessions with members of the team ensure that the patient will be encouraged to eat.

Alcoholism and Drugs

1. The nurse should refrain from judging the patient's drinking habits.
2. The patient should be provided with assistance, including such therapy as Alcoholics Anonymous meetings and rehabilitation centers.
3. The patient should be given intense education on the disease and its complications and treatment.
4. No alcoholic beverage is permitted in the hospital. Abstinence at home is strongly encouraged.
5. The patient should comply with specific usage for any prescription drugs and avoid all others.

Diet Therapy for Transplantation

Candidates need aggressive nutritional support such as is necessary in all major surgery. Thorough nutritional assessment before the surgery is necessary. Patients generally have poor nutritional status and may require enteral or parenteral nutrition before surgery for optimal postoperative results. These patients are given antibiotics before and after surgery to reduce bacterial development. A low-bacteria diet is also recommended before and after surgery.

The essentials of food-handling precautions for transplantation are as follows:

1. Avoid all fermented dairy products such as yogurts and cheeses.
2. Do not eat vegetables, including salads and garnishes, and fruits that are not peeled.
3. Defrost frozen foods in the refrigerator or microwave.
4. Do not use foods kept at room temperature or kept heated for long periods of time.
5. Serve and eat foods quickly following preparation.
6. Cover and freeze leftovers immediately.
7. Use refrigerated leftovers within two days.
8. Keep the preparation and serving area very clean.
9. Be sure that sanitary techniques are maintained throughout, and that food handlers are vigilant about personal habits and dress.

PROGRESS CHECK ON ACTIVITY 1

FILL-IN

Use a separate sheet of paper for your answers.

1. Fill in the sheet marked Exercise 19-1 for a high-carbohydrate, protein, and vitamin diet with moderate fat.

2. Plan a breakfast menu for a diet that is high in calories, carbohydrate, protein, and vitamins, and moderate in fat.

3. Alter this breakfast menu to meet the needs of a client who daily requires 40 g protein and 2 g sodium.

4. Mrs. J. is admitted to the hospital with a diagnosis of infectious hepatitis and is placed in isolation. Her diet prescription is 350 g carbohydrate, 100 g protein, and 100 g easily digested fat. She will receive a therapeutic dose vitamin supplement. Answer the following questions about her diet:

   a. What is the caloric value of her diet? _____

   b. Why were the extra calories ordered? _____

   _____

Exercise 19-1 A practice on the dietary management of selected disorders and nursing implications

Complete the chart by filling in the appropriate information for each column.

Diet	Disease or Condition	Foods Allowed	Foods Limited	Foods Forbidden	Nursing Implications
High-carbohydrate, protein, and vitamin; moderate fat	Hepatitis				
	Early cirrhosis				
	Cancer				
	Marasmus				
	Uncomplicate Postoperative convalescence				

c. Compare the ordered protein intake with the RDAs/DRIs for an adult nonpregnant woman. (See Chapter 9.) _____

_____

d. Why is the extra protein needed? _____

_____

e. What is the role of the extra carbohydrate? ___

_____

_____

f. What is the rationale for the extra vitamins?

_____

_____

g. Which foods should be avoided? _____

_____

_____

h. If Mrs. J. develops ascites, what additional restrictions should be placed on her diet? _____

_____

_____

i. What precautions with the eating utensils will the nurse observe with this patient? _____

_____

j. What other diseases require the diet prescribed for hepatitis? _____

_____

5. List the nine guidelines used to instruct patients, caregivers, and dietary and nursing personnel regarding appropriate food-handling practices before and after a liver transplant.

a. _____

b. _____

c. _____

d. _____

e. _____

f. _____

g. _____

h. _____

i. _____

ACTIVITY 2:

Diet Therapy for Diseases of the Gallbladder and Pancreas

The normal function of the gallbladder is to concentrate and store the bile derived from the liver. The liver produces 600 to 800 milliliters of bile per day, and the gallbladder concentrates and stores 40 to 70 milliliters. When fat enters the duodenum, it stimulates the secretion of a hormone, cholecystokinin, which is carried by the blood to the gallbladder. This hormone directs the gallbladder to contract, so that bile is released into the common duct and then travels to the duodenum. The function of bile is to emulsify fats so that they can be broken down or digested by fat-splitting enzymes, the lipases. Any interference with the flow of bile impairs fat digestion.

Because gallstones may enter the common bile duct and block the flow of the pancreatic juice and enzymes, pancreatitis is a common complication of gallbladder disease. Pancreatitis is a severe disorder, since the enzymes in the immobile juice can cause the pancreas to digest itself. Acute pain and tenderness result, and in critical cases the pancreas may hemorrhage. The treatment of choice is to inhibit the secretion of the enzymes and to treat for shock and renal shutdown. In this case, diet therapy is useful only after the crisis has subsided.

Another causative factor for pancreatitis, especially a chronic condition, is alcoholism. Irrespective of the cause of pancreatitis, dietary treatment and nursing implications are the same.

MAJOR DISORDERS OF THE GALLBLADDER

The two major disorders of the gallbladder are cholecystitis and cholelithiasis. Cholecystitis usually results from a low-grade chronic infection. The major component of bile is cholesterol. When the gallbladder mucosa becomes inflamed or infected, the cholesterol may precipitate, forming gallstones of almost pure cholesterol crystals. Cholelithiasis is an end result of cholecystitis, but a high-fat intake over a long period of time also predisposes to gallstone formation. The body will produce more cholesterol to make more bile to assist in the metabolism of fat.

Treatments and Therapy

Cholecystectomy is the surgical removal of the gallbladder. When a person with cholecystitis or cholelithiasis eats a meal, especially if fat content is high, the gallbladder contracts in response to cholecystokinin stimulation. This causes severe pain, fullness, distention, nausea, and vomiting. Surgery is usually the treatment of choice. However, surgery may be postponed for two reasons: until the inflammation subsides, or until the patient loses weight, if he or she is obese, which many are. In these cases, supportive therapy is largely dietary.

Two recent advances in the removal of gallstones that do not require surgery are being used for selected patients. One, called litholysis, involves the use of either oral doses or direct installation into the gallbladder of certain bile acids that dissolve the stones. The second method, a process called lithotripsy, uses either ultrasonic waves or laser beams to mechanically break the stones into tiny fragments that can then be eliminated.

These methods, and new ones still being developed, are being used successfully for many patients. However, not all patients are candidates for these procedures. Those who have other medical problems, such as people with chronic liver disease or women who are pregnant, are excluded. Additionally, these procedures work only when the stone size is small. Surgery will still be the choice of treatment for many patients.

Regardless of the type of treatment, a low-fat, high-fiber diet is recommended, with caloric reduction, prior to surgery or treatment, if weight loss is needed and the cholecystectomy is not an emergency. Table 19-2 provides a guide for choosing suitable foods, and Table 19-3 lists a sample menu using these foods although the caloric content will require further reduction if weight loss is an objective.

DIET THERAPY FOR GALLBLADDER DISEASE

Dietary fat is reduced to diminish gallbladder contraction, which is responsible for pain and associated symptoms. Fat modification involves only its quantity, approximately 40 to 50 g intake per day. Protein provides only 10%–12% of the daily calories, since most protein foods also contain fats. The remainder of the day's calories should be derived from carbohydrates.

If weight loss is indicated, calories will be reduced accordingly. Use of both the weight-reduction diets discussed in other chapters and the food exchange system is recommended. Caloric intake should not be less than 1200 calories per day. These diets are used only before surgery; otherwise, a patient can be placed on these diets after he or she has completely recovered from surgery. Another consideration is to provide such patients with vitamin K to reduce bleeding.

Restriction of foods that can cause abdominal discomfort, such as gas, is individualized and not implemented randomly.

Because the body manufactures its own cholesterol in amounts several times more than is present in the daily diet, restricting dietary cholesterol to reduce gallstone formation has been questioned. Since cholesterol is manufactured from fat in the diet, lowering total fat intake may prove more effective.

In addition to a comprehensive diet therapy for patients with gallbladder disorder, some suggestions will

TABLE 19-2   Permitted and Prohibited Foods in a Fat-Restricted Diet

Food Group	Foods Permitted	Foods Prohibited
Milk and milk products	Skim milk (fortified with vitamins A and D): fluid, dry powder, and evaporated; yogurt and buttermilk made from skim milk (fortified with vitamins A and D).	Whole milk and all products made from it; low-fat and 2-percent milk and all products made from them; heavy cream, half-and-half, sour cream; cream sauces, nondairy cream substitutes.
Breads and equivalents	Enriched or whole-grain bread; plain buns and rolls; crackers; graham crackers, matzo, melba toast; other varieties not specifically excluded; all cereals that are tolerated by the patient; potatoes except those specifically excluded; rice (brown or white); spaghetti, noodles, macaroni; barley; grits; wild rice; flours (all varieties).	Biscuits, dumplings, corn bread, waffles, pancakes, nut breads, doughnuts, spicy snack crackers, sweet rolls, popovers, French toast, corn chips, muffins, all items made with a large quantity of fat; cereals with nuts and 100 percent bran may be omitted if not well tolerated; fried potatoes, creamed potatoes, potato chips, hash-browned potatoes and potato salad, scalloped potatoes; fried rice, egg noodles, casseroles prepared with cream or cheese sauce; chow mein noodles, bread stuffing; Yorkshire pudding; Spanish rice; fritters; spaghetti with strongly seasoned sauce.
Meats and equivalents	Limited to 4 to 6 oz daily; all lean fresh meat, fish, or poultry (no skin) with fat trimmed; shellfish, salmon, and tuna canned in water; foods may be pan-broiled, broiled, baked, roasted, boiled, stewed, or simmered; soybeans, peas, and meat analogues if tolerated.	Fried, creamed, breaded, or sauteed items; sausage, bacon, frankfurters, ham, luncheon meats, meats with gravy, many processed and canned meats; any seafood packed in oil; nuts, peanut butter, pork and beans.
Cheese and eggs	Any variety not specifically prohibited (2 oz cheese equivalent to 3 oz meat); 1 egg yolk a day, any style, with no fat used in cooking; egg whites may be used as desired; 1 egg yolk equals 1 oz meat.	Any cheese made from whole milk, including cream cheese; any egg that is creamed, deviled, or fried.
Beverages	Most nonalcoholic beverages except those specifically excluded.	All beverages containing chocolate, cream, or whole milk; for example, milk shakes and eggnog, alcoholic beverages if not permitted by doctor.
Fruits and vegetables	All varieties not excluded and tolerated by the patient.	Avocado and any not tolerated by the patient; fried and creamed vegetables, vegetables with cream sauces or fat added; any variety not tolerated.
Soups	Broth, bouillon, or consommé with no fat; fat-free soup stocks; all homemade soups or cream soups made with allowed ingredients; soups made with skim milk, clear soups with permitted vegetables and meats with fat skimmed off; packaged dehydrated soup varieties.	Most commercial soups; any soup made with cream, fat, or whole milk.
Fats	Limited to 2 to 3 tsp per day; all fats and oils (e.g., margarine, butter, shortening, lard); heavy cream (1 tbsp = 1 tsp fat); sour cream or light cream (2 tbsp = 1 tsp fat); cream substitute (4 tsp = 1 tsp fat); salad dressing (1 tbsp = 1 tsp fat); low-calorie dressing in small amounts not counted in fat allowances.	All fats exceeding the 2- to 3-tsp limit, including bacon drippings.
Sweets	Plain sweets, honey, syrup, sugar, molasses, jams, jellies, plain sugar candies, chewing gum, hard candy, marshmallows, gum drops, jelly beans, sour balls, preserves, marmalade, tutti-frutti.	Any candies or sweets made with nuts, coconut, chocolate, cream, whole milk, margarine, butter.

(continues)

TABLE 19-2   (continued)

Food Group	Foods Permitted	Foods Prohibited
Desserts	Sherbet, Jell-O, water ice, fruit-flavored Popsicles and ices; rice, bread, cornstarch, tapioca puddings; plain gelatin, gelatin with fruit added; fruit whips, puddings and custards made with skim milk and egg whites; cookies made with skim milk or egg whites; arrowroot cookies, vanilla wafers, angelfood cake, sponge cake.	Any products made with whole milk, cream, chocolate, butter, margarine, nuts, egg yolks.
Miscellaneous	All herbs and spices tolerated and not specifically excluded; artificial sweetener, baking soda, baking powder.	Any sauces made with fat, oil, cream, or milk; olives, pickles, garlic, chili sauce, chutney, horseradish, relish, Worcestershire sauce.

TABLE 19-3   Sample Menu Supplying 40–45 g of Fat, with 80–90 g of Protein, 260–280 g of Carbohydrate, and 1700–2000 kcal

Breakfast	Lunch	Dinner
Orange juice, ½ c	Beef broth and noodles, ½ c	Tomato juice, ½ c
Oatmeal, cooked, ½ c	Chicken, broiled, 2 oz	Beef, lean, broiled, 3 oz
Egg, poached, 1	Saltines, 4	Potato, baked, small, 1
Raisin toast, 1 slice	Margarine, 1 tsp	Green beans, ½ c
Jam, 2 tsp	Green salad with lemon juice, ½ c	Roll, hard, small, 1
Margarine, 1 tsp	Orange, 1	Butter, 1 tsp
Milk, skim, 1 c	Cola, 8 oz	Gelatin or fruit cocktail, ½ c
Sugar, 2 tsp	Sugar, 2 tsp	Milk, skim, 1 c
Coffee or tea	Coffee or tea	Sugar, 2 tsp
Salt, pepper	Salt, pepper	Coffee or tea
	Salt, pepper	

help to relieve certain symptoms of these patients. Table 19-4 summarizes the information.

OBESITY, DIETING, AND GALLSTONES

Obesity is a strong risk factor for gallstones, especially among women. People who are obese are more likely to have gallstones than people who are at a healthy weight. Body mass index (BMI) can be used to measure obesity in adults. BMI is calculated from this equation:

$$BMI = \frac{Weight\ (kg)}{Height\ (M) \times Height\ (M)}$$

The table in Appendix A calculates BMI for you. A BMI of 18.5 to 24.9 refers to a healthy weight, a BMI of 25 to 29.9 refers to overweight, and a BMI of 30 or higher refers to obese. Also see Chapter 7.

As BMI increases, the risk for developing gallstones also rises. Studies have shown that risk may triple in women who have a BMI greater than 32 compared to those with a BMI of 24 to 25. Risk may increase sevenfold in women with a BMI greater than 45 compared to those with a BMI less than 24.

Researchers have found that people who are obese may produce high levels of cholesterol. This leads to the production of bile containing more cholesterol than it can dissolve. When this happens, gallstones can form. People who are obese may also have large gallbladders that do not empty normally or completely. Some studies have shown that men and women who carry fat around their midsections may be at a greater risk for developing gallstones than those who carry fat around their hips and thighs.

Weight-loss dieting increases the risk of developing gallstones. People who lose a large amount of weight quickly are at greater risk than those who lose weight more slowly. Rapid weight loss may also cause silent gallstones to become symptomatic. Studies have shown that people who lose more than 3 lb per week may have a greater risk of developing gallstones than those who lose weight at slower rates.

TABLE 19-4   Dietary Intervention to Relieve Some Symptoms from Gallbladder Diseases

GI problems	Some suggestions of nutrition intervention and counseling to relieve symptoms
Bloating	1. Eat slow and chew thoroughly. 2. Reduce intake foods with lactose. Take with food commercial preparation capable of digesting lactose. 3. Avoid foods with high contents of fats and/or fiber.
Diarrhea	1. If there is dehydration, standard clear liquids and/or juices, may help to cover loss of fluid and electrolytes. 2. If stool is copious, no food by mouth. If indicated, medical management may be prescribed to compensate for fluid and electrolytes loss. 3. Depending on clinical observation, transition to a modified or regular diet may be prescribed with special consideration to fiber, lactose, fats, and spices.
Gas	1. Modify amount of fiber in the diet. 2. Eat and chew slowly with mouth closed.
Pain	Do not give anything by mouth during the acute phase. When the acute attack has subsided, a clear liquid or fat-free broth may be tried. Tolerance to this regimen can be followed by a low-fat diet. Also, 1. Return to a normal diet when clinical responses so indicate. 2. Avoid or limit high fat or greasy foods including butter, whole milk, certain cheeses, doughnuts, and so on.

A very low-calorie diet (VLCD) allows a person who is obese to quickly lose a large amount of weight. VLCDs usually provide about 800 calories or less per day in food or liquid form, and are followed for 12 to 16 weeks under the supervision of a healthcare provider. Studies have shown that 10%–25% of people on a VLCD developed gallstones. These gallstones were usually silent; they did not produce any symptoms. About one third of the dieters who developed gallstones, however, did have symptoms, and some of these required gallbladder surgery.

Experts believe dieting may cause a shift in the balance of bile salts and cholesterol in the gallbladder. The cholesterol level is increased, and the amount of bile salts is decreased. Following a diet too low in fat or going for long periods without eating (skipping breakfast, for example), a common practice among dieters, may also decrease gallbladder contractions. If the gallbladder does not contract often enough to empty out the bile, gallstones may form.

Weight cycling, or losing and regaining weight repeatedly, may increase the risk of developing gallstones. People who weight cycle, especially with losses and gains of more than 10 pounds, have a higher risk for gallstones than people who lose weight and maintain their weight loss. In addition, the more weight a person loses and regains during a cycle, the greater the risk of developing gallstones.

Why weight cycling is a risk factor for gallstones is unclear. The rise in cholesterol levels during the weight loss phase of a weight cycle may be responsible.

Gallstones are common among people who undergo gastrointestinal surgery to lose weight, also called bariatric surgery. Gastrointestinal surgery to reduce the size of the stomach or bypass parts of the digestive system is a weight loss method for people who have a BMI above 40. Experts estimate that one third of patients who have bariatric surgery develop gallstones. The gallstones usually develop in the first few months after surgery and are symptomatic.

You can take several measures to decrease the risk of developing gallstones during weight loss. Losing weight gradually, instead of losing a large amount of weight quickly, lowers your risk. Experts recommend losing 1–2 lb per week. You can also decrease the risk of gallstones associated with weight cycling by aiming for a modest weight loss that you can maintain. Even a loss of 10% of body weight over a period of 6 months or more can improve the health of an adult who is overweight or obese.

Your food choices can also affect your gallstone risk. Experts recommend including some fat in your diet to stimulate gallbladder contracting and emptying. However, no more than 30% of your total calories should come from fat. Studies have also shown that diets high in fiber and calcium may reduce the risk of gallstone development. Finally, regular physical activity is related to a lower risk for gallstones.

DIET THERAPY FOR ACUTE PANCREATITIS

The aim of diet therapy is to prevent the secretion of pancreatic enzymes. Both food and alcohol stimulate pancreatic secretions. The clinical management procedures of acute pancreatitis are as follows:

1. Initial measures are lifesaving. These include IV or TPN feedings, replacement of fluid and electrolytes, blood transfusions, and drugs for pain and inhibiting gastric secretions. Nasogastric suction may also be used to remove gastric contents. Nothing is given by mouth.

2. As healing progresses, the first oral diet usually consists of clear liquid with amino acids, predigested fats, and other commercial preparations added gradually. The patient progresses to a bland diet given in six small feedings. No stimulants—coffee, caffeine, tea, colas, alcohol—are allowed.

DIET THERAPY FOR CHRONIC PANCREATITIS

The aim of diet therapy is to treat the malabsorption and prevent malnutrition. Diet therapy for chronic pancreatitis usually consists of a bland diet of soft or regular consistency in small meals at frequent intervals (six feedings), and contains no stimulant foods. Pancreatic enzymes are given orally with food. Alcohol is strictly forbidden.

1. Use a low-fat diet.
2. Vitamin and mineral supplementation may be necessary, especially fat-soluble vitamins A, E, and K. B complex vitamins may also be replaced.
3. Tube feedings or TPN may be necessary.

NURSING IMPLICATIONS FOR PATIENTS WITH GALLBLADDER DISORDERS

Responsibilities of nurses treating patients with gallbladder disorders include the following:

1. Evaluate the low-fat diet for adequacy of fat-soluble vitamins and substitute alternate sources of the vitamins, if necessary.
2. Provide instructions on correct methods of food preparation. Discourage use of fats and oils for seasoning and frying foods.
3. Assess the patient's tolerance for foods that cause discomfort and flatulence. Omit those from the diet.
4. Assure nutritional adequacy of a diet with removal of foods not tolerated and substitution of alternate sources as needed.
5. Implement adequate patient education regarding tissue repair after a cholecystectomy.
6. Be alert to the correlation between obesity and gallstones.
7. Be alert to the correlation between dieting and gallstones.

NURSING IMPLICATIONS FOR PATIENTS WITH PANCREATITIS

1. The patient should be taught that no alcohol or caffeine can be tolerated in his or her diet. Sources of caffeine include coffee, tea, and cola beverages.
2. The patient can develop diabetes if the islet cells of the pancreas malfunction. Evaluate frequently for symptoms. If diabetes develops, a calculated diet will be used.

3. Pancreatic enzymes come in capsule and tablet form and should be swallowed whole. They should not be given with hot food or liquids, to avoid breaking their protective coating. They are taken only with meals.
4. The patient with pancreatitis has a poor appetite and may not eat well enough to repair damage done. The patient may not enjoy the type of modifications required. Extra support, encouragement, and counseling are necessary.
5. Be able to supply sources of group support and counseling to patients whose disease is caused by alcoholism: The person who is alcohol dependent cannot usually abstain from alcohol without support.

PROGRESS CHECK ON ACTIVITY 2

FILL-IN

1. Fill in the sheet marked Exercise 19-2 for a low-fat diet.

2. Alter the following day's menu to make it suitable for a patient on a low-fat diet (50 g). Calories are not restricted. Do not change more than is necessary to meet the diet's restriction.

Breakfast
Orange juice

_____

Oatmeal with half-and-half and sugar

_____

Fried egg

_____

Toast with butter and jelly

_____

Coffee

_____

Lunch
Pork chop with dressing

_____

Buttered green beans

_____

Corn on the cob

_____

Roll

_____

Butter

_____

Milk and tea with sugar

_____

Dinner
Spaghetti with meat sauce

_____

Tossed green salad/Italian dressing

_____

French bread/butter

_____

Ice cream with fudge sauce

_____

Red wine

_____

Coffee

_____

3. Write a 1-day menu for a patient who has chronic pancreatitis and has lost 20 lb since the onset two months ago.

4. Risk of gallstone formation can be reduced with:

   a. _____

   b. _____

   c. _____

TRUE/FALSE

Circle T for True and F for False

5. T F People who are obese are more likely to have gallstones than people who are at a healthy weight regardless of where the fat is.

6. T F Weight loss at any rate has no effect on gallstone formation.

7. T F People on a very low-calorie diet (VLCD) have a greater risk of developing gallstones.

8. T F Weight cycling does not increase the risk of developing gallstones.

9. T F Gallstone formation is correlated with obesity and dieting.

REFERENCES

American Dietetic Association. (2006). *Nutrition Diagnosis: A Critical Step in Nutrition Care Process.* Chicago: Author.

Beham, E. (2006). *Therapeutic Nutrition: A Guide to Patient Education.* Philadelphia: Lippincott, Williams and Wilkins.

Bendich, A., & Deckelbaum, R. J. (Eds.). (2005). *Preventive Nutrition: The Comprehensive Guide for Health Professionals* (3rd ed.). Totowa, NJ: Humana Press.

Charlton, M. (2006). Branched-chain amino acid enriched supplements as therapy for liver disease. *Journal of Nutrition, 136*: 295s–298s.

Deen, D., & Hark, L. (2007). *The Complete Guide to Nutrition in Primary Care.* Malden, MA: Blackwell.

DeMeo, M. T. (2001). Pancreatic Cancer and Sugar Diabetes. *Nutrition Reviews, 59*: 112–118.

Eastwood, M. (2003). *Principles of Human Nutrition* (2nd ed.). Malden, MA: Blackwell Science.

Elliot, L., Molseed, L. L., & McCallum, P. (2006). *The Chemical Guide to Oncology Nutrition* (2nd ed.). Chicago: American Dietetic Association.

Escott-Stump, S. (2002). *Nutrition and Diagnosis-Related Care* (5th ed.). Philadelphia: Lippincott, Williams and Wilkins.

Exercise 19-2   A practice on the dietary management of gallbladder disease and nursing implications

Complete the chart by filling in the columns with appropriate information.

Diet	Disease or Condition	Foods Allowed	Foods Limited	Foods Forbidden	Nursing Implications
Low-fat diet	Gallbladder disease				

Hark, L., & Morrison, G. (Eds.). (2003). *Medical Nutrition and Disease* (3rd ed.). Malden, MA: Blackwell.

Ko, A. H. (2007). Pancreatic cancer and medical history in a population-based case-control study in the San Francisco Bay area. *Cancer Causes & Control, 18*: 809–819.

Lieber, C. S. (2000). Alcohol: Its metabolism and interaction with nutrients. *Annual Review of Nutrition, 20*: 395–430.

Lin, Y. (2006). Dietary habits and pancreatic cancer risk in a cohort of middle-aged and elderly Japanese. *Nutrition and Cancer, 56*: 40–49.

Mahan, L. K., & Escott-Stump, S. (Eds.). (2008). *Krause's Food and Nutrition Therapy* (12th ed.). Philadelphia: Elsevier Saunders.

Mann, J., & Truswell, S. (Eds.). (2007). *Essentials of Human Nutrition* (3rd ed.). New York: Oxford University Press.

Marian, M. J., Williams-Muller, P., & Bower, J. (2007). *Integrating Therapeutic and Complementary Nutrition*. Boca Raton, FL: CRC Press.

Mehta, K. (2002). Nonalcoholic fatty liver disease: Pathogenesis and the role of antioxidants. *Nutrition Reviews, 60*: 289–293.

Payne-James, J., & Wicks, C. (2003). *Key Facts in Clinical Nutrition* (2nd ed.). London: Greenwich Medical Media.

Sardesai, V. M. (2003). *Introduction to Clinical Nutrition* (2nd ed.). New York: Marcel Dekker.

Schardt, D. (2004). Not everybody must get stones: How to avoid gallbladder disease. *Nutrition Action Health Letter, 31*: 8–10.

Shils, M. E., & Shike, M. (Eds.). (2006). *Modern Nutrition in Health and Disease* (10th ed.). Philadelphia: Lippincott, Williams and Wilkins.

Thomas, B., & Bishop, J. (Eds.). (2007). *Manual of Dietetic Practice* (4th ed.). Ames, IA: Blackwell.

Webster-Gandy, J., Madden, A., & Holdworth, M. (Eds.). (2006). *Oxford Handbook of Nutrition and Dietetics*. Oxford, London: Oxford University Press.

Zivkovic, A. M. (2007). Comparative review of diets for metabolic syndrome: implications for nonalcoholic fatty liver disease. *American Journal of Clinical Nutrition, 86*: 285–300.

CHAPTER **20**

Diet Therapy for Renal Disorders

Time for completion
Activities: 1 hour
Optional examination: ½ hour

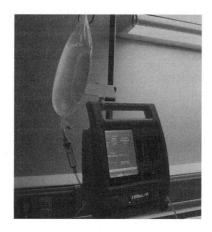

OBJECTIVES

Upon completion of this chapter, the student should be able to do the following:

1. Discuss the use of diet therapy in renal disorders.
2. Describe the therapeutic diets used in renal disorders and the rationale for their use.
3. List appropriate nursing interventions to promote adequate nutrition in a patient with renal disease.

GLOSSARY

Albuminuria: albumin in the urine.
Antigen-antibody response: antigens are those substances that induce an immune response (the foreign invaders); they react with antibodies, which are the immune bodies that destroy the invaders.
Azotemia: nitrogenous compounds in the blood.
BUN: blood urea nitrogen.
CAPD: continuous ambulatory peritoneal dialysis: dialysis performed by the patient in a continuous process.

CCPD: continuous cyclic peritoneal dialysis: dialysis by a machine that performs frequent exchanges of dialysate while the patient is sleeping.

CNS: central nervous system.

Collagen disease: a disease that attacks the connective tissue of the body, such as rheumatoid arthritis, lupus erythematosus, or rheumatic fever.

CRF: chronic renal failure.

Dialysis: the passing of molecules in a solution through a semipermeable membrane, passing from the side with the higher concentration of molecules to the side with the lower concentration (a method used in cases of defective renal function to remove from the blood those elements that are normally excreted).

Diaphoresis: perspiration (sweating), especially profuse perspiration.

Filtration: the process of eliminating certain particles from a solution.

Glomerulus: a small cluster of capillaries encased in a capsule in the kidney; a part of the nephron.

HD: hemodialysis: use of a machine (artificial kidney) outside of the body to remove waste products from the patient's blood.

Hematuria: blood in the urine.

Hyperphosphatemia: high blood phosphate level.

Hypocalcemia: low blood calcium level.

LBV: Low biological value (protein).

Nephron: the basic unit of the kidney. Each nephron can form urine by itself, and each kidney has approximately one million nephrons. Each glomerulus brings blood and waste products to the nephron, which filters it continuously and produces urine, which carries the wastes to be eliminated. Excess sodium, potassium, and chloride are also eliminated in urine, and blood is reabsorbed.

Oliguria: diminished urine secretion in relation to fluid intake (less output than intake).

Oxalate: a salt of oxalic acid. A poisonous acid found in various fruits, vegetables, and metabolism of ascorbic acid. It combines with calcium and is excreted in urine. High concentration may cause urinary calculi.

Proteinuria: presence of proteins in the urine.

Pyuria: presence of pus in the urine.

Renal: pertaining to the kidney.

Renal calculi: formation of mineral stones, usually calcium, in the renal tubules.

SOB: shortness of breath.

Uremia: presence of urinary constituents in the blood.

BACKGROUND INFORMATION

The kidney is an organ of excretion, conversion, secretion, reabsorption, manufacture, and regulation. Its structural and functional unit is the nephron. The nephron has a glomerulus attached to a long tube that empties into collecting ducts. Urine enters via the ureter and leaves at the rate of 1000 to 1500 ml per day. The convoluted tubule, known as Henle's loop, filters blood that circulates through it. It excretes nitrogenous waste: ammonia, urea, uric acid, and creatinine, as well as toxic substances ingested or formed from body metabolism. These substances are excreted in water that is not reabsorbed at the time. The glomerulus holds back in circulation large molecules such as blood proteins. Another function of the kidney is the manufacture of erythropoietin, which stimulates the formation of red blood cells in bone marrow. The kidney also converts inactive vitamin D to the active form the body uses and releases into the blood stream, but does not excrete, thus maintaining the calcium to phosphorus ratio in the bone.

The kidney, along with the lungs, regulates the blood pH by restoring neutrality. This is accomplished by secreting hydrogen ions when there is too much acid, and excreting bicarbonate when it is too alkaline. Electrolytes and other substances such as amino acids, glucose, sodium chloride, and vitamin C are either excreted or reabsorbed, depending upon what the blood needs to maintain homeostasis. The kidney also helps regulate blood pressure.

Each kidney contains over a million nephrons. Loss of half of these, such as donation of a kidney or loss of one in an accident, does not affect kidney function. Kidney function diminishes with age, and the elderly person may have only a one-half to two-thirds filtration rate compared to a young adult. However, kidney function is still adequate unless disease occurs.

Mechanisms of kidney function and the role of nutrition in maintaining them are discussed in the following activities.

ACTIVITY 1:

Kidney Function and Diseases

Because the kidney is such a major factor in the maintenance of body homeostasis, there is little doubt that the consequences are extremely serious any time disease occurs and the kidneys fail. Renal disease can be caused by damage to the kidneys themselves or by other diseases such as diabetes, atherosclerosis, or hypertension.

The most common terms used in describing kidney malfunctioning are hematuria, proteinuria, pyuria, albuminuria, oliguria, azotemia, and uremia. These conditions are dangerous to health.

In addition to excretory functions for maintenance of chemical homeostasis, balancing of body fluids, and maintenance of normal pH, the kidney controls blood pressure. Changes in sodium balance affect blood pressure as well as the rise in renin levels. Renin is a proteolytic enzyme secreted by the kidneys, which acts in blood plasma to form angiotensive II, a powerful vasoconstrictor. This further elevates blood pressure. Most patients with renal disease have hypertension.

The damaged kidney also decreases its production of erythropoietin, which is a critical determinant of erythroid activity. This deficiency results in the severe anemia present in chronic renal disease.

The diseased kidneys will cease to produce the active vitamin D hormone so necessary to maintain the calcium-phosphorus ratio in the bone. Serum phosphorus levels rise as the kidneys are no longer able to excrete phosphorus. Hyperphosphaturia occurs and lowers serum calcium levels. Also, calcium is not absorbed from the gut because calcitrol is not present. Renal osteodystrophy is the result of these imbalances. Osteodystrophy is the condition whereby the bones become soft and calcium is deposited in the soft tissues. It is a common, complex, and usually inevitable outcome of renal disease.

Diseases of the kidney, whether acute or chronic, have many causes. The origin of the disease and the portion of the nephron it affects will determine the symptoms and subsequent treatment. Depending upon the type, kidney disease may produce a nephrotic syndrome with significant protein loss, decreased overall renal function, or a combination of these. Objectives of nutritional care will depend upon the abnormality to be treated. Causes, symptoms, and dietary management of various disorders are described in the following sections.

ACUTE NEPHROTIC SYNDROME

An example of the acute nephrotic syndrome is glomerulonephritis, caused by poststreptococcal infection, which may occur in tonsil, pharynx, or skin. It is most common in children and adolescents. Symptoms vary from mild to severe: fever, discomfort, headache, slight edema, decreased urine volume, mild hypertension, hematuria, proteinuria, and salt and water retention. Prognosis ranges from complete recovery to renal failure.

Dietary management of acute nephrotic syndrome is controversial. Some clinicians prefer restriction of protein, fluid, and sodium intakes, while others do not.

Diet Modification

Acute glomerulonephritis in children is not usually considered crucial unless complications arise. They are generally placed on bed rest with antibiotic drug therapy. The fluid intake will be adjusted to output, including losses from diarrhea and/or vomiting.

Diet therapy may be similar to the initial management of acute renal failure, that is, 25 g of protein (70%–80% HBV) and 500 milligrams of sodium. Fluid permitted varies with the patient. HBV refers to the high biological value of protein. Protein in a restricted diet such as this must be from those foods furnishing the greatest amount of essential amino acids. Milk and eggs are the standard, with meat, fish, and poultry following.

NEPHROTIC SYNDROME

This disorder covers a group of symptoms resulting from kidney tissue damage and impaired nephron function. It may also occur because of other diseases such as diabetes or collagen disease, or from drug reactions, infections, or chemical poisoning. Causes are unknown in some patients. The symptoms are massive edema, proteinuria, and body wasting. Dietary management covers the restoration of fluid and electrolyte balance, reversal of body wasting, and correction of hyperlipidemia, if present.

ACUTE RENAL FAILURE

Acute renal failure includes an abrupt renal malfunction because of infection, trauma, injury, chemical poisoning, severe allergic reaction, or pregnancy. The symptoms are nausea, lethargy, and anorexia. Oliguria may be present at first, followed by diuresis. Azotemia may also be present. Acute renal failure is a life-threatening situation and requires immediate medical management.

Dietary management includes the restoration of fluid and electrolyte balance, elimination of azotemia, and implementation of nutritional rehabilitation. The dietary treatment is similar to that for acute glomerulonephritis. Many patients need dialysis, especially if they are progressing to chronic renal failure.

CHRONIC RENAL FAILURE

Chronic renal failure results from a slow destruction of kidney tubules and may be due to infection, hypertension, hereditary defect, or drugs. Dietary management involves the balancing of fluid and electrolytes, correction of metabolic acidosis, minimization of the toxic effect of uremia, and implementation of nutritional rehabilitation.

PROGRESS CHECK ON BACKGROUND INFORMATION AND ACTIVITY 1

MULTIPLE CHOICE

Circle the letter of the correct answer.

1. The functional unit of the kidney is the:

   a. tubule.
   b. glomerulus.
   c. nephron.
   d. ureter.

2. Approximately how many ml of water leave the body via the kidney per day?

   a. 1000–1500
   b. 2000–2500

c. 500–1000

d. 3000

3. Neutrality is restored to the body by the kidney in which of these ways?

   a. reabsorption of electrolytes

   b. secretion of hydrogen ions

   c. excretion of bicarbonate

   d. all of the above

4. The vitamin whose activity depends upon efficient kidney function is:

   a. ascorbic acid.

   b. B_{12}.

   c. D.

   d. retinol.

5. When a person loses one kidney through accident or donation, kidney function is altered by:

   a. ¼.

   b. ½.

   c. ⅔.

   d. 0.

6. An elderly person's kidney function may be altered by:

   a. 0–¼.

   b. ¼–½.

   c. ½–⅔.

   d. ¾–1.

FILL-IN

The kidney performs six major functions. Name them and give one example of each function.

Function	Example
7. _____	_____
8. _____	_____
9. _____	_____
10. _____	_____
11. _____	_____
12. _____	_____

Name five of the most common terms used in kidney malfunctioning, and define the term.

Term	Definition
13. _____	_____
14. _____	_____
15. _____	_____
16. _____	_____
17. _____	_____

Define:

18. Renin _____

_____

_____

19. Osteodystrophy _____

_____

_____

20. HBV protein _____

_____

_____

ACTIVITY 2:

Kidney Disorders and General Dietary Management

DESCRIPTION AND GENERAL CONSIDERATIONS

As indicated in Activity 1, there are several types of kidney disorders. No matter what type it is, the kidney fails to function properly. A kidney disorder or renal failure may be the result of diseases that involve the nephron, such as untreated glomerulonephritis, insulin-dependent diabetes, infectious renal vascular disease, or congenital abnormalities. The clinical symptoms result from the loss of functioning nephrons and decreased renal blood flow, as well as inability of the kidney to concentrate urine, or to maintain acid-base and electrolyte balance. Dehydration or water toxicity may occur if the amount of ingested fluid is not carefully controlled.

Metabolic acidosis occurs in advanced stages because of reduced excretion of phosphate sulfates and organic acids from food metabolism. These substances increase in body fluids, displacing the bicarbonates.

Sodium balance cannot be maintained by the failing kidney. Any increase in sodium intake will result in edema, as the sodium is not excreted.

Nitrogen retention and anemia, as well as increasing hypertension, are all a direct result of advancing deterioration of the nephrons. Laboratory findings indicate azotemia and elevated BUN, serum creatinine, and uric acid levels.

Depending on the clinical stage, renal failure in any form may lead to acute malnutrition with its myriad symptoms. The health professional will observe weakness, lethargy, fatigue, SOB, oral and GI bleeding, diarrhea, vomiting, CNS involvement, ulceration in the mouth, fetid breath, and increased susceptibility to any infection, as well as the aching and pain in bones and joints due to the osteodystrophy.

DIETARY MANAGEMENT

The dietary management is specific for each type of kidney disorder or renal failure and is usually individualized. However, there are many commonalities in diet therapy, which are discussed in the next section. It provides those general considerations in the dietary management of patients with renal failure. In practice, the attending physician and a registered dietitian individualize the dietary strategies applicable to specific clinical stage and patient conditions.

The following are the general principles of dietary management in renal disease:

1. Achieve a balance between intake and output.
2. Alleviate symptoms.
3. Maintain adequate nutrition.
4. Retard progression of renal failure in order to postpone dialysis.

Diet therapy is focused on controlling five nutrients: protein, sodium, potassium, phosphorus, and fluids. Levels of each nutrient need to be individually adjusted according to progression of the illness, type of treatment being used, and the patient's response to treatment.

Generally the following dietary restrictions apply:

1. Sodium: 1500–3000 mg
2. Potassium: generally no restriction from food sources. Potassium chloride (salt substitutes) may not be used in renal patients.
3. Phosphorus restriction varies. Whenever protein is reduced in the diet, the dietary source of phosphorus falls. Further restriction is usually unwarranted unless serum phosphorus is elevated. As renal disease progresses, and diet alone cannot control phosphorus, phosphate binders become necessary. Calcium-based phosphate binders are recommended and the use of aluminum-based binders contraindicated because of the potential for aluminum toxicity.
4. Protein: 0.6 g/kg body weight is the lowest recommended level plus 24-hour urinary protein loss. For patients at nutritional risk and those who cannot adhere to the diet, raising the protein allowance to 0.7–0.8 g/kg body weight may become necessary. Patients with IDDM are generally recommended to have 0.8 g/kg body weight because insulin deficiency increases the rate of protein degradation. At least 75% of protein should come from HBV protein; the use of eggs should be encouraged because of their high biological quality: high protein foods should be distributed over 24 hours.
5. Calories: adjusted for slow weight gain, maintenance of weight, or slow weight loss as necessary. Calories should be from carbohydrate and fat.
6. Fluid: intake to be calculated. Urine output is useful as a basis for estimating daily fluid needs. Five hundred ml for insensible water loss added to 24-hour urine output is the usual pattern for determining fluid intake.

Individual needs vary. Each person's weight, blood pressure, and urine output must be monitored to determine exact needs. Body weight and blood pressure will increase if the person is retaining sodium (and fluid). The person's weight and blood pressure will fall if sodium intake is too low. Calcium carbonate supplements are sometimes ordered by the doctor. Calcium should be supplemented to 1200–1600 mg/day. Calcium carbonate and calcium acetate are considered the appropriate supplements.

Fat-soluble vitamins are not supplemented. Water-soluble vitamins may require supplementation due to deficiencies arising from anorexia, uremia, and altered metabolism. Treatment with vitamin supplementation is on an individual basis.

NATIONAL KIDNEY FOUNDATIONS

The National Kidney Foundation (www.kidney.org) recommends the following nutritional intakes for two types of kidney patients, among others.

Chronic Renal Insufficiency

Using a patient with a glomerular filtration rate (GFR) of 5–60 ml/min as an example, the nutritional intakes are as follows:

1. Protein: The patient should receive 0.55–0.60 g/kg/day. At least 0.35 g should be derived from those with high biological value (HBV).
2. Energy: The patient should receive at least 35 kcal/kg/day.
3. Phosphorous: The patient should be restricted to 10 or less mg/kg/day.

Acute Renal Failure

The following are recommendations for nutritional intakes for a patient with acute renal failure:

1. Protein: The patient is advised to take in 0.6–0.8 gm/kg body weight (ideal or standard).
2. Sodium: The patient is allowed 1–2 gm/day depending on blood pressure, fluid retention, and status of diuretic phase.
3. Potassium: The patient is allowed 2 gm/day to replace loss from diuretic treatment. The serum phosphorus level should be maintained at less than 5 mEq/l.
4. Phosphorus: Intake is regulated so that an acceptable level is maintained in the serum.
5. Calcium: Intake is regulated so that an acceptable level is maintained in the serum.
6. Fluid: Intake is regulated by output. The replacement for daily loss is accompanied by an addition of 500 ml.

7. Vitamins/minerals: The daily intake is adjusted to reflect patient metabolic status. Patients receiving total parenteral nutrition (TPN) are usually given higher doses of these two nutrients.

8. Fiber: Though an intake of 20–25 gm/day is recommended, the actual intake level will depend on the clinical status of the patient.

Renal Exchange Lists

Refer to Chapter 1 on the use of food exchange lists in general. For the last 25 years, the National Kidney Foundation (NKF) has been the main organization that has gradually developed comprehensive food exchange lists to assist patients with kidney disorders who require a very structured dietary regimen.

For most kidney patients, a diet prescription revolves around five nutritional requirements:

- Calories
- Protein
- Sodium
- Potassium
- Phosphorus

Example: The attending medical team for a patient determines that a nondiabetic kidney patient daily intakes should be:

- Calories: 2100 kcal
- Protein: 60 g
- Sodium: 2 g
- Potassium: 15 or less mg

To comply with this prescription, it will be transformed into a meal plan for breakfast, lunch, and dinner. The information is then provided to the patient. Obviously, the task becomes large when the patient must have a variety of meal plans to avoid eating the same food daily. Currently, there are two ways to make such plans available.

Over the last 25 years, the NKF has systematically developed food exchange lists for kidney patients for the major food groups: milk, meat, starches, vegetables, fruits, and fats. Within each food group, the NKF determines nutrients contributed by one serving of a food item. For example, each serving (e.g., ½ c milk or ¼ c evaporated milk) within the milk group will contribute: 120 kcal, 4 g protein, 80 mg sodium, 185 mg of potassium and 11 mg of phosphorous. Thus the exchange lists for milk group will provide many foods, each serving of which contributes the same amount of nutrients.

Using similar approaches, the nutrients contributed by one serving of a food item in meat, starches, and so on are also determined. Finally, the NKF issues the food exchange lists for all major food groups.

Using such exchange lists, dietitians and other health professionals have developed many meal plans to comply with dietary prescriptions ordered by the health team.

They are then made available to hospitals, medical clinics, community healthcare centers, and so on. These organizations in turn distribute them to the patients.

At the same time, many bookstores sell books devoted entirely to dietary care for kidney patients. Most of them are written by health professionals. Many patients buy such books to have more varieties of meal plans.

At this age of computer technology, there are many types of software available to provide the same information. Using a home computer with such software, a patient can type in his or her dietary prescription and be shown the appropriate meal plans.

NURSING IMPLICATIONS FOR ACTIVITIES 1 AND 2
Caloric Intake

1. Be aware that adequate caloric intake is an important health requirement for renal patients.
2. Plan menus knowing that high caloric intake is difficult to accomplish if grains and starchy vegetables are excluded or severely limited.
3. Use caloric-dense items such as heavy cream, sweets, and carbonated beverages to provide calories when they are needed.

The recommended 30% of total calories from fat with only 10% from saturated fats may not be feasible for patients with renal disease. It may be necessary to abandon fat restrictions in order to meet energy needs and supply enough calories to prevent protein from being used for energy. Complex carbohydrates contain LBV protein, which must be counted as part of the total protein allowance, and so are limited. Saturated fat and cholesterol can be reduced if necessary by using more polyunsaturated and monounsaturated types of fats.

Fluid

1. Apportion the limited fluid intake equally throughout the waking hours.
2. Keep the patient's mouth clean and moist when fluids are restricted.
3. Compensate for diarrhea or diaphoresis by prescribing additional fluid intake.
4. Be aware that proper eating posture is needed for patients with edema and ascites. For example, sitting upright causes discomfort and anorexia for this group of patients.

Diet Compliance

1. Plan diets with the knowledge that patients dislike a diet with little bread, potato, and other low-biological value protein foods. Such diets are unpalatable and

will be further rejected by patients with nausea, vomiting, and anorexia.

2. Realize that when a patient does not comply with a diet, treatment is handicapped and prolonged.

3. Through patient education, help the patient understand the problems and make an effort to comply with the dietary prescription.

PROGRESS CHECK ON ACTIVITY 2

MULTIPLE CHOICE

Circle the letter of the correct answer.

1. Chronic renal failure usually occurs over a long period of time from diseases that affect the nephron. Included are all except which of these diseases?

   a. renal osteodystrophy
   b. congenital abnormalities
   c. untreated glomerulonephritis
   d. insulin-dependent diabetes

2. Reduced secretion of phosphate, sulfates, and organic acids from ingested foods results in:

   a. metabolic alkalosis.
   b. metabolic acidosis.
   c. edema.
   d. ascites.

3. Hypertension in renal failure is usually the result of:

   a. sodium retention.
   b. calcium excretion.
   c. metabolic acidosis.
   d. erythrocyte reduction.

4. General dietary restrictions include which of these nutrients?

   a. calcium, phosphorus, vitamin D
   b. calcium, phosphorus, potassium
   c. sodium, protein, water
   d. all of the above

5. There is an increase in _____ if a patient is retaining sodium.

   a. blood pressure and weight
   b. fluid and acidosis
   c. calcium and appetite
   d. pulse and respiration

SHORT ANSWER

List six nursing implications for patients on a renal diet (two from each category of fluid, calorie, and compliance).

6. _____
7. _____
8. _____
9. _____
10. _____
11. _____

List the four general principles of dietary management in renal disease.

12. _____
13. _____
14. _____
15. _____

ACTIVITY 3:

Kidney Dialysis

DEFINITIONS AND DESCRIPTIONS

Dialysis refers to the diffusion of dissolved particles (solutes) from one side of the semipermeable membrane to the other. Kidney dialysis was started in 1960 and has helped many uremic patients since then. Basically, two kinds of dialysis are used to treat the end stage of renal failure: hemodialysis and peritoneal dialysis.

Hemodialysis, sometimes known as extracorporeal dialysis, uses a machine (artificial kidney) outside the body. Blood is drawn or pumped out of the body and made to circulate through a special machine equipped with a synthetic semipermeable membrane. The dialysate in this case also contains glucose and electrolytes, which resemble concentrations of blood plasma found in the body. Much nitrogenous waste from the patient's blood plasma diffuses into the dialysate. The cleansed blood is returned to the patient's body and the used dialysate is replaced with fresh. The patient undergoes hemodialysis two to four times a week for three to six hours at a time in the hospital or at a dialysis center. Between dialysis treatments, nitrogenous waste products, potassium and sodium, and fluids accumulate, and dietary modifications are necessary to control them. Serum amino acids and water-soluble vitamins are lost in the dialysate, and water-soluble vitamin supplements are necessary.

Peritoneal dialysis may be intermittent or continuous. With intermittent dialysis a catheter is placed in the abdominal cavity and one to two liters of dialysis fluid introduced into the abdominal cavity and removed every hour. This process is repeated until the blood urea drops to normal levels. Loss of blood protein and amino acids are greater in peritoneal dialysis than in hemodialysis.

With continuous ambulatory peritoneal dialysis (CAPD), the patient does his or her own dialysis, and the process is continuous. The fluid (dialysate) is introduced into the peritoneal cavity and remains there for four to six hours, allowing waste products to diffuse into the dialysate. The dialysate is then drained and replaced with fresh fluid. With CAPD, no dietary restriction of fluid, sodium, or potassium is necessary. However, calcium supplements may be needed, and phosphorus is restricted. No phosphate-binding antacids are used. The dialysate contains dextrose, which is absorbed by the body. Calorie control and an exercise program may be needed to prevent excess weight gain. In addition, the extra dextrose can lead to elevated triglycerides and a lower level of high-density lipoproteins (HDLs), increasing the risk of coronary heart diseases. Protein and amino acid losses are minimal and are easily replaced by diet. Continuous cyclic peritoneal dialysis (CCPD) uses a machine that performs frequent exchanges of dialysate while the patient is sleeping. The dialysate is left in place during the day.

Both CAPD and CCPD require that the patients and/or their caregivers receive training in aseptic technique and dialysate exchange, as these treatments are carried out at home.

NURSING IMPLICATIONS FOR ACTIVITY 3
Reluctant Patients

Be aware that patients being transferred from hemodialysis to CAPD are often reluctant to give up their restrictive diets. Explain clearly the possible effects of a restricted diet while on CAPD:

1. Hypotension and dizziness from sodium depletion
2. Nausea, vomiting, irregular heartbeat, and muscle weakness from potassium depletion
3. Dehydration due to rapid fluid removal

Dietary Regime

The following counseling plan is used with success at many clinics as a guide for patients on peritoneal dialysis:

1. High protein: 1.2–1.5 g/kg body weight.
2. Limit phosphorus intake to 1200 mg/day.
   a. Nuts and legumes—one serving/week
   b. Dairy products—½ c daily
   c. Eggs—no more than one
3. High potassium—eat a wide variety of fruits and vegetables daily.
4. High fluid intake to prevent dehydration.
5. Limit or avoid sweets and fats.
6. Control weight. Incorporate the extra calories from dialysate into total calories for the day.
7. Encourage adequate consumption. CAPD patients are often anorexic.

The dietary modifications for patients undergoing hemodialysis differ in several aspects from peritoneal dialysis or CAPD. The differences are as follows:

1. Dietary potassium is controlled. The amount of potassium a person can tolerate will depend on his or her body size, amount of renal function remaining, and whether there is infection or protein catabolism. The physician determines when restrictions are necessary to keep K^+ from rising above safe levels. A daily intake of 1950–3100 mg per day is usually prescribed.
2. Sodium and fluids are regulated to the individual. If the person gains excessive weight between dialysis treatment, they are reduced. No weight gain between treatments indicates that both should be increased.
3. The majority of hemodialysis patients require calcium supplementation.
4. Water-soluble vitamins are supplemented; fat-soluble vitamins are not given routinely.
5. Diabetic patients on hemodialysis require an exchange list different from the American Dietetic Association's exchange lists for meal planning. This is because of the need to control the sodium, potassium, and phosphorus content of the diet; the amount of these nutrients in each food choice must be calculated as well as the usual amount of protein, carbohydrate, and fat. The ADA publishes a guide: *A Healthy Food Guide, Diabetes and Kidney Disease, National Renal Diet*. This guide was compiled by the Renal Dietetic Practice Group of the American Dietetic Association and the National Kidney Foundation, Council on Renal Nutrition. The Kidney Foundation also publishes a brochure on dining out for renal patients. See the References section for addresses.

PATIENT EDUCATION AND COUNSELING

1. The nurse is an integral part of the multidisciplinary health team. Education of the patient involves a full assessment of the individual's nutrition, medical, sociological, economic, and psychological status.
2. Recognize that this is a permanent adjustment for the individual and his or her family, and it will disrupt their lifestyles.
3. As the disease progresses there will be progressively more difficult restrictions. Some patients may adapt, others will not.
4. Emotional support, psychological counseling, and informational support are needed to cope with all the adjustments that must be made.
5. Crises and personal loss are ever-present factors in renal disease.

MAJOR RESOURCES

Apart from hundreds of private and government publications on nutrition, diet, and kidney disorders, two major professional organizations (American Dietetic Association [ADA] and the National Kidney Foundation [NKF]) have developed and distributed guideline documents that are used by professionals and health facilities throughout this country. They are as follows:

1. *A Clinical Guide to Nutrition Care in End-Stage Renal Disease* (3rd edition in progress)
2. *Guidelines for Nutrition Care of Renal Patients,* 3rd edition, 2001.
3. *National Renal Diet: Professional Guide and the National Renal Diet Client Education Guides,* 2002 (update in progress for simplified version of National Renal Diet).

Health professionals should consult these resources in patient care.

TEAMWORK

The dietary treatment of patients with kidney disorders is best done by teamwork as confirmed by the latest clinical observations:

1. The low-protein diets used in renal disease study have been found to be safe for periods of 2 to 3 years. Declines in protein and calorie intake are of concern because of the potential adverse effects of protein calorie malnutrition. Some individuals exhibit low body weight and altered anthropometric and biochemical data. Continuous dietary surveillance is needed, and the diet of patients with end-stage renal disease must be carefully monitored during treatment.
2. Marked improvements in the administration of dialysis has not been matched by the protein and caloric therapy provided to dialysis patients. Intensive assessment and documentation of malnutrition and medical nutrition therapy is highly recommended if the outcomes of dialysis patients are to be positively affected.
3. Malnutrition is an important risk factor for mortality among dialysis patients. Malnutrition is mild to moderate in approximately 33% of dialysis patients and severe in approximately 6%–8%. The underlying causes of malnutrition in this population include low nutrient intake, underlying illnesses, and the dialysis procedure itself.
4. The National Institutes of Health Consensus Development Conference on Morbidity and Mortality of Dialysis brought together experts from a number of disciplines including nephrology, pediatrics, and nutrition to prepare a consensus statement on a number of issues related to dialysis of renal patients. Among their findings, the consensus panel concluded that medical nutrition therapy is critical to the effective treatment of patients with renal disease, and trained dietitians are best suited to provide such nutritional intervention.

In each of these findings, the combined contribution from a nurse and a dietitian in the multidisciplinary team is the most desirable. Qualified dietitians are trained to monitor the nutrition status of dialysis and predialysis patients. The nurse is on the front line to provide clinical observations and to implement nutritional and dietary intervention.

PROGRESS CHECK ON ACTIVITY 3

FILL-IN

Define or describe fully:

1. Dialysis _____

_____

2. Hemodialysis _____

_____

3. Peritoneal dialysis _____

_____

4. Dialysate _____

_____

5. CAPD _____

_____

6. Name the four waste products from the patient's blood that are diffused into the dialysate:

   a. _____

   b. _____

   c. _____

   d. _____

7. Two reliable resources on renal disease information are:

   a. _____

   b. _____

8. Three important guideline documents for health professionals responsible for renal diseases are:

   a. _____

   b. _____

   c. _____

MULTIPLE CHOICE

Circle the letter of the correct answer.

9. Which of these nutrients should be restricted in the diet of the person on CAPD?

   a. sodium
   b. potassium

c. fluid

d. phosphorus

10. The amount of protein needed for a patient on peritoneal dialysis is:

a. 0.4–.6 g/kg body weight

b. 1.0–1.2 g/kg body weight

c. 1.2–1.5 g/kg body weight

d. 0.8 g/kg body weight

11. Effects of a severely restricted diet on a patient with CAPD include all of these except:

a. hemorrhagic shock.

b. nausea and vomiting.

c. heart arrhythmias.

d. dehydration.

12. Caloric control and exercise are necessary for CAPD patients because:

a. patients gain excess weight from being immobilized.

b. fluid is more easily excreted in this way.

c. the dialysate contains absorbable dextrose.

d. amino acids are converted to energy.

MATCHING

Match the food item on the left with its recommendation on the right for a person on peritoneal dialysis. Write the appropriate letter in the space provided.

_____ 13. eggs	a. increase potassium
_____ 14. oranges/bananas	intake
_____ 15. nuts and legumes	b. decrease phosphorus
_____ 16. water	intake
_____ 17. milk	c. increase to prevent
	dehydration
	d. limited to one
	e. limited to ½-cup
	serving

TRUE/FALSE

Circle the letter of the correct answer.

18. T F Dietary treatment of patients with kidney disorders is best done by teamwork of a nurse and a dietitian.

19. T F Low-protein diet can be used by renal disorders patients indefinitely without side effects.

20. T F Malnutrition is an important risk factor for mortality among dialysis patients.

ACTIVITY 4:

Diet Therapy for Renal Calculi

CAUSES OF KIDNEY STONES

Although the basic cause of kidney stones is unknown, there are many direct and indirect contributing factors. These factors include the chemistry of the urine and/or the conditions of the urinary tract.

Calcium Stones

By far the majority of kidney stones—about 96%—are composed of calcium compounds. The calcium usually combines with phosphates or oxalates. Excessive urinary calcium may result from prolonged use of high-calcium foods such as milk and dairy products, from alkali therapy for peptic ulcer, or from continued use of a hard water supply. Also, excess vitamin D may cause increased calcium absorption from the intestine, as well as increased calcium extraction from the bone. Prolonged immobilization such as occurs in body casting, long-term illness, or disability may lead to withdrawal of calcium from the bones and increased calcium in the urine.

Uric Acid Stones

Three percent of kidney stones are uric acid stones, while cystine stones average only 1% (cystine is an amino acid that accumulates in urine from a hereditary disorder). Uric acid stones may come from rapid tissue breakdown (body wasting), prolonged use of high-protein and low-carbohydrate fad diets, and purine breakdown (purine is a body by-product).

Urinary Tract and Stone Formation

Stone formation is facilitated by the following:

1. Concentrated urine (examples include not drinking enough fluid, excessive sweating)

2. Favorable urine acidity (the lower the acidity of the urine, the higher the calcium stone formation; high-acid urine favors uric acid stone formation)

3. Vitamin A deficiency (the resulting changes in the urinary tract tissue favor stone formation)

4. Recurrent urinary tract infections

DIETARY MANAGEMENT

Using diet therapy to manage kidney stones is only part of the medical regimen. The overall dietary treatment is based on the type of stone. Dietary recommendations to treat kidney stones are as follows:

1. Drink a lot of fluid. This will dilute the urine and flush out the stones in some patients. It is ineffective for other patients.

2. Reduce intake of the components of the stones. For example, a calcium stone may be treated with a low-calcium diet. A stone containing primarily phosphorus may be treated with a low-phosphorus diet. The same applies to stones with oxalic acid. When the stone component changes, these therapeutic diets

TABLE 20-1 Daily Meal Planning for a 800-mg Calcium Diet

Food Group	Example	Approximate Calcium Content (mg)
Milk, cheese, eggs	2 c reduced-fat milk	600
Breads and equivalents	3 slices bread	60
Cereals, flours 1 c	Puffed rice	7
Meat, poultry, fish	3 oz chicken; 4 oz lamb; 1½ oz shad, baked	30
Vegetables	½ c beets, cooked; ½ c eggplant, cooked	30
Fruits	½ c applesauce; 2 med. nectarines; 1 med. apple	20
Fats	5–6 servings bacon fat, salad dressings, and others	5
Potatoes and equivalents	½ c noodles	15
Soup (broth of permitted meats or soups made with permitted ingredients)	½ c vegetable-beef	5
Beverages	2–4 servings	10–20
Desserts	1 c flavored gelatin	5
Miscellaneous (sugar, nondairy creamer, sweets, etc.)	No limit	0

simultaneously change the pH (acidity or alkalinity) of the urine as indicated:

Stone Chemistry	Diet Modification	Urinary pH
Calcium	Low calcium (800 mg)	acid ash
Phosphate	Low phosphate (1000 mg)	acid ash
Oxalate	Low oxalate	acid ash

Stones composed of uric acid, cystine, and struvite are unresponsive to diet modifications. Stones composed of calcium oxalate and calcium phosphate are responsive to treatment and diet modification.

3. Change the acidity or alkalinity of the urine by eating certain foods.

To illustrate the use of a low-calcium diet, Tables 20-1 and 20-2 show a meal plan and menu, respectively, for an 800-mg calcium diet. Table 20-3 classifies foods according to their acid-base reactions in the body. The acidity or alkalinity of the urine can be modified by consuming more of the appropriate type of foods.

NURSING IMPLICATIONS

Calcium Intake

1. Although milk can increase an acid urinary pH, it is high in calcium.
2. A low-calcium diet should include foods fortified with vitamin D, which promotes absorption of calcium.
3. Ascertain calcium content of drinking water. If necessary, use packaged beverages or distilled water for drinking and food preparation.

TABLE 20-2 Sample Menu for a 800-mg Calcium Diet

Breakfast
Juice, cranberry, ½ c
Farina, ¼ c
Bread, 1 slice
Margarine, 2 tsp
½ c reduced-fat milk
Salt, pepper; sugar
Imitation cream, nondairy creamer, or coffee whitener
Coffee or tea

Lunch
Soup, tomato, made with milk, ½ c
Chicken, boneless, canned, 3 oz
Mushrooms, canned, ½ c
Bread, 1 slice
Butter or margarine, 2 tsp
Pears, canned, ½ c
Salt, pepper; sugar
Imitation cream, nondairy creamer, or coffee whitener
Coffee or tea

Dinner
Fruit cocktail, canned, ½ c
Veal roast, 3 oz
Potato, baked, med. 1
Cauliflower, cooked, ½ c
Bread, 1 slice
Butter or margarine, 2 tsp
1 c reduced-fat milk
Lemon ice, 1 c
Imitation cream, nondairy creamer, or coffee whitener
Coffee or tea
Salt, pepper; sugar

TABLE 20-3   Classification of Foods According to Their Acid-Base Reactions in the Body

Alkaline-Ash-Forming or Alkaline-Urine-Producing Foods	Acid-Ash-Forming or Acid-Urine-Producing Foods	Neutral Foods
Milk and cream, all types	Meat, poultry, fish, shellfish, cheese, eggs	Butter, margarine, fats and oils (cooking), salad oil, lard
Fruits except plums, prunes, and cranberries	Plums, prunes, cranberries	Cornstarch, arrowroot, tapioca
Carbonated beverages	Corn, lentils	Sugar, honey, syrup
All vegetables except corn and lentils	Bread (especially whole-wheat bread not containing baking soda or powder)	Nonchocolate candy
Chestnuts, coconut, almonds	Cereals, crackers	Coffee, tea
Molasses	Rice, noodles, macaroni, spaghetti	
Baking soda and baking powder	Peanuts, walnuts, peanut butter	
	Pastries, cakes, and cookies not containing baking soda or powder	
	Fats, bacon	

Fluid Intake

1. Warn the patient about dehydration. Prescribe more fluids if the patient perspires heavily or is losing fluid for other reasons.
2. Ascertain the reasons for withholding fluid, such as for scheduled medical tests. Check the validity of the official request.
3. All concerned persons must ensure the patient receives plenty of fluids during the day and the night.

PROGRESS CHECK ON ACTIVITY 4

MULTIPLE CHOICE

Circle the letter of the correct answer.

1. The diet therapy indicated for a patient with calcium phosphate kidney stones is:

   a. low calcium and phosphorus, alkaline ash.
   b. high calcium and phosphorus, acid ash.
   c. low calcium and phosphorus, acid ash.
   d. high calcium and phosphorus, alkaline ash.

2. In planning a diet for a patient with calcium phosphate kidney stones, which of the following foods could you use in unlimited amounts?

   a. fruits
   b. meat
   c. milk
   d. cheese

MATCHING

Match the foods on the left to the type of restriction in an acid-ash diet:

_____ 3. Dried beans   a. unrestricted
_____ 4. Potato   b. partially restricted
_____ 5. Cranberry relish   c. not allowed
_____ 6. Bananas

_____ 7. Egg and cheese omelet
_____ 8. Milk
_____ 9. Carrots
_____ 10. Olives

REFERENCES

American Dietetic Association. (2006). *Nutrition Diagnosis: A Critical Step in Nutrition Care Process*. Chicago: Author.

Axelsson, J. (2004). Truncal fat mass as a contributor to inflammation in end-stage renal disease. *American Journal of Clinical Research, 80*: 1222–1229.

Beauvieux, M. C. (2007). New predictive equations improve monitoring of kidney function in patients with diabetes. *Diabetes Care, 30*: 1988–1994.

Beham, E. (2006). *Therapeutic Nutrition: A Guide to Patient Education*. Philadelphia: Lippincott, Williams and Wilkins.

Buchman, A. (2004). *Practical Nutritional Support Technique* (2nd ed.). Thorofeue, NJ: SLACK.

Caglar, K. (2002). Approaches to the reversal of malnutrition, inflammation, and atherosclerosis in end-stage renal disease. *Nutrition Reviews, 60*: 378–387.

Cheria, G. (2004). Role of L-arginine in the pathogenesis and treatment of renal disease. *Journal of Nutrition, 134*: 2801s–2806s.

Deen, D., & Hark, L. (2007). *The Complete Guide to Nutrition in Primary Care*. Malden, MA: Blackwell.

Eastwood, M. (2003). *Principles of Human Nutrition* (2nd ed.). Malden, MA: Blackwell Science.

Echols, M. S. (Ed.). (2006). *Renal disease*. Philadelphia: Saunders.

Escott-Stump, S. (2002). *Nutrition and Diagnosis-Related Care* (5th ed.). Philadelphia: Lippincott, Williams and Wilkins.

Hark, L., & Morrison, G. (Eds.). (2003). *Medical Nutrition and Disease* (3rd ed.). Malden, MA: Blackwell.

Johansen, K. L. (2006). Association of body size with health status in patients beginning dialysis. *American Journal of Clinical Nutrition, 83*: 543–549.

Mahan, L. K., & Escott-Stump, S. (Eds.). (2008). *Krause's Food and Nutrition Therapy* (12th ed.). Philadelphia: Elsevier Saunders.

Mann, J., & Truswell, S. (Eds.). (2007). *Essentials of Human Nutrition* (3rd ed.). New York: Oxford University Press.

Payne-James, J., & Wicks, C. (2003). *Key Facts in Clinical Nutrition* (2nd ed.). London: Greenwich Medical Media.

Sardesai, V. M. (2003). *Introduction to Clinical Nutrition* (2nd ed.). New York: Marcel Dekker.

Shils, M. E., & Shike, M. (Eds.). (2006). *Modern Nutrition in Health and Disease* (10th ed.). Philadelphia: Lippincott, Williams and Wilkins.

Thomas, B., & Bishop, J. (Eds.). (2007). *Manual of Dietetic Practice* (4th ed.). Ames, IA: Blackwell.

Webster-Gandy, J., Madden, A., & Holdworth, M. (Eds.). (2006). *Oxford Handbook of Nutrition and Dietetics*. Oxford, London: Oxford University Press.

CHAPTER 21

Nutrition and Diet Therapy for Cancer Patients and Patients with HIV Infection

Time for completion
Activities: 1 hour
Optional examination: ½ hour

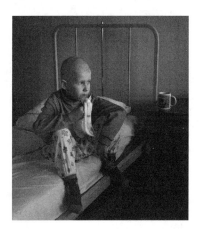

OBJECTIVES

Upon completion of this chapter the student should be able to do the following:

1. Assess a client's nutritional status using physical examination, diet history, and results of laboratory and clinical tests.
2. Identify factors that may alter nutrition.
3. Devise a plan for appropriate diet therapy based on client assessment, the stage of the disease, and its symptoms.
4. Identify the most common causes of malnutrition in patients with cancer or AIDS.
5. Describe measures to enhance food intake and retention.
6. Identify dietary modifications to increase amounts of needed nutrients.

7. Describe methods for the following alterations: modifying consistency, texture, and flavor suitable to the patient's stage of illness and/or treatment; increase the total amount of nutrients; modifications compatible with the client's social, cultural, and ethnic beliefs.
8. In conjunction with the oncology team (doctor, dietitian, pharmacist), implement a nutrition care plan to promote optimal nutrition.
9. Provide nutrition instructions and council to patient, family, and/or significant others of patients with cancer or AIDS.
10. Revise nutrition care plans as situations change.

Optional Objectives for Additional Study

1. Evaluate some unproven nutritional therapies often used by patients with cancer or HIV infections (refer to Chapter 12, Alternative Medicine).
2. Review the essentials of food-handling precautions used for all patients, but especially those with compromised immune systems.
3. Discuss foods and fluids that provide comfort during the terminal phase of cancer or AIDS, and the ethics of decisions sometimes described as "heroic measures."

Glossary

Adenocarcinoma: a cancer that begins in cells that line the internal organs.

AIDS (acquired immunodeficiency syndrome): a deadly viral disease that destroys the body's immune system by invading the helper T lymphocytes.

ARC (AIDS-related complex): the opportunistic infections that begin in a host when the immune system is compromised.

Asthena: lack of strength or energy, debilitation.

B cells: specialized lymphocytes that produce immunoglobulins. They originate in the bone marrow cells and involve many cells in the body in the immune response.

Cachexia: severe malnutrition and emaciation marked by anorexia, unintentional weight loss, loss of muscle and fat stores, anemia, and immunoincompetence.

Candidiasis: infection with the fungus of the genus Candida, appearing as whitish lesions in moist areas of the skin or inner mucous membranes.

Carcinogen: any substance that causes cancer.

Carcinoma: a cancer that begins in the skin or in tissue that lines or covers internal organs. Arises from the surface, glandular, or parenchymal epithelium.

Cellular immunity: specific acquired immunity in which T lymphocytes predominate. A cell-mediated response, they multiply rapidly, engulf, and digest antigens.

Chemotherapy: treatment with anticancer drugs.

Dysgeusia: distortion of the sense of taste.

Gliomas: primary intercranial tumors.

HIV (human immunodeficiency virus): the virus that replicates itself in the T cells and destroys the lymphocyte.

Humoral immunity: specific acquired immunity in which antibodies produced by B lymphocytes and plasma cells predominate. Genetically programmed to recognize antigens and destroy them.

Hypogeusia: reduced taste.

Kwashiorkor: a severe protein deficiency disease.

Leukemia: neoplasm of the blood cells.

Lymphoma: cancer appearing in the lymph nodes, spleen, liver, and bones (Hodgkin's).

Marasmus: a condition characterized by loss of body tissue and strength owing to lack of sufficient caloric intake over a prolonged period.

Metastasis: spread or transfer of cancer from one organ or body part to another not directly connected to the primary site.

Opportunistic infections: infections caused by nondisease-producing organisms when resistance has been decreased by surgery, illness, and other disorders.

Palliative care: care affording relief and comfort, but not cure, usually offered when the patient is terminally ill.

Sarcoma: any malignant tumor of primary tissues other than those listed in carcinoma definition.

Staging: determination of the extent of cancer by the use of exams and diagnostic tests.

Stomatitis: inflammation of the oral mucosa involving the lining of the inside of the cheeks, tongue, palate, floor of the mouth, and gums.

T cells: specialized lymphocytes in the immune response that originate from stem cells in bone marrow and migrate when mature to the thymus gland.

Teratoma: a cancer of mixed components.

Xerostomia: dry mouth.

Background Information

Cancer is a group of more than 100 different diseases. Cancer occurs when cells become abnormal and keep dividing without control or order. Most cancers are named for the type of cell or organ in which they begin (see Glossary). Screening for cancer includes physical examination, laboratory tests and procedures, and the use of imaging modalities to look at internal organs. The most common detection and diagnostic tools are CT (or CAT) scans, MRI, ultrasonography, endoscopy, and biopsy. Common tests include blood and urine tests, Pap smears, mammograms, fecal occult blood, and others as needed. Following the results of the screening, a determination is made of the size and extent of the cancer, and a treatment plan is developed. This process is called staging.

The nutritional status of the individual predicts tolerance and response to therapy. Individuals who do not lose weight have significantly longer survival time than those who do. Malnourished individuals are most susceptible to infection and less likely to tolerate or derive optimal benefits from therapy. Malnutrition is also an important issue in the quality of life of individuals diagnosed with cancer. Many studies indicate that more cancer patients die of malnutrition than from the disease.

Cancer and HIV infections share many similarities in the effects of malnutrition on the disease prognosis, progression, response to therapy, and the quality of life. Death in the individual with HIV syndrome is correlated with the degree of loss of lean body mass, and sustained weight loss is a predictor of progression to AIDS. Numerous studies indicate that malnutrition can predict death from AIDS.

There are myriad nutritional and metabolic changes characteristic of both cancer and AIDS. These changes are directly related to the body's response to the disease, treatment methods, surgical procedures, and psychological and emotional responses of the individual. They will be discussed in detail in Activity 1.

A number of emotional factors contribute to nutritional status, such as depression, guilt, fear, denial, pain, conditioned aversions, and reaction to drugs. Loss of independence creates a major trauma.

Formidable challenges face care providers and caregivers of individuals who have cancer or HIV infections and AIDS. This chapter deals with the nutritional aspects of care.

PROGRESS CHECK ON BACKGROUND INFORMATION

TRUE/FALSE

Circle T for True and F for False.

1. T F Marasmus is a condition characterized by loss of body tissue and strength due to lack of sufficient caloric intake over a prolonged period.
2. T F Kwashiorkor is a common, severe protein deficiency disease in the United States.
3. T F T cells are regular lymphocytes in the immune response that originate from stem cells in bone marrow and migrate when mature to the thymus gland.
4. T F B cells are specialized lymphocytes that produce immunogloblins. They originate in the bone marrow cells and involve many cells in the body in the immune response.
5. T F Palliative care affords relief and comfort, but not cure, offered usually to terminally ill patients.
6. T F Staging is a process to develop a treatment plan based on the results of screening and determination of the size and extent of the cancer.
7. T F Many studies indicate that more cancer patients die of malnutrition than from the disease.
8. T F Loss of independence does not create a major trauma on nutritional status.

MULTIPLE CHOICE

Circle the letter of the correct answer.

9. Screening for cancer includes:

   a. physical examination.
   b. laboratory tests and procedures.
   c. use of imagining modalities to look at internal organs.
   d. all of the above.

10. Common tests for cancer include:

    a. blood and urine tests.
    b. pap smears.
    c. mammograms.
    d. fecal occult blood.
    e. all of the above.

11. The nutritional status of the cancer patient predicts:

    a. tolerance and response to therapy.
    b. susceptibility to infection.
    c. quality of life of individuals.
    d. all of the above.

12. Cancer and HIV infections share many similarities in the effects of malnutrition on:

    a. the disease prognosis and progression.
    b. response to therapy.
    c. the quality of life.
    d. loss of lean body mass and sustained weight loss.
    e. all of the above.

ACTIVITY 1:

Nutrition Therapy in Cancer

Nutrition therapy for cancer patients is highly individualized, depending on the body's response to the disease, the site of the cancer, the type of treatment, and the specific physical and psychological responses of the patient. Myriad metabolic and nutritional changes are characteristic of nearly all cancer patients. These include fatigue, asthenia, cachexia, anorexia, anemia, fluid and electrolyte imbalances, hypogeusia or dysgeusia, xerostomia, dysphagia, esophagitis, malabsorption, stomatitis, nausea and vomiting, fever, altered metabolic rate, negative nitrogen balance, and edema. Infection is not uncommon.

THE BODY'S RESPONSE TO CANCER

The specific type of cancer, and the disease process itself, has profound effects on the entire body system and cause primary nutritional deficiencies. Some examples of the body's responses to several types of cancer are given in the following paragraphs.

Cancers occurring in the gastrointestinal tract or adjacent tissue cause difficulty in ingestion and use of nutrients. Obstruction curtails intake, and malabsorption interferes with digestion of fats and fat-soluble vitamins, especially vitamin D, which in turn leads to decreased metabolism and absorption of calcium, causing osteomalacia. Abdominal tumors may cause fistulas to develop, leading to bypass of the small intestine and consequent malabsorption. Adenocarcinoma of the colon leads to severe electrolyte imbalance. General malabsorption also contributes to fluid and electrolyte imbalance. Vomiting and diarrhea result in loss of water-soluble vitamins.

Intestinal malignancies contribute to hypokalemia. Cancer of the bone, or breast cancer with metastasis to the bone, also lead to hypokalemia. Cancer within the thyroid gland will result in hormonal imbalances. Pancreatic cancer and resulting pancreatectomy lead to the loss of digestive enzymes and diabetes mellitus.

Anorexia, the most common symptom, is related to altered metabolism, type of treatment, or emotional distress. Increased hemolysis, bleeding of lesions, fistulas, and malabsorption of nutrients needed for hemoglobin formation (iron, protein, folic acid, vitamin B_{12}, and vitamin C) lead to severe anemia.

THE BODY'S RESPONSE TO MEDICAL THERAPY

Current cancer therapy takes three major forms: surgery, radiotherapy, and chemotherapy. Sometimes they are used in combination. Nutrition support for these modalities enhances chances of success of the treatments. See Table 21-1.

Surgery

Surgical procedures pose special nutritional problems depending on the site. For example, head and neck surgery or resections greatly affect intake, requiring different feeding methods, feeding intervals, and modifications in oral food preparation.

Nutrition goals for surgical procedures include the following:

1. Provide optimal nutrition preoperatively and maximum support postoperatively to facilitate the healing process and overall body metabolism.
2. Provide specific modifications of the nutrients according to the surgical site and organ function involved.

TABLE 21-1   Common Nutritional Problems Occurring in Cancer Patients with Three Major Treatment Modes

Radiation Therapy (effects depend upon site of irradiation)

Head, neck, or esophagus
1. Anorexia
2. Impaired taste acuity
3. Reduced food intake
4. Tooth decay and gum disease
5. Difficulty swallowing
6. Decreased salivary secretions and taste sensations
7. Sensitivity to texture and temperature of food
8. Inflamed oral mucosa

Abdomen
1. Loss of intestinal villi and absorbing surfaces
2. Vascular changes
3. Inflammation
4. Obstructions
5. Strictures, fistulas
6. Anorexia and nausea
7. Malabsorption
8. Diarrhea

Chemotherapy
1. Interference with production of both white blood cells and red blood cells
2. Nausea, vomiting, stomatitis, anorexia, ulcers, and diarrhea; response of the GI system similar to those that occur in radiotherapy
3. Body fluid and electrolyte disturbances
4. Hair follicle loss

Surgical Therapy (effects site dependent)

GI Tract
1. Impaired food ingestion
2. Malabsorption
3. Potential dumping syndrome
4. Possible low blood glucose following gastric resection
5. Insulin deficiency from resection of the pancreas (diabetes mellitus)
6. Fluid and electrolyte imbalances
7. Head and neck surgery or resection poses special feeding problems: different feeding methods (enteral or parenteral) and feeding intervals, and modifications in oral food preparation.

Radiotherapy

Radiation therapy significantly influences nutritional status, depending on the site and intensity of the treatment.

1. Radiation to the head and neck or esophagus affects oral mucosa, salivary secretions, taste sensation, and sensitivity to temperature and texture of food. The

nutrition plan will include the alterations necessary to overcome these effects.
2. Radiation to the abdomen may produce loss of intestinal villi and absorbing surfaces, vascular changes, ulcer formation, inflammation, obstructions, strictures, and curtailment of food (from anorexia and nausea). Many alterations and modifications in the nutrition plan will be needed to provide aggressive nutrition therapy to these patients.

Chemotherapy

Chemotherapy has the same effect on normal cells as they do on cancer cells. This becomes most apparent in changes in the bone marrow, hair follicles, and GI tract.

1. Bone marrow effects include interference with production of both white and red blood cells, producing anemia, infection, and bleeding.
2. GI effects include nausea, vomiting, stomatitis, anorexia, ulcers, and diarrhea.
3. Hair follicle effects are body hair loss and alopecia.

PLANNING DIET THERAPY

Table 21-2 summarizes the guidelines in planning diet therapy for cancer patients. The objectives of diet therapy are to do the following:

1. Meet the increased metabolic demands of the disease and prevent catabolism of the body tissues.
2. Alleviate symptoms of the disease and its treatment by adapting the food and feeding methods to the individual.

The basis for planning care includes:

1. Thorough personal nutrition assessment
2. Vigorous nutrition therapy to maintain good nutritional status and support
3. Revision of care plan as individual status changes

Major eating problems, as discussed earlier, are:

1. Appetite problems include anorexia caused by systemic effects of cancer and treatment modalities, depression, anxiety, and stress. These problems lead to cancer cachexia.
2. Mouth problems caused by stomatitis, sore mouth, dysgeusia, hypogeusia, low salivary production, and candidiasis often occur.
3. Gastrointestinal problems, in the upper intestine, include nausea, vomiting, bloating, postgastectomy dumping syndrome, and so on. In the lower intestine, diarrhea, constipation, lactose intolerance, and so on occur.

Each of the following factors is related to tissue protein synthesis and energy metabolism. Increased needs for all major nutrients, including fluids, are based on the demands of the disease and treatment. Individual needs may vary, but the general guidelines are the same.

1. Energy: Increase total energy value to prevent excessive weight loss and meet increased metabolic demands. An adult in good nutritional status requires less than 2000 kcalories per day for maintenance. A severely malnourished patient may require 3000 to 4000 kcalories. Carbohydrates should supply most of the energy intake with fat restricted to about 30% of total calories.
2. Protein: Provide additional amino acids and nitrogen for healing and tissue regeneration. An adult in good nutritional status requires less than 80–100 g for maintenance and anabolism. A malnourished patient will need more, depending on individual requirement and treatment(s).
3. Vitamins and minerals: Key vitamins and minerals control energy, protein, and amino acid metabolism. Review Chapters 2 through 6 for specifics. Some characteristics are given here. The B-complex vitamins are coenzymes in protein and energy metabolism. Vitamins A and C are components of tissue structure. Vitamin C is also an antioxidant and functions in immune and enzyme reactions. Vitamin A functions in cell differentiation and protective immunity. Vitamin D has a vital role in the metabolism of calcium and phosphorus in bone and blood serum. Vitamin E protects the integrity of cell walls. Many minerals have structural and/or enzymatic roles in metabolic and tissue building processes.
4. Water is second only to oxygen as the most important nutrient in the human body, and maintenance of the fluid and electrolyte balance is especially crucial in cancer. Review Chapter 6 for the functions and distribution of body water.

Many individuals with cancer or AIDS subscribe to unproven nutritional therapies, from personal beliefs that it will help them take control of their disease, on the advice of family and friends, or information found on Web sites and other media. Herbal remedies, macrobiotic diets, metabolic therapy, and thymus gland extracts are often encountered by the healthcare professional when taking diet histories. Megavitamin and mineral therapies (taking 10 times the RDAs/DRIs) are among the most often used. Vitamins that are popular are A, C, B_{12}, and thiamine, and the minerals iron, zinc, and selenium.

These therapies and others can be harmful, and more details are described in Chapter 12 on alternative medicine.

Special considerations in feeding a cancer patient include the following:

1. Do not provide drinks during meal time if the patient experiences nausea. Separate liquid from solid foods.

TABLE 21-2   General Guidelines for Nutrition Therapy

There are no exact rules for diets for the cancer patient because each is highly individualized. The general guidelines in the following table will be helpful in planning optimal nutrition for a patient, based on the alterations that you find when you assess the needs of the individual.

Alterations

Pain, nausea, decreased taste sensations, diarrhea, fever, decreased appetite, anorexia

Appropriate Interventions

- Small, frequent high-caloric, high-protein meals with snacks between meals and at bedtime.
- Calorie-dense supplements that provide 100% of all required nutrients.
- Milkshakes and custards are good snack foods. Avoid milk products if lactose deficiency or diarrhea is present.
- Increase foods with high liquid content, such as sauces, gravy, or broth if dry mouth is a problem.
- Use appetite stimulants, pain medications, or antiemetics as needed.
- Provide an attractive environment.

Alterations

Diminished taste, unpleasant taste in mouth, food aversions

Appropriate Interventions

- Increase taste sensations: add spices, flavorings such as herbs, lemon, sugar, and wine.
- Remove any foods to which client is adverse. Substitute foods of equal nutrient value.
- Frequent rinsing of mouth, brushing helps.
- Fluids with meals and throughout the day.
- Use temperature extremes (hot/cold) to stimulate taste buds.
- Foods served in attractive environment.
- Eliminate any unpleasant odors.
- Plastic eating utensils may be substituted if client has a metallic taste in mouth.
- Zinc deficiencies sometimes present; supplement may be necessary (doctor's order).

Alterations

Stomatitis, esophagitis, sore mouth

Appropriate Interventions

- Offer frequent small meals and snacks with soft texture, bland, cool to cold.
- Avoid acidic foods and juices, very hot or very cold foods, and spices.
- Avoid hard or irritating foods.
- Use chilled foods and fluids, cooled oral supplements.
- Brush with a soft toothbrush 2–3 times daily.
- Use topical analgesics before meals to decrease pain.
- Sprays, mouthwash, baking soda, or salt rinses used to patient tolerance.

Alteration

Dysphagia

Appropriate Interventions

- Offer small, frequent, high-protein, high-calorie meals, supplemented with calorie-dense high-protein puddings.
- Modify consistency as liquids may be difficult to swallow; soft foods are better tolerated. Liquids can be thickened to semisolid consistency.
- Wait one or two minutes between bites.
- Cool foods are better tolerated.
- Avoid spicy, acidic, or irritating foods.

Alterations

Nausea, vomiting

Appropriate Interventions

- Offer foods cold or room temperature and soft, salty foods as tolerated.
- No greasy, spicy, or rich foods.
- Separate intake of liquids from solids by at least an hour.
- Offer crackers or dry toast.
- Offer high-protein, high-calorie milkshake supplements.
- Use antinausea medications before meals.

Alteration

Constipation

Appropriate Interventions

- Offer high-fiber foods, including fresh fruits and vegetables.
- Offer extra fluids.
- Provide stool softeners when needed.

Alterations

Diarrhea, malabsorption

Appropriate Interventions

- Provide a low-residue diet and supplements.
- Offer small frequent feedings at room temperature.
- Avoid gas-forming, fatty, or high-lactose foods; citrus fruits; alcohol; caffeine; and caffeine-containing beverages.
- Use soy supplement formulas.
- Provide foods high in sodium and potassium (bananas, potatoes, bouillon, Gatorade, etc.).
- Provide foods high in soluble fiber (applesauce, oatmeal, cream of wheat, others).
- Provide 8 c fluid if tolerated.
- Administer antidiarrheal medications.
- Provide multivitamin supplements.

Alteration

Fever

Appropriate Interventions

- Increase fluid volume.
- Use refrigerated foods.
- When planning the diet, include the patient, his or her family members, caregivers, and others who may be able to help with selection of allowed foods. Remember to take into account cultural, ethnic, and religious beliefs.

Source: Adapted from Wilkes, G. M. (1999). Cancer and HIV nutrition (2nd ed.). Sudbury, MA: Jones and Bartlett Publishers.

2. If the patient has diarrhea, avoid the following:
   a. Vitamin C supplements in high dosage
   b. Laxative teas
   c. Foods containing sorbitol such as sugar-free candy and gums
   d. Dairy products rich in lactose
   e. Caffeine
3. If the patient has a decreased appetite, do not recommend large meals.
4. If the patient has oral thrush, avoid the following:
   a. Salty, hot, and/or spicy foods
   b. Acidic foods such as citrus fruits, tomato-based products, vinegar or vinegar-based foods
5. If the patient has difficulty in swallowing, avoid foods that are difficult to swallow. Examples include sticky foods such as peanut butter.
6. If a patient is insulin resistant, avoid a low-fiber diet.
7. If the patient experiences a change in taste sensation, do not use oral supplements in metallic cans.

NURSING IMPLICATIONS

The effectiveness of cancer treatments and patient's subsequent recovery depend in large part upon adequate nutrition. Both are affected by nutrition intake and utilization.

1. Malnutrition in a cancer patient is not inevitable. Most patients can be adequately nourished, if properly planned and executed nutrition therapy is provided.
2. Be aware that nutrition therapy must be proactive. Early assessment, intervention, and continuing preventive measures to prevent malnutrition are mandatory.
3. Nutrition therapy is designed for specific physical and psychological needs and is highly individualized, depending upon the response of each body system to the disease and treatment modality.
4. Nutrition care plans are patient centered: patients need to have some control in planning during disease stages and therapy effects.
5. Anticipate psychosocial situations that relate to appetite, various foods, drug effects, lifestyle, and beliefs of the client.
6. Provide the patients with information regarding symptoms they are experiencing, actions of their drug regimes, and mouth care tips they can do themselves.
7. Make a thorough assessment of energy, protein, electrolyte, fluid, and micronutrient needs of the patient to use as a baseline for planning diet.
8. Nutritional assessment includes physical examination, lab measurements (albumin, lymphocyte count, CBC, nitrogen balance, others), past medical history, present dietary intake (24-hour recall), and any other factors affecting intake.
9. Make revisions in the patient's diet as situations change.
10. Encouragement and support are very helpful. These have a positive effect on a patient's emotional status. They denote caring, comfort, and concern. Emphasize eating to get well, and health and wellness instead of illness.
11. Investigate the use of enteral and/or parenteral methods of feeding if they become necessary. Oral intake is preferred but may not be feasible in some cases.
12. Client education, with the nurse either as the primary teacher or as support teacher in a team effort, is effective in gaining desired goals.
13. Frequent follow-up teaching is desirable.

PROGRESS CHECK ON ACTIVITY 1

FILL-IN

1. Individualized nutrition therapy for cancer patients is dependent on:
   a. _____
   b. _____
   c. _____
   d. _____
   e. _____

2. Name five nutritional changes characteristic of cancer patients:
   a. _____
   b. _____
   c. _____
   d. _____
   e. _____

3. Nutrition goals for surgical procedures include:
   a. _____
   b. _____
   c. _____

4. The basis for planning diet therapy for cancer patients includes:
   a. _____
   b. _____
   c. _____

5. Three major effects of chemotherapy on the body are:
   a. _____
   b. _____
   c. _____

6. Many individuals with cancer or AIDS subscribe to unproven nutritional therapies because of:

   a. _____

   b. _____

   c. _____

7. Three nutritional factors that will improve protein synthesis and energy metabolism are:

   a. _____

   b. _____

   c. _____

8. Three major problems are encountered when planning diets for cancer patients. To what factor(s) are these due?

   a. Appetite problems due to _____
   b. Mouth problems due to _____
   c. GI problems due to _____

9. For each of the alterations listed below, supply at least three appropriate interventions to boost nutritional intake:

   a. decreased appetite, anorexia _____
   b. stomatitis, sore mouth _____
   c. nausea, vomiting _____
   d. dysphagia _____

MULTIPLE CHOICE

Circle the letter of the correct answer.

10. An adult in good nutritional status requires about

    a. 1000 kcalories per day for maintenance
    b. 1500 kcalories per day for maintenance
    c. 2000 kcalories per day for maintenance
    d. 2500 kcalories per day for maintenance

11. An adult in good nutritional status requires about:

    a. 40 to 60 grams of protein for maintenance and anabolism
    b. 60 to 80 grams of protein for maintenance and anabolism
    c. 80 to 100 grams of protein for maintenance and anabolism
    d. 100 to 120 grams of protein for maintenance and anabolism

12. Megavitamin and mineral therapies are among the most often used unproven nutritional therapies. Which of these represents a megadose of vitamin therapy?

    a. 2 times RDA/DRI
    b. 5 times RDA/DRI

    c. 10 times RDA/DRI
    d. 20 times RDA/DRI
    e. none of the above

TRUE/FALSE

Circle T for True and F for False.

13. T F The specific type of cancer and the disease process itself have profound effects on the entire body system and causes primary nutritional deficiencies.

14. T F The development and progress of the disease cancer do not cause primary nutritional deficiencies.

15. T F Hypokalemia can be attributed to intestinal malignancies, cancer of the bone, or breast cancer with metastasis to the bone.

16. T F Breast cancer can be caused by nutritional deficiency.

17. T F Cancer within the thyroid gland will result in hormonal imbalances.

18. T F Pancreatic cancer and resulting pancreatectomy lead to the loss of digestive enzymes and diabetes mellitus.

19. T F Surgical procedures do not pose significant nutritional problems to the cancer patient.

20. T F Radiation therapy significantly influences nutritional status, depending on the site and intensity of the treatment.

21. T F Nutrition plans for patients with radiation therapy usually do not require aggressive nutrition therapy.

22. T F Chemotherapy has the same effect on normal cells as they do on cancer cells.

23. T F Anorexia due to systemic effects of cancer and treatment modalities, depression, anxiety, and stress usually leads to cancer cachexia.

24. T F Increased total energy value prevents excessive weight loss and meets increased metabolic demands.

25. T F Key vitamins and minerals control energy, protein, and amino acid metabolism.

26. T F The B-complex vitamins are coenzymes in protein and energy metabolism.

27. T F Vitamins are not components of tissue structure.

28. T F Many minerals have structural and/or enzymatic roles in metabolic and tissue-building processes.

29. T F Maintaining fluid and electrolyte balance is especially crucial in cancer.

30. T F When taking diet histories, healthcare professionals usually don't encounter the patient's self-prescribed remedies such as macrobiotic diets or metabolic therapy.

31. T F Both vitamin and mineral megadoses are safe at high levels as they are essential nutrients.
32. T F The effectiveness of cancer treatments and patient's subsequent recovery depend in large part upon adequate nutrition intake and utilization.
33. T F Most cancer patients cannot be properly nourished, even when carefully planned and executed therapy is provided.
34. T F Nutrition therapy for all cancer patients is basically the same.
35. T F Nutrition care plans are patient centered; patients need to have some control in planning during disease stages and therapy effects.
36. T F Psychosocial situations are not determinant factors in nutrition therapy.
37. T F Thorough assessment of energy, protein, electrolyte, fluid, and micronutrient needs of the patient should be used as a baseline for planning diet.
38. T F Revisions in the patient's diet as situations change is essential in nutrition therapy.

ACTIVITY 2:

Nutrition and HIV Infections

BACKGROUND

AIDS patients are at high risk for neoplasms. The oncology team is likely to also be involved in the treatment of patients with HIV infection.

Since the discovery of HIV infections and consequent development of AIDS in the early 1980s, much has been learned about retroviruses, immune function, and opportunistic infections. Although many clinicians and HIV specialists and researchers did not recognize the important role that nutrition played in the process, today we know that nutrition has a primary role in the process, progression, and treatment of HIV disease.

There is no dormant phase in HIV infection. Once the virus enters the body, it settles into a pattern in the host cells, replaces the immune system cells, and continues to proliferate. The higher the viral load in the body, the quicker the immune dysfunction occurs and the disease progresses.

Nutrition and immune function are intertwined. Maintenance of optimal nutritional status is not only essential for body stores, but also to the support of medications and other therapies that are used. Food and nutrient interactions with the antiretroviral medications are common, making it difficult for a patient to adhere to the medical regime. However, improvement in nutritional status, especially lean body mass, improves well-being and quality of life, despite the level of HIV in the blood.

The stress response of the body to the immune system's efforts to protect the body is a continuous process, resulting in loss of lean body mass, chronic inflammation, and hypermetabolism. The stress response is also marked by loss of appetite and reduced nutrient intake. Specific factors are discussed later in this chapter.

The clinical course of HIV infection leading to full-blown AIDS varies with each individual. However, the disease goes through three distinct phases: the primary HIV infection and extended incubation period, in which the person is asymptomatic; the second stage in which other illnesses manifest, called the AIDS-related complex (ARC); and the third stage or terminal AIDS.

Primary Stage

Sometimes the person has mild flulike symptoms one or two weeks after exposure and infection, while in others this may not occur. During this stage, the person appears well. This incubation period, while the person is asymptomatic, may last for 8–10 years. It is a crucial period during which the virus grows and multiplies rapidly. Optional nutritional status is essential during this phase, as well as in later stages.

Second Stage

In this stage a group of opportunistic illnesses begin. The HIV infection has killed many of the host's T cells and severely damaged the immune system. Normal infections that usually would not harm the host take root and grow. Symptoms during this period include persistent fatigue, candida (thrush), night sweats, fever, unintentional loss of 10 or more pounds of weight, skin rashes, severe headaches, cough, sore throat and mouth, shortness of breath, and bruises on the skin. Aggressive nutrition therapy during this crucial stage delays the progression of infections.

Final Stage

The terminal stage of HIV infection, or AIDS, is marked by declining T lymphocyte production from the normal level of >1000/mm3. When the count drops to between 200–500/mm3, diseases such as tuberculosis and Kaposi's sarcoma develop. Below 200/mm3, lymphomas, pneumonocystitis, carnii pneumonia, protozoa, and parasites overwhelm the weakened immune system and death follows.

Death in the end stages of HIV syndrome is correlated with the degree of loss of lean body mass. Numerous studies have shown that sustained weight loss is a predictor of progression to AIDS and can predict death from the disease.

BASIC ROLE OF NUTRITION IN HIV INFECTIONS

The goals of nutrition therapy in the care of the AIDS patient are to do the following:

1. Delay the progression of infections and improve the patient's immune system.
2. Prevent the wasting effects of HIV infection—severe involuntary malnutrition and weight loss.
3. Prevent opportunistic diseases.
4. Recognize infections early and provide rapid treatment for an incompetent immune system, which includes infections and cancer.
5. When nutrient needs of HIV/AIDS patients cannot be met by a normal diet, nutrition intervention such as a high-protein, high-calorie diet, and a multivitamin/mineral supplement may be necessary. Low-fat lactose-free oral supplements may be better tolerated than higher-fat supplements.

With the use of protease inhibitors, persons with HIV infections have fewer symptoms and complications from the virus, making nutrition of great importance in stage one. A balanced diet high in protein and calories, modified fat intake of 30% of calories from fat, and daily vitamin and mineral supplements is essential. Maximum nutrient intake enhances immune cell function, delaying the later stages and allowing the person to have a better quality of life.

In the second stage as the disease is progressing, weight loss and malnutrition are prevalent. The body cell count reduction increases the risk of infections and early death, and fatigue and weakness decrease quality of life. These conditions increase the need for extra nutrients and require the whole spectrum of nutritional support. Enteral and parenteral feedings should be considered. Medications to alleviate severe pain, diarrhea, anorexia, nausea, and vomiting should be given. Small, frequent feedings high in quality protein are better tolerated than full meals.

In the last stages, or full blown AIDS, the effects on the GI, neurologic, and pulmonary systems as well as the side effects of medications and altered metabolism present great challenges for both healthcare providers and patients. These complex conditions impair nutritional status and become more difficult to manage as the disease progresses. When the patient is no longer able to eat, enteral tube feedings or parenteral feeding may be used. Ultimately, however, ethical questions about continued feeding efforts must be faced. Answers lie with the patient as long as possible, and with his or her family. The oncology/AIDS team, including physician, nursing personnel, and clinical dietitian, along with the patient and family face these decisions together.

GENERAL GUIDELINES FOR NUTRITION THERAPY IN HIV INFECTIONS

Anorexia and cachexia are the major clinical nutrition alterations in HIV infections and affect all clients with advanced HIV infection or cancer. Cachexia is progressive and occurs despite adequate and supplemental nutrition. It profoundly affects the quality of life and is associated with mortality.

Characteristics of cachexia include anorexia, weakness, early satiety, nonintentional weight loss, loss of muscle and fat stores, decreased mobility and physical activity, nausea, vomiting, dehydration, edema, chronic diarrhea or constipation, pain, fever, night sweats, dysphagia, candidiasis, malabsorption, and dementia. These symptoms have a profound impact on nutrition.

Individual factors that influence food intake include the following:

- Income: Availability of food and the cost of fresh food determine kinds and amounts of food the client purchases.
- Psychosocial factors: The client's beliefs about food, learned food aversions, and social status.
- Dependency issues: The family may support and encourage the client, or they may become alienated.
- Psychological factors: Depression, loss of self-care ability, guilt, low self-esteem, facing the diagnosis of AIDS, and end-of-life measures.
- Ethnic and cultural considerations: HIV/AIDS is poorly understood by many clients not born in the United States, or immigrants. Language barriers present a problem with presenting nutrition and safety measures.

Table 21-1 in Activity 1 (General Guidelines for Nutrition Therapy) is relevant for planning diet for the person with HIV infections. Remember that the diet must be highly individualized. Nutrition interventions specific to the AIDS patient are given in Table 21-3.

NUTRITION IN TERMINAL ILLNESS

Decisions involving nutrition and hydration in terminal patients are becoming more frequent. When a patient is no longer able to eat, enteral or parenteral feedings may be administered. Ethical questions arise concerning this decision: how long to continue the feedings? This is important when the patient is no longer able to make such decisions. In the past, this was a medical issue and the physician providing treatment for a particular patient made the final decision.

Recently, many controversies have developed relating to these issues. In view of this, many states have passed laws requiring hospitals to develop and implement protocols that the care provider team must follow if such medical conditions exist. The patients may or may not be

TABLE 21-3   Nutrition Interventions for AIDS Clients

Careful and thorough assessment and monitoring of the patient's diet by the AIDS team is essential. Finding the cause of underlying malnutrition allows for more appropriate diet therapy.

Assessment of nutritional needs:

- Diet history, past and present, including any self-prescribed nutrition regimes, drug- or alcohol-related medical problems
- Calculation of nutrient intake
- Anthropometric measurements
- Food allergies, intolerances, cultural patterns
- Socioeconomic status, dental health, weight history
- Weight changes, appetite changes
- GI symptoms
- Medication list
- Laboratory reports

In addition to information given in Table 21-2 (Guidelines for Nutrition Therapy), some practical applications specific to AIDS patients are listed here.

- Alteration: nausea

Eliminate strong odors, reduce fat intake, eliminate foods such as fried foods, potato chips, full fat ice cream, fatty beef products, peanuts, doughnuts, and pastries. Substitute foods such as pretzels, saltines, baked or broiled chicken or fish, fat free cookies, sherbets, and sorbets.

- Alteration: diarrhea
  1. Oral feedings preferred, may not have to resort to parenteral feedings.
  2. Diet should be high in soluble fiber, low in lactose, fat, and caffeine.
  3. Avoid dairy products, cow's milk. Try lactose-reduced milk or OTC lactaid tablets, most can tolerate these products.
  4. Offer bananas, rice, applesauce, and tea (commonly called the B.R.A.T. diet), and white toast for a limited time (2–3 days) as this is inadequate nutrition.
  5. Foods rich in soluble fiber help to make the stool firmer. Canned pears, peeled and cooked sweet and white potatoes, cream of wheat, and oatmeal are good sources.
  6. Limit caffeine: regular coffee, colas, tea, Mountain Dew, and chocolate.

If diarrhea is intractable, the use of medium chain triglycerides, elemental formulas (predigested and hydrolyzed products), and fat-soluble vitamins in water-soluble form may be needed.

- Alterations: thrush and dyspnea
  1. The diet should be soft, low acid, low sodium, served at room temperature. Use foods that do not require significant chewing.
  2. Use foods such as macaroni and cheese, yogurt, vanilla pudding, tuna salad, mashed potatoes, rice, noodles, and cream soups.
  3. Add gravies or sauces to any ground meats.
  4. Use straws for liquid (bypasses a sore mouth).

Use of Supplements

The use of supplements should be evaluated. The following is a brief overview of the most frequently used feedings.

- Oral (enteral)

Select one that is balanced in macronutrients (CHO, protein, fat) and calorie-dense (provides the most calories in the smallest volume). When using these supplements, assure adequate hydration with extra water and fluids.

The supplement should be high in protein, CHO, and fat. The fat should be in the form of medium chain tryglycerides (MCT). It should contain soluble fiber, be lactose free, and provide 100% of the U.S. RDA/DRI for vitamins and minerals.

Complete formulas are preferred. Enteral formulas have been developed to target specific problems by reducing the problems of malabsorption.

Some oral formulas containing increased amounts of macronutrients include, but are not limited to, these brand name products:

Ensure plus, Ensure HN, Isocal, Advera, Vivonex, and Boost plus. They come in a variety of flavors and meet all the requirements.

Other preparations that can be obtained at the grocery store are Instant Breakfast, eggnog, and others. Check the labels carefully.

- Tube feedings

Tube feedings can range all the way from blenderized foods prepared from whole foods to commercial formulas.

Several complications can occur, such as diarrhea, fluid and electrolyte imbalances, and hyperglycemia. Blenderized home formulas may not contain balanced nutrients. There is also concern about the safety in handling and storage problems. In the clinical setting, commercial formulas are preferred.

Tube feedings should be monitored closely and frequent lab assessments made.

- Total parenteral nutrition (TPN)

TPN is used when other methods are not suitable. It contains glucose, amino acids, vitamins, trace elements, and often insulin. MCT is administered separately. Because it is hypertonic, it requires frequent monitoring of the blood.

TPN presents an ethical dilemma. It is an invasive procedure, usually administered in the left subclavian vein. It is contraindicated in clients with advanced disease for whom there is no disease reversal.

Source: Adapted from HIV Homecare Handbook, 1999. Daigle, Barbara, Katherine Lasch, Christine McClusky, and Beverly Wancho. Jones and Bartlett Publishers, Sudbury, MA.

involved in this process, depending on their medical status. The legal requirements vary from state to state. This book is not the proper forum to discuss such details. The Internet is the best resource for an interested party to obtain more information.

ALTERNATIVE NUTRITION THERAPIES

As is true of other incurable diseases, many patients will try any alternative that is offered to them, hoping for a miracle. Often cited in treatment for AIDS are alternative nutrition regimes, supposed to boost the immune system, increase enzyme production, prevent further deterioration, create a hostile internal condition to keep the virus from spreading, and restore balance and harmony to the system, to name a few so-called benefits.

Popular among the many such regimes offered is the use of megadoses of vitamin and mineral supplements. For instance, vitamins A, C, and B_{12} and the minerals zinc and selenium are said to strengthen the immune system and enable it to overcome the ravages of the disease. The opposite effect is more likely: excess vitamin C often causes rebound scurvy when discontinued; vitamin A, zinc, and selenium are very toxic when taken in excess over long periods. Excess supplements suppress immune function instead of strengthening it. Laetrile is still around and still touted as a cure for AIDS, as it has been for cancer. Laetrile has never been proven to be beneficial in the treatment of chronic disease. Proponents of laetrile for AIDS treatment also recommend a strict vegan diet, which is totally inadequate in many nutrients and excessive in others. The macrobiotic diet, a longstanding item in the quackery arsenal, produces protein-calorie malnutrition, the opposite effect of what is needed for the AIDS patient.

Many alternative diets, herbs that are toxic to the body, and some supplements are of doubtful value (see Chapter 11, Dietary Supplements, and Chapter 12, Alternative Medicine).

It is important for the nurse to be aware of self-prescribed diets and practices of clients. These practices should be entered as part of the diet history. Develop an understanding of various alternatives, as they are a part of the practitioner's health concerns of each client. Try to provide patients with information regarding the potential harm of self-prescribed nutrition therapies without alienating them. Keep your lines of communication open.

SPECIAL NUTRITIONAL CARE FOR CHILDREN WITH AIDS

Because HIV infections and AIDS are wasting diseases, the child will exhibit the problems and complications similar to those found in adults. Additionally, failure to thrive and impaired brain growth will occur.

The progression and manifestation differ somewhat from adults. The Centers for Disease Control (CDC) developed a system that separates them into four categories based on age, signs, symptoms, or diagnosis.

The severe malnutrition that occurs in children with AIDS affects not only their present condition but also their future growth and development. Nutritional needs are 50%–100% above the RDA/DRI requirements of their age group. Because acute anorexia is also present in children, achieving this necessary increase is a very difficult task. One-on-one support and attention are helpful and needed. Some suggestions for feeding children include the following:

1. Infants: Use kcal-dense formulas, supplements of MCT, or glucose polymers. If the infant is lactose intolerant, as many infants and children with AIDS are, use soy-based formulas and supplements.
2. Children: Use any supplements high in kcal and protein that are tolerated. Use added fats and nutrient-dense snacks. If the child is lactose intolerant, use lactose-free soy milk and/or use Lactaid (a commercial preparation) added to milk products to improve their digestibility. Alternative feeding methods may be considered when a child is unable to eat. Maintain optimal hydration fluids, using available commercial products such as Pedialyte, Gatorade, and so on. Smaller feedings spread throughout the day are usually better accepted. Big doses of patience and love by the person(s) doing the feeding are necessary and increase the child's acceptance. Allow the child to make some food choices. Make food attractive and fun.
3. A word of caution: Although sanitation is very important for all patient feeding, it becomes more so with children who have AIDS. They should never receive unpasteurized products; babies should not be fed directly from the open jar; fruits and vegetables should be peeled and cooked; meats should be well cooked and tender; and all eating utensils should be sanitized before and after using. These precautions are used to avoid bacterial contamination. Salmonella is a particular problem, and it can be deadly in a child who is already compromised.

FOOD SERVICE AND SANITARY PRACTICES

Individuals who serve foods to AIDS patients must be reminded not to discriminate against them. All standard sanitation procedures implemented in the facility against cross-contamination should be complied with whether the patient carries AIDS or any other transmissible disease. For example, articles contaminated with an AIDS patient's emesis, feces, urine, and blood must be decontaminated before being returned for cleaning, as would be the case with any other contaminated patient's discharge ("universal precautions").

Because of impaired immune systems, AIDS patients are unable to fight food-borne infections, which cause severe diarrhea and vomiting. They can be fatal to anyone with HIV infections. The patients must be protected from infection. Food-borne infections occur more frequently among people with HIV infections than in other people. If a facility is not practicing sanitary food preparation, service, and storage, it must do so. Improper food handling is a primary source of bacterial contamination, and personnel should be very careful to follow state and federal laws. Most facilities that serve food are regulated by state and federal laws to implement acceptable food safety and sanitation practices, and these practices become crucial to those serving patients with AIDS.

Because many foreign countries do not have as strict guidelines for food handling, it is better to avoid using imported foods and use only those grown and distributed in the United States. All fresh fruits and vegetables must be thoroughly washed before using. Use only pasteurized products and never serve raw eggs, meat, or fish to the patient. Do not allow such products to be brought in by family and friends. Explain to them the reasons for these rules and the consequences. It is also prudent to inspect any food items being brought from outside the facility before the patient receives them.

NURSING IMPLICATIONS

1. Be supportive and nonjudgmental.
2. Use whatever feeding methods or type of feeding that is most effective.
3. Consider the psychological aspects of feeding: some patients may be willing to fight as long as possible; others are not willing to fight at all.
4. Take advantage of times when the client is pain free to offer food. Feed them any time they feel hungry. Serve foods that require little chewing.
5. Make certain that the environment is free of odors, debris, and clutter and that the tray is attractive and palatable.
6. Serve small, frequent meals of high-protein, high-calorie, nutrient-dense foods. Offer nutrient-dense snacks frequently. Consult with the RD on your team for tips or planning if you need assistance. Be sure to inform dietary personnel if changes are needed.
7. Assistance with eating (buttering, cutting, dipping, and unwrapping) may be needed. Observe the patient to determine if help is wanted or resented.
8. Systemic oral hygiene and topical analgesics should be used as necessary.
9. Encouragement from health personnel is as necessary as that from friends and relatives, so be generous.
10. Be aware of any self-prescribed nutrition therapy and practices of the client. Many of the herbs used are dangerous and have toxic side effects.
11. Educate the patient and all caregivers: use the team's dietitian as a primary teacher or as a consultant for evaluation of your teaching plan.
    a. Teach basic principles of nutrition. Use the food guide pyramid for instructions.
    b. Set realistic goals.
    c. Assess financial resources and living arrangements. Obtain a list of community resources, such as food banks and others.
    d. Adapt foods to differences in lifestyle, cultural and ethnic background, religion, and income.
    e. Assess the client's educational level (can they read, what is their primary language, etc.).
    f. Review safe handling practices.
    g. Include appointments for follow-up teaching in your plan if client will go home between hospital visits.

PROGRESS CHECK ON ACTIVITY 2

MULTIPLE CHOICE

Circle the letter of the correct answer.

1. The stress response to HIV infection is marked by:
    a. loss of appetite and reduced nutrient intake.
    b. loss of lean body mass.
    c. chronic inflammation.
    d. hypermetabolism.
    e. all of the above.

2. Alternative nutrition regimes are supposed to:
    a. boost the immune system.
    b. increase enzyme production.
    c. prevent further deterioration.
    d. create a hostile internal condition to keep the virus from spreading.
    e. restore balance and harmony to the system.
    f. all of the above.

3. T lymphocyte production in HIV infection will drop from normal levels to:
    a. less than 1000/mm3.
    b. less than 800/mm3.
    c. less than 600/mm3.
    d. less than 200/mm3.
    e. none of the above.

FILL-IN

4. The four goals of nutrition therapy for AIDS patients are:
    a. _____
    b. _____
    c. _____
    d. _____

5. Name the three distinct phases of HIV infections. Include manifestations of each phase:

   a. Phase 1: _____

   Manifestations _____

   b. Phase 2: _____

   Manifestations _____

   c. Phase 3: _____

   Manifestations _____

6. For each of the goals listed, supply an appropriate nutritional intervention.

   a. Stop weight loss. _____

   b. Rebuild lean body mass. _____

   c. Minimize malabsorption. _____

   d. Manage the specific problems related to nutrition. _____

      i.   Anorexia _____

      ii. Nausea and vomiting _____

      iii. Severe weight loss _____

      iv. Oral or esophageal lesions _____

      v.   Infection and sepsis _____

7. List five nursing responsibilities pertaining to feeding AIDS patients:

   a. _____

   b. _____

   c. _____

   d. _____

   e. _____

8. Describe the general sanitation techniques to be used by dietary and nursing staff for the protection of staff and patient. _____

   _____

TRUE/FALSE

Circle T for True and F for False.

9. T F Once the HIV virus enters the body, it settles into a pattern in the host cells, replaces the immune system cells, and continues to proliferate. The higher the viral load in the body, the quicker the immune dysfunction occurs and the disease progresses.

10. T F Nutrition and immune function are intertwined.

11. T F Improvement in nutritional status, especially lean body mass, improves well-being and quality of life, despite the level of HIV in the blood.

12. T F Because the primary stage of HIV infection may last for 8–10 years, it is not essential to have optimal nutritional status during this phase.

13. T F Aggressive nutrition therapy during the second stage delays the progression of infections.

14. T F At the terminal stage of HIV infection, or AIDS, the patient has no T lymphocyte production.

15. T F Sustained weight loss is not a predictor of progression to AIDS.

16. T F A balanced diet high in protein and calories, modified fat intake of 20% of calories from fat, and daily vitamin and mineral supplements is essential.

17. T F Medications to alleviate severe pain, diarrhea, anorexia, nausea, and vomiting should not be given to HIV or AIDS patients, because they may be addictive.

18. T F In the last stage, or full-blown AIDS, the patient may no longer be able to eat, and enteral tube feedings or parental feeding may be necessary.

19. T F Anorexia and cachexia are the major clinical nutrition alterations in HIV infections and affect all clients with advanced HIV infection or cancer.

20. T F When nutrition administration becomes invasive and painful, or when the patient feels that he or she is being kept alive by artificial means and life no longer has meaning, it is time to consider the stopping of enteral or parenteral feedings.

21. T F Vitamins A, C, and B_{12} and the minerals zinc and selenium are said to strengthen the immune system and enable it to overcome the ravages of the HIV infection.

22. T F Proponents of laetrile for AIDS treatment also recommend a strict vegan diet, which is totally inadequate in many nutrients and excessive in others.

23. T F Yeast-free diets prevent diseases such as candidiasis.

24. T F The progression and manifestation for children and adults are the same in HIV infections.

25. T F Children with HIV or AIDS should be fed with any supplements high in kcal and protein that are tolerated, as well as use of added fats and nutrient-dense snacks.

26. T F All food and beverages fed to HIV and AIDS patients must be sterile.

27. T F Standard sanitary practices in food preparation must be followed as the HIV-infected or AIDS patients have limited immunity to foodborne infection.

28. T F For patients with HIV infections or AIDS, smaller portions fed at more frequent intervals is not as good as larger portions at less frequent intervals.

REFERENCES

American Dietetic Association & Dieticians of Canada. (2004). Nutrition intervention in the care of persons with human immunodeficiency virus infection: A position paper. *Journal of American Dietetic Association, 104*: 1425–1441.

American Institute for Cancer Research. (2001). *Nutrition and Cancer Prevention: New Insights into the Role of Phytochemcials.* New York: Kluwer Academic.

Baer-Dubowska, W., Bartoszek, A., & Malejka-Giganti, D. (Eds.). (2006). *Carcinogenic and Anticarcinogenic Food Components.* Boca Raton, FL: Taylor and Francis.

Batterham, M. (2001). Nutritional management of HIV/ AIDS in the era of highly active antiretroviral therapy: A review. *Australian Journal of Nutrition and Dietetics, 58*: 211–223.

Beham, E. (2006). *Therapeutic Nutrition: A Guide to Patient Education.* Philadelphia: Lippincott, Williams and Wilkins.

Bendich, A., & Deckelbaum, R. J. (Eds.). (2005). *Preventive nutrition: The Comprehensive Guide for Health Professionals* (3rd ed.). Totowa, NJ: Humana Press.

Brown, D. (2001). Nutritional management of HIV/AIDS in the era of highly active antiretroviral therapy: A review of treatment strategies. *Australian Journal of Nutrition and Dietetics 58*: 224–235.

Buchman, A. (2004). *Practical Nutritional Support Technique* (2nd ed.). Thorofeue, NJ: SLACK.

Cameron, G. T., & Geana, M. V. (2005). Functional foods: Delivering information to the oncology nurse. *Journal of Nutrition, 135*: 1253–1255.

Choudry, H. A., Pan, M., Karinch, A. M., & Souba, W. W. (2006). Branched-chain amino acid-enriched nutritional support in surgical and cancer patients. *Journal of Nutrition, 136*: 314s–318s.

Deen, D., & Hark, L. (2007). *The Complete Guide to Nutrition in Primary Care.* Malden, MA: Blackwell.

Ejaz, S., Lim, C. W., Matsuda, K., & Ejaz, A. (2006). Liminoids as cancer chemopreventive agents. *Journal of Science of Food and Agriculture, 86*: 339–345.

Elliot, L., Molseed, L. L., & McCallum, P. (2006). *The Chemical Guide to Oncology Nutrition* (2nd ed.). Chicago: American Dietetic Association.

Falciglia, G. A., Steward, D. L., Leven, D. L., & Whittle, K. M. (2005). A clinical-based intervention improves diet in patients with head and neck cancer for second primary care. *Journal of American Dietetic Association, 105*: 1609–1612.

Fields-Gradner, C., Salomon, S., & Davis, M. (2003). *Living Well with HIV and AIDS: A Guide to Nutrition.* Chicago: American Dietetic Association.

Gershwin, M. E., Netle, P., & Keen, C. (Eds.). (2004). *Handbook of Nutrition and Immunity.* Totowa, NJ: Humana Press.

Hark, L., & Morrison, G. (Eds.). (2003). *Medical Nutrition and Disease* (3rd ed.). Malden, MA: Blackwell.

Kogut, V., & Luthringer, S. (Eds.). (2005). *Nutritional Issues in Cancer Care.* Pittsburgh: Oncology Nursing Society.

Mahan, L. K., & Escott-Stump, S. (Eds.). (2008). *Krause's Food and Nutrition Therapy* (12th ed.). Philadelphia: Elsevier Saunders.

Marian, M. J., Williams-Muller, P., & Bower, J. (2007). *Integrating Therapeutic and Complementary Nutrition.* Boca Raton, FL: CRC Press.

Mason, J. B., & Nitenberg, G. (Eds.). (2000). *Cancer & Nutrition: Prevention and Treatment.* Basel, NY: Karger.

Moore, M. C. (2005). *Pocket Guide to Nutritional Assessment and Care* (5th ed.). St. Louis, MO: Elvesier Mosby.

Payne-James, J., & Wicks, C. (2003). *Key Facts in Clinical Nutrition* (2nd ed.). London: Greenwich Medical Media.

Physicians Committee for Responsible Medicine. (2002). *Healthy Eating for Life to Prevent and Treat Cancer.* New York: Wiley.

Sardesai, V. M. (2003). *Introduction to Clinical Nutrition* (2nd ed.). New York: Marcel Dekker.

Seifert, C. (2006). Moving beyond the clinic: Nutritional intervention in a human immunodeficiency virus-infected pregnant population. *Journal of American Dietetic Association, 106*: 119–1121.

Shils, M. E., & Shike, M. (Eds.). (2006). *Modern Nutrition in Health and Disease* (10th ed.). Philadelphia: Lippincott, Williams and Wilkins.

Stipanuk, M. H. (Ed.). (2006). *Biochemical, Physiological and Molecular Aspects of Human Nutrition* (2nd ed.). St. Louis, MO: Saunders Elsevier.

Temple, N. J., Wilson, T., & Jacobs, D. R. (2006). *Nutrition Health: Strategies for Disease Prevention* (2nd ed.). Totowa, NJ: Humana Press.

Thomas, B., & Bishop, J. (Eds.). (2007). *Manual of Dietetic Practice* (4th ed.). Ames, IA: Blackwell.

Thorogood, M., Summerbell, C., Brunner, E., Simera, I., & Dowler, E. (2007). A systematic review of population and community dietary interventions to prevent cancer. *Nutrition Research Reviews, 20*: 74–88.

Watson, R. R. (Ed.). (2003). *Functional Foods & Nutraceuticals in Cancer Prevention.* Ames, IA: Iowa State Press.

Webster-Gandy, J., Madden, A., & Holdworth, M. (Eds.). (2006). *Oxford Handbook of Nutrition and Dietetics.* Oxford, London: Oxford University Press.

Whiteside, M. A., Heimberger, D. C., & Johanning, G. L. (2004). Micronutrients and cancer therapy. *Nutrition Reviews, 62*: 142–147.

CHAPTER

22

Diet Therapy for Burns, Immobilized Patients, Mental Patients, and Eating Disorders

Time for completion
Activities: 1½ hours
Optional examination: 1 hour

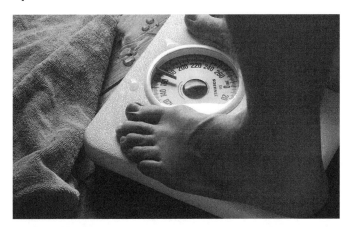

OBJECTIVES

Upon completion of this chapter, the student should be able to do the following:

Burns
1. Describe the severity of a burn by its degree.
2. Define the treatment goals of nutritional care of the burn patient.
3. Calculate the nutrient needs of a burn patient.
4. Recognize the teamwork required for efficient nutritional care.
5. Use aggressive nutritional therapy as a major part of the care of the burn patient.

Immobilized patients
1. Explain the nitrogen balance of such patients.
2. Define the caloric need of such patients.
3. Describe the urinary and bowel functions of such patients.
4. Individualize diet therapy for immobilized patients.

Mental patients

1. Describe the best approach to provide optimal nutritional and dietary care for the patients.
2. Explain their confusion about food and eating.
3. Discuss their mealtime misbehavior.
4. Recognize the reasons mental patients reject food.
5. Present multiple considerations in the dietary care for these patients.

Anorexia nervosa

1. Describe the pathophysiological manifestations of anorexia nervosa and bulimia.
2. Discuss the hospital feeding regime suitable for patient with eating disorders.
3. Recognize the necessity of psychological counseling, and make arrangements for this procedure to use behavior modification as appropriate.

GLOSSARY

Acuity: clearness; acuteness.
Amenorrhea: absence of menstruation.
Cachexia: a profound and marked state of ill health and malnutrition.
Decubitus ulcer: an inflammation, sore, or ulcer in the skin over a bony prominence, most frequently on sacrum, elbows, heels, inner knees, hips, shoulder blades, and ear rims of immobilized patients. Results from prolonged pressure on the part. It is most often seen in the aged, obese, debilitated, or cachectic patient, and those suffering from injuries and infections.
Dehydration: excessive loss of water from body tissues, accompanied by a disturbance in the balance of essential electrolytes.
Delusion: persistent, aberrant belief held by a person even though it is illogical, unique, and probably wrong. There are many kinds.
Dementia: organic loss of intellectual function.
Hydration: level of fluid in the body.
Hypercalcemia: greater than normal amount of calcium in the blood, most often resulting from excessive bone reabsorption and release of calcium.
Mental deviation: of, relating to, or characterized by a disorder of the mind.
Mental disorder: any disturbance of emotional equilibrium manifested in maladaptive behavior and impaired functioning. Caused by genetic, physical, chemical, biological, psychological, social, or cultural factors. Also called emotional illness, mental illness, or psychiatric disorder.
Psychological (aspects): the mental, motivational, and behavioral characteristics and attitudes of an individual or group of individuals.
Rehydration: replacement of fluid level in the body.

BACKGROUND INFORMATION

Space limitation has excluded chapters covering diet therapy for a number of other commonly encountered clinical disorders. This chapter remedies the situation by providing student activities to cover four important clinical subjects not yet addressed. The activities cover burns, immobilized patients, mental patients, and eating disorders.

ACTIVITY 1:

Diet and the Burn Patient

BACKGROUND INFORMATION

A severe burn is perhaps one of the most painful injuries a human being can receive. Burn patients undergo many of the physiological changes experienced by surgical patients. The extent of the burn injury partly determines the dietary care recommended. Nutritional principles for treating burn patients can also be applied to treating other forms of trauma, and vice versa.

The terms *first-*, *second-*, and *third-degree burns* are frequently used to describe the severity of a burn. A first-degree burn is the least severe and is considered only a superficial injury. Third-degree burns, on the other hand, are life threatening, since the skin is totally destroyed and internal organs adversely affected. The degree, or depth, of a burn injury differs by its area, or percentage of the body affected.

The amount of trauma suffered by patients with burns is dependent upon the type of burn (chemical, electrical, and thermal), extent (both depth and area) of the burn injury, and their age. Together these factors determine the likelihood of mortality. Second- and third-degree burns over 15 percent of the total body surface (10 percent in the elderly and children) can result in burn shock because of the quantity of fluid loss. Burns of more than 50 percent of the body surface are frequently fatal, especially in children and the elderly. Burns that involve the face and respiratory tract are most serious; chemical and electrical burns are more difficult to treat than thermal injuries.

NUTRITIONAL AND DIETARY CARE

The goal of treatment is to prevent infection, promote healing, and provide for the body's increased needs for nutrients and fluids. The therapy should continue until an intact skin is achieved and metabolism is normal.

Badly burned patients are extremely unfortunate. They suffer great pain and sometimes face permanent maiming. In addition, they may be extremely anxious about the consequences of plastic surgery and fearful that an altered appearance will alienate their relatives and friends.

In all major burn traumas, body tissues (and thus protein, cells, and protoplasm) are rapidly depleted, as is reserve energy, since the patients usually experience the most severe form of stress experienced by humans. The continuous loss of body tissue and energy may result in death either immediately after the burn or during the "recovery" period. Proper and aggressive nutritional therapy is critical in treating moderately to severely burned patients.

Acute stress rapidly leads to nutritional deficits, which greatly impede the body's efforts to heal damaged tissue and resist bacterial invasion. Proper dietary care can make the difference between life and death. Patients in good nutritional status and with small burns recover because they can eat sufficient food for their needs. However, the survival of an undernourished person suffering a severe burn depends heavily on aggressive nutritional therapy.

The nutritional requirements of burn patients are directly related to the extent and degree of burn. In general, burn patients have more nutritional problems than patients with other kinds of trauma. Since those with large burns have the most difficulty in maintaining an adequate oral intake, they sometimes become debilitated, even in a well-organized and adequately staffed burn center. The nutritional complications of burn victims are worse than those of major surgical patients, since their nutritional therapy is much more than just supportive care.

Many interferences make feeding burn patients difficult. Loss of appetite may occur for many reasons (fear, depression, drug therapy, and so on), making it difficult for patients to eat enough food to meet bodily requirements. An inability to move the head, hands, body, or feet in some patients also makes self-feeding difficult. If pain accompanies any attempt to chew, eat, or swallow, avoidance of food is common. The changing of dressings and skin grafting may also interfere with mealtime. Close supervision and encouragement of the patient are necessary to assure that as many nutrients as possible (especially protein) and optimum calories are ingested.

CALCULATING NUTRIENT NEEDS

This information applies to adult patients only. Consult the references for data applicable to a pediatric patient.

A burn patient has a special need for calories and protein in large amounts to replace fat loss, repair and deposit lean tissues, maintain body functions, and restore water loss. The calorie requirement may be as large as 6000–8000 kcal/d. This energy expenditure increases with the size of the burn and may be 30%–300% above basal levels, and it remains at high levels until grafting is completed. Sources of body weight loss are the breakdown of fat and protein as well as water loss. Food that is consumed provides about 5000–6000 kcal/d, and the breakdown of body fat provides about 1000–2000 kcal/d. A formula to calculate the caloric need of a patient with a burn injury is as follows:

Daily caloric need = 25 kcal/kg body weight
+ 40 kcal/% body surface with burns

In the following example, assume that the patient weighs 75 kg and has 50% of body surface burned.

Daily caloric need = 25 kcal/kg body weight
$\times$ 75 kg body weight + 40 kcal/% body surface with burns
$\times$ 50% body surface with burns
= (25 $\times$ 75 + 40 $\times$ 50) kcal
= 1875 + 2000 kcal
= 3875 kcal (allow 1000 kcal for margin of safety)
= 4500 to 5000 kcal (approximately).

A burn victim needs more protein to cover skin loss, blood protein loss from the burn, and infection.

The following formula is used for calculating the protein needs of a burn patient:

Total daily protein need = 1 g/kg body weight
+ 3 g/% body surface with burns

Assume that an adult patient weighs 75 kg and that 50% of the body surface has burns. The current recommendation for an adult burn patient is 20% of calories from protein (maximum). The calculations are as follows:

Total daily protein need = 1 g/kg body weight
$\times$ 75 kg body weight + 3 g/% body surface with burns
$\times$ 50% body surface with burns
= 75 + 150 g protein
= 225 g protein

A burn patient particularly needs calories and protein. However, in planning menus, fats should provide 30%–40% of total calories, and carbohydrates 45%–55%. A moderate amount of fat is judicious at the beginning, since a large amount of fat tends to satiate the patient and reduce the patient's appetite.

Most clinicians prescribe 2 to 10 times the RDAs/DRIs for water-soluble vitamins for burn patients. Vitamin C is given in amounts 20 to 30 times the RDA/DRI. However, fat-soluble vitamins are usually prescribed guardedly because of potential risks.

The mineral needs of burn patients require attention even after the fluids and electrolytes have been balanced. Body potassium, iron, calcium, zinc, and copper may have been lowered to unacceptable levels and should be monitored daily and replaced as needed.

ENTERAL AND PARENTERAL FEEDINGS

It is almost impossible to feed burn patients three large meals a day that contain up to 6000 kcal with 200 or more grams of protein. Oral feeding (OF) may not be sufficient. For a patient with moderate to severe burns, it is sometimes necessary to use several feeding methods to supply adequate protein and calories. This means enteral feeding (EN) or tube feeding and/or parenteral feeding (PN).

Tube feedings can be used depending on the burn sites. For example, a patient with head and neck burns would not receive EN. Early finding, especially the need for EN, is always an issue with a patient in critical care. It has a different meaning for the medical team in different clinical institutes. The word *early* may mean within a few hours of surgery or injury, while for others, *early* means initiation of feeds within days of surgery or injury. Early feeding also applies to OF, EN, and/or PN.

Early EN has benefits and risks and should be individualized. Tube feeding reaching the bottom of the stomach is ideal in the critically ill because it allows for early initiation of nutrition support, within hours of injury or surgery. Once the feeding is started, it is not necessary to decrease the rate or withhold feedings for medical therapies such as dressing changes, rehabilitative care, surgery, changing intravenous lines, and adjusting supine or prone positioning. Some medical teams prefer the feeding tubes reaching within the stomach itself.

Clinical observations have confirmed that early EN without PN is safe, well tolerated, and costs less. With partial dysfunctional digestive tract, the patient still has the viable option to consume nutrients via the nasoduodenal or nasojejunal delivery.

PN feeding is necessary for some patients with abdominal trauma, persistent intestinal infection or inflammation, severe diarrhea, and other conditions that interfere with digestion and absorption or when sufficient calories and protein cannot be delivered orally or enterally. When PN is used, simultaneous provision of EN feeding whenever feasible is recommended to promote gut function and maintain the mucosal barrier. As the rate of EN feeding is increased the rate of PN is decreased. In general, EN and PN are provided to patients whose digestive tracts are unable to tolerate the volume of feed that is most likely to be large.

PN is used very successfully in restoring balance in and healing severely burned patients. In some burn centers, however, PN is used as little as possible because of the danger of infection, and sometimes the access sites are not available if the patient is burned over a large area of his or her body. This feeding method will definitely be used, however, if EN is unsuccessful, because the nutrition of the patient has the higher priority.

TEAMWORK

The nutritional care of a burn patient requires efficient and conscientious teamwork. Many burn centers have established standard guidelines for dietary care. All team members should follow the individualized plans and goals for a particular patient. All personnel should encourage the patients to eat and provide them with psychological support. The entire health team monitors the progress and status of the patient to be certain that nutritional needs are met. Weight status and caloric intake are the two main criteria used. Weighing is done on a daily basis, as is intake and output, and all pertinent information is carefully recorded so that the diet therapy can be adjusted as needed.

NURSING IMPLICATIONS

Be aware that aggressive nutrition therapy is the major part of care for a burn patient.

1. A loss of more than 10% of preburn body weight places the person at high risk for sepsis and/or death.
2. Peak metabolic needs occur 6–10 days after the injury.
3. Fluid loss is a grave concern immediately after a burn.
4. Replacement of fluid and electrolyte losses is a major concern to prevent hypovolemic shock.
5. Fats, which are calorie dense, help increase caloric intake.
6. The burn patient is thirsty and dehydrated despite the edema that may be present. If NPO (nothing to eat or drink orally), good oral hygiene is necessary.
7. IV solutions of electrolytes, glucose, and especially saline may be necessary. Potassium deficit may occur.
8. Schedule dressing changes, pain medications, and other measures far enough in advance of mealtime that they will not interfere with meals.
9. Foods high in zinc increase wound healing. These include meat, liver, eggs, and seafood.
10. Early ambulation reduces calcium and protein losses due to immobilization.
11. Renal calculi is a common occurrence in the immobilized patient. A generous fluid intake is necessary.
12. "Fast" foods, favorite dishes from home, and any other desired items should be encouraged.
13. Educate the patient and family about the importance of diet to recovery.
14. Tube feedings or TPN, if needed for healing, should be instituted.

PROGRESS CHECK ON ACTIVITY 1

TRUE/FALSE

Circle T for True and F for False.

1. T F Burn patients and surgery patients experience many of the same changes.

2. T   F   A first-degree burn is the most serious of burns.
3. T   F   Acute stress leads to nutritional deficits.
4. T   F   Burn patients have fewer nutritional problems than psychological ones.
5. T   F   Burn patients have little difficulty in maintaining an adequate diet if it is properly prepared and served.

MULTIPLE CHOICE

Circle the letter of the correct answer.

6. The amount of trauma suffered by patients with burns is dependent on:

   a. the type of burn.
   b. previous nutritional status.
   c. age of the person.
   d. all of these.

7. Burns of more than _____ of body surface are often fatal.

   a. 15%
   b. 25%
   c. 50%
   d. 10%

8. Nutritional requirements of burn patients are directly related to:

   a. extent and degree.
   b. type and site.
   c. location and time.
   d. age and previous health.

9. Energy expenditure increases in burn patients range between:

   a. 10%–20%.
   b. 100%–1000%.
   c. 500%–5000%.
   d. 30%–3000%.

FILL-IN

10. List five interferences to successful feeding of burn patients.

    a. _____
    b. _____
    c. _____
    d. _____
    e. _____

11. Identify three sources of body weight loss of burn patients.

    a. _____
    b. _____
    c. _____

SITUATION

12. Lenny Lambrusco, age 10, has received second- and third-degree burns over 40% of his body in an accident. He weighs 77 pounds. Calculate the amount of protein Lenny will need to repair and replace damaged tissue.

13. List five nursing implications for nutrition that must be observed in caring for a burn patient.

    a. _____
    b. _____
    c. _____
    d. _____
    e. _____

ACTIVITY 2:

Diet and Immobilized Patients

INTRODUCTION

A surgical and medical patient may be temporarily immobilized by being confined to bed. Older, chronically ill, disabled, and handicapped patients may be immobilized for many years. Some patients, such as those recovering from strokes, may be gradually rehabilitated, progressing from bed confinement to the use of a wheelchair, crutches, and a cane and finally being able to walk freely. During the immobilization period, there are four important considerations in the patient's nutritional and dietary care: nitrogen balance, calories, calcium intake, and urinary and bowel functions.

NITROGEN BALANCE

Long-term bed confinement causes body muscle to atrophy, even in a healthy person. This process is characterized by a negative nitrogen balance (see Chapter 3). An otherwise healthy person may lose about 2 to 3 g of nitrogen a day given an adequate calorie and protein intake. This means a loss of 13 to 20 g of protein. To compensate for that loss, the person must eat extra protein. A chronically ill person confined to bed will also suffer skin lesions resulting from decubitus ulcers (bedsores). These ulcers may be caused by prolonged pressure on some areas of the skin or an infection that aggravates the sloughing of skin cells. This skin sloughing can also contribute to the negative nitrogen balance. During early immobilization, muscle atrophy and skin sloughing cause a nitrogen loss far exceeding protein intake; this loss cannot be arrested even by a high protein intake. However, over a long period, a high-protein diet can reverse muscle loss and partially maintain the integrity of the skin.

Actual skin breakdown can be avoided only by a combination of a high-protein diet, frequent position adjustment, exercise (whenever feasible), special materials for sheets and bedding, and good hygiene. As debilitated patients stabilize, they excrete less nitrogen and can adapt to the stress of illness. However, tissue atrophy and skin lesions can continue and must be guarded against. Depending on the clinical condition, immobilized patients need 70–120 g of protein a day. In addition, vitamin C intake should be elevated to offset the increased stress.

CALORIES

The caloric intake of an immobilized patient is also very important. It must be continuously monitored and adjusted to the clinical condition of the individual patient. For example, a young athlete suffering from a bone fracture will need a high caloric intake for recovery. Some patients continue to lose weight; some reasons include catabolic and nonspecific effects of trauma and loss of appetite. During the beginning of bed confinement, weight loss may be avoided by a high caloric intake. As the patient's weight stabilizes, the caloric intake must be adjusted to the patient's condition. Patients undergoing physical therapy work hard and may also need a high-calorie diet. But an immobilized patient who is recovering slowly, is quiet, and does very little exercise needs a normal diet or a diet that is slightly low in calories to maintain body weight. Paralyzed patients can gain weight easily because food is their main enjoyment, and they are quite inactive. The excess weight will further limit their activity. To prepare for rehabilitation and a reasonable degree of mobility, paralyzed patients must maintain their ideal weight.

CALCIUM

Bedridden patients have disturbed calcium metabolism, especially patients with bone fractures. Calcium homeostasis is determined by a number of factors: bone integrity, serum calcium, intestinal function, adequacy of active vitamin D, kidney function, and parathyroid activity. Prolonged immobilization may lead to disorders related to excessive calcium: hypercalcemia, hypercalciuria, metastatic calcification of soft tissues such as muscle and kidney, and calcium stone formation in the bladder, kidney, or urinary tract. Characteristic symptoms of hypercalcemia are nausea, vomiting, loss of appetite, excessive thirst, excessive urination, headache, constipation, abdominal pain, listlessness, malaise, dehydration, psychosis, blunting of pain sensations, and coma. If untreated, the condition can lead to kidney failure, high blood pressure, seizures, and hearing loss. The treatment (mainly rehydration) for acute hypercalcemia is as follows: (1) intravenous fluid therapy with saline; (2) intravenous diuretic medications and replacement of all urinary loss of sodium, magnesium, and potassium; (3) replacement of any excessive urine loss by fluid (intravenous saline); and (4) implementation of a low-calcium diet. If there is no response, other modes of therapy are necessary. The long-term treatment for hypercalcemia involves: (1) mobilization as soon as possible; (2) calcium intake kept at 500 to 800 mg/d (a low-calcium diet may not be effective if volume expansion has not been brought under control); and (3) phosphate supplement, which helps some, but not all, patients.

URINARY AND BOWEL FUNCTIONS

An immobilized patient may have problems with the excretory system. The patient should drink a lot of fluid to make certain that the bladder and kidneys are kept clear. In patients with spinal cord injury, the loss of bladder control may expose the genitourinary tract to a higher risk of infection. When there is no hypercalcemia, the immobilized patient may actually have reduced intake and the decreased fluid intake may precipitate formation of calcium stones. Because of the importance of hydration, the patient should be monitored with some recording system either at home or in the hospital. The time and amount of water taken in both beverage and food should be estimated, and the time, frequency, and volume of urination should be recorded.

Bowel movements of immobilized patients pose special problems. Some develop diarrhea and others constipation. Patients must avoid foods that tend to cause gas or indigestion. They should also drink a lot of fluid, eat an adequate amount of fiber, and establish good bowel habits to avoid constipation.

PROGRESS CHECK ON ACTIVITY 2

FILL-IN

1. Four considerations in an immobilized patient's nutritional and diet care are:

   a. _____

   b. _____

   c. _____

   d. _____

2. Actual skin breakdown can be avoided only by a combination of:

   a. _____

   b. _____

   c. _____

   d. _____

   e. _____

3. Calcium homeostasis is determined by factors such as:

   a. _____

   b. _____

   c. _____

   d. _____

   e. _____

   f. _____

4. Diseases related to excessive calcium are:

   a. _____

   b. _____

   c. _____

   d. _____

5. Long-term treatment of hypercalcemia includes:

   a. _____

   b. _____

   c. _____

TRUE/FALSE

Circle T for True and F for False.

6. T F Long-term bed confinement causes body muscle to atrophy with a negative nitrogen loss of at least 2–3 g of nitrogen a day.

7. T F A chronically ill person confined to bed suffers skin lesions resulting from decubitus ulcers (bedsores).

8. T F During early immobilization, atrophy and skin sloughing cause a severe negative nitrogen loss.

9. T F Muscle loss from immobilized patients cannot be reversed.

10. T F Immobilized patients need 70–120 g protein a day with vitamin C supplement.

11. T F Calorie intake of immobilized patients must be adjusted to the clinical conditions of the individual patient.

12. T F Prolonged immobilization may lead to obesity.

13. T F Immobilized patients should drink a lot of fluids to make certain that the bladder and kidneys do not atrophy.

14. T F Intake of fluids for all immobilized patients is basically the same.

15. T F Immobilized patients should avoid foods that tend to produce gas or indigestion.

16. T F Immobilized patients should try to maintain good bowel habits.

ACTIVITY 3:

Diet and Mental Patients

INTRODUCTION

A large number of people in this country are confined to mental institutions—half of all available hospital beds are occupied by such patients. The adequacy of care provided in a mental institution has been subject to public scrutiny for many years. Because of the complex social, political, economic, and medical issues involved, this will be a subject of controversy for many more years.

In many respects, mental patients do not differ from normal people. They need human understanding and a meaningful relationship with their environment and the people around them. They have many of the same attitudes to food as normal people, such as having food preferences and responding to the attractiveness of foods served (see Chapter 14). They need more than a well-balanced diet, however. Food and eating are especially important to them, because they are deprived of many of the other joys of life. Contrary to past belief, proper care can improve nutritional status in these patients, as evidenced by clinical studies.

In planning nutritional and dietary care of a mental patient, a well-coordinated and concerted effort is needed from every member of the health team, which may include a psychiatrist, nurse, social worker, therapist (occupational, physical, or recreational), nutritionist, dietitian, psychologist, clinical specialist, and health aides.

A patient needs total care, which requires several considerations. One is the provision of adequate healthcare facilities and programs. Once a patient has been admitted to an institution, financial problems, family acceptance, and negative social attitudes toward mental illness pose special problems for the patient. Regarding nutritional care, a special diet therapy may be required. The patient's nutritional status and the need for rehabilitation must be evaluated. In addition, feeding a mental patient demands special procedures.

Care in mental institutions varies tremendously. Although each state establishes guidelines for public as well as private mental hospitals, numerous reports have documented substandard or plainly deficient care provided by some institutions, both private and public. Many criticisms are leveled at nutritional care.

In general, these hospitals are crowded and under-budgeted. Food budgets in particular are grossly inadequate. Facilities and equipment are out of date, misused, inadequate, and sometimes even decrepit. This pertains to the kitchen layout, equipment, and serving utensils. Dining environments are unsatisfactory. Dull dining rooms, old and displaced draperies, uncomfortable chairs, and even poor sanitation may add to an already depressing environment.

Staffs are undertrained and too small. This especially applies to dietitians, nurses, nutritionists, and food service managers. Many personnel lack the training for handling feeding difficulties. As a result, nutritional and dietary preparation, planning, and services suffer for severely handicapped patients. For instance, the food texture may be inappropriate for patients having chewing or swallowing difficulties. Cold foods, unattractive meals, over- or undersalted foods, and lack of concern and care in serving may all discourage patients from eating adequately.

Clinical reports indicate that many hospitalized mental patients have an unsatisfactory nutritional status. On one hand, there may be overall undernourishment with overt and covert signs. Emaciated patients may show a lack of interest in food because they are worried, depressed, tense, or anxious, or they may purposefully neglect it. On the other hand, some patients are grossly overweight for similar psychological reasons. They compensate for emotional turmoil by eating constantly.

Patients with an unsatisfactory nutritional status need an understanding and sympathetic staff. Some improvement will always result if they are provided a good, nutritious, balanced diet that is served in an attractive and appetizing manner. These patients need both food and emotional comforts. If they are happy, the undernourished will eat more and the obese less.

There are some basic reasons why mental patients have nutritional and dietary problems. First, they may have eating handicaps, such as being unable to chew, lacking hand and mouth coordination, and experiencing pain in swallowing. The hospital staff may fail to correct these conditions through neglect or understaffing. Second, they may not like the foods they are served. Third, these patients may have abnormal behavioral patterns that inhibit their nutritional intake. The bizarre eating behaviors of some mental patients constitute a major challenge to nurses, dietitians, and aides. A discussion is provided in the following paragraphs.

CONFUSION ABOUT FOOD AND EATING

Patients may be uncertain about eating and unable to decide what and when to eat and with whom. In some cases, the patients forget how to eat foods such as artichokes or grapefruit. Anxiety and hesitation prolong mealtime. These patients cannot be pressured to finish meals even within a reasonable period of time. If hurried, patients may discard the foods, give them to a roommate, or try to bargain with the nurse or dietitian. If the nurse or dietitian knows the reasons behind such behavior, he or she can talk to the patient, help the patient to select menu items, and provide assistance if any difficulty in feeding arises. If a group of patients tends to take a long time to eat, the problem may be solved by letting them eat together at mealtime, thus relieving the nurses from waiting.

MEALTIME MISBEHAVIOR

Mental patients may have many disrupting eating behaviors. These include throwing food and dishes, interfering with other patients' meals, playing with and discarding food, and eating others' leftovers. Patients may also ignore personal cleanliness by spitting out food and catching food thrown in the air. This behavior may result from defective mental coordination or be an expression of a whole spectrum of emotional problems. The appropriate remedy depends on whether mealtime misbehavior results from the mental derangement. If it does not, the nurse and dietitian should apply interpersonal techniques, such as ignoring the behavior. Using plastic or paper utensils reduces danger and the cost of replacing broken items.

FOOD REJECTION

Mental patients may refuse food for many reasons, some of which are familiar and some of which are not. One familiar cause is the side effects of drugs that have been administered. Also, vomiting and food intolerance may make patients afraid to eat. The simplest reason for reduced food intake is that an overweight patient is following a self-imposed regimen of weight reduction.

Reasons for reduced food intake peculiar to mental patients include a malfunctioning hypothalamus. This problem weakens hunger reactions, making the patient want less food. A patient's mental problems may also have caused a loss of coordination, knowledge, or confidence in food acceptance. Refusing food may be a simple rejection of what food represents to or evokes in the patient (such as an event, guilt, or a lost relative). Finally, the patient may be suffering a multitude of psychological problems, such as depression, hearing voices, confusion, hallucinations, and obsession.

A nurse, dietitian, or nutritionist will find several guidelines useful in helping a patient accept food. Frequent communication is highly desirable, because talking demonstrates concern and will thus make a patient feel better. However, this communication should never include accusations of bad behavior in relation to food. Such accusations could cause the patient to reject food again.

It should be ascertained if refusal of food is related to a specific physiological disorder, because some patients may be reluctant to mention it. In some cases, the use of drugs or hormones (such as insulin) may increase a patient's appetite. In others, forced feeding or assistance in eating is required. A patient should never be made to feel guilty or uncomfortable about any extra work that the staff may have to perform to help the patient eat.

If a patient refuses food frequently, the meals missed and the quantity of food involved should be recorded. For instance, a patient may not like to eat at a certain time, and so the feeding time should be adjusted, if possible. Also, an attempt must be made to replace missed meals.

In feeding mental patients, their emotional makeup must be known. Defiance, submission, self-contempt, constant demands for love and affection, and suspicion of food poisoning are some characteristics of a disturbed personality. Concerned staff and volunteers can use appropriate communication to convince patients to eat and enjoy their food, thus improving the quality of patients' lives.

The eating environment must be pleasing, clean, convenient, gay, and comfortable with attractive pictures, paintings, tables, and chairs. Group dining has proved successful in improving the eating habits of patients. They enjoy eating with other patients, relatives, and staff. Thus, arrangements should be made so that they can eat with others at regular intervals. Group dining may be enhanced by having cafeteria-style meals that provide patients with a wide variety of foods.

Other considerations in feeding mental patients are as follows: (1) If the image of a prison or institution can be transformed into that of a clinic, patients show appreciation and improvement. (2) Obesity or weight gain may be the result of extra foods given by relatives and nighttime staff. Such occurrences should be identified and corrected. (3) Keeping a weight record is important to make sure that the patient is not gaining or losing too much weight. (4) Many patients are pleased and feel needed when the hospital pays attention to their birthdays and gives them special treats. The same applies to holidays and festivals. There are some special considerations in the dietary care of elderly mental patients. For example, the psychiatric problems of depression, confusion, anxiety, and suspicion in a mental patient are even more exaggerated when the patient is older. These patients are generally overconcerned about the functions of the alimentary tract. Their worry and concern can aggravate intestinal motility and cause cramps and even distension. Elderly mental patients also tend to need more security and more of their favorite foods. Depression and suspicion that food is poisoned may lead them to refuse food often. As a result of confusion, elderly patients may ignore food altogether.

In the last few years, psychotherapy, drugs (such as sedatives and tranquilizers), and electric shock treatment, which are now standard management programs, have helped some patients to gain a semblance of normalcy in their lives. As a result, many of these patients are no longer institutionalized. Many discharged patients who have an unsatisfactory nutritional status can be taught to nourish themselves adequately. In fact, good nutritional and dietary care with the proper vitamin and mineral supplements may improve a patient's psychological condition. However, many patients receive medications that may harm their nutritional status.

These discharged patients have the same eating problems as those living in the hospital, and they need the same remedies. Because many of these patients still attend treatment centers and clinics and need occasional hospitalization, some nurses and dietitians have succeeded in providing them with sound nutritional education programs. Included in these programs are the following:

1. Teaching some basic facts and skills about food budgeting, purchasing, and preparation. Many of these patients have never cooked before or have not been cooking for a while.
2. Teaching principles of nutritional needs.
3. Teaching known effects of drugs on nutritional status. Practically all mental patients receive some medications; some profound effects of these drugs on nutritional status are discussed in Chapters 10 and 14. Teaching basic facts about food, such as proper sanitation and safety, meal planning, storage, freezing, use of equipment, and so on.

NURSING IMPLICATIONS
General Guidelines

1. Recognize that appropriate nutrition therapy is a major part of care for immobilized and mental patients.
2. The plan of care and approaches may differ. Use whatever method and manner of feeding that is most effective.
3. Check all medications that a patient is receiving; some may interfere with nutritional status. Ask for changes if warranted.
4. Provide nutrition education to patients, family, and caregivers.

Some Specific Considerations

Immobilized Persons

1. Closely monitor hydration. Chart time and amount of fluids ingested (including liquids in foods).
2. Observe the types and amounts of food consumed. Be especially cognizant of protein intake, which should be adjusted to patient's condition. Chart concerns and call attention to M.D. and RD if necessary.
3. Examine patient's skin for signs of decubiti formation, change type of bedding used, and give frequent position adjustments.
4. Increase protein and calorie intake. Add vitamin and mineral supplements if not already part of therapy.
5. Monitor bowel habits (diarrhea or constipation may be present), and adjust diet accordingly.
6. Bedridden patients have disturbed calcium metabolism. Check for symptoms of hypercalcemia and dehydration. Rehydration is critical. A low-calcium diet may be helpful.

7. A reduced caloric intake may be indicated for those who are immobilized for long periods (such as paralyzed patients). Excessive weight gain is common. Identify "extras" brought in by well-meaning family and friends (or staff), and correct. Keep a weight record.

8. Adjust caloric intake to the clinical condition; young people who will be immobilized for short periods of time (such as with fractures) will need a higher calorie diet than those of long-term patients.

Patients with Mental Deviations

The psychological aspects of feeding are very important for this group of patients.

1. Monitor the patient's weight, nutritional status, and mental attitude and be prepared to intervene.

2. The eating environment should be pleasing, clean, comfortable, and attractive.

3. The attitude of staff serving food should be pleasant, cheerful, and helpful.

4. Pay careful attention to what is served: food should be appropriate to the individual patient. For example, a blanket low-sodium diet is unsuitable for all patients.

5. The food should be prepared and served under sanitary conditions. The dietary staff should be clean and neat in appearance.

6. Pay careful attention to patient's needs such as eating handicaps, lack of hand and mouth coordination, chewing and swallowing difficulties, food likes and dislikes, sore mouths, edentulous, and so on.

7. Food should be served either hot or cold, as appropriate, and be seasoned well.

8. Be aware of the patients emotional status, such as confusion, anxiety, suspicion, refusal to eat, and disruptive eating habits:
   a. Techniques: establish communication lines, provide assistance with eating, help with food selection, and use behavioral strategies.
   b. Record meals missed and quantity of uneaten food. Attempt to replace missed meals. Force feeding is a last resort.

9. Special care for the elderly:
   a. All emotional and behavior problems are exaggerated in the elderly, especially depression, anxiety, confusion, suspicion, and refusal to eat.
   b. The elderly are prone to overconcern regarding bowel functions.
   c. Techniques: provide more security, attempt to gain trust, serve more favorite foods, and give verbal reminders that they must eat.

10. Provide nutrition education to patient, family, and/or caregivers. These patients go home, and most need nutrition education on a range of topics, such as what to feed, how much, and sanitation proce-

dures. (See list at the end of this activity for other suggestions.)

11. Enlist the help of the clinical dietitian, if needed for help with planning and handout materials. Group sessions are usually well received. A translator may be needed.

PROGRESS CHECK ON ACTIVITY 3

FILL-IN

1. The health team of a mental patient includes:

   a. _____

   b. _____

   c. _____

   d. _____

   e. _____

   f. _____

   g. _____

   h. _____

   i. _____

2. Criticisms on nutritional care in mental institutions include:

   a. _____

   b. _____

   c. _____

3. Some of the basic reasons why mental patients have nutritional and dietary problems are:

   a. _____

   b. _____

   c. _____

4. General guidelines for nursing immobilized and mental patients:

   a. _____

   b. _____

   c. _____

   d. _____

TRUE/FALSE

Circle T for True and F for False.

5. T F A malfunctioning hypothalamus causes a mental patient to overeat.

6. T F Mental patients' disruptive mealtime behavior is sometimes due to the dining room environment.

7. T F Medications for mental patients may have side effects that cause rejections of food.

8. T F Proper and frequent communication is highly desirable in helping a mental patient accept food.

9. T F Identification of causes for refusal of food is critical in overcoming nutritional and dietary problems in mental patients.

10. T F Physiological and psychological disorders should be separated in treating mental patients' nutritional and dietary problems.

11. T F Group eating is not effective in treating eating problems of mental patients.

12. T F Elderly mental patients should be treated the same way as younger mental patients.

13. T F Psychotherapy, sedatives, tranquilizers, and electric shock treatment are standard management programs used to keep patients under control.

14. T F Good nutritional and dietary care with the proper vitamin and mineral supplements may improve a mental patient's psychological condition.

ACTIVITY 4:

Part I—Eating Disorders: Anorexia Nervosa

BACKGROUND INFORMATION

Anorexia nervosa refers to the clinical condition in which a person voluntarily eats very little food (self-imposed starvation). As a result, there is a large weight loss with all of its concomitant symptoms. The disorder is more common among females, especially teenage girls, although it has been identified in men and older women. Typically the teenage female patient comes from a middle- to upper-middle-class family. Before the problem occurs, the patient is usually healthy and cooperative and has made good progress in school. All indications point to a "model" student and child. Then, the child develops psychological problems leading her to resent her obesity (which may be real or imagined) and embarks on a self-prescribed starvation diet. She continues to abstain from food even when she has achieved an ideal weight. After that, her health deteriorates.

CLINICAL MANIFESTATIONS

The anorexic patient presents several clinical manifestations. Although the desire for food is present, the patient refuses to eat and drink. Occasionally the patient has an uncontrollable urge to gorge, which is followed by self-induced vomiting. Because of this, anorexic patients may lose 25%–35% of their body weight and become emaciated and wasted. Electrolyte imbalances occur, and female anorexic patients develop hair over different parts of their body and cease to menstruate. Also present is decreased body metabolism, cold hands and feet, decreased blood pressure, and decreased sensitivity to insulin. Bone density is compromised, leading to stress fractures, especially in female athletes. The heart muscle becomes thin and weak, the immune system is impaired, anemia develops, insomnia is common, and both men and women lose their sex drives. Anorexic patients exhibit abnormal behavior such as frequent self-induced vomiting, excessive use of cathartics (laxatives), and overexercise (hyperactivity). In some patients, such actions may lead to death.

A number of events can spark the beginning of a voluntary, continuous reduction of food intake. A worsening mother-daughter relationship may set it off, or a sudden, highly emotional conflict between the patient and someone else may do so. Other possible causes are an abrupt failure in schoolwork and the emotional turmoil over beginning or continuing a sexual relationship.

In-depth studies by psychologists and psychiatrists of anorexic patients have indicated a common psychological profile. These patients show a lack of feeling for hunger, satiety, tiredness, and sometimes even physical pain. They generally have a distorted image of their physical size. Some anorexic patients think that they are 40%–60% larger than they, in fact, are. Consequently, they become obsessed with dieting. In addition, these patients commonly feel inadequate in role identity, competence (work or school performance), and effectiveness (in communication, controlling events, etc.). This loss of faith in personal ability leads to an attempt to control the environment by controlling body weight. Food binges, guilt about eating, and a reluctance to admit abnormal food habits are the typical attitudes of anorexic patients toward food.

Treatment for a patient with anorexia nervosa consists of psychotherapy, behavior modification, drug therapy, and hospitalization for refeedings. The treatment objective of diet therapy and hospital feedings is to return the patient to a normal diet and an appropriate, healthy weight. A discussion of rehabilitative measures used in hospitals follows.

HOSPITAL FEEDING

Patients with anorexia nervosa are best hospitalized, because the eating environment can be controlled and family involvement is minimized. Some patients eat better in a hospital because they do not have to make any decisions about what and when to eat. In general, satisfactory care requires careful planning, an experienced staff, and a tremendous amount of concern and understanding.

Once anorexia nervosa has been diagnosed, the first major responsibility of the health team is to develop a dietary and nutrition program. There should be complete understanding and communication among the health team members to avoid any inconsistency or friction. This is important, since the patient may try to manipulate healthcare personnel and parents in order to avoid food intake and secure an opportunity to exercise. Most anorexic patients want to maintain a starved appearance. The nurse can coordinate all activities to assure that the program is implemented. The doctor should describe the treatment procedures to the patient, preferably in the presence of the primary nurse and the dietitian or nutritionist.

Detailed procedures for feeding a hospitalized patient with anorexia nervosa may be obtained from the references at the end of this chapter. General guidelines are given here.

The attending physician will prescribe a diet after studying the patient's condition. Most practitioners start with a diet containing 1000–3000 kcal and progressively increase the intake by 200 kcal every three or four days until the daily intake is adequate for an acceptable weight gain. A liquid diet may be more acceptable to the patient; it appears to have fewer calories. To avoid any misunderstandings, any changes in caloric intake must be made by the doctor or an assigned coordinator in the form of a written request. A cooperative patient can be fed three main meals and occasionally a snack. Elimination of privileges followed by a gradual return of them for compliance is a viable approach. The nurse should be fully informed of the patient's condition, including the treatment protocol. Most importantly, the attending nurse should monitor the patient's eating behavior and pay full attention to the following feeding routines.

1. Check that the foods served comply with the meal plan.
2. Pay attention to the patient's hands constantly.
3. Assume a friendly and supportive attitude so that the patient will not feel spied on.
4. Leave the room only in an emergency, since the patient may try to get rid of some foods.
5. Prevent food disposal by keeping any container (such as a facial tissue box, a wastebasket, or a flower pot) away from the patient during the meal and checking the meal tray after the patient has finished eating. The patient may hide food under napkins or smear it under the bed, on the window sill, and so forth.
6. Permit a maximum of one hour for eating a meal.
7. If feasible, arrange for the patient to eat alone and be monitored by the same nurse.
8. If possible, the patient should wear a pocketless hospital gown while eating.
9. Insist that the patient rest for ½ to one hour after a meal and does not leave the bed, since she may induce vomiting.

Recovery is a long and difficult process that may last from six months to one year or more. About 60%–70% of all patients may recover after several years of treatment; the remaining patients may die. Real recovery is extremely important, since most of these patients tend to be mentally unstable, and the condition will tend to recur at other stressful times in their lives.

NURSING IMPLICATIONS

1. All team members must be consistent and caring in their handling of the feeding routines.
2. Patients may not manipulate or dictate food intake.
3. Feeding periods must be closely supervised.
4. Bathroom privileges must be denied for at least 30 minutes after a meal to prevent self-induced vomiting.
5. Major sleep disturbances that occur early in treatment cease as the patient gains weight.
6. Avoid all conversation related to food or weight gain while the patient is hospitalized, except as it relates to an agreed-upon contract ("You have complied with diet goals this week so you may [have] [get] [do] the reward.").
7. Nutrition education for patient and family can begin when the patient is discharged.
8. Psychological counseling takes precedence over nutritional counseling.

PROGRESS CHECK ON ACTIVITY 4, PART I

MULTIPLE CHOICE

Circle the letter of the correct answer.

1. Clinical manifestations of anorexia nervosa include all except which of these?

   a. disinterest in food
   b. hypotension
   c. hyperactivity
   d. amenorrhea

2. Typical mental attitudes of anorexic patients include:

   a. guilt.
   b. denial.
   c. inadequacy.
   d. all of the above.

3. Prioritize the following treatment measures for an anorexic patient:

   a. diet therapy, drug therapy, psychotherapy
   b. behavior modification, psychotherapy, diet therapy
   c. psychotherapy, behavior modification, drug therapy, hospitalization
   d. hospitalization, drug therapy, diet therapy, psychotherapy

4. The first responsibility of the health team assigned to care for an anorexic patient is to:

   a. remove all sources of stimulation from patient.
   b. develop a satisfactory nutrition program.
   c. implement behavior modification techniques.
   d. assign someone to carefully monitor the patient.

5. The initial diet therapy for an anorexic patient consists of approximately _____ calories.

   a. 1000–2000.
   b. 2000–3000.
   c. 3000–4000.
   d. 4000–5000.

FILL-IN

6. Name five feeding routines that should be observed by the nurse attending a patient with anorexia nervosa.

   a. _____

   b. _____

   c. _____

   d. _____

   e. _____

7. Name five important nursing implications to observe when caring for persons with anorexia nervosa.

   a. _____

   b. _____

   c. _____

   d. _____

   e. _____

ACTIVITY 4:

Part II—Other Eating Disorders

BACKGROUND INFORMATION

As more and more Americans, especially women, strive for the "ideal" body, which is culturally defined as "model" thin, or even thinner, the number of psychological and physical illnesses from eating disorders continues to rise. The trend continues down to the elementary school level, where girls as young as 9 or 10 are beginning to diet. Young boys know that a major criterion for social acceptance is a thin, muscular frame, and so they, too, fall prey to eating disorders. Two widely practiced behaviors for both sexes is cyclic dieting, which leads to the chronic dieting syndrome; and the binge-and-purge syndrome, bulimia nervosa. A brief description of each and some suggestions for dietary management follow.

BULIMIA NERVOSA

This term is descriptive of the pattern of the disease. Huge amounts of food (up to 5000 kcal in a single sitting, eaten rapidly) are consumed. This is followed by feelings of guilt and shame at the loss of control. In response to these feelings and the need to purge the body of this vast intake of food, the person practices self-induced vomiting; uses laxatives, diuretics, or diet pills, and/or engages in strenuous exercise. The effect of these behaviors on the body is very damaging. The effect on the psyche is also damaging, leading to loss of self-esteem and depression. Persons with bulimia usually keep it a guilt-ridden secret until their symptoms become apparent.

Some of the physical symptoms of bulimia include:

1. Blood-shot eyes and broken blood vessels on the face. Decayed teeth and eroded enamel on the teeth from self-induced vomiting. There may also be bruises on the hand that is used to induce the vomiting.
2. Sore throat, swollen salivary glands, and infrequently, esophageal tears or ruptures of the gastric mucosa
3. Intestinal problems from overuse of laxatives.
4. Although fatigue is common, as is cessation of menses, the weight fluctuates. Clients are not usually underweight or, if they are, they will cycle back to their previous weight, and sometimes weigh more than they did previously.

CHRONIC DIETING SYNDROME

This disorder, newly classified by the American Psychiatric Association, is commonly called "compulsive overeating." It is a reaction to psychological stressors, such as anxiety and emotional problems, or a need for comfort. A great deal of compulsive overeating follows very restrictive dieting practices in an attempt to reach an unnatural and unrealistic weight goal. When failure occurs, rebound eating follows. This creates the characteristic weight cycling. Each time a cycle occurs the Basal Metabolic Rate (BMR) drops, and in the next dieting cycle, the weight comes off more slowly than before. Lean body mass is also lost with each cycling, and it is not regained with the refeeding. Body composition is altered.

MANAGEMENT OF BULIMIA AND COMPULSIVE OVEREATING

Managing these eating disorders will require a concerted effort by the health team. As a rule, these clients are not hospitalized; they are managed on an outpatient basis. The approach is individualized to the client, and psychological treatment will be a priority. Clients may receive antidepressant drug therapy along with counseling. Nutrition education and counseling receive high priority. Behavior modification is helpful. Support groups and/or one-on-one counseling in combination with other therapies and follow-up care are needed.

The strategies for nutrition management should include written material such as diet plans and behavioral techniques. The client should keep a journal or log of the food eaten and the things that he or she believes trigger the eating frenzies. Diets should be planned to not go below the average 1200–1500 kcal basal requirements. Foods such as fruits, vegetables, and cereal grains that are high in fiber are emphasized. Clients are advised to use only those foods that are preportioned and only those that are eaten with utensils (not finger foods). The diet should follow the guidelines for nutrient distribution as discussed in Chapters 7 and 14, with 50%–55% complex carbohydrates, protein according to the RDA/DRI for their age and size, and no more than 30% fat.

Students will find that many clients with eating disorders are already knowledgeable about good weight-management practices but are not able to follow them. This is the challenge that health professionals face, but these are serious health matters, and until the societal pressures for excessive thinness are resolved, clients must be assisted to change their individual attitudes and feelings to a healthier outlook.

PROGRESS CHECK ON ACTIVITY 4, PART II

Self-Study

Situation: You have a friend whose 14-year-old daughter is causing her concern. She confides to you the following:

Jenny is so different lately; she has become quite secretive. She has dark circles under her eyes, and her neck looks swollen. I've asked her several times if she's OK, and she says yes, she's just tired. I suppose she is, she eats pretty well and hasn't lost weight, but I think she must have trouble digesting her food. I hear her in the bathroom after meals, and it sounds like she is throwing up, but she says I'm mistaken. Do you think I should force her to go to the doctor, or is this just a phase she's going through?

Based on your present knowledge of eating disorders, and cognizant of the behaviors of adolescents, how will you answer your friend?

REFERENCES

American Dietetic Association. (2006). *Nutrition Diagnosis: A Critical Step in Nutrition Care Process*. Chicago: Author.

Aquilani, R. (2002). Prevalence of decubitus ulcer and associated risk factor in an institutionalized Spanish elderly population. *Nutrition, 1*: 437–438.

Becker, A. E. (2005). Disclosure patterns of eating and weight concern to clinicians, educational professionals, family and peers. *International Journal of Eating Disorders, 38*: 18–23.

Beham, E. (2006). *Therapeutic Nutrition: A Guide to Patient Education*. Philadelphia: Lippincott, Williams and Wilkins.

Buchman, A. (2004). *Practical Nutritional Support Technique* (2nd ed.). Thorofeue, NJ: SLACK.

De Bandt, J. P. (2006). Thermal use of branched-chain amino acids in burn, trauma, and sepsis. *Journal of Nutrition, 136*: 308s–313s.

Deen, D., & Hark, L. (2007). *The Complete Guide to Nutrition in Primary Care*. Malden, MA: Blackwell.

Dickerson, R. N. (2002). Hypocaloric enteral tube feeding in critically ill obese patients. *Nutrition: 18*: 241–246.

Dickerson, R. N. (2002). Estimating energy and protein requirements of thermally injured patients: art or science. *Nutrition, 18*: 439–442.

Frisch, M. J. (2006). Residential treatment for eating disorders. *International Journal of Eating Disorders, 39*: 434–442.

Gonzales-Gross, M. (2005). Nutrition and cognitive impairment in the elderly. *British Journal of Nutrition, 86*: 313–321.

Hark, L., & Morrison, G. (Eds.). (2003). *Medical Nutrition and Disease* (3rd ed.). Malden, MA: Blackwell.

Herrin, M. (2003). *Nutritional Counseling in the Treatment of Eating Disorders*. New York: Brunner-Routledge.

Imbierowicz, K. (2002). High-caloric supplements in anorexia treatment. *International Journal of Eating Disorders, 32*: 135–145.

Kagansky, N. (2005). Poor nutrition habits are predictors of poor outcome in very old hospitalized patients. *American Journal of Clinical Nutrition, 82*: 784–791.

Kim, Y. I. (2001). To feed or not to feed: Tube feeding in patients with advanced dementia. *Nutrition Reviews, 59*: 86–88.

Leppert, S. (2007). Bulk foodservice: A nutrition care strategy for high-risk dementia residents. *Journal of American Dietetic Association, 107*: 814–815.

Mahan, L. K., & Escott-Stump, S. (Eds.). (2008). *Krause's Food and Nutrition Therapy* (12th ed.). Philadelphia: Elsevier Saunders.

Murphy, R. (2004). An evaluation of web-based information. *International Journal of Eating Disorders, 35*: 145–154.

Olmsted, M. P. (2005). Defining remission and relapse in bulimia nervosa. *International Journal of Eating Disorders, 38*: 1–6.

Sallerno-Kennedy, R. (2005). Relationship between dementia and nutrition-related factors and disorders: An overview. *International Journal of Vitamin and Nutrition Research, 75*: 83–95.

Sardesai, V. M. (2003). *Introduction to Clinical Nutrition* (2nd ed.). New York: Marcel Dekker.

Shils, M. E., & Shike, M. (Eds.). (2006). *Modern Nutrition in Health and Disease* (10th ed.). Philadelphia: Lippincott, Williams and Wilkins.

Smith, A. D. (2006). Prevention of dementia: A role for B vitamins. *Nutrition and Health, 18*: 225–226.

Staehelin, H. B. (2005). Micronutrients and Alzheimer's disease. *Proceedings of the Nutrition Society, 64*: 565–570.

Temple, N. J., Wilson, T., & Jacobs, D. R. (2006). *Nutrition Health: Strategies for Disease Prevention* (2nd ed.). Totowa, NJ: Humana Press.

Thomas, B., & Bishop, J. (Eds.). (2007). *Manual of Dietetic Practice* (4th ed.). Ames, IA: Blackwell.

Thomas, D. (2000). The dietitian's role in the treatment of eating disorders. British Nutrition Foundation. *Nutrition Bulletin, 25*: 55–60.

Wasiak, J. (2007). Early and very late enteral nutritional support in adults with burn injury: A systematic review. *Journal of Human Nutrition and Dietetics, 20*: 75–83.

Webster-Gandy, J., Madden, A., & Holdworth, M. (Eds.). (2006). *Oxford Handbook of Nutrition and Dietetics.* Oxford, England: Oxford University Press.

Wray, C. J. (2002). Catabolic response to stress and potential benefits of nutrition support. *Nutrition, 18*: 971–977.

PART —IV

Diet Therapy and Childhood Diseases

CHAPTER **23**

Principles of Feeding a Sick Child

Time for completion
Activities: 1 hour
Optional examination: ½ hour

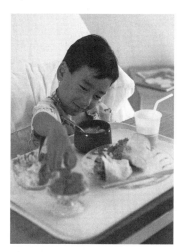

OBJECTIVES

Upon completion of this chapter, the student should be able to do the following:

1. Describe the principles of diet therapy as they apply to sick children.
2. List the major factors that influence the recovery of a sick child.
3. Identify the causes of inadequate nutrient intake in sick children.
4. Assess the nutritional status of a sick child using the accepted standard guidelines.
5. Identify behavioral patterns of the hospitalized child that may interfere with nutrient intake.
6. Describe the measures by which the health team can facilitate a child's recovery from illness.
7. Discuss ways to involve caregivers in the nutritional treatment of a child who is chronically or terminally ill.
8. Explain ways in which a child and his or her caregivers can be encouraged to comply with a modified diet regime.
9. State measures by which the nutrient intake of a sick child can be improved.
10. Identify the conditions for the use of special dietetic products.

GLOSSARY

Anorexia: lack of appetite.

Assessment: to evaluate medical conditions including nutritional status. Other definitions are possible. See Chapter 8.

Casein: milk protein.

Handicap: permanent loss of physical, sensory, or developmental ability (such as mental retardation, behavior disorder, or learning disability).

Lactose: milk sugar.

Low residue: low fiber and other undigestible materials in food. Other definitions are possible. See Chapter 17.

Medium-chain triglycerides (MCT): a form of fat that is better absorbed than regular fats, and used in diseases where there is malabsorption of ingested foods, especially fat.

Metabolic demand: body's demand for both essential nutrients and other substances related to body chemistry such as lactic acid, water and electrolyte balance, and so on.

Methionine: an amino acid.

Regression: retreat from present level of functioning to past levels of behavior.

Rehabilitation: the restoration of eating abilities to preillness levels.

Steatorrhea: a foamy, light-colored, foul-smelling stool consisting primarily of undigested fats.

Terminal illness: any illness of long or short duration with life-threatening outcome.

BACKGROUND INFORMATION

Diseases of infancy and childhood cause distress to all those concerned with the well-being of children. Managing these conditions requires more care than managing similar conditions in adults. Children are particularly vulnerable because their mental and physical development may depend on the proper treatment. Diet and nutritional therapy can play an important role in the full recovery of a sick child.

In spite of advances in pediatric nutrition, we cannot define the absolute nutrient requirements of a child at a particular age. The latest published RDAs/DRIs serve as convenient guidelines, but they do not necessarily correspond to the optimal quantities for children. However, for practical purposes, it is generally agreed that a diet meeting the RDAs/DRIs and based on the basic food groups satisfies the nutritional needs of all growing children. The diet should also be appropriate to a child's age and stage of development. This type of diet is satisfactory for normal and sick children. Details on diet planning are presented in Chapter 1.

Nearly all principles of diet therapy that apply to a sick adult also apply to a young patient. For example, pertinent factors for both groups of patients include personal eating patterns, individual likes and dislikes, and the necessity of frequent diet counseling during a hospital stay. Both children and adults, when ill, encounter the same difficulties in eating well: fatigue, vomiting, nausea, poor appetite, pain from the disease or treatment, drowsiness from medications, fear, anxiety, and so on. Just as with adult patients, the emotional, psychological, social, and physical needs of sick children require careful consideration. In some cases, these may be as important as the attention devoted to the clinical management of the ailment. In general, the principles of feeding a normal child apply more strictly to a sick child.

The nutritional and dietary care of a sick child depends on a number of factors:

1. The disease type, severity, and duration
2. The management strategy (such as the onset of symptoms, the treatment method)
3. The child's age and growth pattern
4. The nutritional status of the child before and during hospitalization
5. The need for rehabilitation

The major reasons why sick children do not have adequate nutritional intake include the following:

1. A malfunctioning gastrointestinal system
2. High metabolic demands from stress and trauma such as fever, infection, burns, or cancer
3. Excessive vomiting and diarrhea
4. Neurological and psychological disturbances that interfere with eating, such as the inability to chew or the fear of food
5. Specific nutritionally related diseases such as disorders of the kidney, liver, or pancreas
   Sometimes a child's failure to eat cannot be traced to any specific reason.

As in the case of an adult patient, the evaluation of the nutritional status of a hospitalized child should include the following tools whenever feasible:

1. Anthropometric measurements: height (length), weight, head circumference, appropriate measurements of the arms, chest, and pelvis, and skin-fold thickness
2. General body signs: muscle tone, activity, movement, posture, condition of the hair, mouth (teeth and gums), skin, ears, eyes
3. Laboratory studies: blood and urine analyses and bone growth assessment using X-rays

There are other considerations that may have an indirect effect on the child's nutritional well-being such as secondhand smoke, lead poisoning, pre- and postnatal cares, and so on.

PROGRESS CHECK ON BACKGROUND INFORMATION

FILL-IN

1. List five illness factors that interfere with adequate nutrient intake.

   a. _____

   b. _____

   c. _____

   d. _____

   e. _____

2. List the three most commonly used guidelines for evaluating nutritional status.

   a. _____

   b. _____

   c. _____

TRUE/FALSE

Circle T for True and F for False.

3. T F The principles of diet therapy apply to children as well as adults.

4. T F Diet therapy is based upon a balanced normal diet.

5. T F The physical needs of the ill child should take precedence over his or her psychosocial needs.

MULTIPLE CHOICE

Circle the letter of the correct answer.

6. The major reasons for development of malnutrition in sick children include all of these except:

   a. increased metabolism.
   b. interferences with digestion and absorption.
   c. constipation.
   d. refusal to eat.

7. The dietary care of a sick child is formulated by using:

   a. the diagnosis of the disease.
   b. the treatment of choice.
   c. evaluation of previous and present nutritional status.
   d. all of the above.

ACTIVITY 1:

The Child, the Parents, and the Health Team

BEHAVIORAL PATTERNS OF THE HOSPITALIZED CHILD

Problems that adult patients have in adjusting to hospitalization are more acute among children. Children are exposed to a totally new environment without the comfort of their parents, especially the mother, and this emotional stress is superimposed upon that caused by the clinical condition. Children may also be frightened by particular treatments and anxious about their outcome. The presence of strangers may also be confusing. Hospitalized children who become psychologically maladjusted may be unable to express themselves well. They need someone whom they trust and can talk to, especially when they have eating problems. In fact, some sick children develop certain undesirable eating habits. On the other hand, for some children with adjustment problems, food is the principal enjoyment.

Quite often children readopt some elementary feeding practices that do not fit their age or stage of development. For example, an older child may ask for a bottle instead of accepting a cup and may refuse to eat chopped foods, preferring liquid or pureed foods. Although fully capable of self-feeding, the child may want to be fed. Some children find reasons to reject food, even if it is their favorite item and served in a familiar manner. They may complain about the size of the portion or the flavor of the food. Some older children may either refuse to eat or eat too much. To help avoid these problems, new routines and ways of eating should not be forced upon these children. Old eating habits should be accommodated when possible.

The degree of feeding problems depends on the age of the child, the disorder, the child's past experience and nutritional status, and the child's social and emotional makeup. Many young patients are cooperative and eat well.

TEAMWORK

To provide optimal nutritional and dietary care for a sick child, the health team, especially the nurse, dietitian, or nutritionist, must like children and be willing to work with them. For example, the nurse becomes familiar with a child's eating habits, preferences, reactions, and remarks about food. Conveying this information to the dietary staff helps them to prepare meals that the child will like. Of course, the parents, especially the mother, can provide much useful information about a child's eating habits. The health team must also occasionally yield to children's unreasonable demands, especially those of terminally ill children.

The nurse probably plays the most important role in ensuring that a child eats the foods that are served. When the nurse relates to the child and is considerate and attentive, the child is most likely to eat well. The nutritionist, dietitian, and doctor depend on the nurse for coordination and provision of optimal dietary care.

In hospitals where dietitians have many other responsibilities, the suggestions, observations, and opinions of the nurses are especially appreciated. A skillful and considerate nurse can help a child to recover more quickly. Apart from ensuring an adequate intake of food, the nurse monitors the fluid consumption of the child and alerts the doctor and dietitian if the intake is poor.

In caring for a sick child, the health team must be fully aware of the anxiety and concern of the parents. Whenever feasible, members of the team should grant parents' requests for additional visiting hours, thereby helping to fulfill the needs of both the parents and the child. Because their child is ill, both parents have a desire to talk with someone knowledgeable about the illness. The nurse, dietitian, or nutritionist should serve as the contact. If the parents want to help in the feeding of their child, they should be encouraged to do so and become members of the health team. Further, the team should keep the parents well informed if they are unable to attend to their child. Parents are likely to be depressed when their child is suffering from a terminal illness, and in these instances the team should involve them in the different facets of clinical care, especially the feeding routine.

In sum, the health team shares the problems of the patient with the family and helps the family to overcome psychological and emotional distress. The parents should be taught to care for the child, and it is important that they trust the doctor and other health personnel. Under some circumstances (such as when the child suffers kidney disease, brain damage, or other special disorders) the team, especially the nurse, can assist the family in obtaining applicable financial aid.

It is very important that the child and parents are counseled together on the child's nutrition and dietary care. Sharing information and experience is important-merely instructing the parents without explanation is not sound nutritional education. During hospital feedings, the nurse can make helpful observations about the parent and child; for example, is the parent forcing the child to eat? How extensive are the child's feeding tantrums and food manipulation? While the child is in the hospital, the parents should be fully informed of the child's progress and adjustment, especially in regard to nutrition and feeding. The mother should implement recommended changes in eating routines after the child has returned home.

NURSING IMPLICATIONS

These nursing implications are applicable to all types of illness in children. Specific measures may be required for specific disorders.

1. Identify eating patterns, such as amounts, times, types of food, ethnic, cultural, and religious observances.
2. Make thorough initial physical assessments and monitor height, weight, and other pertinent data regularly.
3. Calculate caloric, fluid, and nutrient intake, and thoroughly document these. Alert health team members of changes as necessary.
4. Involve the child, parents, and caregivers in feeding and care.
5. Explain all modifications of diet.
6. Give emotional support to the parents of ill children.
7. Establish a relationship of trust with both the parents and the child.
8. Allow for regression during periods of illness.
9. Use play as a teaching strategy when a child's condition permits.
10. Encourage interaction with other children.
11. Help the child to feel safe in the strange and new environment of a hospital.
12. Allow expression of feelings.
13. Provide educational opportunities.
14. Realize the stressors of each age group.
15. Provide the assistance needed for coping with illness or injury.
16. Accept the child's (and parents') negative reactions.
17. Allow choices in food whenever possible.
18. Be honest; for example, don't say, "It will make you well," when it won't.
19. Praise the child when the child does the best he or she can.
20. Expect success; convey the impression to the child that you are confident that the child can eat what he or she needs.
21. Assist in securing financial support and referrals when necessary, such as to state and local agencies and social services.

PROGRESS CHECK ON ACTIVITY 1

FILL-IN

1. List five factors that may interfere with adequate food intake in hospitalized children.

   a. _____

   b. _____

   c. _____

   d. _____

   e. _____

2. Describe the nurse's primary role as a member of the health team in the feeding of sick children.

   _____

   _____

   _____

   _____

   _____

3. List 10 measures that nurses should implement to promote good nutrition in the ill child.

a. _____

b. _____

c. _____

d. _____

e. _____

f. _____

g. _____

h. _____

i. _____

j. _____

ACTIVITY 2:

Special Considerations and Diet Therapy

SPECIAL CONSIDERATIONS

When children are required to eat a modified diet, they may have to be reeducated about eating practices. To do this, the health team must first become familiar with the children's normal ways of eating, upon which the appropriate dietary changes must be based. If a child's hospital stay is long, the nutritional education program may be more aggressive and systematic. Depending on the child's age, teaching aids such as movies, slides, and skits may be used. At the beginning of diet modification, children should be given as much freedom as possible in food selection so that they can adjust to the new nutritional environment. Some children like familiar foods such as peanut butter sandwiches, hamburgers, french fries, puddings, milk, soft drinks, and cookies. If a child is expected to be hospitalized for only a short time and has neither a fluid nor electrolyte imbalance, it may be advisable for the child to eat his or her favorite foods even if they are not nutrient dense. When the child is recovering, the missing nutrients can be made up. A sick child should not be forced into new situations at mealtime, such as having to eat new foods or having to eat foods cooked in an unfamiliar way. Using different utensils than the child is accustomed to and serving a combination of new and familiar foods should also be avoided. A child's attitude toward any change in dietary routine should be carefully noted.

As indicated earlier, a sick child's food preferences should be noted by members of the health team and the parents. It is also advisable to put the list in writing. Children of ethnic origins may require special foods and food preparation. However, even when these preferences are taken into account, a child may find all food served in the hospital undesirable. The child is most likely comparing hospital food to food at home, at fast-food chains, or food served in school. Although the food choices for a sick child are invariably limited, it is extremely important to try to select a diet that has familiar foods that the child will readily eat. Whenever a child does not eat, the reasons should be ascertained and new techniques or approaches found for feeding. The child may simply have a poor appetite or be too sick and anxious to eat. Different methods of food serving may be used, including tube and intravenous (IV) feedings. The oral feeding of a hospitalized child should never be forced. Avoid stern commands such as "Drink your milk," "Eat your fruits and vegetables," "There must be no food left on the plate," and "There will be no dessert until you have finished eating your meat and potatoes." When a child does not eat all the food on the plate, it may mean that the serving size was too large.

Regular hospital procedures such as replacing dressings, giving baths, drawing blood, IV adjustments, drainage, or blood pressure measurements should not interfere with mealtimes. The child should not be exposed to pain or physiotherapy while eating.

Whether a child is sick or well, he or she must eat appropriate amounts and kinds of food. Any nutritional problem may become severe if a child is ill for an extended period of time. Ensuring that a child with a lengthy illness eats a proper amount of food is always a problem demanding constant attention.

There are several ways to improve a child's eating and acceptance of foods. The child can become involved in the food-selection process by being provided with a selective menu, cafeteria-style food service, fast-food counter food service, or a play-setting food service. Children love to get involved and will eat what they have chosen.

Children, (especially anorexic children), generally prefer certain eating practices. First, they like small, frequent meals. Second, they like to eat family style or in groups (especially with other sick children of the same age). Sometimes the dietetic staff can save time by serving all young sick children in one place and at one time. Third, children like to be fed by their parents.

A child's food intake may be improved by:

1. Providing a cheerful eating environment (such as a room having attractive draperies, comfortable chairs and tables, and pleasing paintings), especially when meals are served in a dining room.
2. Serving tasty, attractive foods, using creative menu planning and food-preparation techniques for children with such preferences.
3. Using occasions such as Christmas, Thanksgiving, Halloween, Easter, and birthdays to give surprise parties, which can improve appetites.

DIET THERAPY AND DIETETIC PRODUCTS

The routine house diets (liquid, soft, and so on) described in Chapter 14 are also applicable to children. Many therapeutic diets (for treating diabetes, kidney problems, heart problems, and so on) used to treat adult diseases are also used with children, although some modifications may be necessary. There are a number of home and commercial formulas and diets that are used to feed infants, children, and even adults. Commercially, many companies distribute such formulas to feed infants and children with clinical problems such as low birth weights and a number genetic disorders. Perhaps, the three best known companies specialized in such products are: Mead Johnson, Abbot Nutrition, and Wyeth. Their respective Web sites are: www.meadjohnson.com, www.abbotnutrition.com, and www.wyeth.com. Space limitation does not permit a listing of all relevant products. Table 23-1 presents clinical indications for the use of special dietetic products, examples, and the companies manufacturing them.

To obtain details for such products, the Web sites of the companies are the best resource.

DISCHARGE AND HOME NUTRITIONAL SUPPORT

Planning for home care begins with the decision that the child requires nutrition support at home. Discharge planning is a combined effort of physician, nurse, dietitian, manager, providers of services and supplies, and the company or public agency responsible for payment. Home nutrition supports consist of oral, enteral (tube), and/or parental feedings. Oral feeding is simpler and less complicated. The other two supports require training of the patient and care provider and arrangement for home supplies and services. We will discuss some basic consider-ations in planning and training for home enteral or tube feedings (HEN).

Many members of the healthcare team, including the hospital dietitians, floor nurses, home care nurses, and outpatient dietitians, provide teaching to the patient and caregiver. A simple checklist may resemble the following*:

General Principles

1. Disease process and why HEN is needed
2. Formula type and feeding schedule
3. Clean technique, hand washing, cleaning utensils
4. Preparation and storage of formula, including measuring formula and additives, and mixing formula

Specific Feeding Techniques

1. Preparation of each feeding:
   a. Setting up and filling feeding set
   b. Checking tube placement and gastric residuals
2. Operation of pump
3. Administration of feeding:
   a. Patient position
   b. Flushing the tube
   c. Care of tube and equipment
   d. Skin care

Problem Solving, Monitoring, and Complications

1. Pump, alarms, feeding set
2. Gastrointestinal symptoms
3. Clogged tube
4. Displaced tube, aspiration, peritonitis
5. Nutritional status
6. Blood sugar increase or decrease
7. Fluid balance, intake and output, weight

*Source: Lifshitz F., Finch N, & Lifshitz J. (1991). Children's Nutrition. Sudbury, MA: Jones and Bartlett Publishers.

TABLE 23-1   Indications for the Use of Commercial Formulas: A Partial Listing

Indications	Products
For Healthy Normal and Premature Infants	
Normal infants	Enfamil (Mead Johnson), Similac (Abbot Nutrition)
Low birth weight infants	Enfamil (Mead Johnson), SMA Premie (Wyeth)
For Infants with Clinical Disorders	
Allergy	ProSobee (Mead Johnson), Isomil (Abbot Nutrition)
Electrolyte solutions	Rehydrate (Abbot Nutrition), Resol (Wyeth)
Fat malabsorption	Portagen (Mead Johnson)
Inborn errors of metabolism	
Amino acids	Phenyl-Free 1 (Mead Johnson)
Carbohydrate	ProSobee (Mead Johnson)
Solute regulated	SMA (Wyeth)

8. Assessment of skin at tube site
9. When to call nurse, nutritionist, and/or physician

Space limitation does not permit detailed discussion of other aspects of home nutrition supports.

NURSING IMPLICATIONS

The responsibilities for nurses treating a sick child are as follows:

1. Educate the parents and the child in the use of a modified diet.
2. Do not change harmless eating habits or lifestyles.
3. Base dietary instruction on the child's developmental stage, ability, readiness to learn, and appropriate teaching aids.
4. Make changes slowly, noting and documenting responses.
5. Understand the role of a nurse as the liaison or activities coordinator among the child, caregiver, physician, dietitian, and other health personnel. Be aware that proper coordination assures a well-nourished child.
6. Document reasons for noncompliance, implementation of new strategies, and any dietary revision.
7. Adjust drug administration and treatment or therapies to avoid interference with mealtimes.
8. Relieve nausea and/or pain before meals are served.
9. Use mealtimes for teaching or socializing with other children.
10. Encourage the child to become involved in his or her own care and selection of foods.
11. Provide a clean and cheerful environment for eating.

PROGRESS CHECK ON ACTIVITY 2

Situation

Allen, age 5, is admitted to the hospital with severe burns. He will be in the hospital several weeks. He is withdrawn and eating poorly, and appears very thin. Based on this information, complete the following (use a separate sheet of paper for your responses):

1. Describe data you would collect regarding his eating habits and general nutritional status.
2. Compare nutrient increases needed to the normal growth and development needs of a 5-year-old.
3. List the general diet therapy appropriate for Allen and give rationale.
4. Write a 1-day menu, including snacks, that fit the diet therapy requirements.
5. Allen's previous eating habits have not been ideal and hospitalization has made them worse. Discuss several ways to improve his intake.

REFERENCES

Behrman, R. E., Kliegman, R. M. & Jenson, H. B. (Eds.). (2004). *Nelson Textbook of Pediatrics*. Philadelphia: Saunders.

Berkowitz, C. (2008). *Berkowitz's Pediatrics: A Primary Care Approach* (3rd ed.). Elk Village, IL: American Academy of Pediatrics.

Ekvall, S. W., & Ekvall, V. K. (Eds.). (2005). *Pediatric Nutrition in Chronic Diseases and Developmental Disorders: Prevention, Assessment, and Treatment*. New York: Oxford University Press.

Green, T. P., Franklin, W. H., & Tanz, R. R. (Eds.). (2005). *Pediatrics: Just the Facts*. New York: McGraw-Hill Medical.

Hayman, L. L., Mahon, M. M., & Turners, J. R. (Eds.). (2002). *Health and Behavior in Childhood and Adolescence*. New York: Springer.

Kleinman, R. E. (2004). *Pediatric Nutrition Handbook* (5th ed.). Elk Village, IL: American Academy of Pediatrics.

Lask, B., & Bryant-Waugh, R. (Eds.). (2000). *Anorexia Nervosa and Related Disorders in Childhood and Adolescence*. Hove, East Sussex, UK: Psychology Press.

Lutz, C. A., & Prztulski, K. R. (2006). *Nutrition and Diet Therapy: Evidence-based Applications* (4th ed.). Philadelphia: F. A. Davis.

Mahan, L. K., & Escott-Stump, S. (Eds.). (2004). *Krause's Food and Diet Therapy*. Philadelphia: Saunders.

Nevin-Folino, N. L. (Ed.). (2003). *Pediatric Manual of Clinical Dietetics*. Chicago: American Dietetic Association.

Paasche, C. L., Gorrill, L., & Stroon, B. (2004). *Children with Special Needs in Early Childhood Settings: Identification, Intervention, Inclusion*. Clifton Park: New York: Thomson/Delmar.

Rakel, R. E. (2007). *Textbook of Family Medicine*. Philadelphia: Saunders/Elsevier.

Samour, P. Q., & Helm, K. K. (Eds.). (2005). *Handbook of Pediatric Nutrition* (3rd ed.). Sudbury, MA: Jones and Bartlett Publishers.

Shils, M. E., Shike, M., Ross, A. C., Calallers, B., & Cousins, R. J. (Eds.). (2006). *Modern Nutrition in Health and Disease* (10th ed.). Philadelphia: Lippincott, Williams and Wilkins.

CHAPTER

24

Diet Therapy and Cystic Fibrosis

Time for completion
Activities: 1 hour
Optional examination: ½ hour

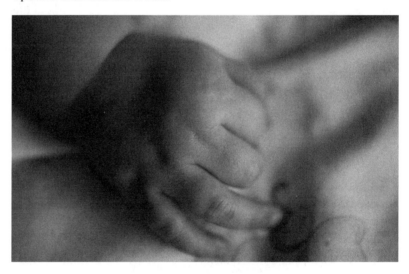

OBJECTIVES

Upon completion of this chapter, the student should be able to do the following:

1. Explain the development of cystic fibrosis:
   a. Incidence/organ involvement
   b. Diagnosis
   c. Clinical manifestations
   d. Symptoms
   e. Prognosis
   f. Treatment
2. Provide the guidelines for dietary management of cystic fibrosis:
   a. Identify the nutritional needs of the patient.
   b. List the nutritional treatment goals.
   c. Describe the diet therapy and rationale for the modification.
   d. Explain at least three methods of improving nutrient intake.
   e. Instruct the child and the family regarding food selection and use of pancreatic enzymes.
   f. Provide adequate support and guidance to the patient's family.

GLOSSARY

Azotorrhea: excess nitrogen in stools.

COPD: chronic obstructive pulmonary disease.

Etiology: the study of all factors involved in the development of a disease, based on usual course of the disease.

Exocrine: process of externally secreting body substances through a duct to the surface of an organ or tissue or into a vessel.

Meconium: a material that collects in the intestines of the fetus and forms the first stools of a newborn (texture is normally thick and sticky; in cystic fibrosis it becomes hard, dry, and tenacious, and the infant is unable to pass it).

Mucus: viscous, slippery secretions of mucous membranes and glands.

Prolapse: falling, sinking, or sliding of an organ from its normal position in the body.

Pulmonary: pertaining to the lungs.

Steatorrhea: excess fat in stools.

Tenacious (adjective): grasping, holding, or immobilizing.

Tenacity (noun): process of grasping, holding, or immobilizing.

Villi (pl): short filaments (or hair tufts) on the inside of the intestine through which digested food substances pass.

Viscid: sticky or glutinous.

BACKGROUND INFORMATION

OCCURRENCE AND TYPE OF DISORDERS

Among Caucasian children, cystic fibrosis (CF) is one of the more frequent and lethal of inherited diseases. It is estimated that about 1 child per 1500 to 3500 live births is affected. Although cystic fibrosis is most common in infants and children, it also occurs in adults. Two major sites of this disease are the exocrine area of the pancreas and the mucous and sweat glands of the body. The mucous glands produce a tenacious and viscid mucous secretion, and an excessive amount of sodium chloride is found in the sweat. The patient may show any or all of the following clinical manifestations:

1. Pulmonary disorder with recurrent infections and other lung trouble leading to COPD
2. Pancreatic insufficiency resulting in a lack of digestive enzymes. Steatorrhea and azotorrhea indicate malabsorption of fat and protein.
3. Excessive electrolytes in sweat, especially chloride
4. Malnutrition
5. Failure to thrive
6. Salt depletion
7. Biliary cirrhosis

CLINICAL SYMPTOMS AND DIAGNOSIS

If the affected child is not treated, overt symptoms occurring during the first year may include any or all of the following:

1. Frequent, large bowel movements with foul odor
2. Substandard weight gain even with good appetite
3. Abdominal bloating
4. Moderate to severe steatorrhea, with stool fat about three to five times normal
5. Frequent and excessive crying
6. Potential sodium deficiency and circulatory collapse resulting from an excessive salt loss in sweat (especially in hot weather)
7. Frequent episodes of pneumonia characterized by coughing and wheezing

This last symptom by itself can indicate cystic fibrosis. At present, the proper diagnosis of a child with cystic fibrosis is determined from clinical symptoms, the level of sodium chloride in the sweat, and X-rays of the chest.

About 8%–12% of CF patients are diagnosed at birth because of a bowel obstruction (meconium ileus) caused by a thickened meconium. There is now a blood-screening assay test that can be done on newborns. The Cystic Fibrosis Foundation (CFF) has approved this method. The diagnosis is confirmed by two positive sweat tests that measure the electrolyte chloride concentration in the body perspiration. A drug, pilocorpine, is given to stimulate perspiration, and the perspiration is collected on a gauze and measured for electrolyte concentration. A chloride measurement of 60 mmol/l is considered positive for CF. This early diagnosis is helpful, since the proper nutritional and dietary care can be instituted early to prevent suffering from undernourishment. In addition, other appropriate medical treatments can be administered. At the time of this writing, improved medical management has permitted an increasing number of patients to survive to adulthood, especially males.

PROGRESS CHECK ON BACKGROUND INFORMATION

FILL-IN

1. List five symptoms of cystic fibrosis that may be observed during the first year of the child's life.

    a. _____

    b. _____

    c. _____

    d. _____

    e. _____

MULTIPLE CHOICE

Circle the letter of the correct answer.

2. The clinical manifestations of cystic fibrosis include all except:

   a. pulmonary infections, malabsorption, and malnutrition.
   b. coronary heart disease, acidosis, and tuberculosis.
   c. failure to thrive and electrolyte imbalance.
   d. steatorrhea, bloating, and circulatory collapse.

3. The three determinations that are made for proper diagnosis of cystic fibrosis are:

   a. chest X-rays, stool cultures, and anthropometric measures.
   b. clinical symptoms, sweat test, and chest X-rays.
   c. saliva test, sweat test, and CAT scan.
   d. all of the above.

4. Which of the following indicators, when present at birth, leads to the diagnosis of cystic fibrosis?

   a. excessive sodium chloride in the sweat
   b. excessive crying and wheezing
   c. meconium ileus
   d. steatorrhea

ACTIVITY 1:

Dietary Management of Cystic Fibrosis

NUTRITIONAL NEEDS AND GOALS OF DIET THERAPY

The nutritional needs of the cystic fibrosis patient must include the following considerations:

1. The problem of recurrent infection is accompanied by defective gastrointestinal functions, increasing the child's nutritional needs.
2. The child needs a working immune defense system for survival. An adequate supply of essential nutrients is necessary to assure sufficient production of antibodies and phagocytic activity of white blood cells.
3. The child suffers from severe malabsorption because of a lack of three pancreatic enzymes: lipase, trypsin, and amylase.

Children with uncontrolled cystic fibrosis have a typical profile. They have a retarded body weight for their age and height, with occasional arrested growth. They are undersized, with a bloated belly and wasted arms and legs, and they appear malnourished. Early diagnosis and management can restore body size and the deposition of muscle and fat. This allows the children to regain a normal appearance, although sexual development may be delayed. However, complete recovery is possible in some cases.

The goals of diet therapy in cases of cystic fibrosis are the following:

1. Improve fat and protein absorption.
2. Decrease the frequency and bulk of stools.
3. Increase the body weight.
4. Control or prevent rectum prolapse.
5. Increase resistance to infection.
6. Control, prevent, or improve associated emotional problems.

General feeding techniques may be used in feeding these children.

USE OF PANCREATIC ENZYMES

Improvements in pancreatic enzyme replacements have greatly benefited the CF child. The new ones are enteric-coated "beads" encased in a capsule. The beads are pH sensitive, dissolving only in an alkaline pH of 6 or more (normal intestinal pH). They will not dissolve in the stomach (which has a pH of 2). Viokase, Catazym, and Pancrease are the most commonly used. They enable the child to eat normally, as the enzyme dosage is large enough to prevent malabsorption. Children under age 10 take the enzyme before meals; older children may take it before or during meals. Infants are given a predigested formula such as Pregestimil. See Table 23-1 (Infant Formulas, Manufacturers, and Uses) for more information.

Enzyme replacement does not always work. Malabsorption may remain because of possible mucosal damage, intestinal gland malfunctioning, and viscid mucous coating the intestinal villi.

GENERAL FEEDING

Feeding a child with cystic fibrosis can be made easier in several ways. Menu planning should be adapted to foods that the child finds acceptable, the clinical condition of the child, and the child's response to enzyme treatment. With the development of better enzyme replacements, the diet for children with CF has improved. A normal diet, with increases in nutrients to prevent weight loss from malabsorption, is now used. It is increased above the RDAs/DRIs for height-weight for age by 20%–50%, depending on the child's condition.

Medium-chain triglycerides (MCTs) facilitate fat absorption, and essential fatty acids prevent linoleic acid deficiency. MCTs used in food preparation can increase energy intake, promote weight gain, and reduce fat malabsorption problems.

Protein malabsorption is mild and usually presents no problem. However, in severe cases the child may lose his or her appetite to the extent that the protein deficiency must be treated. Several procedures can increase the total calorie and protein intake.

One of these involves the addition of dry skim milk powder fortified with fat-soluble vitamins to foods prepared for regular meals. This can be done both at home and in the hospital. It is an inexpensive, easy, and effective way to add calories and protein to the diet. Properly timed snacks at home and in the hospital are also effective, if tolerated. However, the use of pancreatic enzymes must be appropriately scheduled to improve the digestion and absorption of these items.

To assist in increasing the protein-energy value of the diet, the child should be provided with supplements:

1. A mixture of MCTs, oligosaccharides (a carbohydrate chain composed of 4 to 10 glucose segments), beef serum, and protein hydrolysates
2. Commercial nutrient-protein solutions such as Pregestimil, Portagen, and Nutramigen
3. Fat and sugar added to foods if the child can tolerate them
4. Water-miscible vitamins A, D, and E given at one to three times the respective RDAs/DRIs

The CFF has approved for use a high-fat, high-energy supplement to be given orally to CF patients. An 8-ounce serving of the product contains 450 kcal, 13 g protein, 43 g carbohydrate, and 25 g fat. In addition, it contains 2500 IU vitamin A, 15 mg vitamin E, 200 IU vitamin D, and linoleic acid. These micronutrients are important, as they are deficient due to malabsorption of fats. In the study conducted by Rettammel, Marcus, et al., with a grant from the CFF, the patients tolerated the supplement well and showed improved nutritional status. The brand name of the product is Calories Plus. The CFF guidelines for use of Calories Plus recommend its use after attempts to increase weight by normal food intake have been unsuccessful. The guidelines also recommend a gradual increase in amounts given to children younger than 10, to determine how well they tolerate the fat content.

If an infant is being treated, nutritional rehabilitation may require 180–210 kcal/kg/day, while the caloric need of an older child may be 80%–110% above the norm for that age group.

Foods that are not tolerated by the child (such as raw vegetables and high-fat items) must be identified. Some cystic fibrosis patients get diarrhea when they eat rich carbohydrate foods such as fruit, ice cream, or cookies. They may be suffering a temporary carbohydrate intolerance when this occurs. Lactase deficiency, which occurs in about 1%–10% of the patients, is to blame. Special formulas that are lactose free can be used for as long as the intolerance persists.

A high ambient temperature may cause a child with cystic fibrosis to lose electrolytes through sweating. Salty foods such as peanuts, potato chips, and other items will alleviate the problem if the foods are tolerated.

FAMILY INVOLVEMENT AND FOLLOW-UP

Parents and caregivers involved in the feeding and care of the child with CF will need extensive dietary education and counseling, especially in the use of supplement and enzyme therapy. The child's family should become involved as early as possible. Merely handing the mother a list of foods is not sufficient dietary education, since it could result in the child being fed a lopsided diet that omits some major food groups. Without appropriate instruction, family members cannot easily make substitutions for various foods (such as for fat), and they may not assess the nutritional intake correctly. Furthermore, concessions may have to be made to the child's demands occasionally if an appropriate diet is to be implemented effectively.

The dietitian, nutritionist, and nurse must work with the family (especially the primary food provider). The essentials of the Food Guide Pyramid should be taught, as well as techniques of substituting acceptable nutritious replacements for high-fat and poorly tolerated food items. It should be emphasized that dietary planning for a cystic fibrosis child takes into consideration the following factors:

1. The food preferences of the child
2. Appropriate supplements and amounts to be given
3. Changes in appearance
4. Maintenance of a food record for reference so that the nutritional status of the child can be assessed and the nurse or dietitian can make suggestions

A prescheduled procedure (weekly or monthly checkup) should be used to follow up on the progress of a child being treated for cystic fibrosis. An evaluation of nutritional status should be made that includes height, weight, skin-fold measurement, and bone age. The information obtained should then be compared with standard values. Some practitioners recommend continuing this evaluation for five years. The child's dietary intake and the nutritional education of the family should also be assessed. If the condition of a child who has been feeling well and who has had a good appetite should suddenly deteriorate, immediate investigation and referral is necessary. Complications such as infection or the ineffectiveness of the diet may cause sudden changes. Arrangements can be made so that such evaluations, assessments, investigations, referrals, and emergency handling can be done by a clinic, family physician, or other health professional (nutritionist, dietitian, nurse, or public health worker).

NUTRITIONAL AND DIETARY MANAGEMENT AT DIFFERENT STAGES OF CHILDHOOD

Infant

1. Pancreatic enzymes are given an hour or so before feedings, milk or otherwise.
2. Depending on the clinical status, initial feedings may include milk (breast or formula). Special commercial formula may also be used, including Alimentum (Ross) or Pregestimil (Mead Johnson).
3. Vitamins may be added as supplements.
4. A source of fluoride may be needed.
5. Extra salt will be needed as determined by the extent of perspiration.
6. Standard solid foods are introduced as recommended for normal infants. If high-calorie feedings are needed, design meal plans accordingly. Also consider the special need for salt.
7. Participation in available community programs is essential. Appropriate public and private programs such as WIC (Women, Infants, Children) programs, well-baby clinics, clinics for children with special needs, and special county programs for cystic fibrosis children may be available.

Toddler

1. Continue with normal prescription of pancreatic enzymes.
2. Inform parents about the reduction in growth and appetite.
3. Offer standard age-designed diets for normal toddlers.
4. Schedule regular meals and snacks.
5. Discourage sweetened beverages and constant snacking.
6. Continue vitamin and fluoride supplements if indicated. Consider the need for high salt intake.
7. Continue participation in community programs.

Age Groups: Preschool, Child Care, and School

1. Provide a normal diet for age groups when at home. Discourage sweetened beverages and continue vitamin supplements if indicated.
2. Continue with prescribed consumption of pancreatic enzymes.
3. When at child care center or schools, note the following:
   a. Parents have no control over what the child eats.
   b. For most children, inform the care provider or school of the special nutritional and dietary need.
   c. In most cases, the prescribed diet should be high in calories, protein and salt.

d. The care provider or school should be alerted to the prescription of pancreatic enzymes.

Adolescent

This age group is independent and can usually take care of their nutritional and dietary needs at home or at school. However, note the following:

1. If applicable, they should learn to prepare easy high-calorie foods.
2. Part of the calories may come from snacks and/or fast foods.
3. Limit sweetened beverages.
4. They should learn, preferably from the health professions, about the significance of:
   a. High caloric take
   b. Pancreatic enzymes preparation
   c. Vitamin and salt supplements
   d. Growth spurt for adolescents and preadolescents

NURSING IMPLICATIONS

The responsibilities of the nurse for treating a child with cystic fibrosis are as follows:

1. Maintain adequate nutrition:
   a. Provide diet high in carbohydrate and protein; supplement diet to increase intake.
   b. Provide altered forms of fat as necessary.
   c. Assure adequate salt intake.
   d. Administer pancreatic enzymes with meals and snacks.
   e. Administer water-soluble vitamin and iron supplements.
2. Promote growth and development by encouraging optimal nutrition.
3. Provide support to the family, including references, resources, support groups, and counseling.
4. Educate the child and the family:
   a. Provide accurate information regarding diet and rationale.
   b. Teach the use of and proper administration of pancreatic enzymes.
   c. Promote eating at the table to improve posture and lung expansion.
   d. Encourage good dental hygiene; cystic fibrosis children may have unhealthy teeth because of deficiencies in nutrition.
   e. Encourage high fluid intake to assist in liquefying secretions.
   f. Encourage optimal nutritional status as a means of preventing rectal prolapse.
   g. Employ strategies to improve child's appetite.

PROGRESS CHECK ON ACTIVITY 1

Situation

Susie is a 10-year-old girl with cystic fibrosis who is hospitalized with a severe upper respiratory infection. She has poor muscle development and tires easily. She is 42 inches tall and weighs 50 pounds. Based on your knowledge of growth and development patterns in children and the etiology of cystic fibrosis, answer the following questions:

1. Are Susie's height and weight appropriate for her age? Explain. _____

    _____

    _____

    _____

    _____

2. Susie has chronic diarrhea, and is acting lethargically. To what factors would each of these deviations be attributed? _____

    _____

    _____

    _____

    _____

3. List the diet modifications and the reasons they are necessary for restoring adequate nutrition to Susie.

    _____

    _____

    _____

    _____

4. Susie's appetite is very poor. List several things you can do to tempt her to eat. _____

    _____

    _____

    _____

    _____

5. Outline a day's food plan for Susie. Check the amount of protein and calories by calculating the total food values. _____

    _____

    _____

    _____

    _____

REFERENCES

American Dietetic Association. (2006). *Nutrition Diagnosis: A Critical Step in Nutrition Care Process.* Chicago: Author.

Baker, S. S., Baker, R. D. & Davis, A. M. (Eds.). (2007). *Pediatric Nutrition Support.* Sudbury, MA: Jones and Bartlett Publishers.

Behrman, R. E., Kliegman, R. M., & Jenson, H. B. (Eds.). (2004). *Nelson Textbook of Pediatrics.* Philadelphia: Saunders.

Berkowitz, C. (2008). *Berkowitz's Pediatrics: A Primary Care Approach* (3rd ed.). Elk Village, IL: American Academy of Pediatrics.

Borowitz, D. (2002). Consensus report on nutrition for pediatric patients with cystic fibrosis. *Journal of Pediatric Gastroenterology and Nutrition, 35*: 246–259.

Chinuck, R. S. (2007). Appetite stimulants in cystic fibrosis: A systematic review. *Journal of Human Nutrition and Dietetics, 20*: 526–537.

Deen, D., & Hark, L. (2007). *The Complete Guide to Nutrition in Primary Care.* Malden, MA: Blackwell.

Ekvall, S. W., & Ekvall, V. K. (Eds.). (2005). *Pediatric Nutrition in Chronic Diseases and Developmental Disorders: Prevention, Assessment, and Treatment.* New York: Oxford University Press.

Kleinman, R. E. (2004). *Pediatric Nutrition Handbook* (5th ed.). Elk Village, IL: American Academy of Pediatrics.

Madarasi, A. (2000). Antioxidant status in patients with cystic fibrosis. *Annals of Nutrition and Metabolism, 44*(5, 6): 207–211.

Mahan, L. K., & Escott-Stump, S. (Eds.). (2008). *Krause's Food and Nutrition Therapy* (12th ed.). Philadelphia: Elsevier Saunders.

Massimini, K. (2000). *Genetic Disorders Sourcebook: Basic Consumer Information About Hereditary Diseases and Disorders, Including Cystic Fibrosis, Down Syndrome* (2nd ed.). Detroit, MI: Omnigraphics.

Nevin-Folino, N. L. (Ed.). (2003). *Pediatric Manual of Clinical Dietetics.* Chicago: American Dietetic Association.

Paasche, C. L., Gorrill, L., & Stroon, B. (2004). *Children with Special Needs in Early Childhood Settings: Identification, Intervention, Inclusion.* Clifton Park: NY: Thomson/Delmar.

Powers, S. W. (2003). A comparison of nutrient intake between infants and toddlers with and without cystic fibrosis. *Journal of American Dietetic Association, 103*: 1620–1625.

Samour, P. Q., & Helm, K. K. (Eds.). (2005). *Handbook of Pediatric Nutrition* (3rd ed.). Sudbury, MA: Jones and Bartlett Publishers.

Shils, M. E., & Shike, M. (Eds.). (2006). *Modern Nutrition in Health and Disease* (10th ed.). Philadelphia: Lippincott, Williams and Wilkins.

Thomas, B., & Bishop, J. (Eds.). (2007). *Manual of Dietetic Practice* (4th ed.). Ames, IA: Blackwell.

Trabulsi, J. (2007). Evaluation of formulas for calculating total energy requirements of preadolescent children with cystic fibrosis. *American Journal of Clinical Nutrition, 85*: 144–151.

Wailoo, K. (2006). *The Troubled Dream of Genetic Medicine: Ethnicity and Innovation in Tay-Sachs, Cystic Fibrosis, and Sickle Cell Disease.* Baltimore: John Hopkins University Press.

Wiedemann, B. (2007). Evaluation of body mass index percentiles for assessment of malnutrition in children with cystic fibrosis. *European Journal of Clinical Nutrition, 61*: 759–768.

Diet Therapy and Celiac Disease

Time for completion
Activities: 1 hour
Optional examination: ½ hour

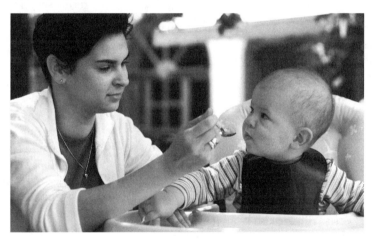

OBJECTIVES

Upon completion of this chapter, the student should be able to do the following:

1. Describe the etiology of celiac disease.
2. Explain the role of gluten in the pathophysiology of celiac disease.
3. Identify the sources of gluten.
4. Plan a gluten-free diet.
5. Provide adequate substitutes in the diet that enable the individual with celiac disease to meet his or her RDAs/DRIs.
6. Teach parents or caregivers the specifics of dietary control and methods of dietary compliance.
7. Alert adults with celiac disease of the necessity of strict adherence to the diet and methods of dietary compliance.

GLOSSARY

Atrophy: decrease in size of a developed organ or tissue; wasting.
Cheilosis: cracking open and dry scaling of the lips and angles of the mouth.
Emaciation: a wasted condition of the body; excessively lean.

Enteropathy: any disease of the intestine, such as celiac disease.

Glossitis: inflammation of the tongue.

Hyperosmolarity: abnormally high (increased) concentration of a solution.

Jejunum: part of the small intestine that extends from the duodenum to the ileum of the intestine; jejunal: of, or relating to the jejunum.

Lumen: the cavity or channel within a tube or tubular organ, as in blood vessel or intestine.

Macrocytic anemia: anemia marked by abnormally large red blood cells.

Microcytic anemia: anemia marked by abnormally small red blood cells.

Villi: threadlike projections covering the lining of the small intestine and serving as sites for the absorption of nutrients.

BACKGROUND INFORMATION

Part of the information in this chapter has been modified from the fact sheet on celiac disease distributed by the National Institute of Health (www.nih.gov).

Celiac disease results from a patient's sensitivity to a flour protein (gluten). Flour is made up of about 10% protein. Celiac disease has many names: gluten (or gluten-induced) enteropathy, nontropical sprue, and celiac sprue. This disease tends to run in families.

A jejunal biopsy of a patient with celiac disease invariably shows mucosal atrophy of the small intestine. The cells, instead of being columnar, are squamous (flat). These abnormal cells secrete only small amounts of digestive enzymes. Villi are also lacking in the intestine.

Medical records indicate that before the cause of celiac disease was identified, only children were suspected to have this disease. At present, adults with symptoms and positive identification from intestinal biopsy are classified as having adult celiac disease, especially if they respond to gluten-free diets.

Apart from using the references at the end of this chapter to find more details on celiac disease, the private organizations list below are an excellent source for details on the disorder.

1. Celiac Disease Foundation. www.celiac.org
2. Celiac Sprue Association/USA Inc. www.csaceliacs.org

ACTIVITY 1:

Dietary Management of Celiac Disease

SYMPTOMS

The symptoms exhibited by a patient with celiac disease are diarrhea, steatorrhea, two to four bowel movements daily, loss of appetite and weight, emaciation; and in children, failure to thrive (such children typically have "pot bellies"). Children's growth is retarded because of the incompetent mucosa, which causes severe malabsorption. When the fat is not absorbed, it is moved to the large intestine and becomes emulsified by bile and calcium salts. The odor of the stool is caused by large amounts of fatty acids. The unabsorbed carbohydrates are fermented by the bacteria in the large intestine, producing gas and occasional abdominal cramps. Hyperosmolarity induces the colon to secrete water and electrolytes into the lumen. The patient may show many malnutrition symptoms, including bone pain and tetany, anemia, rough skin, and lowered prothrombin time. Most adult patients have iron and folic acid deficiencies, with microcytic and macrocytic anemias. Symptoms such as cheilosis and glossitis, caused by water-soluble vitamin deficiencies, may also be present.

Dermatitis herpetiformis (DH) is a severe, itchy, blistering skin manifestation of celiac disease. Not all people with celiac disease develop dermatitis herpetiformis. The rash usually occurs on the elbows, knees, and buttocks. Unlike other forms of celiac disease, the range of intestinal abnormalities in DH is highly variable, from minimal to severe. Only about 20% of people with DH have intestinal symptoms of celiac disease.

To diagnose DH, the doctor will test the person's blood for autoantibodies related to celiac disease and will biopsy the person's skin. If the antibody tests are positive and the skin biopsy has the typical findings of DH, patients do not need to have an intestinal biopsy. Both the skin disease and the intestinal disease respond to a gluten-free diet and recur if gluten is added back into the diet. In addition, the rash symptoms can be controlled with medications such as dapsone (4′,4′diamino-diphenylsuphone). However, dapsone does not treat the intestinal condition, and people with DH should also maintain a special diet as explained below.

PRINCIPLES OF DIET THERAPY

The basic principle of diet therapy for celiac disease is to exclude all foods containing gluten—chiefly buckwheat, malt, oats, rye, barley, and wheat. The patient's response to such a regimen is dramatic. A child shows improvement in one to two weeks, while an adult takes one to three months for visible improvement. In either case, symptoms gradually disappear. With the child patient, there is weight gain and thriving, and diarrhea and steatorrhea clear up. The mucosal changes will also return to normal after a gluten-free diet. The degree of improvement is directly related to the extent the patient adheres to the diet. The therapy can be proven to be curing the disease if symptoms reappear when the patient returns to a regular diet.

For most people, following this diet will stop symptoms, heal existing intestinal damage, and prevent further damage. Improvements begin within days of starting the diet. The small intestine is usually completely healed in 3 to 6 months in children and younger adults and within 2 years for older adults. Healed means a person now has villi that can absorb nutrients from food into the bloodstream.

To stay well, people with celiac disease must avoid gluten for the rest of their lives. Eating any gluten, no matter how small an amount, can damage the small intestine. The damage will occur in anyone with the disease, including people without noticeable symptoms. Depending on a person's age at diagnosis, some problems will not improve, such as delayed growth and tooth discoloration.

Some people with celiac disease show no improvement on the gluten-free diet. This condition is called unresponsive celiac disease. The most common reason for poor response is that small amounts of gluten are still present in the diet. Advice from a dietitian who is skilled in educating patients about the gluten-free diet is essential to achieve the best results.

Rarely, the intestinal injury will continue despite a strictly gluten-free diet. People in this situation have severely damaged intestines that cannot heal. Because their intestines are not absorbing enough nutrients, they may need to receive nutrients directly into their bloodstream through a vein, or intravenously. People with this condition may need to be evaluated for complications of the disease.

Table 25-1 lists those foods that are permitted or prohibited in a gluten-restricted diet. Table 25-2 provides a sample meal plan for such a diet.

PATIENT EDUCATION

After celiac disease has been diagnosed, patients should be educated about its cause and treatment. Patients who understand this illness are much more likely to follow a prescribed diet. They should first be taught that adherence to a gluten-free or gluten-restricted diet is essential. If the patients also have lactose intolerance (as is sometimes the case), the necessity of avoiding milk and milk products must also be emphasized.

Patients should be forewarned of the great difficulty in following a gluten-restricted diet. Buckwheat, malt, oats, barley, rye, and wheat all contain gluten and are extensively used in different food products. Patients must therefore be taught to read all labels on prepared and packaged foods to ascertain if they contain gluten. Gluten-free wheat products are commercially available for those on special diets. In addition, potato, rice, corn, soybean flours, and tapioca may be substituted.

If a patient is already malnourished when treatment begins, an aggressive nutritional rehabilitation regimen should be instituted. This includes high amounts of calories, protein, vitamins, and minerals. It should also provide fluids and electrolyte compensation (with special attention to potassium, magnesium, and calcium). Medium-chain triglycerides (MCTs) should also be included. A gluten-restricted diet may be deficient in thiamin (vitamin B_1) and should include vitamin supplements.

All patients should be taught to plan their menus in accordance with some food guides to achieve their daily RDAs. Health professionals should help the patient in this planning.

NURSING IMPLICATIONS

The responsibilities of the nurse to patients with celiac disease are listed below.

1. Emphasize to parents and child the importance of complying with diet therapy to treat the disease.
2. Explain the disease etiology to the parents, especially the specific role of gluten in the pathophysiology.
3. Advise the patient and parents regarding the necessity of reading all food labels carefully.
4. Explain the necessity of any other restrictions that may be placed on the diet owing to the child's condition, such as low-residue, lactose-free diets.
5. Recommend that the diet be continued for a lifetime.
6. Provide a gluten-free diet tailored to the child's appetite and capacity to absorb; emphasize suitable substitutes.
7. Arrange for conferences with the dietitian, caregiver, child, and nurse to coordinate care.
8. Administer aqueous vitamin-mineral supplements as ordered; request prescription for supplements if child's intake is poor.
9. Monitor fluid and food intake carefully, and document well.
10. Teach parents or caregivers specifics of dietary control; provide a written list of common food sources of gluten.
11. Emphasize other dietary principles, such as high-calorie, high-protein, low-residue diets.
12. Emphasize the importance of good health in preventing infections, the dangers of fasting, and drug and food interactions.
13. Make referrals for financial aid or additional dietary counseling, and follow up after patient is discharged.
14. Assist the parents and the child in adjusting to life-long regimes; be positive about dietary treatment.
15. Recommend the now-available home test kit for gluten detection.

TABLE 25-1   Foods Permitted and Prohibited in a Gluten-Restricted Diet

Food Group	Foods Permitted	Foods Prohibited
Meat, poultry	Those prepared without prohibited grains or their flours	All products using prohibited flours, including Swiss steak, chili con carne, commercial sausages (e.g., weiners), gravies, sauces, stews, batter, stuffings, croquettes
Fish	All fish and shellfish containing no restricted grains or their flours	Any product made with the restricted grains and flours, e.g., wheat-flour-breaded fish sticks and shrimp
Cheese	All not specifically prohibited	Processed cheese and cheese spread prepared with gluten as a stabilizer
Eggs	All frozen and fresh eggs and egg substitutes without restricted grains or their flours	All others
Textured vegetable proteins	All those made from soy ingredients	All others
Milk, milk products	Milkshakes, milk, cream, buttermilk, plain yogurt, cheese, cream cheese, processed cheese foods, cottage cheese	Malted milk
Fats, oils	Butter, margarine, cream and cream substitutes; bacon; olive oil, vegetable oil, salad oil; vegetable (hydrogenated) shortening; mayonnaise	Salad dressings thickened with wheat or rye products; cream, butter, white sauce made with forbidden flour
Cereals	All cereals made from corn and rice, e.g., Sugar Pops, Rice Krispies, Corn Chex, Corn Flakes, Puffed Rice, Frosted Flakes, Cream of Rice, grits, hominy, and cornmeal	All cereals containing prohibited grains, e.g., Cream of Wheat
Bread	Muffins, pone, and corn bread prepared without wheat flour; rolls, muffins, and breads prepared with cornmeal, cornstarch, lima bean flour, and arrowroot; rice pancakes; products made with low-gluten wheat starch	All products made from prohibited grains, e.g., sweet rolls, crackers, muffins, prepared mixes, bread crumbs, commercial yeast breads
Vegetables, vegetable juices	All vegetables and juices; sauces made with potato flour or cornstarch may be used	Vegetables prepared with cracker crumbs, bread, or cream sauces thickened with prohibited flours or cereals
Fruits, fruit juices	All fruits and juices	Fruit sauces thickened with prohibited grains
Potatoes or substitutes	Potatoes, rice, grits, corn, sweet potatoes, dried peas and beans	Pasta
Sweets	All unless specifically prohibited	Candies and chocolate syrup with bases made from prohibited grains
Soups	Cream or vegetable soups thickened with cornstarch or potato flour; meat stock; clear broths	Milk and cream soups; bouillon cubes or powdered soups; canned soups; soups with prohibited grain products; soups thickened with wheat flour
Beverages	Coffee, tea, cocoa, chocolate, carbonated beverages, milk, Kool-Aid	Ale, beer, malted milk; instant cocoa, coffee, or tea; cereal beverages; milk shakes; others including Ovaltine, Postum
Desserts	Products made with permitted grains; plain or fruit-flavored gelatin; homemade ice, ice cream, sherbet, Popsicles, cornstarch, rice and tapioca puddings; cakes, pies, and cookies, using water, sugar, and fruits	All products made with prohibited grains, e.g., pastries (cakes), desserts (ice cream cones, sherbet), prepared mixes
Miscellaneous	Herbs, pepper, olives, salt, vinegar, catsup, pickles, relishes, spices, sauces prepared from permitted grains and their flours; peanut butter, nuts, flavoring extracts, popcorn	Creamed and scalloped foods; au gratin dishes, rarebit; fritters, timbales, malt products, prepared mixes of all kinds; condiments prepared with gluten base

TABLE 25-2   Sample Meal Plan for a Gluten-Restricted Diet

Breakfast	Lunch	Dinner
Juice	Meat	Meat, fish, or poultry
Cereal, hot or dry*	Potato	Potato
Scrambled egg(s)	Vegetable	Vegetable
Corn bread (special)	Salad with dressing	Juice
Margarine	Fruit or dessert	Fruit or dessert
Jelly	Corn bread	Corn bread
Milk	Margarine	Margarine
Coffee or tea	Milk	Milk
Sugar	Beverage	Beverage
Cream	Cream	Cream
Salt, pepper	Sugar	Sugar
	Salt, pepper	Salt, pepper

*From permitted cereals. See Table 22-1.

PROGRESS CHECK ON ACTIVITY 1

MULTIPLE CHOICE

Circle the letter of the correct answer.

1. Gluten is found in:

   a. wheat, rye, oats, barley.
   b. rice, potato, corn, beans.
   c. milk and meat.
   d. all of the above.

2. Jane has been diagnosed as having celiac disease. Which of the following snacks would be suitable for her to have in nursery school?

   a. malted milk shake
   b. popcorn and apple slices
   c. hot dog with catsup
   d. graham crackers and peanut butter

3. Diet therapy for celiac disease is continued:

   a. indefinitely.
   b. until patient is middle-aged.
   c. through prepubertal growth spurt.
   d. for at least six weeks.

Situation

Mrs. Jones, age 30, was recently diagnosed as having adult celiac disease, and her physician ordered a gluten-free diet. She recognizes you as a health professional and states that she is quite apprehensive about her diet. Counsel her regarding the following:

4. Explain what gluten is and why it is restricted.

   _____

   _____

   _____

   _____

5. Because Mrs. Jones works outside the home, she will be eating lunch away from home. Provide lunch suggestions that conform to her diet.

   _____

   _____

   _____

   _____

6. Name at least six typical foods containing gluten for Mrs. Jones. _____

   _____

   _____

   _____

   _____

7. List the cereal grains that can be used on Mrs. Jones's diet. _____

   _____

   _____

   _____

8. Name at least five hidden food sources of gluten.

   _____

   _____

_____

_____

9. Mrs. Jones states that she is also lactose intolerant. What additional foods must be omitted from her diet? _____

_____

_____

_____

_____

10. Would you recommend that Mrs. Jones add medium-chain triglycerides to her diet? Explain.

_____

_____

_____

_____

OPTIONAL EXERCISE

Write down all the foods you ate yesterday. Change the menu to make it gluten free.

_____

_____

_____

_____

_____

_____

ACTIVITY 2:

Screening, Occurrence, and Complications

SCREENING

Screening for celiac disease involves testing asymptomatic people for the antibodies to gluten. Americans are not routinely screened for celiac disease. However, because celiac disease is hereditary, family members—particularly first-degree relatives—of people who have been diagnosed may need to be tested for the disease. About 10% of an affected person's first-degree relatives (parents, siblings, or children) will also have the disease. The longer a person goes undiagnosed and untreated, the greater the chance of developing malnutrition and other complications.

In Italy, where celiac disease is common, all children are screened by age 6 years so that even asymptomatic disease is caught early. In addition, Italians of any age are tested for the disease as soon as they show symptoms.

As a result of this vigilance, the time between when symptoms begin and the disease is diagnosed is usually only 2 to 3 weeks. In the United States, the time between the first symptoms and diagnosis averages about 10 years.

According to the NIH, data on the prevalence of celiac disease is spotty. In Italy about 1 in 250 people, and in Ireland about 1 in 300 people, have celiac disease. Recent studies have shown that it may be more common in Africa, South America, and Asia than previously believed.

Until recently, celiac disease was thought to be uncommon in the United States. However, studies have shown that celiac disease is very common. Recent findings estimate about 2 million people in the United States have celiac disease, or about 1 in 133 people. Among people who have a first-degree relative diagnosed with celiac disease, as many as 1 in 22 people may have the disease.

Celiac disease could be underdiagnosed in the United States for a number of reasons:

- Celiac symptoms can be attributed to other problems.
- Many doctors are not knowledgeable about the disease.
- Only a handful of U.S. laboratories are experienced and skilled in testing for celiac disease.

More research is needed to find out the true prevalence of celiac disease among Americans.

COMPLICATIONS

Damage to the small intestine and the resulting problems with nutrient absorption put a person with celiac disease at risk for several diseases and health problems:

- Lymphoma and adenocarcinoma are types of cancer that can develop in the intestine.
- Osteoporosis is a condition in which the bones become weak, brittle, and prone to breaking. Poor calcium absorption is a contributing factor to osteoporosis.
- Miscarriage and congenital malformation of the baby, such as neural tube defects, are risks for untreated pregnant women with celiac disease because of malabsorption of nutrients.
- Short stature results when childhood celiac disease prevents nutrient absorption during the years when nutrition is critical to a child's normal growth and development. Children who are diagnosed and treated before their growth stops may have a catch-up period.
- Seizures, or convulsions, result from inadequate absorption of folic acid. Lack of folic acid causes calcium deposits, called calcifications, to form in the brain, which in turn cause seizures.

NURSING IMPLICATIONS

Some points in patient counseling:

1. People with celiac disease cannot tolerate gluten, a protein in wheat, rye, barley, and possibly oats.

2. Celiac disease damages the small intestine and interferes with nutrient absorption.

3. Treatment is important because people with celiac disease could develop such complications as cancer, osteoporosis, anemia, and seizures.

4. A person with celiac disease may or may not have symptoms.

5. Diagnosis involves blood tests and biopsy.

6. Because celiac disease is hereditary, family members of a person with celiac disease may need to be tested.

7. Celiac disease is treated by eliminating all gluten from the diet. The gluten-free diet is a lifetime requirement.

PROGRESS CHECK ON ACTIVITY 2

TRUE/FALSE

Circle T for True and F for False.

1. T F About 10% of an celiac-affected person's first-degree relatives (parents, siblings, or children) will also have the disease.

2. T F Celiac disease is usually diagnosed in the first 6 months of life.

3. T F Gluten is a protein found in rye, wheat, oats, and rice.

4. T F Celiac disease damages the small intestine and interferes with nutrient absorption.

5. T F People with celiac disease can develop such complications as cancer, osteoporosis, anemia, miscarriage, congenital malformation of the baby, short stature, convulsions, and seizures.

6. T F Diagnosis involves blood tests such as antibody tests against gluten and biopsy.

7. T F Persons diagnosed with celiac disease must stay on a gluten-free diet the rest of their lives.

FILL-IN

8. Celiac disease could be underdiagnosed in the United States for a number of reasons:

    a. _____

    b. _____

    c. _____

REFERENCES

Behrman, R. E., Kliegman, R. M., & Jenson, H. B. (Eds.). (2004). *Nelson Textbook of Pediatrics.* Philadelphia: Saunders.

Biagi, F. (2004). A milligram of gluten a day keeps the mucosal recovery away: A case report. *Nutrition Reviews, 62*: 360–363.

Bonci, L. (2003). *American Dietetic Association Guide to Better Digestion.* New York: John Wiley & Sons.

Buchman, A. (2004). *Practical Nutritional Support Technique* (2nd ed.). Thorofeue, NJ: Slack.

Collin, P. (2004). It is the compliance, not milligrams of gluten, that is essential in the treatment of celiac disease. *Nutrition Reviews, 62*: 490–491.

Collin, P. (2007). Safe gluten threshold for patients with Celiac Disease: some patients are more tolerant than others. *American Journal of Clinical Nutrition, 86*: 260.

Fasano, A., Troncone, R., & Branski, D. (2008). *Frontiers in Celiac Disease.* Basel, Switzerland: S. Karger AG.

Green, P. H. R., & Jones, R. (2006). *Celiac Disease: A Hidden Epidemic.* New York: HarperCollins.

Hansen, D. (2006). Clinical benefit of a gluten-free diet in type 1 diabetic children with screen-detected celiac disease: A population-based screening study with 2-years follow-up. *Diabetes Care, 29*: 2452–2456.

Hark, L., & Morrison, G. (Eds.). (2003). *Medical Nutrition and Disease* (3rd ed.). Malden, MA: Blackwell.

Hartmann, G. (2006). Rapid degradation of gliadin peptides toxic for celiac disease patients by proteases from germinating cereals. *Journal of Cereal Science, 44*: 368–371.

Hay, D. W. (2001). *Blackwell's Primary Care Essentials: Gastrointestinal Diseases.* Ames, IA: Blackwell.

Hornell, A. (2005). Effect of a gluten-free diet on gastrointestinal symptoms in celiac disease. *American Journal of Clinical Nutrition, 81*: 1452–1453.

Kleinman, R. E. (2004). *Pediatric Nutrition Handbook* (5th ed.). Elk Village, IL: American Academy of Pediatrics.

Kliegman, R. M., Greenbaum, L. A., & Lye, P. S. (Eds.). (2004). *Practical Strategies in Pediatric Diagnosis and Therapy* (2nd ed.). Philadelphia: Elsevier Saunders.

Lee, A. R. (2005). Celiac disease: Detection and treatment. *Topics in Clinical Nutrition, 20*: 139–145.

Lee, A. R. (2007). Economic burden of a gluten-free diet. *Journal of Human Nutrition and Dietetics, 20*: 323–430.

Libonati, C. J. (2007). *Recognizing Celiac Disease: Signs, Symptoms, Associated Disorders and Complications.* Fort Washington, PA: Gluten Free Works.

Lowdon, J. (2007). Celiac disease and dietitians: Are we getting it right. *Journal of Human Nutrition and Dietetics, 20*: 401–402.

Mahan, L. K., & Escott-Stump, S. (Eds.). (2008). *Krause's Food and Nutrition Therapy* (12th ed.). Philadelphia: Elsevier Saunders.

Malkin-Washeim, D. L. (2006). Type 1 diabetes and celiac disease: An overview. *Topics in Clinical Nutrition, 21*: 341–354.

McGough, N. (2005). Celiac disease: A diverse clinical syndrome caused by intolerance of wheat, barley, and rye. *Proceedings of the Nutrition Society, 64*: 434–450.

Mendoza, N. (2005). Celiac disease: An overview. *Nutrition and Food Science, 35*: 156–162.

Mistkovitz, P., & Betancourt, M. (2005). *The Doctor's Guide to Gastrointestinal Health Preventing and Treating Acid Reflux, Ulcers, Irritable Bowel Syndrome, Diverticulitis, Celiac Disease, Colon Cancer, Pancreatitis, Cirrhosis, Hernias and More.* Hoboken, NJ: Wiley.

Nevin-Folino, N. L. (Ed.). (2003). *Pediatric Manual of Clinical Dietetics.* Chicago: American Dietetic Association.

Niewinski, M. M. (2008). Advances in celiac disease and gluten-free diet. *Journal of American Dietetic Association, 108*: 661–672.

Paasche, C. L., Gorrill, L., & Stroon, B. (2004). *Children with Special Needs in Early Childhood Settings: Identification, Intervention, Inclusion.* Clifton Park: NY: Thomson/Delmar.

Patrias, K., Willard, C. C., & Hamilton, F. A. (2004). *Celiac Disease January 1986 to March 2004, 2382 citations.* Bethesda, MD: United States National Library of Medicine, National Institutes of Health, Health & Human Services.

Patwari, A. K. (2005). Catch-up growth in children with late-diagnoses celiac disease. *British Journal of Nutrition, 94*: 437–442.

Peraaho, M. (2004). Oats can diversify a gluten-free diet in celiac disease and dermatitis herpetiform. *Journal of American Dietetic Association, 104*: 1148–1150.

Rostom, A., Dube, C., Cranney, A., Saloojee, N., Sy, R., Garritty, C. et al. (Eds.). (2004). *Celiac Disease.* Rockville, MD: Agency for Health Research and Quality.

Samour, P. Q., & Helm, K. K. (Eds.). (2005). *Handbook of Pediatric Nutrition* (3rd ed.). Sudbury, MA: Jones and Bartlett Publishers.

Seraphin, P. (2002). Mortality in patients with celiac disease. *Nutrition Reviews, 60*: 116–118.

Shils, M. E., & Shike, M. (Eds.). (2006). *Modern Nutrition in Health and Disease* (10th ed.). Philadelphia: Lippincott, Williams and Wilkins.

Stepniak, D. (2006). Enzymatic gluten detoxification: The proof of the pudding is in the eating. *Trends in Biotechnology, 24*: 433–434.

Storsrud, S. (2003). Beneficial effects of oats in the gluten-free diet of adults with special reference to nutrient status, symptoms and subjective experiences. *British Journal of Nutrition, 90*: 101–107.

Sverker, A. (2005). 'Controlled by food': Lived experiences of celiac disease. *Journal of Human Nutrition and Dietetics, 18*: 171–180.

Sverker, A. (2007). Sharing life with a gluten-intolerant person: The perspective of close relatives. *Journal of Human Nutrition and Dietetics, 20*: 412–422.

Thomas, B., & Bishop, J. (Eds.). (2007). *Manual of Dietetic Practice* (4th ed.). Ames, IA: Blackwell.

Webster-Gandy, J., Madden, A., & Holdworth, M. (Eds.). (2006). *Oxford Handbook of Nutrition and Dietetics.* Oxford, London: Oxford University Press.

Wiesser, H. (2008). The biochemical basis of celiac disease. *Cereal Chemistry, 85*: 1–13.

Williamson, D. (2002). Celiac disease. *Molecular Biotechnology, 22*: 293–299.

Yucel, B. (2006). Eating disorders and celiac disease: A case report. *International Journal of Eating Disorders, 39*: 530–532.

CHAPTER

26

Diet Therapy and Congenital Heart Disease

Time for completion
Activities: 1 hour
Optional examination: ½ hour

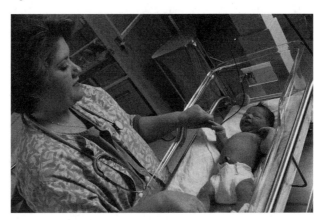

OBJECTIVES

Upon completion of this chapter, the student should be able to do the following:

1. Describe the effects of congenital heart disease upon the nutritional status of children.
2. List three reasons for growth retardation in a child with congenital heart disease.
3. Identify the four major nutritional problems to be considered for patients with congenital heart disease.
4. Explain the appropriate diet therapy for congenital heart disease, and give supporting rationale.
5. Describe formulas and supplements used for infants with congenital heart disease.
6. Evaluate the introduction of solid foods and precautions used when feeding.
7. Compare the feeding problems encountered in a child with a defective heart to those of normal children.
8. Describe methods of maintaining optimum nutritional status in the hospitalized child.
9. Teach parents and the child the principles of feeding and eating when congenital heart disease is present.
10. Describe appropriate discharge procedures.

GLOSSARY

Congenital: present at birth

Cyanotic: condition exhibiting bluish discoloration of the skin and mucous membranes due to excessive concentrations of reduced hemoglobin or extensive oxygen extraction.

Dehydration: excessive loss of water from body tissue, accompanied by imbalance of electrolytes, especially sodium, potassium, and chloride (dehydration is of particular concern among infants and young children).

Diuretic: a drug or other substance that promotes the formation and excretion of urine.

Milliequivalent (mEq): the number of grams of solute dissolved in one milliliter of normal solution.

Milliliter: a metric unit of measurement of volume.

Milliosmol (mosm): a unit of measure representing the concentration of an ion in solution.

Renal: of or pertaining to the kidney.

Respiration (breathing): exchange of carbon dioxide and oxygen in the lungs.

Respiratory distress: inability of the infant to make the exchange, characterized by rapid breathing, grunting on expiration, and other severe symptoms.

Solute: any substance dissolved in a solution.

BACKGROUND INFORMATION

Part of the information in this section has been modified from the fact sheets on congenital heart disease published and distributed by the National Institute of Health (www.nih.gov).

Congenital heart defects are problems with the heart's structure that are present at birth. These defects can involve the interior walls of the heart, valves inside the heart, or the arteries and veins that carry blood to the heart or out to the body. Congenital heart defects change the normal flow of blood through the heart because some part of the heart didn't develop properly before birth.

There are many different types of congenital heart defects. They range from simple defects with no symptoms to complex defects with severe, life-threatening symptoms. They include simple ones such as a hole in the interior walls of the heart that allows blood from the left and right sides of the heart to mix, or a narrowed valve that blocks the flow of blood to the lungs or other parts of the body.

Other defects are more complex. These include combinations of simple defects, problems with the blood vessels leading to and from the heart, and more serious abnormalities in how the heart develops.

Congenital heart defects are the most common type of birth defect, affecting 8 of every 1000 newborns. Each year, more than 35,000 babies in the United States are born with congenital heart defects. Most of these defects are simple conditions that are easily fixed or need no treatment.

A small number of babies are born with complex congenital heart defects that need special medical attention soon after birth. Over the past few decades, the diagnosis and treatment of these complex defects has greatly improved.

As a result, almost all children with complex heart defects grow to adulthood and can live active, productive lives because their heart defects have been effectively treated.

Most people with complex heart defects continue to need special heart care throughout their lives. They may need to pay special attention to certain issues that their condition could affect, such as health insurance, employment, pregnancy and contraception, and preventing infection during routine health procedures. Today in the United States, about 1 million adults are living with congenital heart defects.

Many congenital heart defects have few or no symptoms. A doctor may not even detect signs of a heart defect during a physical exam.

Some heart defects do have symptoms. These depend on the number and type of defects and how severe the defects are. Severe defects can cause symptoms, usually in newborn babies. These symptoms can include:

- Rapid breathing
- Cyanosis (a bluish tint to the skin, lips, and fingernails)
- Fatigue (tiredness)
- Poor blood circulation

Congenital heart defects don't cause chest pain or other painful symptoms.

Abnormal blood flow through the heart caused by a heart defect will make a certain sound. Your doctor can hear this sound, called a heart murmur, with a stethoscope. However, not all murmurs are a sign of a congenital heart defect. Many healthy children have heart murmurs.

Normal growth and development depend on a normal workload for the heart and normal flow of oxygen-rich blood to all parts of the body. Babies with congenital heart defects may have cyanosis or tire easily when feeding. Sometimes they have both problems. As a result, they may not gain weight or grow as they should.

Older children may get tired easily or short of breath during exercise or activity. Many types of congenital heart defects cause the heart to work harder than it should. In severe defects, this can lead to heart failure, a condition in which the heart can't pump blood strongly throughout the body. Symptoms of heart failure include:

- Fatigue with exercise
- Shortness of breath
- A buildup of blood and fluid in the lungs
- A buildup of fluid in the feet, ankles, and legs

Congenital heart disease can retard a child's growth in a number of ways. First, it can cause the child to eat too little. The child may voluntarily reduce food intake in order to reduce the workload of the heart. Or, the child can become listless because of rapid respiration and a lack of oxygen, thus reducing the child's ability to eat an adequate amount of food. A second reason for growth retardation is a high body metabolic rate caused by the increased nutrient needs of the organs and tissues and elevated body temperature and thyroid activity. A third reason for growth retardation is a high loss of body nutrients owing to inadequate intestinal absorption, excessive urine output, and the presence of hemorrhages or open wounds. It is not known how a heart defect can cause all these clinical problems.

The only cure for congenital heart disease is successful surgery, performed during early or late infancy.

Although corrective surgery can be successful, the mortality rate is high for small children. However, if death is imminent because of heart failure, high-risk surgery is indicated. It is therefore of paramount importance that infants with heart disease are provided adequate nutrition so that surgery can be performed when their growth reaches a body weight of 30 to 50 pounds. This must be accomplished despite the diminished nutrient supply to cells because of the decreased oxygen supply that results from a defective heart.

ACTIVITY 1:

Dietary Management of Congenital Heart Disease

There are no standard recommendations for the nutritional care of children with congenital heart disease. Each patient requires an individualized plan designed by the physician and implemented by the dietitian with the assistance of the attending nurse. Therefore, the information in Activity 1 must be interpreted as such. Guided by your instructor, use the references at the end of this chapter to obtain more details and analyses.

MAJOR CONSIDERATIONS IN DIETARY CARE

There are four major considerations in feeding children with congenital heart disease. One is caloric need. Because of the expected retardation of growth caused by the clinical condition, the child's caloric need is higher than the RDAs. For example, if the RDA of calories for a normal child is 100 kcal/pound, the need for a patient with congenital heart disease may be 130 to 160 kcal/pound.

A second concern is renal load. The child may have difficulty handling any large renal load of solutes. A large renal load may be caused by excessive electrolytes or dehydration, which can result from an insufficient fluid intake.

The third consideration is food intolerance. A large amount of simple sugars may produce diarrhea, the fat in regular milk and food may cause steatorrhea, and food ingestion may cause abdominal discomfort.

The fourth major consideration is vitamin and mineral need. Vitamin and mineral deficiencies have been documented in infants with congenital heart disease. Because of the small quantity of food consumed, the child's intake of these nutrients must be carefully monitored.

FORMULAS AND REGULAR FOODS

An infant with congenital heart disease is usually fed a special formula, although regular foods are sometimes used. The formula should be high in calories but contain only the minimal amount of protein and electrolytes needed for growth without causing kidney overload. Some guidelines are as follows: 8%–10% of the daily calories should come from protein; 35%–65% from carbohydrate; and 35%–50% from fat. Infants under 4 months old should get 1.8–2.0 g of protein per 100 kcal, and infants 4–12 months old should receive 1.65–1.75 g of protein per 100 kcal.

Some clinicians prefer special low-electrolyte, low-protein formulas supplemented with fat or carbohydrate solution. The preparer adds supplements to these formulas, which are commercially available. Other clinicians recommend using formulas with 25–30 kcal/oz, and diluting accordingly. The solute load of such preparations must be calculated, and their effects on the child carefully monitored. Sometimes the prepared formulas are supplemented with a limited amount of solid foods that is not adequate to support growth by itself. Some clinicians have good experience with Wyeth's SMA and Ross's Similac PM 60/40 (Chapter 20).

If formulas are not used, the calorie and sodium contents, digestibility, and renal solute load of the foods fed to the child must be appropriate. Carbohydrate and fat do not affect the solute load. Clinical practice has established that 1 milliosmol (mosm) of solute is formed by 1 milliequivalent (mEq) of sodium, potassium, and chloride, and that 1 g of dietary protein provides about 4 mosm of renal solute load. If the infant is given regular food, the diet should begin with easily digested and accepted items such as fruit, with cereal or unsalted vegetables included later.

Certain precautions are important in feeding a child with congenital heart disease. If the child is given any high-caloric supplement, small amounts should be used, at least at the beginning, as large portions can produce diarrhea and reduce appetite. If the child is eating moderately to considerably less than the calculated amount, he or she is especially susceptible to folic acid deficiency. Since many nonprescription vitamin supplements for children do not contain folic acid, it is important to obtain a proper preparation. The child may also require iron and calcium supplementation.

Table foods may be introduced when the child is over 5½ to 6½ months old. Very small servings of chopped, mashed, or pureed cereal, fruits, potato, and meat with vegetables can be served, all prepared without salt. The amount of meat should be limited to less than 1 oz a day if the child's condition is poor.

Sodium intake must be carefully considered. Most commercial strained baby foods, especially meat and vegetable items, contain a large amount of sodium and are usually not suitable. If they are used, their sodium contents must be ascertained and the effects monitored. Home-prepared baby foods must be properly selected and quantified and prepared without salt. The child's need for sodium is a delicate balance between too much, which is bad for the heart, and too little, which affects growth. For example, if the child suffers any clinical symptoms of heart failure, dietetic low-sodium formulas may be indicated. If diuretics are used to remove body sodium, all complications associated with their usage must be monitored and corrected. The child's intake of sodium should be less than 8 mEq per day.

Fluid intake should also be carefully monitored because children with heart disease can lose much water from fever, high environmental temperature, diarrhea, vomiting, and rapid respiration. Thus, children with congenital heart disease need more water than normal children of the same age. Both urine and solute level should be monitored to assure that patients drink enough fluid and are not overloaded with solutes. An acceptable urine solute load is 400 mosm per liter.

MANAGING FEEDING PROBLEMS

Feeding children with congenital heart disease also poses problems. A child may lose his or her appetite or become tired, thus reducing food intake. Of course, food intake may be inadequate owing to the regular feeding problems of normal children. For example, if the parents force a child to eat, the child may stubbornly refuse. The child may cry and become cyanotic, which can frighten some parents. If a child does not enjoy eating and the parents do not know what to do, the child's eating problems can be perpetuated.

Educating parents of children with congenital heart disease is important. The parents should become familiar with the basic eating pattern of a normal child and all associated feeding problems. They should also become familiar with managing a child with feeding problems that may be psychological. For example, they can learn to anticipate the problems, to be aware of their child using food as a weapon, to avoid overconcern for their child, to be consistent in their management, and to avoid being manipulated by the child.

In addition to learning how to cope with normal feeding problems, the parents should learn about feeding difficulties related to the heart condition, such as vomiting, gagging, and regurgitation. They should learn such techniques as massaging and stimulation of the child's gums, lips, and tongue to increase the child's sucking ability. They should also learn to evaluate the child's responses such as tiredness, resting, amount of formula consumed over a fixed period, and complexion after eating. At the same time, they should seek professional help to make sure that their child is adequately nourished.

DISCHARGE PROCEDURES

When a child with congenital heart disease is discharged from the hospital, certain procedures must be followed by the health professionals. The child's nutritional status must be studied periodically. The child's family background and daily routine, especially the eating pattern of the entire family, should be evaluated, and preparations should be made for meeting the child's nutritional needs (the role of the caretaker, the times when the child can be fed, the frequency of the child's visits to the clinic). The parental food preparer should be completely familiar with the nutritional and dietary care of the child. If the parents are unable to cope with the different methods of combining or preparing formulas, they should be taught easier feeding methods. A list of low-sodium, nondietetic products such as sugar, cereal, fruits, and vegetables should be provided. If diarrhea and steatorrhea occur, medium-chain triglycerides can be used and the consumption of simple sugars can be reduced.

NURSING IMPLICATIONS

Nursing responsibilities for treating a child with congenital heart disease are listed below:

1. Adjust the diet to the child's condition and capabilities.
2. Avoid extremes of temperature in the child's environment.
3. Maintain optimum nutrition with a well-balanced diet.
4. Discourage consumption of food with high salt content; do not add salt to any foods.
5. Encourage potassium-rich foods to prevent depletion.
6. If supplements are used, mix them in juice to hide their taste.
7. Request iron supplements as needed to correct anemia.
8. Provide consistent discipline from infancy to prevent behavior problems such as overdependency and manipulation.
9. Feed the child slowly; administer small and frequent meals.

10. Encourage the anorexic child to eat.
11. Delay self-feeding to minimize exertion.
12. Stay calm.

PROGRESS CHECK ON ACTIVITY 1

MATCHING

Match the factors in dietary care in the column at the left to the appropriate nutritional alteration at the right:

1. renal overload/dehydration
2. high metabolic rate
3. poor food intake
4. food intolerances/ malabsorption

  a. 130–160 kcal per lb body weight
  b. monitor fluid intake
  c. low in sugar, moderate fat
  d. adjust diet

MULTIPLE CHOICE

Circle the letter of the correct answer.

5. The effects of congenital heart disease on the nutritional status of a child include all but:

a. growth retardation.
b. esophageal varices.
c. lack of energy.
d. inadequate absorption.

6. Congenital heart disease can retard a child's growth by:

a. elevating body temperature.
b. increasing thyroid activity.
c. decreasing intestinal absorption.
d. all of the above.

7. Energy supplements suitable for infants with congenital heart defects include:

a. MCT oil and corn oil.
b. Karo syrup.
c. pablum and albumin.
d. a and b.

8. Guidelines for nutrient distribution for the infant with congenital heart disease should be in the range of:

a. 50% carbohydrate, 20% protein, 30% fat.
b. 35%–65% carbohydrate, 10% protein, 35%–50% fat.
c. 30% carbohydrate, 30% protein, 60% fat.
d. none of the above.

9. The electrolytes that must be closely monitored in the diet when congenital heart disease is present are:

a. sodium, chloride, and potassium.
b. calcium, iron, and iodine.
c. carbohydrate, protein, and fat.
d. phosphorus, magnesium, and calcium.

10. The child with congenital heart disease is especially susceptible to which of the following vitamin deficiencies?

a. ascorbic acid
b. linoleic acid
c. folic acid
d. amino acid

FILL-IN

11. Write a 1-day menu for a 6½-month-old child with congenital heart disease who has just been introduced to solid foods. _____

_____

_____

_____

_____

_____

12. List five feeding problems of children with congenital heart disease, and ways to overcome them.

a. _____

b. _____

c. _____

d. _____

e. _____

13. List five ways the nurse/healthcare provider can maintain optimal nutrition in a child with congenital heart disease.

a. _____

b. _____

c. _____

d. _____

e. _____

14. Name three discharge procedures to be followed when a child with congenital heart disease is going home.

a. _____

b. _____

c. _____

REFERENCES

Allen, H. D., Driscoll, D. J., Shaddy, R. E., & Feltes, T. F. (2007). *Moss and Adams' Heart Disease in Infants, Children, and Adolescents* (7th ed.). Philadelphia: Lippincott, Williams and Wilkins.

American Dietetic Association. (2006). Nutrition diagnosis: A critical step in nutrition care process. Chicago: Author.

Bader, R., Hornberger, L. K., & Huhta, J. C. (2008). *The Perinatal Cardiology Handbook.* Philadelphia: Elsevier Saunders.

Behrman, R. E., Kliegman, R. M., & Jenson, H. B. (Eds.). (2004). *Nelson Textbook of Pediatrics.* Philadelphia: Saunders.

Berkowitz, C. (2008). *Berkowitz's Pediatrics: A Primary Care Approach* (3rd ed.). Elk Village, IL: American Academy of Pediatrics.

Buchman, A. (2004). *Practical Nutritional Support Technique* (2nd ed.). Thorofeue, NJ: SLACK.

Deen, D., & Hark, L. (2007). *The Complete Guide to Nutrition in Primary Care.* Malden, MA: Blackwell.

Driscoll, D. J. (2006). *Fundamentals of Pediatric Cardiology.* Philadelphia: Lippincott, Williams and Wilkins.

Ekvall, S. W., & Ekvall, V. K. (Eds.). (2005). *Pediatric Nutrition in Chronic Diseases and Developmental Disorders: Prevention, Assessment, and Treatment.* New York: Oxford University Press.

Hosenpud, J. D., & Greenberg, B. H. (2006). *Congestive Heart Failure.* Philadelphia: Lippincott, Williams and Wilkins.

Johnson , W. H., Jr., & Moller, J. H. (2001). *Pediatric Cardiology.* Philadelphia: Lippincott, Williams and Wilkins.

Kleinman, R. E. (2004). *Pediatric Nutrition Handbook* (5th ed.). Elk Village, IL: American Academy of Pediatrics.

Mahan, L. K., & Escott-Stump, S. (Eds.). (2008). *Krause's Food and Nutrition Therapy* (12th ed.). Philadelphia: Elsevier Saunders.

Nevin-Folino, N. L. (Ed.). (2003). *Pediatric Manual of Clinical Dietetics.* Chicago: American Dietetic Association.

Nydegger, A. (2006). Energy metabolism in infants with congenital heart disease. *Nutrition, 22*: 697–704.

Paasche, C. L., Gorrill, L., & Stroon, B. (2004). *Children with Special Needs in Early Childhood Settings: Identification, Intervention, Inclusion.* Clifton Park: NY: Thomson/Delmar.

Park, M. K. (2008). *Pediatric Cardiology for Practitioners* (5th ed.). Philadelphia: Mosby/Elsevier.

Payne-James, J., & Wicks, C. (2003). *Key Facts in Clinical Nutrition* (2nd ed.). London: Greenwich Medical Media.

Samour, P. Q., & Helm, K. K. (Eds.). (2005). *Handbook of Pediatric Nutrition* (3rd ed.). Sudbury, MA: Jones and Bartlett Publishers.

Sardesai, V. M. (2003). *Introduction to Clinical Nutrition* (2nd ed.). New York: Marcel Dekker.

Shils, M. E., & Shike, M. (Eds.). (2006). *Modern Nutrition in Health and Disease* (10th ed.). Philadelphia: Lippincott, Williams and Wilkins.

Thomas, B., & Bishop, J. (Eds.). (2007). *Manual of Dietetic Practice* (4th ed.). Ames, IA: Blackwell.

Vetter, V. L. (2006). *Pediatric Cardiology.* Philadelphia: Elsevier Science Health.

Webster-Gandy, J., Madden, A., & Holdworth, M. (Eds.). (2006). *Oxford Handbook of Nutrition and Dietetics.* Oxford, London: Oxford University Press.

CHAPTER **27**

Diet Therapy and Food Allergy

Time for completion
Activities: 1½ hours
Optional examination: 1 hour

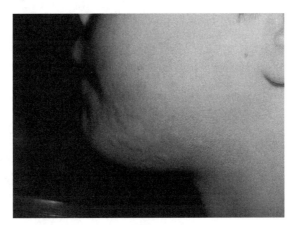

OBJECTIVES

Upon completion of this chapter the student should be able to do the following:

1. Identify the most common food allergens.
2. Differentiate between food allergy and food intolerance.
3. Describe the symptoms and management of food allergies.
4. Identify testing that is used to diagnose and confirm food allergies.
5. Name the most common food offenders and their expected symptoms.
6. Explain how nutritional status is affected by food allergies.
7. Educate children and their caregivers about the management of allergies while maintaining adequate nutrition.

GLOSSARY

Angioedema: swelling and spasm of the blood vessels, resulting in wheals.
Asthma: "panting," respiratory spasm and wheezing in an attempt to get more air.
Bronchitis: inflammation of the mucous membranes of one of the tubes leading to the lung.
Challenge diet: a diet designed to elicit a reaction by deliberately feeding a person certain ingredients, assuming the person is reactive to them.

Dermatitis: inflammation of the skin with symptoms such as itching, redness, and so on.

Eczema: acute or chronic inflammation of skin and immediately underneath it, with symptoms such as pus, discharge, and itching.

Elimination diet: a diet with certain ingredients removed, assuming a person is reactive to such ingredients. The disappearance of symptoms assumes that the person is reactive to the missing ingredients.

Immunoglobulin (Ig): one of a family of proteins that are capable of forming antibodies.

Mastitis: inflammation of the breasts.

Purpura: a variety of symptoms; for example, hemorrhage into skin.

Urticaria: eruption of the skin with severe itching.

Wheals: *see* Urticaria.

BACKGROUND INFORMATION

Allergy refers to an excess sensitivity to substances or conditions such as food; hair; cloth; biological, chemical, or mechanical agents; emotional excitement; extremes of temperature; and so on. The hypersensitivity and abnormal reactions associated with allergies produce various symptoms in affected people. The substance that triggers an allergic reaction is called an allergen or antigen, and it may enter the body through ingestion, injection, respiration, or physical contact.

In food allergies, the offending substance is usually, though not always, a protein. After digestion, it is absorbed into the circulatory system, where it encounters the body's immunological system. If this is the first exposure to the antigen, there are no overt clinical signs. Instead, the presence of an allergen causes the body to form immunoglobulins (Ig): IgA, IgE, IgG, and IgM. The organs, tissues, and blood of all healthy people contain antibodies that either circulate or remain attached to the cells where they are formed. When the body encounters the antigen a second time, the specific antibody will complex with it. Because the resulting complexes may or may not elicit clinical manifestations, merely identifying a specific immunoglobulin in the circulatory system will not indicate whether a person is allergic to a specific food antigen.

The human intestine is coated by the antibody IgA, which protects a person from developing a food allergy. However, infants under 7 months old have a lower amount of intestinal IgA. The mucosa thus permits incompletely digested protein molecules to enter. These can then enter the circulation and cause antibodies to form.

Children can also develop a food allergy called the "delayed allergic reaction" or "hypersensitivity." The classic sign of this is the tension-fatigue syndrome. Children with the syndrome have a dull face, pallor, infraorbital circles, and nasal stuffiness. A delayed food-allergy symptom is more difficult to diagnose than an immediate one.

Although food allergy is not age specific, it is more prevalent during childhood. Because a reaction to food can impose stress and interfere with nutrient ingestion, absorption, and digestion, the growth and development of children with food allergies can be delayed. Half of the adult patients with food allergy claim that they had a childhood allergy as well. Apparently, a childhood food allergy rarely disappears completely in an adult. If a newborn baby develops hypersensitivity in the first five to eight days of life, the pregnant mother was probably eating a large quantity of potentially offending foods, such as milk, eggs, chocolate, or wheat. The child becomes sensitized in the womb, and the allergic tendency may either continue into adult life or gradually decrease.

In clinical medicine, it is extremely important to differentiate food allergy from food intolerance. The former relates to the immunosystem of the body, while the latter is the direct result of maldigestion and malabsorption due to a lack of intestinal enzyme(s) or an indirect intestinal reaction because of psychological maladjustment.

ACTIVITY 1:

Food Allergy and Children

SYMPTOMS AND MANAGEMENT

About 2%–8% of all Americans have some form of food allergy. The clinical management of food allergy is controversial and has many problems. For instance, a food allergy is influenced by the amount of allergen consumed, whether the allergen is cooked or raw, and the cumulative effects from successive ingestions of the allergen. A person with a food allergy also tends to be allergic to one or more of the following: pollen, mold, wool, cosmetics, dust, and other inhalable items. Because these substances are so common, they are difficult to avoid.

Other difficulties in allergy management are as follows:

1. If a person is allergic to a food, even a very small amount can produce a reaction.
2. Some patients allergic to an item at one time are not allergic at another.
3. Some patients react to an allergen only when they are tired, frustrated, or emotionally upset.
4. Although protein is suspected to be the substance most likely to cause allergy, people can be allergic to almost any food chemical.

In managing patients with food allergy, there are two basic objectives. First, the offending substance must be identified. Patients should then be placed on a monitored antiallergic diet to assure adequate nutrient intake, especially young patients whose growth and development may be adversely affected by the allergy.

The clinical reactions of patients allergic to a food vary from relatively mild ones such as skin rash, itchy eyes, or headache to more severe ones such as abdominal cramps, diarrhea, vomiting, and loss of appetite. Other symptoms include cough, asthma, bronchitis, purpura, urticaria, dermatitis, and various problems affecting the digestive tract (vomiting, colic, ulceration of colon, etc.). In children, undernutrition and arrested development may occur.

MILK ALLERGY

Many individuals of all ages develop an allergy as well as an intolerance to milk and milk products. The reaction may occur when a person is sick (e.g., with infection, alcoholism, surgery, or trauma); thus, dietitians and nurses should always check to see whether a patient can tolerate milk. If the intolerance is due to a reduced activity of lactase, proper dietary therapy can be implemented.

Someone allergic to milk must also avoid many foods containing milk products. Ingesting regular homogenized fresh milk can damage the digestive mucosa of some susceptible individuals, especially children. The damaged cells bleed continuously but only minute amounts of blood are lost. The result is occult blood loss in the stool and iron-deficiency anemia. Professionals do not agree about whether this phenomenon is an allergic reaction. In rare cases, penicillin used in cows to prevent or control mastitis may leave a residue in milk. Consequently, some individuals who are allergic to the penicillin may have an allergic reaction to the inoculated cow's milk.

Breastmilk is much preferred over cow's milk for feeding a baby in a family whose members have allergies. Cow's milk contains the protein beta-lactoglobulin, which may trigger an allergic reaction, while breastmilk does not. If an infant has symptoms of milk allergy, special formulas with soy or another protein source as a base can be safely substituted for milk.

However, breastfeeding does have one major problem when it is used to prevent an infant from having an allergic reaction to cow's milk. If the child is also allergic to substances such as cheese, crab, or chocolate, the mother can in effect feed them to her child via breastmilk if she ingests them herself. Therefore, the breastfed child may show allergic reactions.

DIAGNOSIS AND TREATMENT

Food allergies are difficult to test for and subsequently to diagnose and confirm. Furthermore, patients with an allergic reaction to one food may in reality be allergic to many others that contain a common ingredient. Or, when an infant is allergic to a formula, it is usually assumed that the protein is responsible. In reality, it could be the vegetable oil base.

When food allergy is suspected in a child, the parents, nurse, and dietitian or nutritionist should work together to identify the culprit. The child's reactions to food coloring and additives (which are found in many processed foods) and salicylate-related chemicals should also be noted. Unless the culprit is one of the common offenders, it is difficult for the physician to make an accurate diagnosis because of the many different components in a child's diet.

The National Institute of Health and the Department of Health and Human Services has made the following recommendations about diagnosis of a food allergy.

After ruling out food intolerances and other health problems, your healthcare provider will use several steps to find out if you have an allergy to specific foods.

Detailed History

A detailed history is the most valuable tool for diagnosing food allergy. Your provider will ask you several questions and listen to your history of food reactions to decide if the facts fit a food allergy. The following are samples of such questions:

1. What was the timing of your reaction?
2. Did your reaction come on quickly, usually within an hour after eating the food?
3. Did allergy medicines help? Antihistamines should relieve hives, for example.
4. Is your reaction always associated with a certain food?
5. Did anyone else who ate the same food get sick? For example, if you ate fish contaminated with histamine, everyone who ate the fish should be sick.

Diet Diary

Sometimes your healthcare provider can't make a diagnosis solely on the basis of your history. In that case, you may be asked to record what you eat and whether you have a reaction. This diet diary gives more detail from which you and your provider can see if there is a consistent pattern in your reactions.

Elimination Diet

The next step some healthcare providers use is an elimination diet. In this step, which is done under your provider's direction, certain foods are removed from your diet. You don't eat a food suspected of causing the allergy, such as eggs. You then substitute another food-in the case of eggs, another source of protein.

Your provider can almost always make a diagnosis if the symptoms go away after you remove the food from your diet. The diagnosis is confirmed if you then eat the food and the symptoms come back. You should do this only when the reactions are not significant and only under healthcare provider direction.

Your provider can't use this technique, however, if your reactions are severe or don't happen often. If you have a severe reaction, you should not eat the food again.

Skin Test

If your history, diet diary, or elimination diet suggests a specific food allergy is likely, your healthcare provider will then use either the scratch or the prick skin test to confirm the diagnosis.

During a scratch skin test, your healthcare provider will place an extract of the food on the skin of your lower arm. Your provider will then scratch this portion of your skin with a needle and look for swelling or redness, which would be a sign of a local allergic reaction.

A prick skin test is done by putting a needle just below the surface of your skin of the lower arm. Then, a tiny amount of food extract is placed under the skin.

If the scratch or prick test is positive, it means that there is IgE on the skin's mast cells that is specific to the food being tested. Skin tests are rapid, simple, and relatively safe. You can have a positive skin test to a food allergen, however, without having an allergic reaction to that food. A healthcare provider diagnoses a food allergy only when someone has a positive skin test to a specific allergen and when the history of reactions suggests an allergy to the same food.

Blood Test

Your healthcare provider can make a diagnosis by doing a blood test as well. Indeed, if you are extremely allergic and have severe anaphylactic reactions, your provider can't use skin testing because causing an allergic reaction to the skin test could be dangerous. Skin testing also can't be done if you have eczema over a large portion of your body.

Your healthcare provider may use blood tests such as the RAST (radioallergosorbent test) and newer ones such as the CAP-RAST. Another blood test is called ELISA (enzyme-linked immunosorbent assay). These blood tests measure the presence of food-specific IgE in your blood. The CAP-RAST can measure how much IgE your blood has to a specific food. As with skin testing, positive tests do not necessarily mean you have a food allergy.

Double-Blind Oral Food Challenge

The final method healthcare providers use to diagnose food allergy is double-blind oral food challenge.

Your healthcare provider will give you capsules containing individual doses of various foods, some of which are suspected of starting an allergic reaction. Or your provider will mask the suspected food within other foods known not to cause an allergic reaction. You swallow the capsules one at a time or swallow the masked food and are watched to see if a reaction occurs.

In a true double-blind test, your healthcare provider is also "blinded" (the capsules having been made up by another medical person). In that case your provider does not know which capsule contains the allergen.

The advantage of such a challenge is that if you react only to suspected foods and not to other foods tested, it confirms the diagnosis. You cannot be tested this way if you have a history of severe allergic reactions.

In addition, this testing is difficult because it takes a lot of time to perform and many food allergies are difficult to evaluate with this procedure. Consequently, many healthcare providers do not perform double-blind food challenges.

This type of testing is most commonly used if a healthcare provider thinks the reaction described is not due to a specific food and wishes to obtain evidence to support this. If your provider finds that your reaction is not due to a specific food, then additional efforts may be used to find the real cause of the reaction.

NURSING IMPLICATIONS

The nurse should be aware of the following principles when caring for children with allergies:

1. Diet therapy is used to identify allergic reactions and also to avoid these reactions.
2. Newborns of parents with allergies should be protected from potential allergens in breastmilk.
3. Breastmilk is the best food for a potentially allergic infant.
4. Pregnant women with a family history of allergies should avoid foods known to be allergens to reduce the risk of sensitizing the infant.
5. Solid foods should be introduced one at a time and evaluated over several days before adding another.
6. Delay introduction of solid foods in an infant's diet to reduce absorption of potential allergens in an immature GI tract.
7. Appropriate substitutions or supplementation of an allergic child's diet is essential to prevent malnutrition created by gaps in permitted foods.
8. Children who are allergic to eggs should never be immunized with vaccines grown on chick embryo.
9. Diabetic children allergic to pork are unable to use insulin made from hog pancreas.
10. Children with allergens should wear medical alert tags.
11. Allergens are usually (though not always) proteins.
12. Raw foods are more likely to be allergens than cooked ones.
13. Parents and children should read all labels carefully and be taught to look for hidden sources of the allergen.

14. Foods that cause immediate allergic reactions in susceptible individuals are eggs, seafood, nuts (especially peanuts), and berries.
15. Foods that cause delayed reactions are wheat, milk, legumes, corn, white potatoes, chocolate, and oranges (citrus).
16. Patients who are allergic to a specific food will react to other foods in the same family.
17. Foods that cause allergic responses may be reintroduced at a later time because children tend to outgrow food allergies.
18. Differentiate between food allergies and food intolerance. The treatments are very different.

PROGRESS CHECK ON BACKGROUND INFORMATION AND ACTIVITY 1

FILL-IN

1. Define allergy. _____

2. Name the substance(s) that trigger allergic reactions. _____

3. Describe how IgA, IgE, IgG, and IgM are formed in the body. _____

4. What is the delayed allergic reaction syndrome? _____

5. Describe the difference between a food allergy and a food intolerance. _____

6. Identify six major problems that arise in regard to management of food allergies.
   a. _____
   b. _____
   c. _____
   d. _____
   e. _____
   f. _____

7. Name the two basic diet objectives in allergy management.
   a. _____
   b. _____

8. Why is breastmilk preferred over cow's milk for feeding infants? _____

9. Identify the two types of tests available for diagnosing children.
   a. _____
   b. _____

ACTIVITY 2:
Common Offenders

Although a food allergy rarely constitutes a serious, life-threatening concern, it results in chronic illness for many sufferers. This problem can be significantly eliminated if one is alert to the most common allergens and the manifestations of allergic reaction.

COMMON ALLERGENS
Cow's Milk

The allergen in cow's milk is probably the most common. A susceptible person may be allergic to whole, skimmed, evaporated, or dried milk, as well as to milk-containing products such as ice cream, cheese, custard, cream and creamed foods, and yogurt. Milk allergy can range from a mild to a severe stage. As a result, for those with more severe form of milk allergy, even butter and bread can create a reaction. Symptoms can include either or both constipation and diarrhea, abdominal pain, nasal and bronchial congestion, asthma, headache, foul breath, sweating, fatigue, and tension.

Kola Nut Products

Chocolate (cocoa) and cola (a source of caffeine) are products obtained from the kola nut, as indicated in most health documents issued by government agencies, both state and federal. However, botanically, the kola nut associated with cocoa is common in South America and the kola nut associated with cola is common in Africa. An allergy to one almost always means an allergy to the other as well. Symptoms most commonly include headache, asthma, gastrointestinal allergy, nasal allergy, and eczema. As far as the patients and doctors are concerned, the question of the source (Africa or South America) of kola nut is moot.

Corn

Because corn syrup is widely used commercially, corn allergy can result from a wide variety of foods. Candy, chewing gum, prepared meats, cookies, rolls, doughnuts, some breads, canned fruits, jams, jellies, some fruit juices, ice cream, and sweetened cereals often contain corn syrup. Additionally, whole corn, cornstarch, corn flour, corn oil, and cornmeal can cause allergic reactions to such foods as cereals, tortillas, tamales, enchiladas, soups, beer, whiskey, fish sticks, and pancake or waffle mixes.

Symptoms can be bizarre, ranging from allergic tension to allergic fatigue. Headache can take the form of migraine.

Eggs

Those with severe allergy to eggs can react to even their odor. Egg allergy can also cause reaction to vaccines, since they are often grown on chicken embryo. Allergic reactions are generally to such foods as eggs themselves, baked goods, candies, mayonnaise, creamy dressings, meat loaf, breaded foods, and noodles.

Symptoms can be widely varied, as with milk. Egg allergy often results in urticaria (hives) though, like chocolate, larger amounts are usually necessary to produce that symptom. Other symptoms include headache, gastrointestinal allergy, eczema, and asthma.

Peas (Legumes)

The larger family of plants that are collectively known as peas include peanuts, soybeans, beans, and peas. Peanuts tend to be the greatest offender, and dried beans and peas cause more difficulties than fresh ones. Products that can cause selected allergy reaction are honey (made from the offending plants) and licorice, a legume. Soybean allergy presents a problem similar to corn owing to its widespread use in the form of soybean concentrate or soybean oil.

Legume allergies can be quite severe, even resulting in shock. They commonly cause headache and can be especially troublesome for asthma patients, urticaria patients, and angioedema sufferers.

Citrus Fruits

Oranges, lemons, limes, grapefruit, and tangerines can cause eczema and hives, and often, asthma. They commonly cause canker sores (aphthous stomatitis). Although citrus fruit allergy does not cause allergy to artificial orange and lemon-lime drinks, if patients are allergic to citric acid in the fruits then they will also react to tart artificial drinks and may also react to pineapple.

Tomatoes

This fruit, commonly called a vegetable, can cause hives, eczema, and canker sores. It can also cause asthma. In addition to its natural form, it can be encountered in soups, pizza, catsup, salads, meat loaf, and tomato paste or tomato juice.

Wheat and Other Grains

Wheat, rice, barley, oats, millet, and rye are known allergens, with wheat the most common of the group. Wheat occurs in many dietary products. All common baked goods, cream sauce, macaroni, noodles, pie crust, cereals, chili, and breaded foods contain wheat.

Reaction to wheat and its related grains can be severe. Asthma and gastrointestinal disturbances are the most common reactions.

Spices

Of various spices that can cause allergic reaction, cinnamon is generally the most potent. It can be found in catsup, chewing gum, candy, cookies, cakes, rolls, prepared meats, and pies. Bay leaf allergy generally occurs as well, since this spice is related to cinnamon. Pumpkin pie reactions are common owing to their high cinnamon content. Other spices most frequently mentioned as allergens are black pepper, white pepper, oregano, the mints, paprika, and cumin.

Artificial Food Colors

Although various artificial food colors have been implicated in such problems as hyperactive syndrome in children, as allergens the two most common offenders are amaranth (red dye) and tartrazine (yellow dye). Amaranth is most often encountered, but reactions to tartrazine tend to be more severe. Food colors occur in carbonated beverages, some breakfast drinks, bubble gum, flavored ice foods, gelatin desserts, and such medications as antibiotic syrups.

OTHER FOOD ALLERGENS

Any food is capable of producing an allergic reaction. However, those offenders often mentioned after the top 10 are pork and beef, onion and garlic, white potatoes, fish, coffee, shrimp, bananas, and walnuts and pecans.

Vegetables, other than those already mentioned, rarely cause allergic reactions. Fruits that usually are safe include cranberries, blueberries, figs, cherries, apricots, and plums. Chicken, turkey, lamb, and rabbit have proven to be the safest meats. Tea, olives, sugar, and tapioca are also relatively safe foods, although some herbal teas can cause unique difficulties.

PEANUT ALLERGY AND DEATHS

Peanut allergy is probably the most serious among children and teenagers. Two examples of death from peanut allergy are provided here.

Death of a Cadet in Australia

On June 6, 2008, the *Sydney Morning Herald* of Australia reported the following:

Nathan Francis, a 13-year-old cadet associated with the Australian Defense Force (ADF), died from eating a military ration pack meal. This occurred on March 30, 2007, when the teenager from Melbourne was participating in an army cadet unit west of Victoria. The meal contains peanuts as one of the ingredients. The boy suffered an allergic shock.

The Australia occupation health and safety authority claimed that the ADF was not offering adequate measures to provide health and safety protection for its cadets.

Death of a Teenager in Canada

On April 16, 2007, the *Victoria Times-Colonist* of British Columbia, Canada, reported the following:

Carley Kohnen, a 13-year-old, died at Summit Park, Victoria. She died from an anaphylactic shock brought about by an allergic reaction to a food ingredient she ate. In this case, while visiting a mall with some friends, she ate a burrito. She suffered from an allergy to dairy products and peanuts while they were on the way to the park. The offending ingredients were most likely from the burrito.

Normally, she carries an auto-injector just in case an allergic shock occurs. Unfortunately, she left it in her locker at school. Her shock required medical treatment immediately, and she died because there was very little time for help to arrive.

Unfortunately, severe food allergy is a problem with teenagers in Canada and the United States. Legal, medical, and educational authorities in both countries are considering the most effective ways to counteract such medical problems. In some situations, food with a peanut ingredient is banned from all public and private schools.

PROGRESS CHECK ON ACTIVITY 2

MULTIPLE CHOICE

Circle the letter of the correct answer.

1. The most common offender to trigger allergies is:

    a. wheat.
    b. cow's milk.
    c. corn.
    d. eggs.

2. The most common artificial food colors to trigger allergies in susceptible children include:

    a. amaranth and tantrazine.
    b. tyrosine and amaranth.
    c. chlorophyll and rubella.
    d. melanine and xanthine.

3. Egg allergies can cause reaction to vaccines because:

    a. egg yolk is a very common allergen in children.
    b. egg forms a complex with the drug causing the reaction.
    c. the vaccine is grown on a chicken embryo.
    d. all of the above

TRUE/FALSE

Circle T for True and F for False.

4. T F   Allergic reactions to chocolate include asthma and eczema.
5. T F   Corn allergies do not develop from ingestion of corn syrup.
6. T F   People with severe allergies to eggs can react to their odor.
7. T F   Legume allergies are not usually as severe as milk allergies.
8. T F   Citrus allergy sufferers usually do not react to artificial citrus flavors.
9. T F   The most common grain allergen is wheat.
10. T F   The most potent spice allergen is ginger.

ACTIVITY 3:

Inspecting Foods to Avoid Allergic Reactions

Each year the Food and Drug Administration (FDA) receives reports of consumers who experienced adverse reactions following exposure to an allergenic substance in foods. Food allergies are abnormal responses of the immune system, especially the production of allergen-specific IgE antibodies to naturally occurring proteins in certain foods that most individuals can eat safely. Frequently such reactions occur because the presence of the allergenic substance in the food is not declared on the food label. Current regulations require that all added ingredients be declared on the label, yet there are a number of issues that have arisen in connection with undeclared allergens that are not clearly covered by label regulations.

To protect the consumers, both adults and children, the FDA has asked its food inspectors to pay attention to the following when inspecting an establishment that manufactures processed food products.

1. Products that contain one or more allergenic ingredients, but the label does not declare the ingredient in the ingredient statement.
2. Products that become contaminated with an allergenic ingredient due to the firm's failure to exercise adequate control procedures, for example, improper rework practices, allergen carryover due to use of common equipment and production sequencing, and inadequate cleaning.

3. Products that are contaminated with an allergenic ingredient due to the nature of the product or the process, for example, use of common equipment in chocolate manufacturing where interim wet cleaning is not practical and only dry cleaning and product flushing is used.

4. A product containing a flavor ingredient that has an allergenic component, but the label of the product only declares the flavor, for example, natural flavor. Under current regulations, firms are not required to declare the individual components of flavors, certain colors, and spices. However, firms are encouraged to specifically label allergenic components and ingredients that are in spices, flavors, and colors.

5. Products that contain a processing aid that have an allergenic component, but the label does not declare it. Processing aids that contain allergenic ingredients are not exempt from ingredient declaration.

FDA believes there is scientific consensus that the following foods can cause serious allergic reactions in some individuals and account for more than 90% of all food allergies:

- Peanuts
- Soybeans
- Milk
- Eggs
- Fish
- Crustacea (e.g., shrimp)
- Tree nuts
- Wheat

Each FDA food inspector is asked to pay special attention to the following:

1. Product development: Determine whether the firm identifies potential sources of allergens starting in the product development stage.

2. Receiving: Determine whether the firm uses allergenic ingredients and how they are stored.

3. Equipment: Try to inspect the equipment before processing begins and document the adequacy of clean up.

4. Processing: Determine what control measures, if any, are used by the firm to prevent the contamination of products that do not contain allergens.

The inspection is especially concerned about the labeling that will be checked as follows:

1. Determine if finished product label controls are employed; for example, how are labels delivered to the filling and/or packaging area?

2. Determine if product labels with similar appearances but different ingredients are controlled to ensure that the correct label is applied to correct product.

3. Determine if finished product packages are inspected prior to distribution to ensure that an allergen-

containing product is labeled properly, or that labels are inspected during production. Is that inspection documented?

4. Determine if secondary ingredients are incorporated in the final product ingredient statement, for example, the raw material mayonnaise, which contains eggs, oil, and vinegar.

5. Determine if the firm uses a statement such as "This product was processed on machinery that was used to process products containing (allergen)" or a statement such as "may contain (allergen)" if the firm uses shared equipment for products that contain and products that do not contain allergens. Any other such statement? Ask the firm why they believe they have to use the advisory statement.

6. Determine if the finished product label reflects any advisory statements that were on the raw material labels, for example, "This product was processed on machinery that was used to process products containing (allergen)."

7. Determine if the firm has a system to identify finished products made with rework containing allergenic ingredients. Does the final product label identify the allergens that may have been in the reworked product?

Although some labels do not state allergic ingredients, most do. Therefore, if your child has a food allergy, the best prevention method is to read the label of any food product that will be consumed by the child.

PROGRESS CHECK ON ACTIVITY 3

TRUE/FALSE

Circle T for True and F for False.

1. T F Food allergies are abnormal responses of the immune system, especially the production of allergen-specific IgE antibodies to naturally occurring proteins in certain foods that most individuals can eat safely.

2. T F Frequently food allergic reactions occur because the allergenic substance originates from the food itself.

3. T F The FDA inspector is especially concerned about the labeling of products with a statement such as "This product was processed on machinery that was used to process products containing (allergen)" or a statement such as "may contain (allergen)."

FILL-IN

4. Name the eight foods that the scientific community believes account for more than 90% of all food allergies:

a. _____

b. _____

c. _____

d. _____

e. _____

f. _____

g. _____

h. _____

REFERENCES

Accetta, D. (2007). *Medical Encyclopedia: Food Allergy.* Bethesda, MD: National Library of Medicine, National Institutes of Health.

Behrman, R. E., Kliegman, R. M., & Jenson, H. B. (Eds.). (2004). *Nelson Textbook of Pediatrics.* Philadelphia: Saunders.

Boguniewicz, M. (2008). Allergenic diseases, quality of life, and the role of the dietitian. *Nutrition Today, 43*: 6–10.

Cappellano, K. L. (2008). Food allergy and intolerance: The nuts and bolts of detection and management. *Nutrition Today, 43*: 11–14.

Dean, T. (2007). Government advice on peanut avoidance during pregnancy: Is it followed correctly and what is the impact on sensitization. *Journal of Human Nutrition and Dietetics, 20*: 95–99.

Fu, T. J., & Gendel, S. M. (Eds.). (2002). *Genetically Engineered Foods: Assessing Potential Allergenicity.* New York: New York Academy of Sciences.

Grimshaw, K. E. C. (2006). Dietary management of food allergy in children. *Proceedings of the Nutrition Society, 65*: 412–417.

Hardman, G. (2007). Dietary advice based on food-specific IgG results. *Nutrition and Food Science, 37*: 16–23.

Joneja, J. M. V. (2003). *Dealing with Food Allergies: A Practical Guide to Detecting Culprit Foods and Eating a Healthy, Enjoyable Diet.* Boulder, CO: Bull.

Kleinman, R. E. (2004). *Pediatric Nutrition Handbook* (5th ed.). Elk Village, IL: American Academy of Pediatrics.

Mahan, L. K., & Escott-Stump, S. (Eds.). (2008). *Krause's Food and Nutrition Therapy* (12th ed.). Philadelphia: Elsevier Saunders.

Maintz, L. (2007). Histamine and histamine intolerance. *American Journal of Clinical Nutrition, 85*: 1185–1196.

Maleki, S. J., Burks, A. W., & Helm, R. M. (Eds.). (2006). *Food Allergy.* Washington, DC: ASM Press.

Melina, V., Stepaniak, J., & Aronson, D. (2004). *Food Allergy Survival Guide: Surviving and Thriving with Food Allergies and Sensitivities.* Summertown, TN: Healthy Living.

Meredith, C. (2005). Allergenic potential of novel foods. *Proceedings of the Nutrition Society, 64*: 487–490.

Metcalfe, D. D., Sampson, H., & Simon, R. (2008). *Food Allergy: Adverse Reactions to Food and Food Additives* (3rd ed.). Ames, IA: Blackwell.

Mills, C., Wichers, H., & Hoffmann-Sommergruber, K. (Eds.). (2007). *Managing Allergens in Food.* Boca Raton, FL: CRC Press.

Mills, E. N. C., & Shewry, P. R. (Eds.). (2004). *Plant Food Allergens.* Malden, MA: Blackwell Science.

Paasche, C. L., Gorrill, L., & Stroon, B. (2004). *Children with Special Needs in Early Childhood Settings: Identification, Intervention, Inclusion.* Clifton Park: NY: Thomson/Delmar.

Samartin, S. (2001). Food hypersentivity. *Nutrition Research, 21*: 473–497.

Samour, P. Q., & Helm, K. K. (Eds.). (2005). *Handbook of Pediatric Nutrition* (3rd ed.). Sudbury, MA: Jones and Bartlett Publishers.

Sarkar, S. (2007). Probiotic therapy for gastro-intestinal allergenic infants: A preliminary review. *British Food Journal, 109*: 481–492.

Shils, M. E., & Shike, M. (Eds.). (2006). *Modern Nutrition in Health and Disease* (10th ed.). Philadelphia: Lippincott, Williams and Wilkins.

Staden, U. (2007). Specific oral tolerance induction in food allergy in children: Efficacy and clinical patterns of reactions. *Allergy, 62*: 1261–1269.

Thom, D. (2002). *Coping with Food Intolerances* (4th ed.). New York: Sterling.

Thomas, B., & Bishop, J. (Eds.). (2007). *Manual of Dietetic Practice* (4th ed.). Ames, IA: Blackwell.

Vileg-Boerstra, B. J. (2006). Dietary assessment in children adhering to a food allergen avoidance diet for allergy prevention. *European Journal of Clinical Nutrition, 60*: 1384–1390.

CHAPTER

28

Diet Therapy and Phenylketonuria

Time for completion
Activities: 1 hour
Optional examination: ½ hour

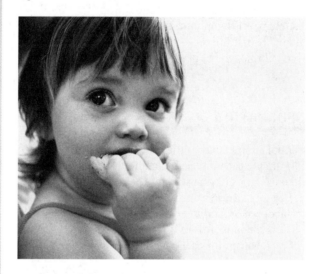

OBJECTIVES

Upon completion of this chapter, the student should be able to do the following:

1. Explain the etiology of phenylketonuria (PKU).
2. Identify a method of diagnosing PKU.
3. Relate the symptoms of untreated PKU.
4. Describe the dietary management of PKU:
   a. Requirements
   b. Restrictions
   c. Appropriate supplements
5. Evaluate the controversies regarding terminating diet therapy and restricted diet during pregnancy.
6. Discuss the responsibilities of the health team for follow-up care in monitoring the progress of a PKU child.
7. List health team interventions appropriate to successful dietary management of PKU children.
8. Provide information to caregivers on diet management, resources, and counseling as necessary.

GLOSSARY

Casein hydrolysate: principal protein of milk, partially digested.

Eczema: a superficial inflammatory process of the skin marked by redness, itching, scaling, sometimes weeping and oozing.

Electroencephalogram (EEG): the recording of changes in the electrical potential of the brain by evaluating the brain waves.

Fibrinogen: a protein in the blood necessary for clotting.

Mental retardation: significantly subaverage general intellectual functioning existing along with deficits in adaptive behavior, which manifests itself during the developmental period.

Phenylketonuria (PKU): an inborn error of amino acid metabolism.

Plasma: fluid portion of the blood in which corpuscles are suspended.

Reticulosarcoma: a type of malignant tumor; a lymphoid neoplasm; also called "stem cell" lymphoma and "undifferentiated malignant" lymphoma.

Serum: plasma from which fibrinogen has been removed in the process of clotting.

BACKGROUND INFORMATION

Each of the 8 to 10 essential amino acids in the human body is metabolized via a unique pathway. Some infants are born with a defect in one of the enzyme systems that regulate one or more of these pathways. As a result, if the amino acid is not metabolized properly, certain products may accumulate in the blood or urine. If this occurs, an inborn error of metabolism for that particular amino acid results.

One example of faulty protein metabolism involves phenylalanine and tyrosine. Although both substances are essential amino acids, the body derives part of its tyrosine needs from phenylalanine with the help of a certain enzyme (phenylalanine hydroxylase). A newborn may have no or very low activity of this enzyme, and as a result the body is unable to change phenylalanine to tyrosine. Consequently the chemicals phenylalanine, phenylpyruvic acid, and other metabolites accumulate. If they exceed certain levels in the blood, they cross the brain barriers (membranes), and the child suffers mental retardation. It is currently believed that one in 25,000 live births in the United States inherits this disorder, commonly referred to as phenylketonuria (PKU), which causes a high level of phenylpyruvic acid in the urine. Immediately after birth the baby appears normal, but the child soon becomes slightly irritable and hyperactive. The urine has a musty odor.

If the disorder is not diagnosed and treated, the child will develop aggressive behavior, unstable muscular and nervous systems, eczema, convulsions, and seizures. Since tyrosine is responsible for making pigments, its decreased supply results in decreased coloration, with such effects as decreased body pigmentation, blue eyes, a fair complexion, and blond hair in Caucasian patients. Some patients develop reticulosarcoma-like skin lesions. Severe mental retardation may result. The accumulation of chemicals in the blood interferes with the normal development of the central nervous system and the brain. Some young children show abnormal electroencephalograms. In spite of all these adverse symptoms, the child shows a normal birth weight.

A method of diagnosing PKU in newborns was developed in the 1960s, and its use has since become widespread. The method, known as the Guthrie test, involves analyzing blood drawn from the child's heel. A normal infant's blood contains about 1 to 2 mg of phenylalanine/100 ml of plasma, while that of a PKU child is about 15 to 30 mg/100 ml plasma. However, a positive Guthrie test does not necessarily indicate PKU, because transient high blood phenylalanine may occur in some infants; thus, additional tests are required for confirmation.

The Guthrie test is normally done before the baby is removed from the nursery, 2 to 5 days after birth. At 1 month of age, the test is repeated, especially for babies who show high blood phenylalanine during the first blood screening. A blood level of over 4 mg phenylalanine/100 ml plasma may indicate that additional tests are needed. A level of 20 mg/100 ml positively indicates PKU.

All states and U.S. territories screen for PKU, whether voluntary or mandatory. Babies are screened before discharge from the hospital. Although the principles of the test are the same as it was discovered in 1960, the technique of analysis is faster, easier, and more accurate.

PROGRESS CHECK ON BACKGROUND INFORMATION

MULTIPLE CHOICE

Circle the letter of the correct answer.

1. PKU may be defined as an inborn error of metabolism because:

   a. amino acids have a separate pathway from other nutrients.
   b. there is a defect in the enzyme system that regulates certain amino acids.
   c. the amino acids accumulate in the urine.
   d. the mother's diet was very low in amino acids.

2. The absent or limited enzyme that causes the symptoms of PKU to develop is:

   a. lactase-galactase.
   b. gliadin.
   c. phenylalanine hydroxylase.
   d. phenylpyruvic acid.

3. The level of phenylalanine in a normal baby's blood is _____/100 ml plasma, while in that of a PKU baby it is _____/100 ml plasma.

    a. 1–2 mg; 15–30 mg
    b. 12–15 mg; 30–40 mg
    c. 30–40 mg; 65–75 mg
    d. 10–20 mg; 50–100 mg

4. The most prominent symptom of untreated PKU is:

    a. aggressive behavior.
    b. decreased skin coloration/skin lesions.
    c. convulsions.
    d. severe mental retardation.

5. The diagnostic test for PKU is done:

    a. one month after birth.
    b. two to five days after birth.
    c. at birth.
    d. any time before the first year.

TRUE/FALSE

Circle T for True and F for False.

6. T F A positive reaction to a Guthrie test always indicates that a baby has PKU.
7. T F It is voluntary in the United States that all states screen new babies for PKU.

ACTIVITY 1:

Phenylketonuria and Dietary Management

TREATMENT AND REQUIREMENT

The dietary management for PKU children consists of rigidly restricting phenylalanine intake. This special, low-phenylalanine diet starts immediately after diagnosis. If treatment starts after retardation has already occurred, normal mental ability may not return completely, but there will be no further deterioration and no recurrence of symptoms. Although the intake of phenylalanine must be restricted, these children still need a minimal amount of the amino acid for growth and development, in addition to an adequate supply of all other essential nutrients.

A newborn child needs about 65 to 90 mg of phenylalanine per kilogram of body weight, while a 2-year-old needs 20 to 25 mg. Thus, an infant should be provided with enough phenylalanine to maintain a level of 2–6 mg/dl of blood, based on tolerance, or 60 mg/kg/day. The protein should be 3.0–3.5 g/kg and the caloric intake of at least 110 cal/kg. Any formula used should have at least 90% of phenylalanine removed; meaning 90% of protein for the infant should come from specialized infant formula. If a particular level of intake raises serum levels to abnormally high concentrations, the level must be lowered. Conversely, the serum level must not be allowed to fall below acceptable limits.

LOFENALAC AND PHENYLALANINE FOOD EXCHANGE LISTS

Since phenylalanine is an essential amino acid, it is found in most animal products, including milk, which is the main nutritional component of an infant's diet; thus, milk has to be specially processed to remove part or all of the phenylalanine. For many years most practitioners have used the commercial powder Lofenalac (Mead Johnson). It is a special low-protein powder containing casein hydrolysate with about 95% of the phenylalanine removed. It is also supplemented with vitamins and minerals. Although Lofenalac is still widely used, Mead Johnson has developed several new products with some modifications. For ease of discussion, we will continue to use Lofenalac as an illustration and a product of choice.

There are also formulas that are age related: Analog, Maxamaid, and Maximum, from Scientific Hospital Supplies; and the 1993 Metabolic Formula System from Ross Laboratories.

Because Lofenalac contains less than 1% phenylalanine, it cannot support normal growth and development of a child. As a result, specified amounts of natural foods are commonly provided to increase the child's phenylalanine intake, such as evaporated or whole milk. As the child grows, additional solid foods are given. Close monitoring of the child's nutrient intake is essential. Table 28-1 compares the phenylalanine, calorie, and protein content of Lofenalac with that of evaporated and whole milk. Table 28-2 describes the phenylalanine, energy, and protein intake for a PKU patient under 1 year old.

TABLE 28-1 Calorie, Phenylalanine, and Protein Contents of Lofenalac and Milk

Food	Amount	Kilocalories	Protein (g)	Phenylalanine (g)
Lofenalac	10 g	45.4	1.5	0.008
Milk				
Evaporated	29–30 g (1 oz)	44.0	2.2	106
Whole	29–30 g (1 oz)	19.7	1.1	51

TABLE 28-2   Suggested Phenylalanine, Energy, and Protein Intakes per Day for PKU Patients under One Year Old

Amount of Nutrient Needed per Kilogram Body Weight				Lofenalac		Milk (oz)	
Age (months)*	Phenylalanine (mg)	Protein (g)	Kilocalories	Protein Provided by Product to Child's Need (%)	Measures† Permitted per Kilogram Body Weight	Whole	Evaporated
0–2½	85	4.4	125	85	2½–3	2–4	1–3
2½–6½	65	3.3	115	85	2–2½	2–4	1–2½
6½–9½	45	2.5	105	90	1½–2	1½–2½	½–1½
9½–12	32	2.5	105	90	1½–2	½–1½	½–1

Note: the child may or may not need additional foods. See text.
*The separation between age groups is not exact.
†One measure equals 1 tbsp, containing about 10 g of powder.
An example: a one-month-old child is permitted 2 to 4 oz whole milk (or 1 to 3 oz evaporated milk) and 2½ to 3 measures of Lofenalac per kilogram body weight per day.

To provide the PKU child with regular food, the phenylalanine, protein, and calorie contents of regular foods must be known. As a result, young children's foods are grouped into exchange lists, each of which contains food items that contribute equivalent amounts of phenylalanine.

Currently, both U.S. Public Health Service and private medical centers use the dietary guidelines for management of PKU. Dietary management has two purposes: an appropriate substitute for milk (especially for the infant) and guidelines for adding solid foods. Lofenalac is the milk substitute most generally used in the United States. It contains approximately 5% phenylalanine. Other products that are phenylalanine free can be used by older children and pregnant mothers. This allows them a wider variety of foods before they reach the limits of the phenylalanine allowance in their diet.

Caregivers, nurses, and physicians must bear the primary responsibility for providing and continuing care so that the child with PKU will grow and develop normally. This requires a coordinated effort of understanding the absolute necessity of following the diet carefully. Patience is very important as counseling, guidance, and education are provided. Teaching guides and materials are available to help in planning and follow-up. Home health nurses may provide follow-up care and reinforcement. Social services and support groups are also good adjuncts to assist in the vigilance required.

SPECIAL CONSIDERATIONS

When feeding a patient with PKU, several considerations should be kept in mind. First, calories and taste should be varied. Second, special low-protein products are available and can also be used to advantage. Request a list from dietitians or nurses. Third, patients should avoid meat and dairy products (except the permitted milk).

Fourth, the feeding regimen must be consistent with the age and development of the child, and the food quantity and texture must be adjusted to the child's eating ability. Fifth, the nutritional adequacy of the child's diet should be constantly evaluated, using the RDAs/DRIs as a guide. Table 28-3 lists some common baby foods along with their nutritional values, and Table 28-4 offers a child's sample menu.

One of the most controversial issues in treating a child with PKU is the uncertainty about when to terminate dietary restrictions. Some children are put on a normal diet at the age of five, when further mental progress may require additional phenylalanine. Other clinicians keep the child on a phenylalanine-restricted diet indefinitely. There is no known age when the diet can be safely discontinued. Developmental problems occur in older children and adolescents who have discontinued the diet.

It should be noted that if a restrictive diet is discontinued, the child and family go through a very important transition period. The parents and the child will need time and patience to adapt to this sudden exposure to meat and a whole variety of other foods.

Successful management of PKU babies over the years has allowed them to attain normal growth and develop into healthy adults. Now the young women are having babies of their own. The pregnant woman with PKU is at high risk, but the fetal risks are even higher. The major hazards to the fetus are congenital deformities and mental retardation. Untreated PKU during a pregnancy also leads to higher rates of stillbirth and/or prematurity.

In the United States, thousands of women of childbearing age have had their PKU successfully treated. Most discontinued their special diet in childhood when their doctors determined that it was safe to do so.

If these young women are eating a normal diet, their blood phenylalanine levels are very high when they become pregnant. During pregnancy, high blood levels of

TABLE 28-3 Contents of Calories, Protein, and Phenylalanine in Some Selected Foods

Food	Phenylalanine (mg)	Protein (g)	Kilocalories
Gerber's strained and junior vegetables			
Carrots, 5 tbsp	15	0.5	21
Sweet potatoes, 1½ tbsp	15	0.3	15
Gerber's strained and junior fruits			
Applesauce, 7 tbsp	10	0.2	81
Apricots with tapioca, 8 tbsp	10	0.5	88
Orange-pineapple juice, 11 tbsp	10	0.8	41
Peaches, 3 tbsp	10	0.3	35
Gerber's baby cereals			
Barley cereal, 1¼ tbsp	18	0.4	11
Rice with mixed fruit (in jar), 1¼ tbsp	18	0.3	13
Rice with strawberries, 2¼ tbsp	18	0.5	21
Total	124	3.8	326

phenylalanine in the mother can cause serious problems in the fetus such as mental retardation, a small head size at birth, heart defects, and low birth weight.

Fortunately, most of the clinical problems can be prevented in babies of women with PKU if proper precautions are taken by these pregnant women:

1. Resume their special diets at least three months before pregnancy and continue the diet throughout pregnancy.
2. Undergo weekly blood tests throughout pregnancy to monitor blood phenylalanine levels assuming that high levels will be treated by the obstetrician.

Obviously, undiagnosed PKU in a pregnant woman can pose a risk to her baby. Careful screening and counseling is necessary for identified PKU-potential mothers. Their pregnancies should be carefully planned, and they should be on a restricted phenylalanine diet. Since PKU diets are low in protein, their diet must be strictly constructed and monitored by a clinical dietitian throughout the pregnancy. Low-phenylalanine formulas and food products become the mainstay of the diet.

Many authorities strongly recommend that PKU children, especially girls, remain on their diets throughout life. In this way, some of the dangers of pregnancy can be minimized.

FOLLOW-UP CARE

The health team must monitor progress after a child is placed on a phenylalanine-restricted diet. During the first few weeks of the diet, the child's blood should be tested twice a week. After the child has been on the diet for a brief period and his or her clinical condition has improved and stabilized, blood tests should be performed

TABLE 28-4 Sample Menu Plan for a 9-Month-Old Child with PKU

Breakfast
Lofenalac formula, 6 oz
Rice with strawberries, Gerber's baby cereal, 2¼ tbsp
Carrots, Gerber's strained and junior vegetables, 5 tbsp

Midmorning Feeding
Peaches, Gerber's strained and junior fruit, 3 tbsp

Lunch
Lofenalac formula, 6 oz
Cereal, barley, Gerber's baby cereal, 1¼ tbsp
Apricots with tapioca, Gerber's strained and junior fruit, 8 tbsp
Orange-pineapple juice, Gerber's strained and junior fruit, 5 tbsp

Midafternoon Feeding
Applesauce, 7 tbsp

Dinner
Lofenalac formula, 6 oz
Rice with mixed fruit (in jar), Gerber's baby cereal, 1¾ tbsp
Sweet potatoes, Gerber's strained and junior vegetables, 1½ tbsp

Bedtime Feeding
Lofenalac formula, 6 oz
Orange-pineapple juice, Gerber's strained and junior fruit, 6 tbsp

weekly until the child is 1 year old. Later, the toddler's blood should be tested once every 2 to 3 weeks. When all symptoms have disappeared and the child has adapted to the diet, the blood tests can be done monthly.

The dietary supply and blood levels of phenylalanine are strongly correlated with the height and weight gains of the child. If children get an insufficient amount of phenylalanine, they will become lethargic, have stunted growth, and lose their appetite. More severe effects include mental retardation, clinical deterioration (fever, coma), and even death. Also, when children with PKU become sick or have infections, blood phenylalanine may rise to unacceptable levels.

DRUG THERAPY

In December 2007, the U.S. Food and Drug Administration approved Kuvan (sapropterin dihydrochloride), the first drug of its kind approved to slow the effects of PKU. The drug has different effects on babies with PKU. It is estimated that it is effective in about 1 out of every 12,000 to 15,000 live births in the United States.

Kuvan must be used in combination with a phenylalanine-restricted diet. A patient can override the effects of Kuvan by not following a restricted diet. Patients being treated with Kuvan must have their blood phenylalanine levels monitored frequently by their physicians or other healthcare professional to ensure their its levels are in the normal range.

NURSING IMPLICATIONS

Nursing responsibilities for treating a child with PKU are as follows:

1. Be aware that dietary management is the only treatment for children with PKU.
2. The diet for PKU must meet two criteria:
   a. It must meet the child's nutritional needs for growth and development.
   b. It must maintain phenylalanine levels within a safe range.
3. The diet therapy is very strict and presents difficulties to the families or caregivers.
4. Lofenalac and Phenyl-Free are very expensive; financial aid may be required. Funding sources should be furnished to the parents.
5. Frequent monitoring of urinary and blood levels of phenylalanine are necessary.
6. Careful dietary records as well as height and weight records must be maintained to monitor diet adequacy.
7. While brain damage is irreversible, diet therapy will limit its progress.
8. Restricting phenylalanine in older children with PKU is beneficial in improving behavior and motor ability, as well as decreasing eczema. Poor bone growth and impaired mental abilities have also been documented in those whose diets were discontinued early.

9. The meaning of the treatment must be explained to the health team and the parents. Successful control of PKU requires that the family learn to:
   a. plan the baby's diet.
   b. monitor food intake.
   c. take blood samples.
   d. keep accurate records of intake and state of health.
   e. cope with normal developmental stages.
10. Therapeutic communication is necessary to allow parents to voice feelings of guilt, fear, and frustration and to attain a healthy outlook.
11. Provide information on:
    a. signs of inadequate phenylalanine intake: anorexia, vomiting, listlessness.
    b. situations that require increased amounts of phenylalanine, such as during periods of rapid growth and during febrile illnesses.
    c. possible deficiencies in other nutrients: intake of manganese, zinc, and niacin may be low when the primary protein source is synthetic.
12. Closely monitor hemoglobin levels, since protein is severely restricted.
13. Lofenalac provides 454 calories, 15 g protein, 60 g carbohydrate, and 18 g fat per 100 mg powder.
14. Special products such as low-protein flour, cookies, pasta, and other bakery items can be purchased to augment this severe diet and increase carbohydrate intake.
15. Recognize that primary diet teaching may require the services of a specialist, and the nurse may prefer to reinforce the teaching and encourage compliance.
16. Counsel family members that the current practice is long-term dietary management so that they will be prepared for the process.
17. When solid foods are added to the child's diet (at about 6 months of age) parents and caregivers will need a low-phenylalanine food exchange list.

PROGRESS CHECK ON ACTIVITY 1

MULTIPLE CHOICE

Circle the letter of the correct answer.

1. The objectives of dietary management of the child with phenylketonuria (PKU) include:

   a. lowering phenylalanine content to the minimum requirement for growth by calculating the diet for phenylalanine content.
   b. removing all milk and milk products from the diet.
   c. removing all protein foods from the diet.
   d. all of the above.

2. From the following list of lunch menus, choose the one most appropriate for a PKU youngster who is 2-½ years old:

   a. 2 tbsp roast beef, ½ slice bread, ¼ c green beans, ½ banana, ½ c Lofenalac
   b. 1 hard-boiled egg, raw carrot sticks, 2 Ritz crackers, 1 pear half, ½ c Lofenalac
   c. ¼ c sliced beets, ¼ c green beans, 3 tbsp boiled potato, ½ c Lofenalac vanilla pudding with whipped topping, apple juice
   d. 4 potato chips, 1 graham cracker with butter, ½ c Lofenalac vanilla pudding, 8 oz cola

3. In which of the following persons with PKU could the diet be safely liberalized?

   a. pregnant female
   b. 20-year-old male
   c. 4-year-old female
   d. 2-year-old male

4. The young parents of an infant consistently forget to give the child the required milk allowance in addition to his Lofenalac. The following may be expected:

   a. The child will become allergic to milk.
   b. The child's growth and development will be retarded.
   c. The child will develop a lactose intolerance.
   d. The child will become hyperactive.

5. If dietary treatment starts after mental retardation occurs, the following may be expected:

   a. The brain will continue its deterioration.
   b. No further deterioration will take place.
   c. The mental retardation will be reversed and the child will become normal.
   d. Physical growth will be retarded.

6. Phenylalanine may not be omitted from the infant's diet because:

   a. as an essential amino acid, it must be supplied by diet or the infant will fail to develop.
   b. the electrolytes of the body will be in negative balance.
   c. it must be in the diet to produce tyrosine.
   d. the child will get bradycardia.

7. The diet of the PKU child must be calculated for:

   a. phenylalanine, tyrosine, and histamine.
   b. protein, carbohydrate, and fat.
   c. phenylalanine, protein, and calories.
   d. calcium, iron, and ascorbic acid.

8. Techniques that promote compliance when feeding a PKU child include:

   a. varying taste by using allowed flavorings and seasonings.
   b. using low-protein grain products for variety.
   c. adjusting quantity and texture to child's eating ability.
   d. all of the above.

9. Insufficient phenylalanine will result in which of the following symptoms?

   a. stunted growth
   b. anorexia, lethargy
   c. mental retardation
   d. all of the above

TRUE/FALSE

Circle T for True and F for False.

10. T F Feeding must be consistent with age and development.
11. T F Nutritional adequacy must be constantly evaluated.
12. T F Meat and milk are not used in the diet plan for PKU, except for a small quantity of evaporated milk daily.
13. T F PKU is a self-limiting disorder—the child will "grow out of it" as he or she grows up.

FILL-IN

14. List five steps necessary to the planning of an adequate diet for PKU.

    a. _____
    b. _____
    c. _____
    d. _____
    e. _____

15. Describe three ways to vary calories and taste in a PKU diet without unbalancing it.

    a. _____
    b. _____
    c. _____

REFERENCES

American College of Medical Genetics. (2005). Newborn screening: Toward a uniform screening panel and system. Final Report. See www.ACMG.net.

Anonymous. (2003). What you need to know about phenylketonuria. (2003). *Nursing Times, 99*(30): 26.

Behrman, R. E., Kliegman, R. M., & Jenson, H. B. (Eds.). (2004). *Nelson Textbook of Pediatrics.* Philadelphia: Saunders.

Cederbaum, S. (2002). Phenylketonuria: An update. *Current Opinion in Pediatrics, 14*(6): 702.

Clark, J. T. R. (2006). *A Clinical Guide to Inherited Metabolic Diseases* (3rd ed.). Cambridge, UK: Cambridge University Press.

Clarke, J. T. (2003). The Maternal Phenylketonuria Project: A summary of progress and challenges for the future. *Pediatrics, 112*(6 Pt 2): 1584.

de Baulny, H. O., Abadie, V., Feillet, F., & de Parscau, L. (2007). Management of phenylketonuria and hyperphenylalaninemia. *Journal of Nutrition, 137*(6 Suppl 1): 1561S, 1573S.

Ekvall, S. W., & Ekvall, V. K. (Eds.). (2005). *Pediatric Nutrition in Chronic Diseases and Developmental Disorders: Prevention, Assessment, and Treatment.* New York: Oxford University Press.

Food and Drug Administration (FDA). (2007). FDA approves kuvan for treatment of phenylketonuria. See www.FDA.gov.

Greene, A. (2007). *Medical Library—Phenylketonuria.* Bethesda, MA: National Library of Medicine and National Institute of Health.

Kaye, C. I., & American Academy of Pediatrics Committee on Genetics. (2006). Newborn Screening Fact Sheets. Pediatrics, 118: e934–963.

Kleinman, R. E. (2004). *Pediatric Nutrition Handbook* (5th ed.). Elk Village, IL: American Academy of Pediatrics.

Koch, R., & de la Cruz, F. (2003). The Maternal Phenylketonuria Collaborative Study: New Developments and the Need for New Strategies—Preface. *Pediatrics,* 112: (6).

Koch, R. et al. The Maternal Phenylketonuria International Study: 1984–2002. (2003). *Pediatrics,* 112(6): 1523–1529.

Litcher, M. G. (2004). *Gale Encyclopedia of Medicine—Phenylketonuria.* Farmington Hills, MI: Gales Group.

Lucas, B. L., Feucht, A., & Grieger, L. E. (Eds.). (2004). *Children with Special Health Care Needs.* Revised edition. Chicago: American Dietetic Association.

National Institutes of Health. (2000). Consensus development statement. Phenylketonuria: Screening and management. Washington, D.C. See www.NIH.gov.

Nevin-Folino, N. L. (Ed.). (2003). *Pediatric Manual of Clinical Dietetics.* Chicago: American Dietetic Association.

Paasche, C. L., Gorrill, L., & Stroon, B. (2004). *Children with Special Needs in Early Childhood Settings: Identification, Intervention, Inclusion.* Clifton Park: NY: Thomson/Delmar.

Parker, J. N., & Parker, P. M. (Eds.). (2002). *The Official Parent's Sourcebook of Phenylketonuria.* San Diego, CA: Icon Health.

Parker, P. M. (2007). *Phenylketonuria—A Bibliography and Dictionary for Physicians, Patients, and Genome Researchers.* San Diego, CA: Icon Health.

Samour, P. Q., & Helm, K. K. (Eds.). (2005). *Handbook of Pediatric Nutrition* (3rd ed.). Sudbury, MA: Jones and Bartlett Publishers.

Surendran, S., & Surendran, S. (Eds.). (2007). *Neurochemistry of Metabolic Diseases—Lysosomal Storage Diseases, Phneylketonuria and Canavan Disease.* Trivandrum, Kerada India: Transworld Research Network.

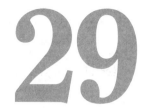

CHAPTER

Diet Therapy for Constipation, Diarrhea, and High-Risk Infants

Time for completion
Activities: 1 hour
Optional examination: ½ hour

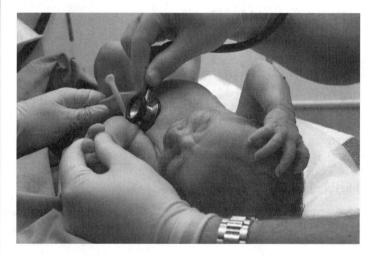

OBJECTIVES

Upon completion of this chapter the student should be able to do the following:

1. Describe the normal patterns and characteristics of bowel movements in infants and young children.
2. Identify deviations from normal when:
   a. constipation is the problem.
   b. diarrhea is the problem.
3. Identify the major causes of constipation and diarrhea.
4. List the major purposes of diet therapy for constipation and diarrhea in infants and children.
5. Identify the types of feedings necessary to meet the goals of diet therapy in these disorders.
6. Describe the strategies the health professional would teach caregivers to prevent further problems.
7. Name the categories of high-risk infants requiring specialized nutritional therapy.

8. Describe the types of feedings necessary to meet the individual needs of each infant.
9. Exhibit proficiency in the selection of formulas and recommended feeding methods.
10. Teach all caregivers the pertinent facts they must know in order to adequately nourish their high-risk infant.

GLOSSARY

Benign: not malignant, not recurrent.

Electrolyte: a chemical substance that, when dissolved in water or melted, dissociates into electrically charged particles (ions).

Fiber (dietary): that portion of undigested foods that cannot be broken down by enzymes, so it passes through the intestine and colon undigested.

Immune (immunological): highly resistant to a disease because of developed antibodies, or development of immunologically competent cells, or both.

Meconium: mucilaginous material in the intestine of the full-term fetus.

Mucilage: aqueous solution of a gummy substance.

Osmolarity: concentrating a solution in terms of osmoles of solutes per liter of solution (osmolality).

Osmosis: passage of a solvent from a solution of lesser to one of greater solute concentration when separated by a membrane.

Prematurity: underdevelopment; born or interrupted before maturity or occurring before the proper time.

Residue: that which remains in the intestine after the removal of other substances; a remainder.

Suppository: a medicated mass used for introduction into the rectum, urethra, or vagina.

BACKGROUND INFORMATION

Space limitation has excluded chapters covering diet therapy for a number of other clinical disorders of infancy and childhood. This chapter remedies the situation by providing student activities to cover three important clinical subjects not yet discussed: constipation, diarrhea, and high-risk infants.

The student should use the references provided at the end of this chapter to obtain more details to supplement the activities provided.

ACTIVITY 1:

Constipation

BACKGROUND INFORMATION

Patterns of bowel movements among children and infants vary. If a child is active, passes a soft to slightly compact stool, gains weight progressively, shows normal development, and is free from any known clinical disorder, the mother has no reason to worry.

A newborn may have a constipation problem that is most likely the result of plugging by meconium. Constipation in an older infant is usually due to a change in the type of feeding. An anatomical defect may also be a cause, but this is rare. There are several ways to recognize the presence of constipation in a young infant:

1. A change in the stool (number, consistency, texture, appearance)
2. Pain in the infant when defecating
3. Distended abdomen with or before every bowel movement
4. Very black or bloody stools

The constipation of many newborns disappears shortly after discharge from the hospital. If this does not occur, the mother should consult her pediatrician.

INFANTS

Constipation in a baby may be caused by a change in diet. Some babies develop constipation when breastfeeding is replaced with formula (homemade or commercial). Characteristic signs include the face turning red, straining, and the legs turned upward while defecating, even though the child may pass a soft stool. The doctor will evaluate the child after being informed of the symptoms. The doctor first looks for any obstruction that may require special medical attention. If no obstruction is found, the mother should be advised of the benign nature of the constipation and told that the child's bowel habits will return to normal after it adapts to the new formula. Actually, the stools of some infants change from soft to hard even if they are not constipated.

Other babies develop constipation when they are switched from liquid or strained food to solid food. The signs of such constipation vary. In some infants, a day with normal bowel movements is followed by one with none. In others, the passing of hard stools is accompanied by crying and intense straining. Many of these cases are of unknown origin. A typical cause is excessive water absorption (reabsorption) by the colon, resulting in dry stools and constipation. The anal passage may be stretched, causing pain and bleeding if there is an open wound. The child passes red stools, which are easily observed on toilet paper. The management of this form of constipation consists of a reduction in milk intake and an increased intake of juices, fruits, and fluids. Some clinicians may prescribe enemas, laxatives, and suppositories, such as a glycerin suppository. The dosage and frequency of application of these drugs must be determined with care.

Home remedies have no scientific evidence; however, adding sugar to the gut will draw water in to increase osmotic load and will create softer stools. No studies have examined how much sugar would be needed.

Infants older than 6 months may benefit from drinking prune juice or increasing appropriate high-fiber foods such as whole grain breads and cereals, fruit, vegetables, and cooked legumes.

YOUNG CHILDREN

Constipation in children under 4 or 5 years old is of two types: psychological and anatomical. The latter refers to a defect in the muscles regulating the defecation process. In some children under 2 years old, any initial sign of constipation can create a psychological barrier to defecation. When children start passing hard stools, they experience some pain, so they subsequently strain to retain the stools in order to reduce the pain. The accumulated feces become larger and harder, causing more pain in subsequent defecations. Some parents report that their children turn red in the face, strain, and arch their backs during bowel movement. Although toilet trained, they soil their pants frequently and are reluctant to go to the bathroom. Some parents complain that these children are lazy. In this case, the parental attitudes make the constipation problem worse. This psychological barrier to bowel movement can be difficult to overcome.

On the other hand, constipation in some children results from fecal impaction, which may develop for a number of reasons. For instance, children between the ages of five and eight may develop constipation because they consider visiting the bathroom a waste of time. How are older children with a constipation problem managed? The basic principles are similar to those for an adult. If the parents consult a physician, the doctor may need to study the problem and advise the parents about what actions to take.

As a start, the parents may help the child initiate a good bowel movement by using an enema. The dose, which may be large at the beginning, may be used until a defecation pattern of three to five times a day is established. Mineral oil is not recommended for young children. The child should be put on a conditioning schedule, such as 10 to 20 minutes daily on the toilet. The child should also be encouraged to have bowel movements as frequently as possible. At the same time, milk intake may be reduced to 60%–80% of normal, and the intake of fruits, juices, and bran cereals increased. A diet high in fiber and fluid should be designed for future use to aid in regulation.

NURSING IMPLICATIONS

Healthcare personnel should do the following:

1. Be aware of the signs and symptoms of constipation in the infant.

2. Be prepared to counsel parents about the possible reasons for constipation in their child.

3. Consult the physician regarding the diagnosis of constipation in any given infant before educating the parents.

4. Expect that signs of constipation may be different for individual infants.

5. Teach the caregivers the necessity of precision of dosage and monitoring of any drugs prescribed by a physician.

6. If the infant is on solid food, food sources that relieve constipation in adults will also, in smaller proportions, help the child to defecate.

7. Be alert for psychological problems that prevent defecation in the young child.

8. Assist the caregivers to help the child initiate regular bowel habits.

PROGRESS CHECK ON ACTIVITY 1

MULTIPLE CHOICE

Circle the letter of the correct answer.

1. All except which of these characteristics indicate that a child is not constipated?

   a. steady weight gain
   b. good appetite
   c. one to three bowel movements daily
   d. active

2. Newborns' constipation problems are most likely the result of a(n):

   a. change in feeding.
   b. anatomical defect.
   c. clinical disorder.
   d. change in routine.

3. Safe food(s) that may be used to combat constipation in infants include:

   a. prune juice.
   b. 1 tsp sugar/4 oz of formula.
   c. strained apricots.
   d. all of the above.

4. Recommended treatment for dry, hard stools in an infant is to:

   a. increase formula feedings.
   b. increase fluids.
   c. increase laxative intake.
   d. increase activity level.

5. Two types of constipation common in children under 5 years old are:

   a. physiological and psychological.
   b. anatomical and environmental.
   c. psychological and anatomical.
   d. environmental and physiological.

FILL-IN

6. Fecal impaction in children is usually the result of:

   _____

   _____

7. Name four ways a parent may assist the child to initiate regular elimination habits.

   a. _____

   b. _____

   c. _____

   d. _____

8. Name five nursing responsibilities in dealing with the problem of constipation in the infant and young child.

   a. _____

   b. _____

   c. _____

   d. _____

   e. _____

ACTIVITY 2:

Diarrhea

FECAL CHARACTERISTICS AND CAUSES OF DIARRHEA

The stools of infants change with age and development, as indicated in Table 29-1. It is important for parents to recognize a child's normal feces. Children with diarrhea have an abnormally frequent evacuation of watery (and sometimes greasy and/or bloody) stools. Diarrhea is frequent among infants and children and can be a very distressing condition. In chronic cases, it may last for weeks or months, while the child continues to grow normally.

Chronic diarrhea may be a symptom of a disease. In general, diarrhea is classified as acute or chronic according to its stool, profile, cause, or site of clinical defect. There are a number of common causes of diarrhea in infants and children:

1. It can be due to a specific clinical disorder.
2. Bacterial contamination of formulas or foods can cause food poisoning.
3. Some youngsters develop diarrhea because of intestinal reactions to certain foods such as sugars, fats (too little or too much), milk, and eggs.

TREATMENT AND CAUTION

The initial management of diarrhea in children involves two steps. The clinician's first and major objective is to restore fluid and electrolyte balance by oral or IV therapy, since a child is highly susceptible to dehydration. Subsequently, the clinician determines if the child can be managed adequately by oral nourishment without parenteral feeding, which requires hospitalization.

If a child's diarrhea is accompanied by mild to moderate dehydration with persistent vomiting, hospitalization for parenteral fluid therapy is indicated. In general, it is feasible to provide oral fluids and electrolytes for children with mild diarrhea or children recovering from severe diarrhea. If diarrhea is mild to moderate and the patient shows normal clinical signs otherwise and is not dehydrated, most physicians prescribe outpatient therapy consisting of an oral hypotonic solution of glucose and electrolytes.

In caring for an infant with diarrhea, the major concern is supplying an adequate supply of fluid and electrolytes. Some readily available regular and commercial solutions are listed in Table 29-2. Because milk contains too many electrolytes, especially sodium, most clinicians do not recommend it at the beginning of treatment. All other solutions listed in the table may be initially fed to a child with diarrhea. To prevent gas from being trapped and the accompanying discomfort, some soda drinks can be decarbonated. Gelatin should be made in half strength

TABLE 29-1   Fecal Characteristics of Infants

Age (months)	Diet	Fecal Characteristics			Number of Bowel Movements Daily
		pH	Color	Texture	
0–4	Home or commercial formulas	6–8	Pale yellow to light brown	Compressed, solid	2–3
	Breast milk	< 6	Yellow to golden	Like cream or ointment	2–4
4–12	Regular foods and/or milk	Variable	Intensified yellow	Harder	1–3
Over 12	Regular foods and/or milk	Variable	Similar to adult, i.e., highly variable (yellow to black)	Similar to adult, i.e., highly variable (soft to very hard)	Similar to adult, i.e., highly variable (1–4)

to avoid aggravating dehydration. Kool-Aid and unflavored gelatin should not be used, since they contain few electrolytes.

After about two days of fluid and electrolyte support as described, the diarrhea should subside somewhat. At this stage, the child should be given a diluted regular infant formula, for example, one fourth, one third, or even one half of normal strength. Additional calories are supplied by adding corn syrup (1 tsp per 3 oz of formula) or using a supplemental feeding of strained baby cereals and fruits.

Recent concern has been expressed about the common practice of eliminating milk, eggs, and wheat to reduce diarrhea in a young patient. Although some pediatric patients benefit from this treatment, the attending physician must be alert to (1) potential undernutrition that may occur if the elimination diet is prolonged, and (2) the possibility that the child has celiac disease (see Chapter 26). An elimination diet may mask this disorder.

The initial treatment for diarrhea in children over 1 year old consists of giving clear liquids such as diluted broth, fruit juices, soft drinks, gelatin dessert, and popsicles. After the diarrhea has subsided, a low-residue diet may be used. Subsequent management is the same as that for an adult (see Chapter 17). Once the condition has stabilized, a regular diet appropriate to the child's age can be implemented.

NURSING IMPLICATIONS

Healthcare personnel should do the following:

1. Be able to recognize normal fecal characteristics of infants.
2. Differentiate between acute and chronic diarrhea.
3. Develop care plans to meet the individual child's problems:
   a. Replace fluid and electrolytes.
   b. Restore adequate nutrition orally or parenterally.
4. Be familiar with common beverages and foods that can be used for treating diarrhea.
5. Alert the physician to observed potential problems if the child is on an elimination diet for a prolonged period.
6. Select a low-residue diet as the diet therapy of choice after acute symptoms have subsided.

PROGRESS CHECK ON ACTIVITY 2

FILL-IN

1. On what three bases is diarrhea classified as acute or chronic?

   a. _____

   b. _____

   c. _____

2. Name three common causes of diarrhea in children.

   a. _____

   b. _____

   c. _____

3. Describe the two steps in the dietary management of children with diarrhea.

   a. _____

   b. _____

TABLE 29-2   Calorie, Sodium, and Potassium Contents of Some Preparations for Treating Diarrhea

Beverage	mg Sodium/100 ml	mg Potassium/ 100 ml	kcal/100 ml
Milk, whole	50	144	62
Milk, skim	52	145	36
Apple juice, canned or bottled	1	101	47
Grape juice, canned or bottled	2	116	66
Orange juice, from concentrate	1	202	49
7-Up	10	Trace	40
Coca-Cola	1	52	44
Pepsi-Cola	15	3	46
Ginger ale	8	Trace	35
Root beer	13	2	41
Flavored gelatin	54	Trace	59
Pedialyte	69	78	20
Lytren	69	98	30

4.* Name three beverages with a high-sodium content suitable for the treatment of diarrhea.

   a. _____

   b. _____

   c. _____

5.* Name three beverages with a high-potassium content suitable for the treatment of diarrhea.

   a. _____

   b. _____

   c. _____

6. Name two well-known commercial preparations suitable for the treatment of diarrhea.

   a. _____

   b. _____

7. Describe three ways to increase caloric content of a recovering child's food intake. Assume the child is 6 months old.

   a. _____

   b. _____

   c. _____

*See answer sheet (Table 29-2)

ACTIVITY 3:

High-Risk Infants

BACKGROUND INFORMATION

Five major categories of infants are considered high risk at birth: those of low birth weight, those born prematurely with complications, those delivered by diabetic mothers, those who are critically ill, and those with birth defects. These newborns are unable to function properly as normal infants and need special help.

Drug use during pregnancy, especially the use of the so-called recreational drugs, causes many birth defects and developmental problems. Cocaine (crack) use is related to prematurity, placenta detachment, intrauterine growth retardation, and low birth weight (LBW). The infant may be paralyzed, have uncontrolled jerking movement, and/or have permanent physical and mental retardation. The use of opiates and barbiturates produce an addicted infant who must go through the painful, sometimes fatal withdrawal process. Amphetamine use causes behavioral abnormalities and central nervous system damage.

The most widely used drug during pregnancy is alcohol, and it is a leading cause of mental retardation. It is especially devastating to the fetus in the first trimester and leads to fetal alcohol syndrome (FAS) in the infant.

The classic symptoms of FAS are facial abnormalities, brain damage, and physical and mental retardation. While the subclinical effects from the fetal alcohol effect (FAE) are not as readily identified, prenatal consumption of alcohol produces children with some brain damage, learning disabilities, and behavior problems, which make school and social situations very difficult for the child. One of the major criteria for survival is proper nutrition, without which the child may die.

There is considerable controversy over what constitutes a low birth weight or prematurity. In this text, a premature infant is defined as one born before the 37th or 38th week of gestation. Standard charts show the expected infant weight at different gestational ages. If weight is unacceptably low for gestational age, the infant is small for date (SFD) or small for gestational age (SGA). These infants have suffered intrauterine retardation but may be either full term or premature. A low birth weight (LBW) infant weighs 2500 g (5-½ lb) or less. These infants may be premature, small for gestational age, and/or small for date. They account for 60%–70% of all cases of newborn mortality after birth; about 5%–10% of live births are of low birth weight. Infants weighing less than 1500 g (3.3 lb) at birth are considered to have very low birth weight (VLBW).

NUTRIENT NEEDS

The caloric need of the high-risk infant is definitely higher than that of a normal infant: about 100 to 130 kcal/kg/d. This is about three to four times that of an adult and twice that of a normal infant.

The estimated protein need of the high-risk child is 3 to 4 g/kg/d. Excessive protein is undesirable, since it can increase blood amino acids and nitrogen; however, a premature infant may require the essential amino acids tyrosine and cystine.

A high-risk infant needs a large amount of fluid for a number of reasons. First, the child has a high body water content. Second, the ambient temperature may be too high, causing increased evaporation for the small patient. Vomiting or diarrhea, if present, may result in a loss of intestinal fluid. The child's kidney is unable to concentrate urine, resulting in more fluid loss. If the child undergoes any form of treatment that causes body evaporation, such as photo or radiant heat therapy, its need for fluid will be further increased.

One way to assure that a child gets enough fluid is to measure the intake and output of fluid, monitor overt clinical signs of dehydration, and analyze urine osmolality, using blood sodium and nitrogen levels as guides. Extra fluid may be given orally (water, milk, or 10% glucose) or intravenously (10% glucose).

High-risk infants have special needs for calcium, iron, and vitamin K. If the intake of these nutrients is inadequate, appropriate supplementation is needed.

INITIAL FEEDINGS

The first feeding should be given to a high-risk infant several hours after birth, when the child is given fluid and calories. A normal-term infant receives the first feeding two to four hours after birth, as does a baby weighing at least 1500 g with a gestational age of 33 or 34 weeks and without any complications such as respiratory difficulty and infection. In general, this latter baby receives smaller but more frequent feedings than a normal child.

If an infant has complications, weighs less than 1500 g, and has a gestational age of less than 33 weeks, the feeding practice is more cautious and varies with the infant and the doctor's evaluation. Depending on the practitioner, the child may be fed in one of two ways. In one, only 10% glucose is given intravenously with no other nourishment until the infant stabilizes, usually 3 days later, at which time oral or tube feedings or total parenteral nutrition is used. Some practitioners prefer direct oral feeding within the first 12 to 24 hours. If oral feeding is not feasible, total parenteral nutrition is started at the beginning of the second day.

USE OF BREASTMILK OR FORMULAS

The decision of whether to nurse or formula-feed a high-risk infant depends partly on the degree of risk. Babies of nearly normal size may respond well to breastmilk. Breastmilk permits satisfactory growth for infants weighing more than 1500 g, especially because of the quality of fat and protein, the solute load, and immunological protection provided. In some circumstances, breastmilk produces less necrotizing enterocolitis than formulas. The mother should be actively encouraged to breastfeed if the child can suck and weighs over 2000 g. If the child is unable to breastfeed, the mother can provide milk by expressing breast milk either manually or with a breast pump. Advice from a lactation consultant should be sought. The milk is then given to the child by tube, gavage, bottle, or dropper. This procedure can also strengthen the mother's emotional attachment to the child. The milk should be fresh, unheated, unrefrigerated, and less than 8 to 10 hours old.

Although breastmilk has certain advantages, it does not provide enough protein to enable some high-risk infants to grow. To supplement the low supply of protein in breast milk, a breastfed child can be given some concentrated or standard formulas. Neither regular formulas nor breastmilk alone is adequate for growth for most high-risk infants.

There are no readily available "standard" formulas for low-birth-weight or high-risk infants, since their requirements for nutrients are unknown. The best guide is to use the estimated nutrient needs as described earlier. However, most standard formulas are high in protein, calories, and calcium. The smaller the child, the more unsatisfactory these formulas are. Some clinicians propose that the formula should contain 80–100 kcal/100 ml and 2.6–3.0 g of protein/100 kcal (ideally 2.8 g).

Some clinics and hospitals use defined-formula diets containing glucose, amino acids, minerals, vitamins, and medium-chain triglycerides (or no fat). Some infants respond favorably when fed these diets, while others do not. The major problems with these defined-formula diets are their high solute load and excessive nitrogen. Since infant response to any method of feeding varies, the high-risk baby's growth must be closely monitored. In addition to the type of formula chosen, its dilution must be carefully considered. The concentration, calories, protein, and fluid of a high-risk baby's formula should all be sufficient but within the eating and digestive capacity of the child. Whereas a normal child is usually provided about 67 kcal/100 ml (20 kcal/oz) of milk, a high-risk infant needs about 80–100 kcal/100 ml (25–30 kcal/oz) of milk. And although a normal child drinks about 100 ml/kg of milk, a high-risk infant may need as much as 200 ml/kg. If the formula is too concentrated, the excessive osmotic load can be harmful to the gastrointestinal tract and the kidney.

The decision to use breastmilk or infant formulas is determined by many factors including the clinical condition of the infant and the potential benefits and concerns offered by each feeding method. The following gives one advantage and one disadvantage of each method of feeding.

- Human milk—The nutrients are readily absorbed. Milk volume production may be inadequate to nourish the infant.
- Formulas for premature infants—Protein is at a higher concentration than in a standard infant formula to meet the patient's higher protein need. The amount of feeding must be increased slowly for the very low birth weight infant.
- Premature discharge or transition formulas—Formulas have the nutrient composition that is between the concentrated premature formulas and the standard infant formula. The infant should weigh at least 1.8 kg when this formula is prescribed.
- Standard discharged infant formulas—Prescribed for infants reaching certain clinical criteria. It is inadequate for a premature infant.
- Elemental infant formulas—It is specifically designed for infants with intestinal disorders, and its nutrient contents are inadequate for premature infants.
- Soy formulas—This should not be used unless prescribed by attending physician.

PREMATURE BABIES: AN ILLUSTRATION

A general discussion has been presented on the nutritional supports for high-risk infants including premature babies. This section provides specifics for a premature infant.

The attending physician routinely places a newly born premature infant in the neonatal intensive care unit (NICU) of the hospital with three objectives:

1. Carefully monitor fluid and electrolytes (sodium, potassium, etc.) balance and nutritional status, with proper intervention when indicated.
2. The use of an incubator or a medical warmer minimizes caloric needs.
3. When the environmental air is moist and warm, the body temperature fluctuates less with a minimal loss of body water.

The clinical condition of a premature baby will lead to the following feeding problems:

1. Inability to coordinate sucking, breathing, and swallowing interferes with proper bottle or breastfeeding.
2. The small patient may suffer disorders of the circulatory and respiratory systems, leading to decreased oxygen levels, gagging, blood infection, and so on. As a result, the baby may be unable to receive oral feeding through the nipple.
3. Preemies are most likely small and sick. Their nutrition and fluid requirements have to be met by using the following progressive methods:
   a. Initially, intravenous feeding is used.
   b. The next stage uses enteral or tube feedings. The baby is given the nourishment slowly.
   c. Oral feeding is not used until clinical conditions permit. At this stage, bottle or breastfeeding may be used. Most infants prefer a bottle with a large hole in the nipple.

After a baby is fed, sleep or a satisfactory rest is a good sign, accompanied daily by 1–6 bowel movements and 5–9 urinations (wet diapers with or without stool). The health team is always alert to the following:

1. Constant vomiting can be serious.
2. Stools watery or bloody is another warning.

One major clinical concern is fluid balance in a premature baby from the following perspectives:

1. The loss of water through skin and respiratory routes is higher in a preterm than a full-term baby.
2. The premature baby's urinary system, especially the kidneys, is unable to regulate the proper amount of water lost.
3. A decrease or an increase of body water may result.

The health team takes precaution as follows:

1. The patient's urine is monitored to assure balance of fluid intake and output.
2. Body electrolytes are monitored by scheduled testings for their blood levels.

The storage of nutrients of a preterm infant is not adequate for normal sustenance because the accumulation of nutrients in the womb has been shortened. Nutritional supplements become a necessity. Apart from the previous discussion on the use of breastmilk or formulas for high-risk infants, a discussion on specific recommendations in feeding a premature infant with breastmilk or commercial formulas is described below:

1. Breastmilk is usually recommended if the infant's clinical conditions permit. There is some evidence that breastmilk may prevent sudden infant death syndrome and may minimize infections. A supplement should provide additional calories, protein, vitamins, and selected minerals such as calcium and iron. Some label this supplement as "human milk fortified." This supplementation may have to be continued at home after discharge.
2. Commercial and customized formulas are available for those infants not suitable for feeding with breastmilk. The nutritional contents of most of them are satisfactory. Again, a supplement may be needed to provide extra nutrients such as vitamins and minerals. This may have to be continued at home after discharge.
3. When the infant's clinical conditions permit, he or she will be fed standard infant formulas. The health team may provide extra guidelines once it is decided to use a standard formula.

The caloric needs of premature infants to achieve the proper growth rate are estimated as follows:

1. Those without major health problems may need 90–130 calories/kg/day.
2. Those with serious health problems may need 150–185 calories/kg/day.

The health team evaluates the baby's weight gain according to the following:

1. The infant is weighed every day after birth.
2. Most infants lose weight (water) during the few days after birth.
3. Weight gain starts after the initial loss of weight.
4. The pattern of weigh gain is predictable according to body size, prematurity, and clinical status. For example, the baby may gain $\frac{1}{6}$ to $\frac{1}{5}$ oz (~ 6 g) daily for a baby 25 weeks old. For a large baby, 34 weeks old, weight gain can be 20 g or $\frac{7}{10}$ oz daily.
5. Health teams use different criteria to determine a satisfactory weight gain for the baby confined in a hospital. Most use the average goal of 0.2–0.3 oz gain per lb body weight per day.
6. It is a standard practice that if the record shows a steady weight gain, the health team will recommend a date of hospital discharge. Otherwise, the infant is not discharged.

NURSING IMPLICATIONS

Health personnel should do the following:

1. Be alert to the five major categories of infants at risk at birth and be prepared to provide the specialized nutrition needed on an individual basis.
2. Recognize the physiological feeding problems of a high-risk infant:
   a. Protein deficit and risk of overload
   b. Increased fluid needs: fluctuating body temperature, inability to concentrate urine
   c. Need for increased calories
   d. Graduated vitamin and mineral needs
3. Be proficient in the use of feeding methods recommended by the practitioner.
4. Encourage mothers of high-risk infants to breastfeed unless mother or baby has medical problems.
5. Be familiar with the types and dilutions of formulas suitable for high-risk infants, depending upon their size and weight.
6. Closely monitor infant response to feedings.
7. Be prepared to teach all caregivers the proper feeding techniques, prescribed formulas, signs, and symptoms of acceptance and any other pertinent facts.
8. Follow up for further evaluation.

PROGRESS CHECK ON ACTIVITY 3

MULTIPLE CHOICE

Circle the letter of the correct answer.

1. The SGA infant is:
   a. full term but underweight.
   b. premature but small for date.
   c. either full term or premature.
   d. any child who weighs less than 6 lb.
2. LBW infants account for _____ % of all live births.
   a. 60–70
   b. 20–30
   c. 1–2
   d. 5–10
3. Caloric needs of the high-risk infant are:
   a. twice those of a normal infant.
   b. three to four times those of a normal infant.
   c. approximately six times those of a normal infant.
   d. the same as those of the normal infant; they have little movement.
4. High-risk infants need large amounts of fluid for all except which of these reasons?
   a. They require extra essential amino acids.
   b. They have a larger body water content than normal infants.

   c. Their kidneys can't concentrate urine.
   d. They have increased water evaporation.
5. First feedings for high-risk infants include:
   a. TPN.
   b. fluid with extra calories.
   c. 10% glucose IVs.
   d. no food or fluid until stabilized.

FILL-IN

6. What are the criteria for breastfeeding a high-risk infant? _____

   _____

   _____

7. Describe the procedure for feeding breastmilk to an infant who cannot nurse. _____

   _____

   _____

   _____

8. Describe the four most appropriate guides for meeting nutrient needs of high-risk infants.
   a. _____
   b. _____
   c. _____
   d. _____
9. What is a defined formula? _____

   _____

   _____

REFERENCES

Adamkin, D. H. (2006). Feeding problems in the late preterm infant. *Clinics in Perinatology, 33*: 831–837.

Adamkin, D. H. (2006). Nutrition management of the very low-birthweight infant. *NeoReviews, 7*: e602–e614.

American Dietetic Association. (2006). *Nutrition Diagnosis: A Critical Step in Nutrition Care Process.* Chicago: Author.

Behrman, R. E., Kliegman, R. M., & Jenson, H. B. (Eds.). (2004). *Nelson Textbook of Pediatrics.* Philadelphia: Saunders.

Berkowitz, C. (2008). *Berkowitz's Pediatrics: A Primary Care Approach* (3rd ed.). Elk Village, IL: American Academy of Pediatrics.

Crowley, E. (2008). Evidence of a role of cow's milk consumption in chronic functional constipation in children: Systematic review of the literature from 1980–2006. *Nutrition & Dietetics, 65*: 29–35.

Ekvall, S. W., & Ekvall, V. K. (Eds.). (2005). *Pediatric Nutrition in Chronic Diseases and Developmental Disorders: Prevention, Assessment, and Treatment.* New York: Oxford University Press.

Green, T. P., Franklin, W. H. & Tanz, R. R. (Eds.). (2005). *Pediatrics: Just the Facts.* New York: McGraw-Hill Medical.

Hark, L., & Morrison, G. (Eds.). (2003). *Medical Nutrition and Disease* (3rd ed.). Malden, MA: Blackwell.

Kleinman, R. E. (2004). *Pediatric Nutrition Handbook* (5th ed.). Elk Village, IL: American Academy of Pediatrics.

Kliegman, R. M., Behrman, R. E., Jenson, H. B., & Stanton, B. F. (2004). *Nelson Textbook of Pediatrics* (17th ed.). Philadelphia: Saunders.

Loening-Bauke, V. (2001). Controversies in the management of the chronic constipation. *Journal of Pediatric Gastroenterology and Nutrition, 32*(Suppl. 1): s38–s39.

Mahan, L. K., & Escott-Stump, S. (Eds.). (2008). *Krause's Food and Nutrition Therapy* (12th ed.). Philadelphia: Elsevier Saunders.

Nevin-Folino, N. L. (Ed.). (2003). *Pediatric Manual of Clinical Dietetics.* Chicago: American Dietetic Association.

Paasche, C. L., Gorrill, L., & Stroon, B. (2004). *Children with Special Needs in Early Childhood Settings: Identification, Intervention, Inclusion.* Clifton Park: NY: Thomson/Delmar.

Paulo, A. Z. (2006). Low-dietary fiber intake as a risk factor for recurrent abdominal pain in children. *European Journal of Clinical Nutrition, 60*: 823–827.

Rigo, J., & Senterre, J. (2006). Nutritional needs of premature infants: Current issues. *Journal of Pediatrics, 149*(Suppl): S80–S88.

Salvatore, S. (2007). Nutritional options for infant constipation. *Nutrition, 23*: 615–616.

Samour, P. Q., & Helm, K. K. (Eds.). (2005). *Handbook of Pediatric Nutrition* (3rd ed.). Sudbury, MA: Jones and Bartlett Publishers.

Appendices

Weights for Adults

TABLE A-1   Body Mass Index for Adults: Principles and Applications

What is BMI?

Body Mass Index or BMI (WT/HT2), based on an individual's height and weight, is a helpful indicator of obesity and underweight in adults.

Determine BMI

BMI can be determined by looking it up on one or more tables, using a hand-held calculator, or using the Internet Web calculator. Only the tables are presented in this Appendix.

Application

BMI compares weight to body fat but cannot be interpreted as a certain percentage of body fat. The relation between fatness and BMI is influenced by age and gender. For example, women are more likely to have a higher percent of body fat than men for the same BMI. At the same BMI, older people have more body fat than younger adults.

BMI is used to screen and monitor a population to detect risk of health or nutritional disorders. In an individual, other data must be used to determine if a high BMI is associated with increased risk of disease and death for that person. BMI alone is not diagnostic.

How does BMI relate to health among adults?

A healthy BMI for adults is between 18.5 and 24.9. BMI ranges are based on the effect body weight has on disease and death.

A high BMI is predictive of death from cardiovascular disease. Diabetes, cancer, high blood pressure and osteoarthritis are also common consequences of overweight and obesity in adults. Obesity itself is a strong risk factor for premature death.

BMI Cutpoints for Adults

We interpret BMI values for adults with one fixed number, regardless of age or sex, using the following guidelines:

* Underweight BMI less than 18.5

* Overweight BMI of 25.0 to 29.9

* Obese BMI of 30.0 or more

For more information about overweight among adults, see: *Clinical Guidelines on the Identification, Evaluation, and Treatment of Overweight and Obesity in Adults.* Bethesda, MD: NHLBI, 1998.

Source: United States Department of Health and Human Services, Centers for Disease Control and Prevention, National Center for Chronic Disease Prevention and Health Promotion. Division of Nutrition and Physical Activity.

Body Mass Index Table

To use the table, find the appropriate height in the left-hand column labeled Height. Move across to a given weight. The number at the top of the column is the BMI at that height and weight. Pounds have been rounded off.

BMI	19	20	21	22	23	24	25	26	27	28	29	30	31	32	33	34	35
Height (inches)	Body Weight (pounds)																
58	91	96	100	105	110	115	119	124	129	134	138	143	148	153	158	162	167
59	94	99	104	109	114	119	124	128	133	138	143	148	153	158	163	168	173
60	97	102	107	112	118	123	128	133	138	143	148	153	158	163	168	174	179
61	100	106	111	116	122	127	132	137	143	148	153	158	164	169	174	180	185
62	104	109	115	120	126	131	136	142	147	153	158	164	169	175	180	186	191
63	107	113	118	124	130	135	141	146	152	158	163	169	175	180	186	191	197
64	110	116	122	128	134	140	145	151	157	163	169	174	180	186	192	197	204
65	114	120	126	132	138	144	150	156	162	168	174	180	186	192	198	204	210
66	118	124	130	136	142	148	155	161	167	173	179	186	192	198	204	210	216
67	121	127	134	140	146	153	159	166	172	178	185	191	198	204	211	217	223
68	125	131	138	144	151	158	164	171	177	184	190	197	203	210	216	223	230
69	128	135	142	149	155	162	169	176	182	189	196	203	209	216	223	230	236
70	132	139	146	153	160	167	174	181	188	195	202	209	216	222	229	236	243
71	136	143	150	157	165	172	179	186	193	200	208	215	222	229	236	243	250
72	140	147	154	162	169	177	184	191	199	206	213	221	228	235	242	250	258
73	144	151	159	166	174	182	189	197	204	212	219	227	235	242	250	257	265
74	148	155	163	171	179	186	194	202	210	218	225	233	241	249	256	264	272
75	152	160	168	176	184	192	200	208	216	224	232	240	248	256	264	272	279
76	156	164	172	180	189	197	205	213	221	230	238	246	254	263	271	279	287

TABLE A-3   Body Mass Index Table (Second Part)

Body Mass Index Table

To use the table, find the appropriate height in the left-hand column labeled Height. Move across to a given weight. The number at the top of the column is the BMI at that height and weight. Pounds have been rounded off.

BMI	36	37	38	39	40	41	42	43	44	45	46	47	48	49	50	51	52	53	54
Height (inches)	Body Weight (pounds)																		
58	172	177	181	186	191	196	201	205	210	215	220	224	229	234	239	244	248	253	258
59	178	183	188	193	198	203	208	212	217	222	227	232	237	242	247	252	257	262	267
60	184	189	194	199	204	209	215	220	225	230	235	240	245	250	255	261	266	271	276
61	190	195	201	206	211	217	222	227	232	238	243	248	254	259	264	269	275	280	285
62	196	202	207	213	218	224	229	235	240	246	251	256	262	267	273	278	284	289	295
63	203	208	214	220	225	231	237	242	248	254	259	265	270	278	282	287	293	299	304
64	209	215	221	227	232	238	244	250	256	262	267	273	279	285	291	296	302	308	314
65	216	222	228	234	240	246	252	258	264	270	276	282	288	294	300	306	312	318	324
66	223	229	235	241	247	253	260	266	272	278	284	291	297	303	309	315	322	328	334
67	230	236	242	249	255	261	268	274	280	287	293	299	306	312	319	325	331	338	344
68	236	243	249	256	262	269	276	282	289	295	302	308	315	322	328	335	341	348	354
69	243	250	257	263	270	277	284	291	297	304	311	318	324	331	338	345	351	358	365
70	250	257	264	271	278	285	292	299	306	313	320	327	334	341	348	355	362	369	376
71	257	265	272	279	286	293	301	308	315	322	329	338	343	351	358	365	372	379	386
72	265	272	279	287	294	302	309	316	324	331	338	346	353	361	368	375	383	390	397
73	272	280	288	295	302	310	318	325	333	340	348	355	363	371	378	386	393	401	408
74	280	287	295	303	311	319	326	334	342	350	358	365	373	381	389	396	404	412	420
75	287	295	303	311	319	327	335	343	351	359	367	375	383	391	399	407	415	423	431
76	295	304	312	320	328	336	344	353	361	369	377	385	394	402	410	418	426	435	443

Menus for a Healthy Diet

TABLE B-1   TLC Sample Menu: Traditional American Cuisine, Male, 25–49 Years

Breakfast
Oatmeal (1 cup)
    Fat-free milk (1 cup)
    Raisins (¼ cup)
English muffin (1 medium)
    Soft margarine (2 tsp)
    Jelly (1 Tbsp)
Honeydew melon (1 cup)
Orange juice, calcium fortified (1 cup)
Coffee (1 cup) with fat-free milk (2 Tbsp)

Lunch
Roast beef sandwich
    Whole-wheat bun (1 medium)
    Roast beef, lean (2 oz)
    Swiss cheese, low fat (1 oz slice)
    Romaine lettuce (2 leaves)
    Tomato (2 medium slices)
    Mustard (2 tsp)
Pasta salad (1 cup)
    Pasta noodles (¾ cup)
    Mixed vegetables (¼ cup)
    Olive oil (2 tsp)
Apple (1 medium)
Iced tea, unsweetened (1 cup)

Dinner
Orange roughy (3 oz) cooked with olive oil (2 tsp)
    Parmesan cheese (1 Tbsp)
Rice (1½ cup) ⟶   *For a higher fat alternative, substitute 1/3 cup of unsalted peanuts,
Corn kernels (½ cup)   chopped (to sprinkle on the frozen yogurt) for 1 cup of the rice.
    Soft margarine (1 tsp)
Broccoli (½ cup)
    Soft margarine (1 tsp)
Roll (1 small)
    Soft margarine (1 tsp)
Strawberries (1 cup) topped with low-fat frozen yogurt (½ cup)
Fat-free milk (1 cup)

Snack
Popcorn (2 cups) cooked with canola oil (1 Tbsp)
Peaches, canned in water (1 cup)
Water (1 cup)

Nutrient Analysis

Calories	2523	Total fat, % calories	28
Cholesterol (mg)	139	Saturated fat, % calories	6
Fiber (g)	32	Monounsaturated fat, % calories	14
Soluble (g)	10	Polyunsaturated fat, % calories	6
Sodium (mg)	1800	Trans fat (g)	5
		Omega 3 fat (g)	0.4
Carbohydrates, % calories	57	Protein, % calories	17

*Higher Fat Alternative

Total fat, % calories	34

No salt is added in recipe preparation or as seasoning.
The sample menu meets or exceeds the Daily Reference Intake (DRI) for nutrients.

Source: National Cholesterol Education Program, Adult Treatment Panel III Report, 2001. National Institutes of Health, Washington, D.C.

TABLE B-2   TLC Sample Menu: Traditional American Cuisine, Female, 25–49 Years

Breakfast
Oatmeal (1 cup)
    Fat-free milk (1 cup)
    Raisins (¼ cup)
Honeydew melon (1 cup)
Orange juice, calcium fortified (1 cup)
Coffee (1 cup) with fat-free milk (2 Tbsp)

Lunch
Roast beef sandwich
    Whole-wheat bun (1 medium)
    Roast beef, lean (2 oz)
    Swiss cheese, low fat (1 oz slice)
    Romaine lettuce (2 leaves)
    Tomato (2 medium slices)
    Mustard (2 tsp)
Pasta salad (½ cup)
    Pasta noodles (¼ cup)
    Mixed vegetables (¼ cup)
    Olive oil (1 tsp)
Apple (1 medium)
Iced tea, unsweetened (1 cup)

Dinner
Orange roughy (2 oz) cooked with olive oil (2 tsp)
    Parmesan cheese (1 Tbsp)
Rice (1 cup) ───────────▶   *For a higher fat alternative, substitute 2 Tbsp of unsalted peanuts,
    Soft margarine (1 tsp)   chopped (to sprinkle on the frozen yogurt) for ½ cup of the rice.
Broccoli (½ cup)
    Soft margarine (1 tsp)
Strawberries (1 cup) topped with low-fat frozen yogurt (½ cup)
Water (1 cup)

Snack
Popcorn (2 cups) cooked with canola oil (1 Tbsp)
Peaches, canned in water (1 cup)
Water (1 cup)

Nutrient Analysis

Calories	1795	Total fat, % calories	27
Cholesterol (mg)	115	Saturated fat, % calories	6
Fiber (g)	28	Monounsaturated fat, % calories	14
Soluble (g)	9	Polyunsaturated fat, % calories	6
		Trans fat (g)	2
Sodium (mg)	1128	Omega 3 fat (g)	0.4
Carbohydrates, % calories	57	Protein, % calories	19

*Higher Fat Alternative

Total fat, % calories	33

No salt is added in recipe preparation or as seasoning.
The sample menu meets or exceeds the Daily Reference Intake (DRI) for nutrients.

Source: National Cholesterol Education Program, Adult Treatment Panel III Report, 2001. National Institutes of Health, Washington, D.C.

TABLE B-3   TLC Sample Menu: Southern Cuisine, Male, 25–49 Years

Breakfast
Bran cereal (¾ cup)
    Banana (1 medium)
    Fat-free milk (1 cup)
Biscuit, made with canola oil (1 medium)
    Jelly (1 Tbsp)
    Soft margarine (2 tsp)
Honeydew melon (1 cup)
Orange juice, calcium fortified (1 cup)
Coffee (1 cup) with fat-free milk (2 Tbsp)

Lunch
Chicken breast (3 oz), sautéed with canola oil (2 tsp)
Collard greens (½ cup)
    Chicken broth, low sodium (1 Tbsp)
Black-eyed peas (½ cup)
Corn on the cob (1 medium) ⟶ *For a higher fat alternative, substitute ¼ cup of unsalted almond slices
    Soft margarine (1tsp)   for the corn on the cob. Sprinkle the almonds on the rice.
Rice, cooked (1 cup)
    Soft margarine (1 tsp)
Fruit cocktail, canned in water (1 cup)
Iced tea, unsweetened (1 cup)

Dinner
Catfish (3 oz) coated with flour and baked with canola oil (½ Tbsp)
Sweet potato (1 medium)
    Soft margarine (2 tsp)
Spinach (½ cup)
    Vegetable broth, low sodium (2 Tbsp)
Corn muffin (1 medium), made with fat-free milk and egg substitute
    Soft margarine (1 tsp)
Watermelon (1 cup)
Iced tea, unsweetened (1 cup)

Snack
Bagel (1 medium)
Peanut butter, reduced fat, unsalted (1 Tbsp)
Fat-free milk (1 cup)

Nutrient Analysis

Calories	2504	Total fat, % calories	30
Cholesterol (mg)	158	Saturated fat, % calories	5
Fiber (g)	52	Monounsaturated fat, % calories	13
Soluble (g)	10	Polyunsaturated fat, % calories	9
Sodium (mg)	2146	Trans fat (g)	6
Carbohydrates, % calories	59	Protein, % calories	18

*Higher Fat Alternative

Total fat, % calories	34

No salt is added in recipe preparation or as seasoning.
The sample menu meets or exceeds the Daily Reference Intake (DRI) for nutrients.

Source: National Cholesterol Education Program, Adult Treatment Panel III Report, 2001. National Institutes of Health, Washington, D.C.

TABLE B-4   TLC Sample Menu: Southern Cuisine, Female, 25–49 Year

Breakfast
Bran cereal (¾ cup)
    Banana (1 medium)
    Fat-free milk (1 cup)
Biscuit, low sodium and made with canola oil (1 medium)
    Jelly (1 Tbsp)
    Soft margarine (1 tsp)
Honeydew melon (½ cup)
Coffee (1 cup) with fat-free milk (2 Tbsp)

Lunch
Chicken breast (2 oz) cooked with canola oil (2 tsp)
Corn on the cob (1 medium) ⟶ *For a higher fat alternative, substitute ¼ cup of unsalted almond slices
    Soft margarine (1 tsp)   for the corn on the cob. Sprinkle the almonds on the rice.
Collards greens (½ cup)
    Chicken broth, low sodium (1 Tbsp)
Rice, cooked (½ cup)
Fruit cocktail, canned in water (1cup)
Iced tea, unsweetened (1 cup)

Dinner
Catfish (3 oz), coated with flour and baked with canola oil (½ Tbsp)
Sweet potato (1 medium)
    Soft margarine (2 tsp)
Spinach (½ cup)
    Vegetable broth, low sodium (2 Tbsp)
Corn muffin (1 medium), made with fat-free milk and egg substitute
    Soft margarine (1 tsp)
Watermelon (1 cup)
Iced tea, unsweetened (1 cup)

Snack
Graham crackers (4 large)
Peanut butter, reduced fat, unsalted (1 Tbsp)
Fat-free milk (½ cup)

Nutrient Analysis

Calories	1823	Total fat, % calories	30
Cholesterol (mg)	131	Saturated fat, % calories	5
Fiber (g)	43	Monounsaturated fat, % calories	14
Soluble (g)	8	Polyunsaturated fat, % calories	8
Sodium (mg)	1676	Trans fat (g)	3
		Omega 3 fat (g)	0.4
Carbohydrates, % calories	59	Protein, % calories	18

*Higher Fat Alternative

Total fat, % calories	35

No salt is added in recipe preparation or as seasoning.
The sample menu meets or exceeds the Daily Reference Intake (DRI) for nutrients.

Source: National Cholesterol Education Program, Adult Treatment Panel III Report, 2001. National Institutes of Health, Washington, D.C.

TABLE B-5   TLC Sample Menu: Asian Cuisine, Male, 25–49 Years

Breakfast
Scrambled egg whites (¾ cup liquid egg substitute)
    Cooked with fat-free cooking spray ————▶ *For a higher fat alternative, cook egg whites
English muffin (1 whole)   with 1 Tbsp of canola oil.
    Soft margarine (2 tsp)
    Jam (1 Tbsp)
Strawberries (1 cup)
Orange juice, calcium fortified (1 cup) ————▶ **If using higher fat alternative, eliminate orange juice.
Coffee (1 cup) with fat-free milk (2 Tbsp)

Lunch
Tofu Vegetable stir-fry
    Tofu (3 oz)
    Mushrooms (½ cup)
    Onion (¼ cup)
    Carrots (½ cup)
    Swiss chard (1 cup)
    Garlic, minced (2 Tbsp)
    Peanut oil (1 Tbsp)
    Soy sauce, low sodium (2½ tsp)
Rice, cooked (1 cup)
Vegetable egg roll, baked (1 medium)
Orange (1 medium)
Green tea (1 cup)

Dinner
Beef stir-fry
    Beef tenderloin (3 oz)
    Soybeans, cooked (¼ cup)
    Broccoli, cut in large pieces (½ cup)
    Carrots, sliced (½ cup)
    Peanut oil (1 Tbsp)
    Soy sauce, low sodium (2 tsp)
Rice, cooked (1 cup)
Watermelon (1 cup)
Almond cookies (2 cookies)
Fat-free milk (1 cup)

Snack
Chinese noodles, soft (1 cup)
    Peanut oil (2 tsp)
Banana (1 medium)
Green tea (1 cup)

Nutrient Analysis

Calories	2519	Total fat, % calories	28
Cholesterol (mg)	108	Saturated fat, % calories	5
Fiber (g)	37	Monounsaturated fat, % calories	11
Soluble (g)	15	Polyunsaturated fat, % calories	9
Sodium (mg)	2268	Trans fat (g)	3
Carbohydrates, % calories	57	Protein, % calories	18

*Higher Fat Alternative

Total fat, % calories	32

No salt is added in recipe preparation or as seasoning.
The sample menu meets or exceeds the Daily Reference Intake (DRI) for nutrients.

**Because canola oil adds extra calories, the orange juice is left out of the menu.

Source: National Cholesterol Education Program, Adult Treatment Panel III Report, 2001. National Institutes of Health, Washington, D.C.

TABLE B-6   TLC Sample Menu: Asian Cuisine, Female, 25–49 Years

Breakfast
Scrambled egg whites (½ cup liquid egg substitute)
    Cooked with fat-free cooking spray ⟶ *For a higher fat alternative, cook egg whites with
English muffin (1 whole)   1 Tbsp of canola oil.
    Soft margarine (2 tsp)
    Jam (1 Tbsp)
Strawberries (1 cup)
Orange juice, calcium fortified (1 cup) ⟶ **If using higher fat alternative, eliminate orange juice.
Coffee (1 cup) with fat-free milk (2 Tbsp)

Lunch
Tofu Vegetable stir-fry
    Tofu (3 oz)
    Mushrooms (½ cup)
    Onion (¼ cup)
    Carrots (½ cup)
    Swiss chard (½ cup)
    Garlic, minced (2 Tbsp)
    Peanut oil (1 Tbsp)
    Soy sauce, low sodium (2½ tsp)
Rice, cooked (½ cup)
Orange (1 medium)
Green tea (1 cup)

Dinner
Beef stir-fry
    Beef tenderloin (3 oz)
    Soybeans, cooked (¼ cup)
    Broccoli, cut in large pieces (½ cup)
    Peanut oil (1 Tbsp)
    Soy sauce, low sodium (2 tsp)
Rice, cooked (½ cup)
Watermelon (1 cup)
Almond cookie (1 cookie)
Fat-free milk (1 cup)

Snack
Chinese noodles, soft (½ cup)
    Peanut oil (1 tsp)
Green tea (1 cup)

Nutrient Analysis

Calories	1829	Total fat, % calories	28
Cholesterol (mg)	74	Saturated fat, % calories	6
Fiber (g)	26	Monounsaturated fat, % calories	11
Soluble (g)	10	Polyunsaturated fat, % calories	9
Sodium (mg)	1766	Trans fat (g)	3
Carbohydrates, % calories	56	Protein, % calories	18

*Higher Fat Alternative

Total fat, % calories	33

No salt is added in recipe preparation or as seasoning.
The sample menu meets or exceeds the Daily Reference Intake (DRI) for nutrients.

**Because canola oil adds extra calories, the orange juice is left out of the menu.

Source: National Cholesterol Education Program, Adult Treatment Panel III Report, 2001. National Institutes of Health, Washington, D.C.

TABLE B-7   TLC Sample Menu: Mexican-American Cuisine, Male, 25–49 Years

Breakfast
Bean tortilla
    Corn tortilla (2 medium)
    Pinto beans (½ cup) ——————▶ *For a higher fat alternative, cook beans with canola oil
    Onion (¼ cup), tomato, chopped (¼ cup)   (1 Tbsp).
    Jalapeno pepper (1 medium)
    Sauté with canola oil (1 tsp)
Papaya (1 medium) ——————▶ **If using higher fat alternative, reduce papaya serving to
Orange juice, calcium fortified (1 cup)   ½ medium fruit.
Coffee (1 cup) with fat-free milk (2 Tbsp)

Lunch
Stir-fried beef
    Sirloin steak (3 oz)
    Garlic, minced (1 tsp)
    Onion, chopped (¼ cup)
    Tomato, chopped (¼ cup)
    Potato, diced (¼ cup)
    Salsa (¼ cup)
    Olive oil (2 tsp)
Mexican rice
    Rice, cooked (1 cup)
    Onion, chopped (¼ cup)
    Tomato, chopped (¼ cup)
    Jalapeno pepper (1 medium)
    Carrots, diced (¼ cup)
    Cilantro (2 Tbsp)
    Olive oil (1 Tbsp)
Mango (1 medium)
Blended fruit drink (1 cup)
    Fat-free milk (1 cup)
    Mango, diced (¼ cup)
    Banana, sliced (¼ cup)
    Water (¼ cup)

Dinner
Chicken fajita
    Corn tortilla (2 medium)
    Chicken breast, baked (3 oz)
    Onion, chopped (2 Tbsp)
    Green pepper, chopped (¼ cup)
    Garlic, minced (1 tsp)
    Salsa (2 Tbsp)
    Canola oil (2 tsp)
Avocado salad
    Romaine lettuce (1 cup)
    Avocado slices, dark skin, California type
    (1 small)
    Tomato, sliced (¼ cup)
    Onion, chopped (2 Tbsp)
    Sour cream, low fat (1½ Tbsp)
Rice pudding with raisins (¾ cup)
Water (1 cup)

Snack
Plain yogurt, fat free, no sugar added (1 cup)
    Mixed with peaches, canned in water (½ cup)
Water (1 cup)

Nutrient Analysis

Calories	2535	Total fat, % calories	28
Cholesterol (mg)	158	Saturated fat, % calories	5
Fiber (g)	48	Monounsaturated fat, % calories	17
Soluble (g)	17	Polyunsaturated fat, % calories	5
Sodium (mg)	2118	Trans fat (g)	<1
Carbohydrates, % calories	58	Protein, % calories	17

*Higher Fat Alternative

Total fat, % calories	33

No salt is added in recipe preparation or as seasoning.
The sample menu meets or exceeds the Daily Reference Intake (DRI) for nutrients.

**Because the peanuts add extra calories, the papaya serving is reduced in the menu.

Source: National Cholesterol Education Program, Adult Treatment Panel III Report, 2001. National Institutes of Health, Washington, D.C.

TABLE B-8   TLC Sample Menu: Mexican-American Cuisine, Female, 25–49 Years

Breakfast
Bean tortilla
    Corn tortilla (1 medium)
    Pinto beans (¼ cup)
    Onion (2 Tbsp), tomato, chopped (2 Tbsp), jalapeno pepper (1 medium)
    Sauté with canola oil (1 tsp)
Papaya (1 medium) ⎯⎯⎯⎯⎯⎯⎯➤ **If using higher fat alternative, eliminate papaya.
Orange juice, calcium fortified (1 cup)
Coffee (1 cup) with fat-free milk (2 Tbsp)

Lunch
Stir-fried beef
    Sirloin steak (2 oz)
    Garlic, minced (1 tsp)
    Onion, chopped (¼ cup)
    Tomato, chopped (¼ cup)
    Potato, diced (¼ cup) ⎯➤*For a higher fat
    Salsa (¼ cup)   alternative,
    Olive oil (1½ tsp)   substitute ½ cup of
Mexican rice (½ cup)   unsalted peanut
    Rice, cooked (½ cup)   halves for the
Onion, chopped (2 Tbsp)   potatoes.
    Tomato, chopped (2 Tbsp)
    Jalapeno pepper (1 medium)
    Carrots, diced (2 Tbsp)
    Cilantro (1 Tbsp)
    Olive oil (2 tsp)
Mango (1 medium)
    Blended fruit drink (1 cup)
    Fat-free milk (1 cup)
    Mango, diced (¼ cup)
    Banana, sliced (¼ cup)
    Water (¼ cup)

Dinner
Chicken fajita
    Corn tortilla (1 medium)
    Chicken breast, baked (2 oz)
    Onion, chopped (2 Tbsp)
    Green pepper, chopped (2 Tbsp)
    Garlic, minced (1 tsp)
    Salsa (1½ Tbsp)
    Canola oil (1 tsp)
Avocado salad
    Romaine lettuce (1 cup)
    Avocado slices, dark skin, California type
    (½ small)
    Tomato, sliced (¼ cup)
    Onion, chopped (2 Tbsp)
    Sour cream, low fat (1½ Tbsp)
Rice pudding with raisins (½ cup)
Water (1 cup)

Snack
Plain yogurt, fat free, no sugar added (1 cup)
    Mixed with peaches, canned in water (½ cup)
Water (1 cup)

Nutrient Analysis

Calories	1821	Total fat, % calories	26
Cholesterol (mg)	110	Saturated fat, % calories	4
Fiber (g)	35	Monounsaturated fat, % calories	15
Soluble (g)	13	Polyunsaturated fat, % calories	4
Sodium (mg)	1739	Trans fat (g)	<1
Carbohydrates, % calories	61	Protein, % calories	17

*Higher Fat Alternative

Total fat, % calories	34

No salt is added in recipe preparation or as seasoning.
The sample menu meets or exceeds the Daily Reference Intake (DRI) for nutrients.

**Because the peanuts add extra calories, the papaya is left out of the menu.

Source: National Cholesterol Education Program, Adult Treatment Panel III Report, 2001. National Institutes of Health, Washington, D.C.

Drugs and Nutrition

ALLERGIES

Antihistamines are used to relieve or prevent the symptoms of colds, hay fever, and allergies. They limit or block histamine, which is released by the body when we are exposed to substances that cause allergic reactions. Antihistamines are available with and without a prescription (over-the-counter). These products vary in their ability to cause drowsiness and sleepiness.

Antihistamines

Some examples are:

Over the Counter:
brompheniramine / DIMETANE, BROMPHEN
chlorpheniramine / CHLOR-TRIMETON
diphenhydramine / BENADRYL
clemastine / TAVIST

Prescription:
fexofenadine / ALLEGRA
loratadine / CLARITIN (now available over the counter)
cetirizine / ZYRTEC
astemizole / HISMANAL

Interaction

Food: It is best to take prescription antihistamines on an empty stomach to increase their effectiveness.
Alcohol: Some antihistamines may increase drowsiness and slow mental and motor performance. Use caution when operating machinery or driving.

ARTHRITIS AND PAIN
Analgesic / Antipyretic

They treat mild to moderate pain and fever. An example is: acetaminophen / TYLENOL, TEMPRA

Interactions

Food: For rapid relief, take on an empty stomach because food may slow the body's absorption of acetaminophen.
Alcohol: Avoid or limit the use of alcohol because chronic alcohol use can increase your risk of liver damage or stomach bleeding. If you consume three or more alcoholic drinks per day talk to your doctor or pharmacist before taking these medications.

Non-Steroidal Anti-Inflammatory Drugs (NSAIDS)

NSAIDs reduce pain, fever, and inflammation.

Some examples are:
aspirin / BAYER, ECOTRIN
ibuprofen / MOTRIN, ADVIL
naproxen / ANAPROX, ALEVE, NAPROSYN
ketoprofen / ORUDIS
nabumetone / RELAFEN

Interaction

Food: Because these medications can irritate the stomach, it is best to take them with food or milk.
Alcohol: Avoid or limit the use of alcohol because chronic alcohol use can increase your risk of liver damage or stomach bleeding. If you consume three or more alcoholic drinks per day talk to your doctor or pharmacist before taking these medications. Buffered aspirin or enteric coated aspirin may be preferable to regular aspirin to decrease stomach bleeding.

Corticosteroids

They are used to provide relief to inflamed areas of the body. Corticosteroids reduce swelling and itching, and help relieve allergic, rheumatoid, and other conditions.

Some examples are:
methylprednisolone / MEDROL
prednisone / DELTASONE
prednisolone / PEDIAPRED, PRELONE
cortisone acetate / CORTEF

Interaction

Food: Take with food or milk to decrease stomach upset.

Narcotic Analgesics

Narcotic analgesics are available only with a prescription. They provide relief for moderate to severe pain.

APPENDICES

Codeine can also be used to suppress cough. Some of these medications can be found in combination with non-narcotic drugs such as acetaminophen, aspirin, or cough syrups. Use caution when taking these medications: take them only as directed by a doctor or pharmacist because they may be habit forming and can cause serious side effects when used improperly.

Some examples are:
codeine combined with acetaminophen / TYLENOL #2, #3, & #4
morphine / ROXANOL, MS CONTIN
oxycodone combined with acetaminophen / PERCOCET, ROXICET
meperidine / DEMEROL
hydrocodone with acetaminophen / VICODIN, LORCET

Interaction

Alcohol: Avoid alcohol because it increases the sedative effects of the medications. Use caution when motor skills are required, including operating machinery and driving.

ASTHMA
Bronchodilators

Bronchodilators are used to treat the symptoms of bronchial asthma, chronic bronchitis, and emphysema. These medicines open air passages to the lungs to relieve wheezing, shortness of breath, and troubled breathing.

Some examples are:
theophylline / SLO-BID, THEO-DUR, THEO-DUR 24, UNIPHYL,
albuterol / VENTOLIN, PROVENTIL, COMBIVENT
epinephrine / PRIMATENE MIST

Interactions

Food: The effect of food on theophylline medications can vary widely. High-fat meals may increase the amount of theophylline in the body, while high-carbohydrate meals may decrease it. It is important to check with your pharmacist about which form you are taking because food can have different effects depending on the dose form (e.g., regular release, sustained release or sprinkles). For example, food has little effect on Theo-Dur and Slo-Bid, but food increases the absorption of Theo-24 and Uniphyl which can result in side effects of nausea, vomiting, headache, and irritability. Food can also decrease absorption of products like Theo-Dur Sprinkles for children.

Caffeine: Avoid eating or drinking large amounts of foods and beverages that contain caffeine (e.g., chocolate, colas, coffee, and tea) because both oral bronchodilators and caffeine stimulate the central nervous system.

Alcohol: Avoid alcohol if you're taking theophylline medications because it can increase the risk of side effects such as nausea, vomiting, headache and irritability.

CARDIOVASCULAR DISORDERS

There are numerous medications used to treat cardiovascular disorders such as high blood pressure, angina, irregular heart beat, and high cholesterol. These drugs are often used in combination to enhance their effectiveness. Some classes of drugs can treat several conditions. For example, beta blockers can be used to treat high blood pressure, angina, and irregular heart beats. Check with your doctor or pharmacist if you have questions on any of your medications. Some of the major cardiovascular drug classes are:

Diuretics

Sometimes called "water pills," diuretics help eliminate water, sodium, and chloride from the body. There are different types of diuretics.

Some examples are:
furosemide / LASIX
triamterene / hydrochlorothiazide / DYAZIDE, MAXZIDE
hydrochlorothiazide / HYDRODIURIL
triamterene / DYRENIUM
bumetamide / BUMEX
metolazone / ZAROXOLYN

Interaction

Food: Diuretics vary in their interactions with food and specific nutrients. Some diuretics cause loss of potassium, calcium, and magnesium. Triamterene, on the other hand, is known as a "potassium-sparing" diuretic. It blocks the kidneys' excretion of potassium, which can cause hyperkalemia (increased potassium). Excess potassium may result in irregular heartbeat and heart palpitations. When taking triamterene, avoid eating large amounts of potassium-rich foods such as bananas, oranges and green leafy vegetables, or salt substitutes that contain potassium.

Beta Blockers

Beta blockers decrease the nerve impulses to the heart and blood vessels. This decreases the heart rate and the workload of the heart.

Some examples are:
atenolol / TENORMIN
metoprolol / LOPRESSOR
propranolol / INDERAL
nadolol / CORGARD

Interaction

Alcohol: Avoid drinking alcohol with propranolol / INDERAL because the combination lowers blood pressure too much.

Nitrates

Nitrates relax blood vessels and lower the demand for oxygen by the heart.

Some examples are:
isosorbide dinitrate / ISORDIL, SORBITRATE
nitroglycerin / NITRO, NITRO-DUR, TRANSDERM-NITRO

Interaction

Alcohol: Avoid alcohol because it may add to the blood vessel-relaxing effect of nitrates and result in dangerously low blood pressure.

Angiotensin Converting Enzyme (ACE) Inhibitors

ACE inhibitors relax blood vessels by preventing angiotensin II, a vasoconstrictor, from being formed.

Some examples are:
captopril / CAPOTEN
enalapril / VASOTEC
lisinopril / PRINIVIL, ZESTRIL
quinapril / ACCUPRIL
moexipril / UNIVASC

Interactions

Food: Food can decrease the absorption of captopril and moexipril. So take captopril and moexipril one hour before or two hours after meals. ACE inhibitors may increase the amount of potassium in your body. Too much potassium can be harmful. Make sure to tell your doctor if you are taking potassium supplements or diuretics (water pills) that may increase the amount of potassium in your body. Avoid eating large amounts of foods high in potassium such as bananas, green leafy vegetables, and oranges.

HMG-CoA Reductase Inhibitors

Otherwise known as "statins," these medications are used to lower cholesterol. They work to reduce the rate of production of LDL (bad cholesterol). Some of these drugs also lower triglycerides. Recent studies have shown that pravastatin can reduce the risk of heart attack, stroke, or miniature stroke in certain patient populations.

Some examples are:
atorvastatin / LIPITOR
cerivastatin / BAYCOL
fluvastatin / LESCOL
lovastatin / MEVACOR
pravastatin / PRAVACHOL
simvastatin / ZOCOR

Interactions

Alcohol: Avoid drinking large amounts of alcohol because it may increase the risk of liver damage.
Food: Lovastatin (Mevacor) should be taken with the evening meal to enhance absorption.

Anticoagulants

Anticoagulants help to prevent the formation of blood clots.

An example is:
warfarin / COUMADIN

Interactions

Food: Vitamin K produces blood-clotting substances and may reduce the effectiveness of anticoagulants. So limit the amount of foods high in vitamin K (such as broccoli, spinach, kale, turnip greens, cauliflower, and brussel sprouts).
High doses of vitamin E (400 IU or more) may prolong clotting time and increase the risk of bleeding. Talk to your doctor before taking vitamin E supplements.

INFECTIONS
Antibiotics and Antifungals

Many different types of drugs are used to treat infections caused by bacteria and fungi. Some general advice to follow when taking any such product is:

- Tell your doctor about any skin rashes you may have had with antibiotics or that you get while taking this medication. A rash can be a symptom of an allergic reaction, and allergic reactions can be very serious.
- Tell your doctor if you experience diarrhea.
- If you are using birth control, consult with your health care provider because some methods may not work when taken with antibiotics.
- Be sure to finish all your medication even if you are feeling better.
- Take with plenty of water.

Antibacterials

Penicillin

Some examples are:
penicillin V / VEETIDS
amoxicillin / TRIMOX, AMOXIL
ampicillin / PRINCIPEN, OMNIPEN

Interaction

Food: Take on an empty stomach, but if it upsets your stomach, take it with food.

Quinolones

Some examples are:

ciprofloxacin / CIPRO
levofloxacin / LEVAQUIN
ofloxacin / FLOXIN
trovafloxacin / TROVAN

Interactions

Food: Take on an empty stomach one hour before or two hours after meals. If your stomach gets upset, take it with food. However, avoid calcium-containing products like milk, yogurt, vitamins or minerals containing iron, and antacids because they significantly decrease drug concentration.

Caffeine: Taking these medications with caffeine-containing products (e.g., coffee, colas, tea, and chocolate) may increase caffeine levels, leading to excitability and nervousness.

Cephalosporins

Some examples are:

cefaclor / CECLOR, CECLOR CD
cefadroxil / DURICEF
cefixime / SUPRAX
cefprozil / CEFZIL
cephalexin / KEFLEX, KEFTAB

Interaction

Food: Take on an empty stomach one hour before or two hours after meals. If your stomach gets upset, take with food.

Macrolides

Some examples are:

azithromycin / ZITHROMAX
clarithromycin / BIAXIN
erythromycin / E-MYCIN, ERY-TAB, ERYC
erythromycin + sulfisoxazole / PEDIAZOLE

Interaction

Food: Take on an empty stomach one hour before or two hours after meals. If your stomach gets upset, take with food.

Sulfonamides

An example is:

sulfamethoxazole + trimethoprim / BACTRIM, SEPTRA

Interaction

Food: Take on an empty stomach one hour before or two hours after meals. If your stomach gets upset, take with food.

Tetracyclines

Some examples are:

tetracycline / ACHROMYCIN, SUMYCIN
doxycycline / VIBRAMYCIN
minocycline / MINOCIN

Interaction

Food: Take on an empty stomach one hour before or two hours after meals. If your stomach gets upset, take with food. However, it is important to avoid taking tetracycline / ACHROMYCIN, SUMYCIN with dairy products, antacids and vitamins containing iron because these can interfere with the medication's effectiveness.

Nitroimidazole

An example is:

metronidazole / FLAGYL

Interaction

Alcohol: Avoid drinking alcohol or using medications that contain alcohol or eating foods prepared with alcohol while you are taking metronidazole and for at least three days after you finish the medication. Alcohol may cause nausea, abdominal cramps, vomiting, headaches, and flushing.

Antifungals

Some examples are:

fluconazole / DIFLUCAN
griseofulvin / GRIFULVIN
ketoconazole / NIZORAL
itraconazole / SPORANOX

Interactions

Food: It is important to avoid taking these medications with dairy products (milk, cheeses, yogurt, ice cream), or antacids.

Alcohol: Avoid drinking alcohol, using medications that contain alcohol, or eating foods prepared with alcohol while you are taking ketoconazole/NIZORAL and for at least three days after you finish the medication. Alcohol may cause nausea, abdominal cramps, vomiting, headaches, and flushing.

MOOD ORDERS

Depression, Emotional, and Anxiety Disorders

Depression, panic disorder, and anxiety are a few examples of mood disorders—complex medical conditions with varying degrees of severity. When using medications to treat mood disorders it is important to follow your doctor's instructions. Remember to take your dose as directed even if you are feeling better, and do not stop unless you consult your doctor. In some cases it may take several weeks to see an improvement in symptoms.

Monomine Oxidase (MAO) Inhibitors

Some examples are:
 phenelzine / NARDIL
 tranylcypromine / PARNATE

Interactions

MAO Inhibitors have many dietary restrictions, and people taking them need to follow the dietary guidelines and physician's instructions very carefully. A rapid, potentially fatal increase in blood pressure can occur if foods or alcoholic beverages containing tyramine are consumed while taking MAO Inhibitors.

Alcohol: Do not drink beer, red wine, other alcoholic beverages, non-alcoholic and reduced-alcohol beer and red-wine products.

Food: Foods high in tyramine that should be avoided include:

- American processed, cheddar, blue, brie, mozzarella and Parmesan cheese; yogurt, sour cream.
- Beef or chicken liver; cured meats such as sausage and salami; game meat; caviar; dried fish.
- Avocados, bananas, yeast extracts, raisins, sauerkraut, soy sauce, miso soup.
- Broad (fava) beans, ginseng, caffeine-containing products (colas, chocolate, coffee, and tea).

Anti-Anxiety Drugs

Some examples are:
 lorazepam / ATIVAN
 diazepam / VALIUM
 alprazolam / XANAX

Interactions

Alcohol: May impair mental and motor performance (e.g., driving, operating machinery).

Caffeine: May cause excitability, nervousness, and hyperactivity and lessen the anti-anxiety effects of the drugs.

Antidepressant Drugs

Some examples are:
 paroxetine / PAXIL
 sertraline / ZOLOFT
 fluoxetine / PROZAC

Interactions

Alcohol: Although alcohol may not significantly interact with these drugs to affect mental or motor skills, people who are depressed should not drink alcohol.

Food: These medications can be taken with or without food.

STOMACH CONDITIONS

Conditions like acid reflux, heartburn, acid indigestion, sour stomach, and gas are very common ailments. The goal of treatment is to relieve pain, promote healing, and prevent the irritation from returning. This is achieved by either reducing the acid the body creates or protecting the stomach from the acid. Lifestyle and dietary habits can play a large role in the symptoms of these conditions. For example, smoking cigarettes and consuming products that contain caffeine may make symptoms return.

Histamine Blockers

Some examples are:
 cimetidine / TAGAMET or TAGAMET HB
 famotidine / PEPCID or PEPCID AC
 ranitidine / ZANTAC or ZANTAC 75
 nizatadine / AXID OR AXID AR

Interactions

Alcohol: Avoid alcohol while taking these products. Alcohol may irritate the stomach and make it more difficult for the stomach to heal.

Food: Can be taken with or without regard to meals.

Caffeine: Caffeine products (e.g., cola, chocolate, tea, and coffee) may irritate the stomach.

DRUG-TO-DRUG INTERACTIONS

Not only can drugs interact with food and alcohol, they can also interact with each other. Some drugs are given together on purpose for an added effect, like codeine and acetaminophen for pain relief. But other drug-to-drug interactions may be unintended and harmful. Prescription drugs can interact with each other or with over-the-counter (OTC) drugs, such as acetaminophen, aspirin, and cold medicine. Likewise, OTC drugs can interact with each other.

Sometimes the effect of one drug may be increased or decreased. For example, tricyclic antidepressants such as amitriptyline (ELAVIL), or nortriptyline (PAMELOR) can decrease the ability of clonidine (CATAPRES) to lower blood pressure. In other cases, the effects of a drug can increase the risk of serious side effects. For example, some antifungal medications such as itraconazole (SPORANOX) and ketoconazole (NIZORAL) can interfere with the way some cholesterol-lowering medications are broken down by the body. This can increase the risk of a serious side effects.

Doctors can often prescribe other medications to reduce the risk of drug-drug interactions. For example, two cholesterol-lowering drugs—pravastatin (PRAVACHOL) and fluvastatin (LESCOL)—are less likely to interact with antifungal medications. Be sure to tell your doctor about all medications—prescription and OTC—that you are taking.

Source: Food and Drug Administration and the National Consumers League 1998.

APPENDIX D

CDC Growth Charts

TABLE D-1   Boys: Birth to 36 Months Weight-for-Age

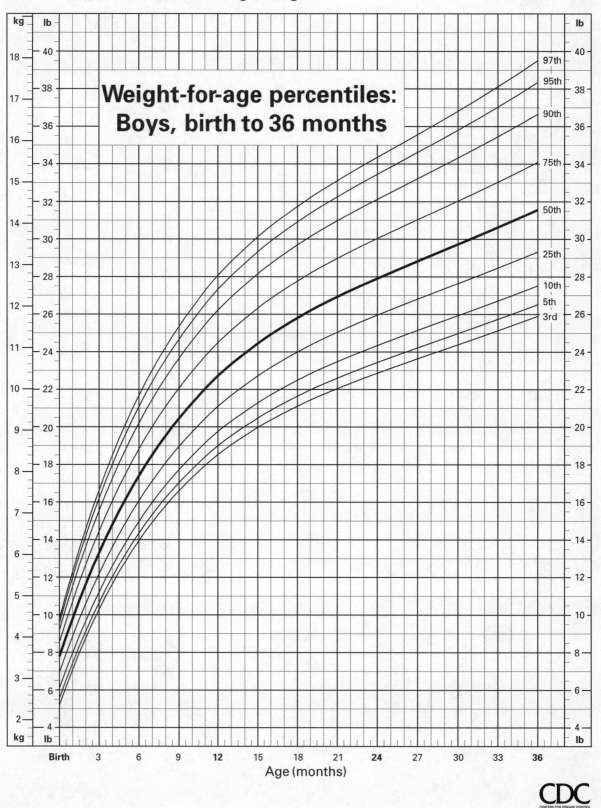

Weight-for-age percentiles: Boys, birth to 36 months

Source: Developed by the National Center for Health Statistics in collaboration with the National Center for Chronic Disease Prevention and Health Promotion (2000).

TABLE D-2   Girls: Birth to 36 Months Weight-for-Age

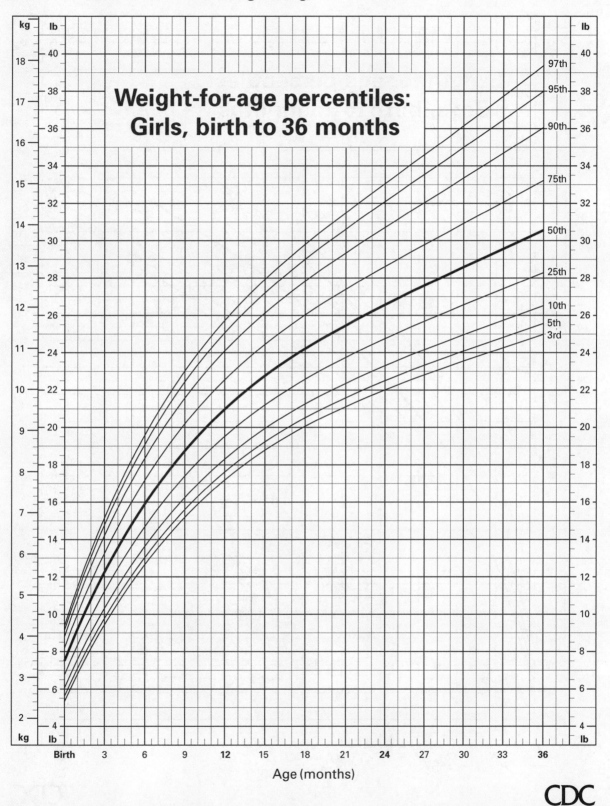

**Weight-for-age percentiles:
Girls, birth to 36 months**

Source: Developed by the National Center for Health Statistics in collaboration with the National Center for Chronic Disease Prevention and Health Promotion (2000).

TABLE D-3   Boys: Birth to 36 Months Length-for-Age

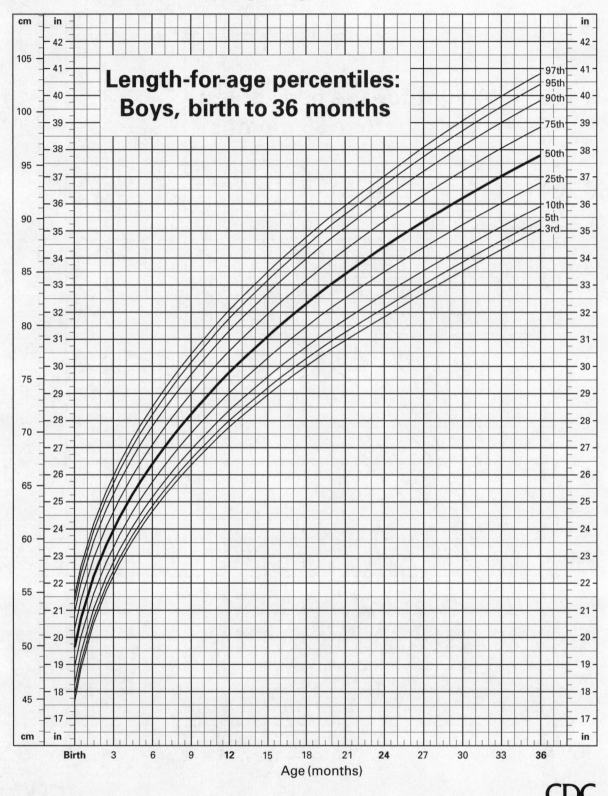

Length-for-age percentiles: Boys, birth to 36 months

Source: Developed by the National Center for Health Statistics in collaboration with the National Center for Chronic Disease Prevention and Health Promotion (2000).

TABLE D-4   Girls: Birth to 36 Months Length-for-Age

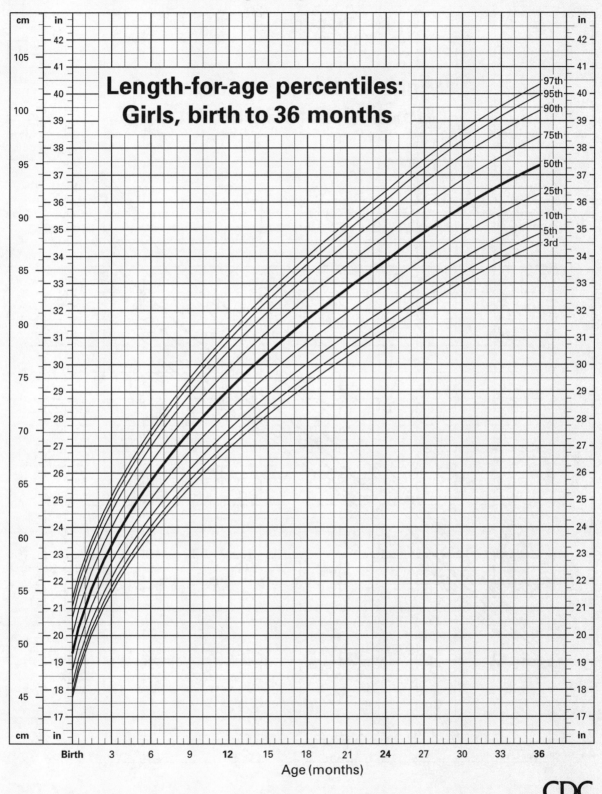

Length-for-age percentiles: Girls, birth to 36 months

Age (months)

CDC
CENTERS FOR DISEASE CONTROL AND PREVENTION

Source: Developed by the National Center for Health Statistics in collaboration with the National Center for Chronic Disease Prevention and Health Promotion (2000).

TABLE D-5   Boys: Birth to 36 Months Weight-for-Length

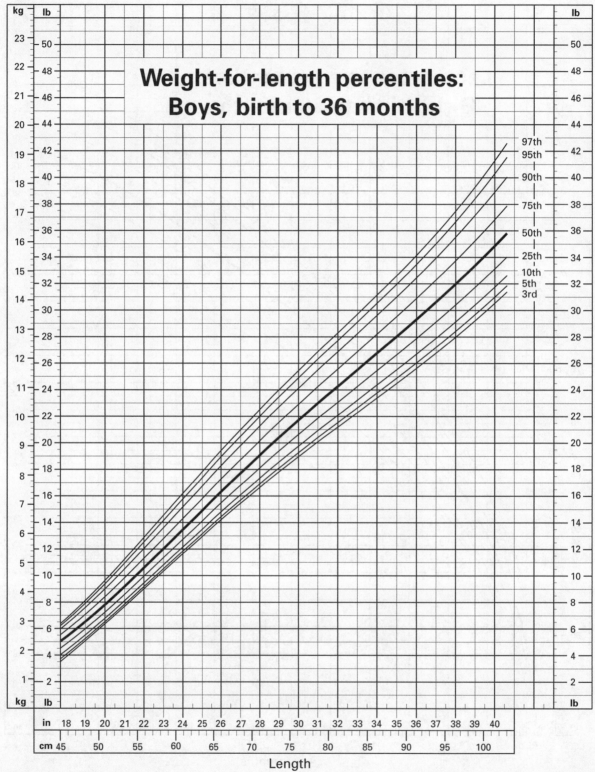

Weight-for-length percentiles:
Boys, birth to 36 months

Length

Revised and corrected June 8, 2000.

Source: Developed by the National Center for Health Statistics in collaboration with the National Center for Chronic Disease Prevention and Health Promotion (2000).

TABLE D-6   Girls: Birth to 36 Months Weight-for-Length

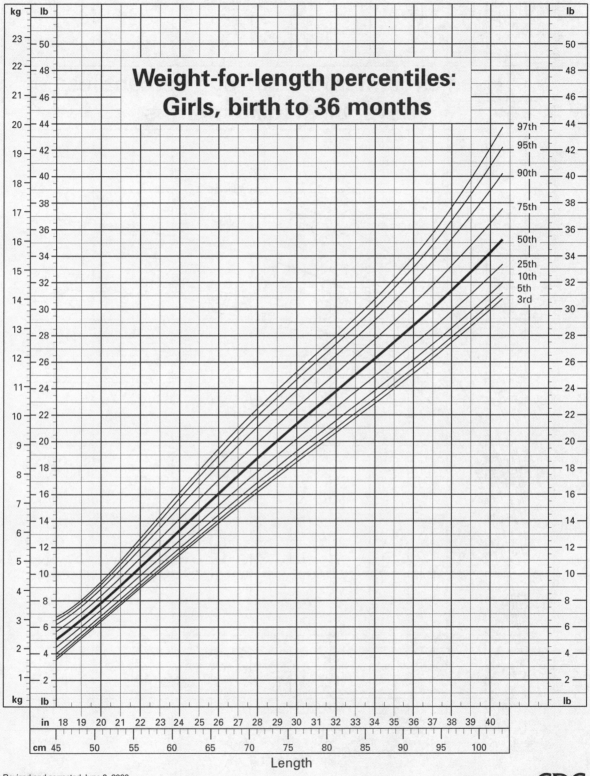

Weight-for-length percentiles: Girls, birth to 36 months

Length

Revised and corrected June 8, 2000.

Source: Developed by the National Center for Health Statistics in collaboration with the National Center for Chronic Disease Prevention and Health Promotion (2000).

TABLE D-7   Boys: Birth to 36 Months Head Circumference-for-Age

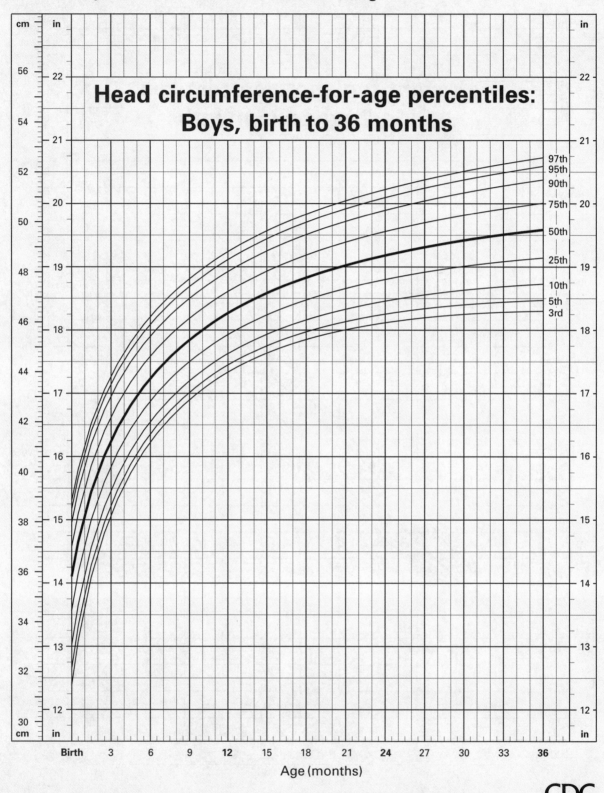

Head circumference-for-age percentiles:
Boys, birth to 36 months

Source: Developed by the National Center for Health Statistics in collaboration with the National Center for Chronic Disease Prevention and Health Promotion (2000).

TABLE D-8   **Girls: Birth to 36 Months Head Circumference-for-Age**

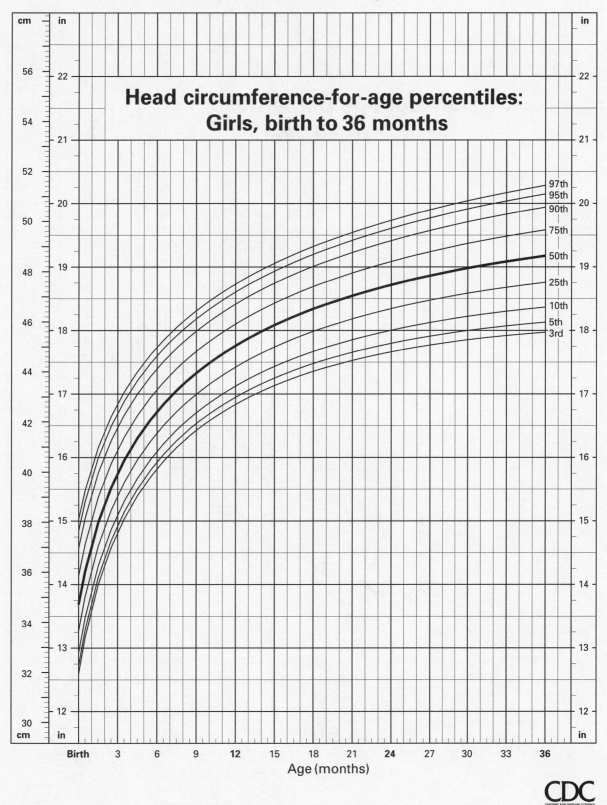

Head circumference-for-age percentiles:
Girls, birth to 36 months

Age (months)

Source: Developed by the National Center for Health Statistics in collaboration with the National Center for Chronic Disease Prevention and Health Promotion (2000).

TABLE D-9 Boys: 2 to 20 Years Weight-for-Age

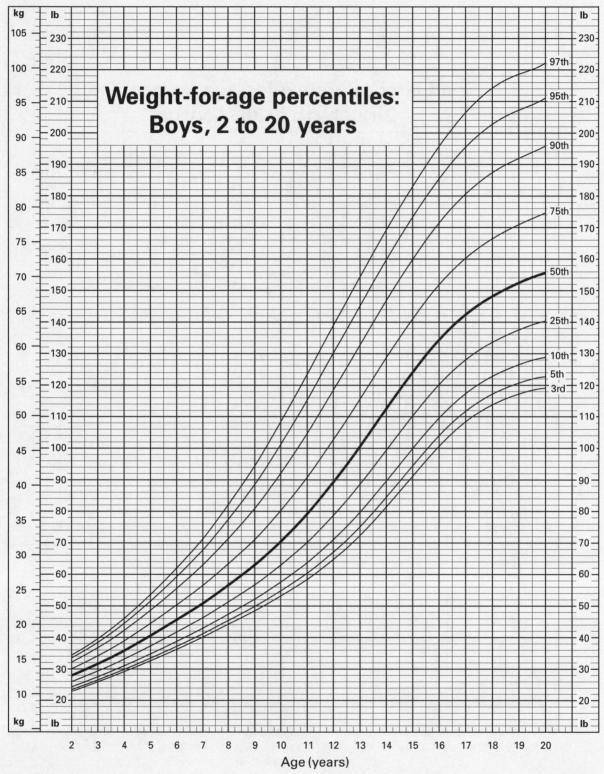

Weight-for-age percentiles: Boys, 2 to 20 years

Source: Developed by the National Center for Health Statistics in collaboration with the National Center for Chronic Disease Prevention and Health Promotion (2000).

TABLE D-10   Girls: 2 to 20 Years Weight-for-Age

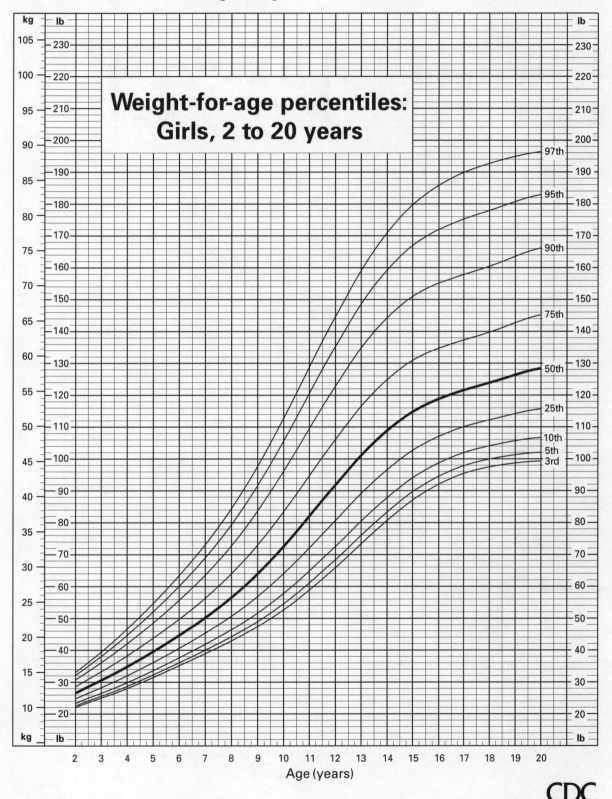

Weight-for-age percentiles: Girls, 2 to 20 years

CDC
CENTERS FOR DISEASE CONTROL AND PREVENTION

Source: Developed by the National Center for Health Statistics in collaboration with the National Center for Chronic Disease Prevention and Health Promotion (2000).

TABLE D-11   Boys: 2 to 20 Years Stature-for-Age

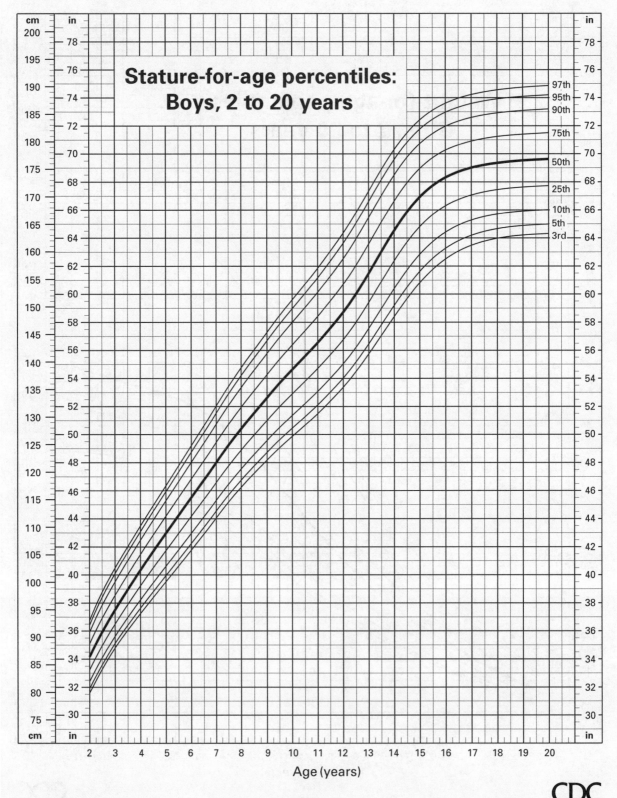

Stature-for-age percentiles:
Boys, 2 to 20 years

Age (years)

CDC

Source: Developed by the National Center for Health Statistics in collaboration with the National Center for Chronic Disease Prevention and Health Promotion (2000).

TABLE D-12   Girls: 2 to 20 Years Stature-for-Age

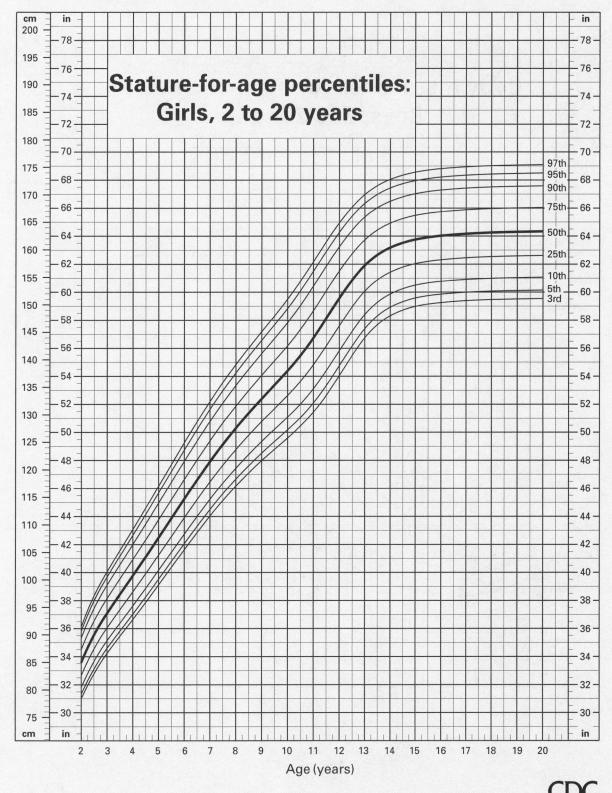

Stature-for-age percentiles:
Girls, 2 to 20 years

Source: Developed by the National Center for Health Statistics in collaboration with the National Center for Chronic Disease Prevention and Health Promotion (2000).

TABLE D-13   Boys: 2 to 20 Years Body Mass Index-for-Age

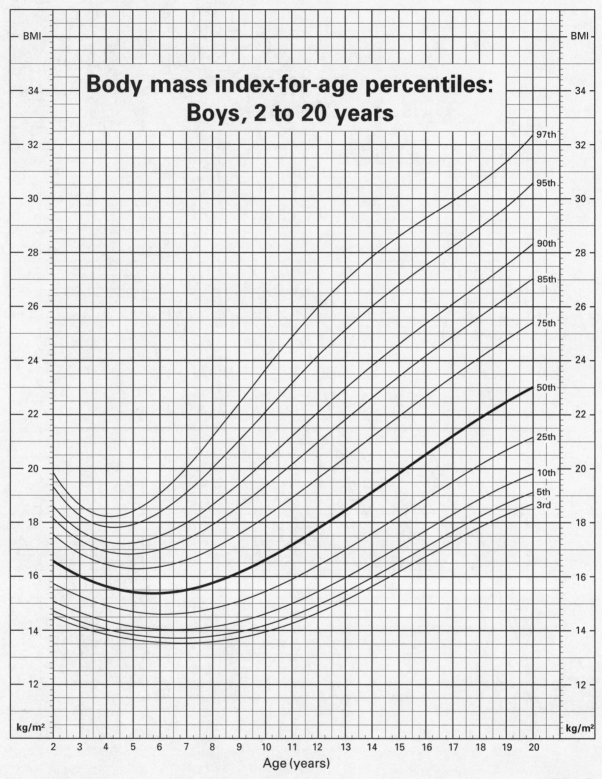

Body mass index-for-age percentiles:
Boys, 2 to 20 years

Source: Developed by the National Center for Health Statistics in collaboration with the National Center for Chronic Disease Prevention and Health Promotion (2000).

TABLE D-14   Girls: 2 to 20 Years Body Mass Index-for-Age

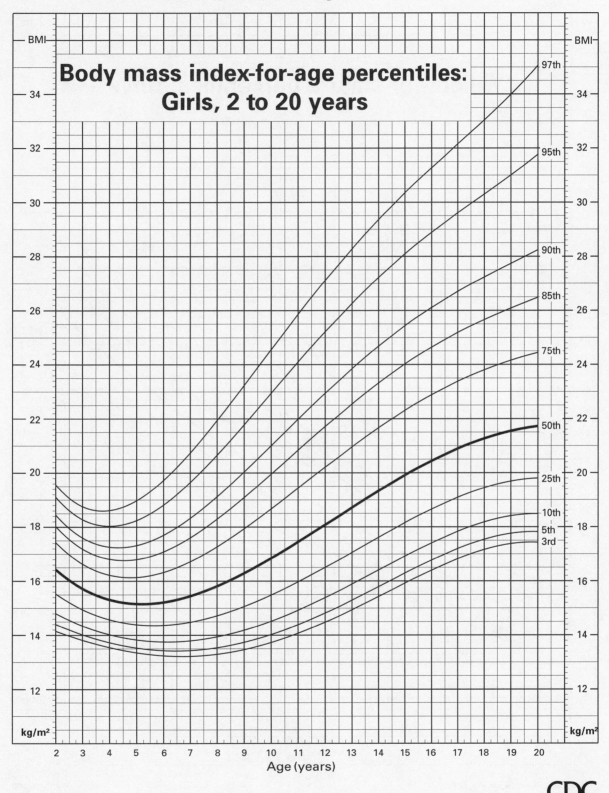

Body mass index-for-age percentiles:
Girls, 2 to 20 years

Source: Developed by the National Center for Health Statistics in collaboration with the National Center for Chronic Disease Prevention and Health Promotion (2000).

TABLE D-15   Boys: 2 to 5 Years Weight-for-Stature

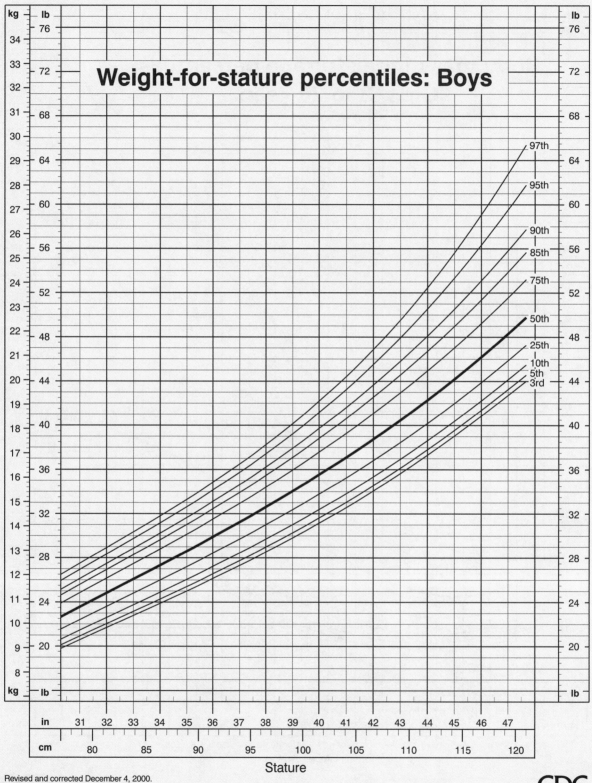

Weight-for-stature percentiles: Boys

Stature

Revised and corrected December 4, 2000.

Source: Developed by the National Center for Health Statistics in collaboration with the National Center for Chronic Disease Prevention and Health Promotion (2000).

TABLE D-16   Girls: 2 to 5 Years Weight-for-Stature

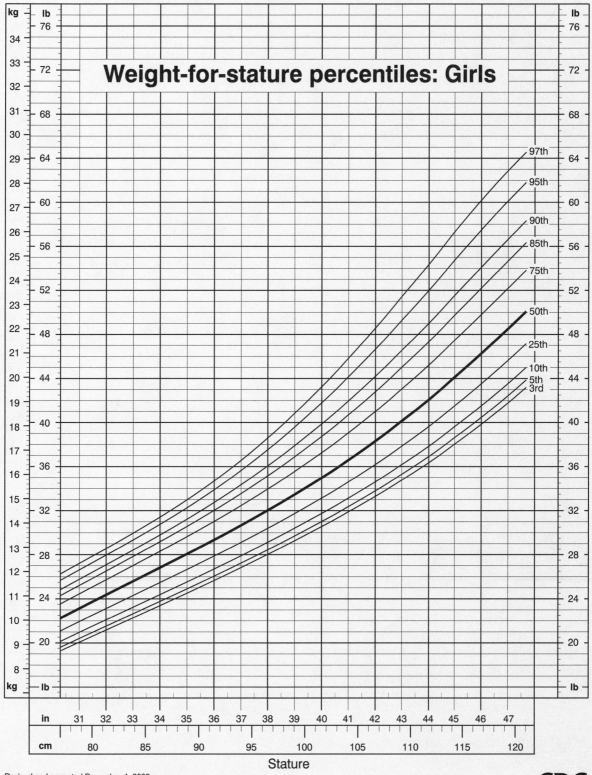

Weight-for-stature percentiles: Girls

Revised and corrected December 4, 2000.

Source: Developed by the National Center for Health Statistics in collaboration with the National Center for Chronic Disease Prevention and Health Promotion (2000).

Weights and Measures

TABLE E-1 Common Weights and Measures

Measure	Equivalent	Measure	Equivalent
3 tsp	1 tbsp	1 fl oz	28.35 g
2 tbsp	1 oz	½ c	120 g
4 tbsp	¼ c	1 c	240 g
8 tbsp	½ c	1 lb	454 g
16 tbsp	1 c		
	1 g	1 ml	
2 c	1 pt	1 tsp	5 ml
4 c	1 qt	1 tbsp	15 ml
4 qt	1 gal	1 fl oz	30 ml
1 tsp	5 g	1 c	240 ml
1 tbsp	15 g	1 pt	480 ml
1 oz	28.35 g	1 qt	960 ml
	1 L	1000 ml	

TABLE E-2 Weights and Measures Conversions

U.S. System to Metric		Metric to U.S. System	
U.S. Measure	**Metric Measure**	**Metric Measure**	**U.S. Measure**
Length		Length	
1 in	25.0 mm	1 mm	0.04 in
1 ft	0.3 m	1 m	3.3 ft
Mass		Mass	
1 g	64.8 mg	1 mg	0.015 g
1 oz	28.35 g	1 g	0.035 oz
1 lb	0.45 kg	1 kg	2.2 lb
1 short ton	907.1 kg	1 metric ton	1.102 short tons
Volume		Volume	
1 cu in	16.0 cm3	1 cm^3	0.06 in^3
1 tsp	5.0 ml	1 mL	0.2 tsp
1 tbsp	15.0 ml	1 mL	0.07 tbsp
1 fl oz	30.0 ml	1 mL	0.03 oz
1 c	0.24 L	1 L	4.2 c
1 pt	0.47 L	1 L	2.1 pt
1 qt (liq)	0.95 L	1 L	1.1 qt
1 gal	0.004 m^3	1 m^3	264.0 gal
1 pk	0.009 m^3	1 m^3	113.0 pk
1 bu	0.04 m^3	1 m^3	28.0 bu
Energy		Energy	
1 cal	4.18 J	1 J	0.24 cal

Temperature

To convert Celsius degrees into Fahrenheit, multiply by $\frac{9}{5}$ and add 32.

To convert Fahrenheit degrees into Celsius, subtract 32 and multiply by $\frac{5}{9}$. For example:

$$30°C = (30 \times \frac{9}{5} + 32)°F = (54 + 32)°F = 86°F \qquad 90°F = (90 - 32) \times \frac{5}{9}°C = 58 \times \frac{5}{9}°C = 32.2°C$$

Food Exchange Lists

SOURCE AND CREDITS

The information in this appendix has been derived from the September 2007 edition of the Food Exchanges Lists for Diabetes and is used with the permission of the American Dietetic Association. For ease of reference, it will be referred to as the Lists throughout this appendix.

When professionals apply the tables in this appendix, they follow the comprehensive guidelines presented in the original booklet. Students and nonprofessionals should not apply the tables in this appendix without the supervision of one or both of the following:

1. The instructor using this book
2. A registered dietitian

For the permission to include the data in this appendix, the publisher and the authors express their appreciation to:

1. The American Diabetes Association, Inc., and the American Dietetic Association
2. Those individual professionals who reviewed and updated the original document:
   - Madelyn L Wheeler, MS, RD, FADA
   - Anne Daly, MS, RD
   - Alison Evert, MS, RD
   - Marion Franz, MS, RD
   - Patti Geil, MS, RD
   - Lea Ann Holzmeister, RD
   - Karmeen Kulkami, MS, RD
   - Emily Loghmani, MS, RD
   - Tami A. Ross, RD

As discussed in Chapter 18, the principles of using the List are the same for the 2003 and 2007 editions. However, the 2007 list contains more than 700 foods and the levels of the major nutrients are also provided for each food. In view of the size of the Lists, it will not be reproduced here. Instead, a number of selected foods are presented.

BACKGROUND

Planning is based on this specifically prepared nutrient database of almost 700 foods. The serving sizes of the foods in each list (starches, fruits, milks, vegetables, meats, fats, etc.) reflect the mean macronutrient and energy values for each of the groups in this database.

Foods included are those commonly eaten by a majority of individuals in the United States. Many are core foods in the U.S. food supply, while some foods represent ethnic or other eating preferences (e.g., vegetarian). In almost all instances, the foods from each list are based on commercially prepared products rather than homemade recipes, because of the extreme variability of the latter. Wherever possible, nutrition values represent generic rather than name brand, or are an average of several nationally available name brands. Some foods may be in the database in more than one form. Vegetables, for example, are fresh raw as well as fresh or frozen cooked, and canned. Some foods are in two lists (e.g., beans, peas, and lentils), and some are in two lists but in different serving sizes (peanut butter, for example).

The first column of each of the tables indicates the source of the nutrient data.

1. The most common source of energy and nutrient values for foods is the United States Department of Agriculture (USDA) Nutrient Database for Standard Reference.[a] It is the foundation for most food composition databases in the public and private sectors and is identified by the USDA 5-digit number beginning with a 0, 1, 2, or 4.
2. Some foods are from the USDA's Food and Nutrient Database for Dietary Studies[b] and are identified by a 5-digit number starting with 5, 7, or 9.
3. The other main source is an average of nutrition facts from food labels of similar foods and is designated "Label."
4. Occasionally nutrition information was obtained from a recipe and is designated "Recipe." Recipes used for the List are on file with this data.

---

[a]USDA, Agricultural Research Service, 2006. USDA National Nutrient Database for Standard Reference, Release 19. Nutrient Data Laboratory Home Page. http://www.ars.usda.gov/ba/bhnrc/ndl. Accessed August 17, 2007.

[b]USDA Food and Nutrient Database for Dietary Studies, 1.0. (2004). Beltsville, MD: Agricultural Research Service, Food Surveys Research Group. http://www.barc.usda.gov/ bhnrc/foodsurvey/fields_ intro.html. Accessed August 17, 2007.

The food names and serving size columns cross-reference the same designations in the List. The fourth column, grams per serving, is the metric weight of the portion, providing more definition for words such as "medium," as well as providing specifics for those who are doing carbohydrate gram counting as a meal planning method. The rest of the columns represent the energy and nutrients used in the Nutrition Facts portion of food labels. Polyunsaturated and monounsaturated fatty acids are included because of the configuration of the fat list. The following abbreviations are used:

SFA = saturated fatty acids trans = trans-fatty acids
PUFA = polyunsaturated fatty acids
MUFA = monounsaturated laity acids
chol = cholesterol
sod = sodium
carb = carbohydrate
pro = protein
ETOH = 200 proof alcohol

LIST CATEGORIES

The Lists include the following:

Starch list
  Bread
  Cereals and grains
  Crackers and snacks
  Starchy vegetables
  Beans, peas, and lentils
Sweets, desserts, and other carbohydrates list
  Beverages, sodas, and energy/sports drinks
  Brownies, cake, cookies, gelatin, pie, and pudding
  Candy, spreads, sweets, sweeteners, syrups, and toppings
  Condiments and sauces
  Doughnuts, muffins, pastries, and sweet breads
  Frozen bars, frozen desserts, frozen yogurt, and ice cream
  Granola bars, meal replacement bars/shakes, and trail mix
Fruit list
  Fruits
  Fruit juices
Vegetables (nonstarchy) list
Meat and meat substitutes list
  Lean meat
  Medium-fat meat
  High-fat meat
  Plant-based proteins (for beans, peas, and lentils, see starch list)
Milk list
  Fat-free and low-fat milk
  Reduced fat

Whole milk
  Dairy-like foods
Fat list
  Monounsaturated fats list
  Polyunsaturated fats list
  Saturated fats list
Fast-foods list
  Breakfast sandwiches
  Main dishes/entrees
  Oriental
  Pizzas
  Sandwiches
  Salads
  Sides/appetizers
  Desserts
Combination foods list
  Entrees
  Frozen entrees/meals
  Salads (deli style)
  Soups
Free foods list
  Low carbohydrate foods
  Modified-fat foods with carbohydrate
  Condiments
  Free snacks
  Drinks/mixes
Alcohol list

Table F-1 presents an example of nutrient data for each of the entries above.

MEASUREMENT, NUTRIENTS, AND LISTS

To apply information in the lists in this appendix, we need the two groups of data presented in Tables F-2 and F-3.

The following provides some example of foods in the Lists including name of food, serving size, and exchanges. It is important to realize that none of the nutrient data in Table F-1 is presented. If the levels of sodium and fat are important to the patient a healthcare provider will provide details about the nutrient data of the foods. For details, your instructors can provide assistance.

Starch List

Serving size for one exchange for some examples in this list is:

1. ½ c of cooked cereal, grain, or starchy vegetable
2. ½ c of cooked rice or pasta
3. 1 oz of a bread product, such as 1 slice of bread
4. ¾ to 1 oz of most snack foods (some snack foods may also have added fat)

One starch exchange equals 15 g of carbohydrate, 3 g of protein, 0–1 g of fat, and 80 calories.

TABLE F-1   An Example of Nutrient Data for Each List and Sub-list from the 2007 Food Exchange Lists

Source Food[a]	Serving Size	Grams per serving	Cal	Fat (g)	SFA (g)	Trans (g)	PUFA (g)	MUFA (g)	Chol (mg)	Sod (mg)	Carb (g)	Fiber (g)	Sugars (g)	Pro (g)
Starch														
Breads														
18069 Bread, white	1 sl	28	69	1.2	0.3	ND	0.5	0.2	0	134	12.4	0.6	1.0	2.0
Cereals														
08065 Rice krispies	0.75 c	20	77	0.3	0.1	ND	0.1	0.1	0	191	17.4	0.1	1.8	1.2
Grains/Rice/Pasta														
20121 Spaghetti, cooked, firm	0.33 c	48	85	0.3	0	ND	0.1	0	0	0	13.1	0.8	0.6	2.2
Crackers/Snacks														
19050 Tortilla chips	0.75 oz	21	82	0.8	0	ND	0	0	0	111	18.0	3.0	0.1	2.2
Starchy vegetables														
11367 Potato, white, peeled, cooked	3 oz	85	73	0.1	0	0	0	0	0	4	17.0	1.5	1.4	1.5
Beans/Peas/Lentils														
16038 Beans, navy, cooked	½ c	91	129	0.5	0.1	ND	0.2	0	0	1	23.9	5.8	2.0	7.9
Sweets, Desserts and other carbohydrates														
Beverages, Sodas, and Energy/Sports Drinks														
Label Sports drink	1 c	237	50	0	0	0	0	0	0	110	14.0	0	14	0
Brownie, Cake, Cookies, Gelatin, Pie, and Pudding														
Brownie, small, unfrosted	1 (1-¾ sq. ⅞" high)	28	115	4.6	1.2	ND	0.6	2.5	5	88	18.1	0.6	10.4	1.4
Candy, Spreads, Sweets, Sweeteners, Syrups, and Toppings														
19129 Syrup, pancake type, regular Jelly	1 T	20	50	0	0	0	0	0	0	34	13.2	0	9.5	0
Condiments and Sauces														
06150 Barbecue sauce, bottled	3 T	52	79	0.2	0	0	0.1	0	0	587	19.0	0.3	13.7	0
Doughnuts, Muffins, Pastries, and Sweet Breads														
Doughnut, yeast type, glazed	1 (3-¾" diameter)	60	239	11.5	3.3	ND	1.7	6.0	18	232	30.4	1.3	11.7	3.7
Frozen Bars, Frozen Desserts, Frozen Yogurt, and Ice Cream														
Label Ice cream	½ c	72	165	10.0	4.5	ND	0.4	2.7	23	102	15.0	0	1.5	3.0
Granola Bars, Meal Replacement Bars/Shakes, and Trail Mix														
19015 Granola bar	1 bar (1 oz)	28	134	5.6	1.0	ND	3.4	1.2	0	83	18.3	1.5	6.5	2.9
Fruits														
Fresh/Canned/Dried Fruits														
09266 Pineapple, fresh	0.75 c	116	56	0.1	0	0	0	0	0	1	14.7	1.6	10.8	0.6
Fruit juices														
09294 Prune juice	0.33 c	84	59	0	0	0	0	0	0	3	14.7	0.9	11.3	0.5
Vegetables														
11283 Onions, fresh, cooked	½ c	105	46	0.2	0	0	0.1	0	0	3	10.7	1.5	6.5	1.4
Meats and Meat Substitutes														
Lean Meats														
05220 Turkey breast (cutlet), no skin, roasted	1 oz	28	38	0.2	0.1	ND	0.1	0	23	15	0	0	0	8.5
Medium Fat Meats														
13150 Beef, short ribs, cooked	1 oz	28	84	5.1	2.2	ND	0.2	2.3	26	16	0	0	0	8.7
High Fat Meats														
07064 Pork sausage, cooked	1 oz	28	104	8.8	3.1	ND	1.1	3.9	23	366	0.3	0	0.3	5.6
Plant-Based Proteins (for Beans, Peas, and Lentils, see Starch List)														
16126 Tofu, firm	4 oz (½ c)	114	80	4.7	1.0	ND	2.0	1.4	0	14	1.9	1.0	0.7	9.3

continues

[a]The "source food" is indicated by:
• an identification number followed by the name of a food; OR
• the word label followed by the name of a food
The meaning of these two items is explained under the section background for the Food Exchange Lists.

TABLE F-1 (continued)

Source Food[a]	Serving Size	Grams per serving	Cal	Fat (g)	SFA (g)	Trans (g)	PUFA (g)	MUFA (g)	Chol (mg)	Sod (mg)	Carb (g)	Fiber (g)	Sugars (g)	Pro (g)
Milk														
Fat-free milks/low-fat milks														
01088 Buttermilk, low-fat (1%)	1 c	245	98	2.2	1.3	0	0.1	0.6	10	257	11.7	0	11.7	8.1
Reduced-fat milks														
01079 Milk, reduced-fat (2%)	1 c	244	130	5.0	3.0	0	0.2	1.4	20	130	12.0	0	12.0	8.1
Whole milks														
01077 Milk, whole	1 c	244	150	8.0	5.0	0.2	0.5	2.0	33	120	12.0	0	12.0	8.0
Dairy-like foods														
Label Yogurt and juice blend	1 c	236	115	4.1	0.5	0.0	2.5	1.0	0	55	34.0	0	32.0	3.0
Fats														
Monounsaturated fats														
16098 Peanut butter	1.5 T	8	48	4.2	0.8	0.0	1.2	2.0	0	40	1.5	0.5	0.6	2.0
Polyunsaturated fats														
04510 Oil, safflower	1 t	4	40	4.5	0.3	ND	3.4	0.6	0	0	0	0	0	0
Saturated fats														
04002 Bacon grease	1 t	4	39	4.3	2.0	ND	0.5	1.9	4	0	0	0	0	0
Fast foods														
Breakfast sandwiches														
Label Sausage biscuit sandwich	1 biscuit	137	493	34.0	10.0	4.5	3.3	14.2	28	1136	34.0	0.7	3.0	13.0
Main Dishes/Entrees														
Label Chicken nuggets	1 serving; ~6 nuggets	93	263	16.5	3.3	0.8	5.4	6.8	38	624	14.7	0	0	14.7
Oriental														
Label Fried rice, no meat	½ c	98	173	5.9	1.1	0	2.6	1.5	47	376	24.0	1.5	0	5.4
Pizzas														
Label Cheese/pepperoni pizza, regular crust	1 sl (⅛, 14″ pizza)	117	321	13.6	5.6	0.1	2.4	4.3	32	795	34.7	1.6	4.0	14.0
Sandwiches														
21118 Hot dog with bun, plain	1	98	242	14.5	5.1	ND	1.7	6.9	44	670	18.0	1.0	2.7	10.4
Salads														
21052 Salad, side (no dressing or cheese)	1 serving	138	22	0.1	0	0	0	0	0	36	4.4	0.8	3.0	1.7
Sides/Appetizers														
Label Onion rings. Breaded, fried French fries	3 oz serving	94	340	18.0	3.8	3.7	0.8	7.5	1	608	40.0	1.0	4.0	4.0
Desserts														
Label Milkshake, any flavor	1 small serving, ~12 oz	363	500	12.5	10.0	1.7	0.6	3.5	47	230	85.0	1.3	38.0	13.7
Combination foods														
Entrees														
22570 Lasagna with meat and sauce	1 c	227	293	11.4.	5.0	ND	0.6	3.7	43	776	27.9	3.4	10.7	19.4
Frozen Entrees/Meals														
Label Pot pie, double crust	1 pie (7 oz)	198	390	21.3	6.7	ND	4.5	8.9	54	778	39.3	2.7	1.3	9.7
Salads (Deli-Style)														
Label Coleslaw, deli style	½ c	100	130	7.0	1.0	ND	4.1	1.5	5	160	16.0	2.0	14.0	1.0
Soups														
06402 Soup, bean	1 c	247	116	1.5	0	ND	0.5	0.5	0	1198	19.8	4.4	3.3	5.6
Free foods														
Low carbohydrate foods														
Modified fat foods with carbohydrate														
Condiments														
06150 Barbecue sauce	2 t	12	1	0	0	0	0	0	0	130	4.2	0.1	3.0	0
01069 Creamer, non-dairy, powder	1 T	4	22	1.4	1.3	ND	0	0	0	7	2.2	0	2.2	0.2
Free snacks														
Drinks/mixes														
18228 Saltine-type crackers, free food size	2 crackers	6	26	0.7	0.1	0.2	0.1	0.4	0	64	4.3	0.2	0	0.8
11457 Spinach, fresh, raw	1 c	30	7	0	0	0	0	0	0	24	1.1	0.7	0.1	0.9
14355 Tea, brewed	1 c													
Alcohol														
14096 Wine, red (14.0% alcohol)	5 fl oz	148	106	0	0	0	0	0	0	7	2.5	0	2.5	0.3

TABLE F-2   Common Measurements

3 tsp = 1 tbsp	4 oz = ½ c
4 tbsp = ¼ c	8 oz = 1 c
5-⅓ tbsp = ⅓ c	1 c = ½ pint

One starch exchange equals 15 g of carbohydrate, 3 g of protein, 0–1 g of fat, and 80 calories.

Bread

Bagel, 4 oz	¼ (1 oz)
Bread, reduced-calorie	2 slices (1-½ oz)
Bread, white, whole wheat, pumpernickel, rye	1 slice (1 oz)
Bread sticks, crisp, 4 in. × ½ in.	4 (⅔ oz)
English muffin	½
Hot dog bun or hamburger bun	½ (1 oz)
Naan, 8 × 2 in.	¼
Pancake, 4 in. across, ¼ in. thick	1
Pita, 6 in. across	½
Roll, plain, small	1 (1 oz)
Raisin bread, unfrosted, 1 slice	1 slice (1 oz)
Tortilla, corn, 6 in. across	1
Tortilla, flour, 6 in. across	1
Tortilla, flour, 10 in. across	2 ½
Waffle, 4 in. square or across, reduced-fat	1

Cereals and Grains

Bran cereals	½ c
Bulgur	½ c
Cereals, cooked	½ c
Cereals, unsweetened, ready-to-eat	¾ c
Cornmeal (dry)	3 tbsp
Couscous	⅓ c
Flour (dry)	3 tbsp
Granola, low-fat	¼ c
Grape-Nuts	¼ c
Grits	½ c
Kasha	½ c
Millet	¼ c
Muesli	¼ c
Oats	½ c
Pasta	⅓ c
Puffed cereal	1 ½ c
Rice, white or brown	⅓ c
Shredded Wheat	½ c
Sugar-frosted cereal	½ c
Wheat germ	3 tbsp

One starch exchange equals 15 g of carbohydrate, 3 g of protein, 0–1 g of fat, and 80 calories.

TABLE F-3   The Amount of Macronutrients in One Serving of Each Food Represented in Each Food Group or List

Groups/Lists	Carbohydrate (grams)	Protein (grams)	Fat (grams)	Calories
Carbohydrate Group				
Starch	15	3	0–1	80
Sweets, desserts, and other carbohydrates list	15	varies	varies	varies
Fruit	15	—	—	60
Vegetables (non-starchy)	5	2	—	25
Meat and meat substitutes				
Lean	—	7	0–3	35–55
Medium-fat	—	7	5	75
High-fat	—	7	8	100
Plant-based protein	varies	varies	varies	varies
Milk				
Fat-free and low-fat	12	8	0–3	90
Reduced-fat	12	8	5	120
Whole	12	8	8	150
Dairy-like foods	varies	varies	varies	varies
Fats	—	—	5	45
Fast foods	varies	varies	varies	varies
Combination foods	varies	varies	varies	varies
Free food	varies	varies	varies	varies

Crackers and Snacks

Animal crackers	8
Graham cracker, 2 1-in. square	3
Matzoh	¾ oz
Melba toast	4 slices
Oyster crackers	24
Popcorn (popped, no fat added, or low-fat microwave)	3 c
Pretzels	¾ oz
Rice cakes, 4 in. across	2
Saltine-type crackers	6
Snack chips, fat-free or baked (tortilla, potato)	15–20 (¾ oz)
Whole wheat crackers, no fat added	2–5 (¾ oz)

Starchy Vegetables

Baked beans	⅓ c
Corn	½ c
Corn on cob, large	½ cob (5 oz)
Mixed vegetables with corn, peas, or pasta	1 c
Peas, green	½ c
Plantain	½ c
Potato, boiled	½ c or ½ medium (3 oz)
Potato, baked with skin	¼ large (3 oz)
Potato, mashed	½ c
Squash, winter (acorn, butternut, pumpkin)	1 c
Yam, sweet potato, plain	½ c

Beans, Peas, and Lentils

Count as 1 starch exchange, plus 1 very lean meat exchange.

Beans and peas (garbanzo, pinto, kidney, white, split, black-eyed)	½ c
Lima beans	⅔ c
Lentils	½ c
Miso	3 tbsp

Sweets, Desserts, and Other Carbohydrates List

In general one exchange equals 15 grams of carbohydrate, or 1 starch, or 1 fruit, or 1 milk. In view of the wide variety of foods covered in this list, exchanges per serving will vary. In the following, foods are selected from different groups within the list and the possible exchanges per serving are indicated. Note each food contributes multiple types of exchanges.

Fruit List

In general, one fruit exchange is:

1. 1 small fresh fruit (4 oz)
2. ½ c of canned or fresh fruit or fruit juice
3. ¼ c of dried fruit

One fruit exchange equals 15 g of carbohydrate and 60 calories. The weight includes skin, core, seeds, and rind.

TABLE F-4   Number of Exchanges Represented by Each Serving of Selected Foods

Food	Serving Size	Exchanges per Serving
Angel food cake, unfrosted	1/12 cake (about 2 oz)	2 carbohydrates
Brownie, small, unfrosted	2 in. square (about 1 oz)	1 carbohydrate, 1 fat
Cake, unfrosted	2 in. square (about 1 oz)	1 carbohydrate, 1 fat
Cake, frosted	2 in. square (about 2 oz)	2 carbohydrates, 1 fat
Cookie or sandwich cookie with creme filling	2 small (about 2/3 oz)	1 carbohydrate, 1 fat
Cookies, sugar-free	3 small or 1 large (3/4–1 oz)	1 carbohydrate, 1–2 fats
Cranberry sauce, jellied	1/4 c	1/2 carbohydrates
Cupcake, frosted	1 small (about 2 oz)	2 carbohydrates, 1 fat
Doughnut, plain cake	1 medium (1/2 oz)	1/2 carbohydrates, 2 fats
Doughnut, glazed	3/4 in. across (2 oz)	2 carbohydrates, 2 fats
Energy, sport, or breakfast bar	1 bar (1/3 oz)	1/2 carbohydrates, 0–1 fat
Energy, sport, or breakfast bar	1 bar (2 oz)	2 carbohydrates, 1 fat
Fruit cobbler	1/2 c (3-1/3 oz)	3 carbohydrates, 1 fat
Fruit juice bars, frozen, 100% juice	1 bar (3 oz)	1 carbohydrate
Fruit snacks, chewy (pureed fruit concentrate)	1 roll (3/4 oz)	1 carbohydrate
Fruit spreads, 100% fruit	1-1/2 Tbs	1 carbohydrate
Gelatin, regular	1/2 c	1 carbohydrate
Gingersnaps	3	1 carbohydrate
Granola or snack bar, regular or low-fat	1 bar (1 oz)	1/2 carbohydrates
Honey	1 tbsp	1 carbohydrate
Ice cream	1/2 c	1 carbohydrate, 2 fats
Ice cream, light	1/2 c	1 carbohydrate, 1 fat
Ice cream, low-fat	1/2 c	1/2 carbohydrates
Ice cream, fat-free, no sugar added	1/2 c	1 carbohydrate
Jam or jelly, regular	1 tbsp	1 carbohydrate
Milk, chocolate, whole	1 c	2 carbohydrates, 1 fat
Pie, fruit, 2 crusts	1/6 of 8 in. commercially prepared pie	3 carbohydrates, 2 fats
Pie, pumpkin or custard	1/8 of 8 in. commercially prepared pie	2 carbohydrates, 2 fats
Pudding, regular (made with reduced-fat milk)	1/2 c	2 carbohydrates
Pudding, sugar-free or sugar-free and fat-free (made with fat-free milk)	1/2 c	1 carbohydrate
Reduced-calorie meal replacement (shake)	1 can (10–11 oz)	1/2 carbohydrates, 0–1 fat
Rice milk, low-fat or fat-free, plain	1 c	1 carbohydrate
Rice milk, low-fat, flavored	1 c	1/2 carbohydrates
Salad dressing, fat-free	1/4 c	1 carbohydrate
Sherbet, sorbet	1/2 c	2 carbohydrates
Spaghetti or pasta sauce, canned	1/2 c	1 carbohydrate, 1 fat
Sports drinks	8 oz (about 1 c)	1 carbohydrate
Sugar	1 tbsp	1 carbohydrate
Sweet roll or Danish	1 (2-1/2 oz)	2-1/2 carbohydrates, 2 fats
Syrup, light	2 tbsp	1 carbohydrate
Syrup, regular	1 tbsp	1 carbohydrate
Syrup, regular	1/4 c	4 carbohydrates
Vanilla wafers	5	1 carbohydrate, 1 fat
Yogurt, frozen	1/2 c	1 carbohydrate, 0–1 fat
Yogurt, frozen, fat-free	1/3 c	1 carbohydrate
Yogurt, low-fat with fruit	1 c	3 carbohydrates, 0–1 fat

Fruit

Apple, unpeeled, small	1 (4 oz)
Applesauce, unsweetened	½ c
Apples, dried	4 rings
Apricots, fresh	4 whole (5-½ oz)
Apricots, dried	8 halves
Apricots, canned	½ c
Banana, small	1 (4 oz)
Blackberries	¾ c
Blueberries	¾ c
Cantaloupe, small	⅓ melon (11 oz) or 1 c cubes
Cherries, sweet, fresh	12 (3 oz)
Cherries, sweet, canned	½ c
Dates	3
Figs, fresh	½ large or 2 medium (3-½ oz)
Figs, dried	1 ½
Fruit cocktail	½ c
Grapefruit, large	½ (11 oz)
Grapefruit sections, canned	¾ c
Grapes, small	17 (3 oz)
Honeydew melon	1 slice (10 oz) or 1 c cubes
Kiwi	1 (3-½ oz)
Mandarin oranges, canned	¾ c
Mango, small	½ fruit (5-½ oz) or ½ c
Nectarine, small	1 (5 oz)
Orange, small	1 (6-½ oz)
Papaya	½ fruit (8 oz) or 1 c cubes
Peach, medium, fresh	1 (4 oz)
Peaches, canned	½ c
Pear, large, fresh	½ (4 oz)
Pears, canned	½ c
Pineapple, fresh	¾ c
Pineapple, canned	½ c
Plums, small	2 (5 oz)
Plums, canned	½ c
Plums, dried (prunes)	3
Raisins	2 tbsp
Raspberries	1 c
Strawberries	1-¼ c whole berries
Tangerines, small	2 (8 oz)
Watermelon	1 slice (13-½ oz) or 1-¼ c cubes

Fruit Juice

Apple juice/cider	½ c
Cranberry juice cocktail	⅓ c
Cranberry juice cocktail, reduced-calorie	1 c
Fruit juice blends, 100% juice	⅓ c
Grape juice	⅓ c
Grapefruit juice	½ c
Orange juice	½ c
Pineapple juice	½ c
Prune juice	⅓ c

Vegetable (Nonstarchy) List

In general, one vegetable exchange is:

- ½ c of cooked vegetables or vegetable juice
- 1 c of raw vegetables

One vegetable exchange (½ c cooked or 1 c raw) equals 5 g of carbohydrate, 2 g of protein, 0 g of fat, and 25 calories.

Artichoke, cooked	½
Artichoke hearts, canned, drained	½
Asparagus, frozen, cooked	½ c
Beans (green, wax, Italian)	½ c
Bean sprouts, fresh, cooked	½ c
Beets, canned, drained	½ c
Broccoli, fresh, cooked	½ c
Brussels sprouts, frozen, cooked	½ c
Cabbage, fresh, cooked	½ c
Carrots, fresh, cooked, strips or slices	½ c
Cauliflower, frozen, cooked	½ c
Celery, fresh, raw, strips	1 c
Collard greens, fresh cooked	½ c
Cucumber, with peel,	1 c
Eggplant, fresh, cooked, 1-in. cubes	½ c
Green onions (spring) or scallions,	1 c
Kohlrabi, fresh, cooked	½ c
Leeks, fresh, cooked	½ c
Mixed vegetables (without corn, peas, or pasta)	½ c
Mushrooms, fresh	1 c
Okra, fresh, cooked	½ c
Onions, fresh	1 c
Pea pods (snow), fresh	1 c
Peppers, green bell, raw, slices	1 c
Radishes	1 c
Sauerkraut, canned, rinsed, drained	½ c
Spinach, canned, drained	½ c
Squash, summer, fresh, cooked	½ c
Tomatoes, canned, regular	½ c
Tomatoes, raw	1 c
Tomato sauce	½ c
Turnips, fresh, cooked, diced	½ c
Vegetable juice	½ c
Water chestnuts, canned, drained	½ c
Zucchini, raw, slices	1 c

Meat and Meat Substitutes List

Meat and meat substitutes that contain both protein and fat are on this list. In general, one meat exchange is:

1 oz of meat, fish, poultry, or cheese
½ c of beans, peas, or lentils

Lean Meat and Substitutes

One exchange equals 0 g of carbohydrate, 7 g of protein, 0–3 g of fat, and 35–50 calories.

Beef, chuck, pot roast, lean only, cooked	1 oz
Beef, frank steak, lean, cooked	1 oz
Beef, rib roast, lean, roasted	1 oz
Catfish, cooked	1 oz
Cheese, American, fat-free	1 slice
Cheese, mozzarella, fat-free	1 oz
Chicken breast, meat only, cooked	1 oz
Chicken, dark meat, no skin, roasted	1 oz
Clams, fresh, cooked	1 oz
Cod fillet, cooked	1 oz
Cottage choose, creamed, 4.5% milk fat	0.25 c
Crab, steamed	1 oz
Flounder, cooked	1 oz
Egg white	2
Ham, boiled lean deli, sandwich type	1 oz
Ham, canned, fully cooked	1 oz
Hot dog or frankfurter	1 oz
Lamb leg, sirloin, roast, lean	1 oz
Liver, chicken, cooked	1 oz
Lobster, fresh, steamed	1 oz
Oysters, cooked	6 medium
Pork chop, cooked	1 oz
Rabbit, cooked	1 oz
Salmon, fresh, broiled or baked	1 oz
Sardines, packed in oil, drained	2 small
Sausage, smoked	1 oz
Scallops, fresh steamed	1 oz
Shrimp, fresh, cooked in water	1 oz
Steak, porterhouse, lean, broiled	1 oz
Steak, T-bone, lean, broiled	1 oz
Trout, cooked	1 oz
Tuna, fresh, cooked	1 oz
Turkey breast (cutlet), no skin, roasted	1 oz
Turkey ham	1 oz
Veal roast	1 oz

Medium-Fat Meat

One exchange equals 0 g of carbohydrate, 7 g of protein, 5 g of fat, and 50–75 calories.

Beef patty, ground regular, pan broiled (75% lean)	1 oz
Beef, prime rib, roasted	1 oz
Cheese, mozzarella (part skim milk)	1 oz
Cheese, string	1 oz
Chicken, meat and skin, fried, flour-coated	1 oz
Corned beef brisket, cooked	1 oz
Duck, wild, meat and skin, (not cooked)	1 oz
Egg, fresh	1
Fish, fried, cornmeal coating	1 oz
Lamb, ground, broiled	1 oz
Meatloaf	1 oz
Pork, Boston blade, roasted	1 oz
Sausage, hard	1 oz

Plant-Based Proteins

For beans, peas, and lentils, see starch list.

Since the contribution of one serving of each of the following foods may vary with the formulation for its manufacture, you instructor will provide assistance on this issue.

Breakfast patty, meatless (soy-based)	1 patty (1-½ oz)
Cashew butter, plain	1 tbsp
Frankfurter (hot dog), meatless (soy-based)	1 frankfurter (1-½ oz)
Meatless burger (soy-based)	1 patty (3 oz)
Meatless "beef" crumbles (soy-based)	2 oz
Peanut butter, smooth or crunchy	1 tbsp
Tofu, firm	4 oz (½ c)

Milk List

One milk exchange equals 12 g of carbohydrate and 8 g of protein.

Fat-Free and Low-Fat Milk

There are 0–3 g fat per serving.

Fat-free milk	1 c
1/2% milk	1 c
1% milk	1 c
Buttermilk, low-fat or fat-free	1 c
Evaporated fat-free milk	½ c
Fat-free dry milk	⅓ c dry
Soy milk, low-fat or fat-free	1 c
Yogurt, fat-free, flavored, sweetened with nonnutritive sweetener and fructose	⅔ c (6 oz)
Yogurt, plain fat-free	⅔ c (6 oz)

Reduced-Fat

There are 5 g fat per serving.

2% milk	1 c
Acidophilus milk, 2%	1 c

Whole Milk

There are 8 g fat per serving.

Whole milk	1 c
Evaporated whole milk	½ c
Yogurt, plain	
(made from whole milk)	¾ c

Dairy-Like Foods

Nutrient levels vary. Instructor will provide assistance.

Eggnog, whole milk	½ c
Soy milk, regular, plain	1 c
Yogurt with fruit,	
low-fat, container, 6 oz	1

Fat List

In general, one fat exchange is:

1. 1 tsp of regular margarine or vegetable oil
2. 1 tbsp of regular salad dressings

Monounsaturated Fats List

One fat exchange equals 5 g fat and 45 calories.

Avocado, medium	2 tbsp (1 oz)
Oil (canola, olive, peanut)	1 tsp
Olives: ripe (black)	8 large
green, stuffed	10 large
Nuts: almonds, cashews	6 nuts
mixed (50% peanuts)	6 nuts
peanuts	10 nuts
pecans	4 halves
Peanut butter, smooth or crunchy	½ tbsp
Sesame seeds	1 tbsp
Tahini or sesame paste	2 tsp

Polyunsaturated Fats List

One fat exchange equals 5 g fat and 45 calories.

Margarine: stick, tub, or squeeze	1 tsp
lower-fat spread	
(30% to 50% vegetable oil)	1 tbsp
Mayonnaise: regular	1 tsp
reduced-fat	1 tbsp
Nuts: walnuts, English	4 halves
Oil (corn, safflower, soybean)	1 tsp
Salad dressing: regular	1 tbsp
reduced-fat	2 tbsp
Miracle Whip salad dressing:	
regular	2 tsp
reduced-fat	1 tbsp
Seeds: pumpkin, sunflower	1 tbsp

Saturated Fats List

One fat exchange equals 5 g of fat and 45 calories.

Bacon, cooked	1 slice
	(20 slices/lb)
Bacon, grease	1 tsp
Butter: stick	1 tsp
whipped	2 tsp
reduced-fat	1 tbsp
Chitterlings, boiled	2 tbsp (½ oz)
Coconut, sweetened, shredded	2 tbsp
Coconut milk	1 tbsp
Cream, half and half	2 tbsp
Cream cheese: regular	1 tbsp (½ oz)
reduced-fat	1-½ tbsp (¾ oz)
Shortening or lard	1 tsp
Sour cream: regular	2 tbsp
reduced-fat	3 tbsp

Fast-Foods List

Because of variations in nutrient contents of fast foods, exchanges per serving are expressed in a combination, e.g., one serving of pizza (with meat) may provide 2-½ carbohydrate exchanges plus 2 medium-fat meat exchanges. Your instructor will provide you with guidance. The following food samples do not provide exchanges per serving.

Breakfast Sandwiches

Egg, cheese, meat,	
English muffin sandwich	1 sandwich
Sausage biscuit sandwich	1 biscuit

Main Dishes/Entrees

Burrito, beef and beans (fast food)	1 serving
	(about 8 oz)
Chicken breast, breaded and fried	1 serving
	(about 5 oz)
Chicken nuggets	1 serving
	(~6 nuggets)

Oriental

Beef, chicken, or shrimp with	
vegetable and sauce	1 c (about 5 oz)
Fried rice, no meat	0.5 c
Noodles and vegetables in sauce	
(chow/lo mein)	1 c

Pizzas

Cheese/pepperoni pizza,	
regular crust	1 slice (⅛ of a
	14″ pizza)
Cheese/vegetarian pica,	
thin crust	1 slice (¼ of a
	12″ pizza)

Sandwiches

Hamburger, regular plain	1 sandwich
Hot dog with bun, plain	1 hot dog
Submarine sandwich	1 sub (6″)
Taco, hard or soft shell	1 small

Salads

Salad, main dish (grilled chicken, no dressing)	1 serving
Salad, side (no dressing or cheese)	1 serving

Sides/Appetizers

French fries, restaurant style	1 large serving (about 7)
Nachos with cheese	1 small serving (about 4)
Onion rings, breaded, fried	1 serving (about 3 oz)

Desserts

Milkshake, any flavor	1 small (about 12 oz)
Soft-serve cone, regular	1

Combination Foods List

Many of the foods we eat are mixed together in various combinations. These combination foods do not fit into any one exchange list. Often it is hard to tell what is in a casserole dish or prepared food item. This is a list of exchanges for some typical combination foods. This list will help you fit these foods into your meal plan. Ask your instructor for information about other combination foods.

Entrees

Spaghetti, sauce, meatballs	1 c
Chili with beans	1 c
Macaroni and cheese	1 c (8 oz)
2 carbohydrates, 2 medium-fat meats	
Tuna or chicken salad	½ c (3-½ oz)
½ carbohydrate, 2 lean meats, 1 fat	

Frozen Entrees/Meals

Dinner-type meal, frozen	generally 14–17 oz
3 carbohydrates, 3 medium-fat meats, 3 fats	
Meatless burger, vegetable and starch-based	3 oz
1 carbohydrate, 1 lean meat	
Pizza, meat topping, thin crust	¼ of 10″ (5 oz)
2 carbohydrates, 2 medium-fat meats, 2 fats	

Pot pie	1 (7 oz)
2 ½ carbohydrates, 1 medium-fat meat, 3 fats	

Soups

Bean	1 c
1 carbohydrate, 1 very lean meat	
Cream of mushroom (made with water)	1 c (8 oz)
1 carbohydrate, 1 fat	
Split pea (made with water)	½ c (4 oz)
1 carbohydrate	
Tomato (made with water)	1 c (8 oz)
1 carbohydrate	

Free Foods List

A *free food* is any food or drink that contains less than 20 calories or less than 5 g of carbohydrate per serving. Foods with a serving size listed should be limited to 3 servings per day. Be sure to spread them out throughout the day. If you eat all 3 servings at one time, it could affect your blood glucose level. Foods listed without a serving size can be eaten as often as you like.

Low Carbohydrate Foods

Candy, hard, sugar-free, small size	1 candy
Gelatin dessert, sugar-free	½ c
Carrots, fresh cooked	¼ c
Chewing gum, regular	1 stick
Cucumber, with peel	½ c
Jam or jelly, low or reduced sugar	2 tsp
Sugar substitute (Splenda sucralose)	1 packet
Syrup, sugar-free	2 tbsp

Modified-Fat Foods with Carbohydrate

Cream cheese, fat-free	1 tbsp (½ oz)
Creamer, nondairy, liquid	1 tbsp
Creamers, nondairy, powdered	2 tsp
Mayonnaise, reduced-fat	1 tsp
Margarine spread, reduced-fat	1 tsp
Salad dressing, fat-free or low-fat	1 tbsp
Sour cream, fat-free, reduced-fat	1 tbsp
Whipped topping, regular	1 tbsp

Condiments

Catsup, tomato	1 tbsp
Horseradish	1 tbsp
Lemon juice	1 tbsp
Pickle relish	1 tbsp
Pickles, sweet (bread and butter)	2 slices
Salsa	¼ c
Soy sauce, regular or light	1 tbsp
Vinegar	1 tbsp

Free Snacks

Blueberries, fresh, free food size	¼ c
Cheese, fat-free, free food size	½ c
Lean meat, cooked, free food size	½ oz
Popcorn, light free food size	1 c
Vanilla wafers, free food size	1

Drinks/Mixes

Bouillon, broth, consomme	
Bouillon or broth, low-sodium	
Carbonated or mineral water	
Club soda	
Cocoa powder, unsweetened	1 tbsp
Coffee	
Diet soft drinks, sugar-free	
Drink mixes, sugar-free	
Tea	
Tonic water, sugar-free	

Seasonings

Be careful with seasonings that contain sodium or are salts, such as garlic or celery salt and lemon pepper.

Flavoring extracts
Garlic
Herbs, fresh or dried
Pimento
Spices
Tabasco or hot pepper sauce
Wine, used in cooking
Worcestershire sauce

Alcohol

Beer, regular (4.9%)	1 can (12 oz)
Rum, 80 proof	1.5 fl oz
Wine, white	5 fl oz

Answers to Progress Checks

CHAPTER 1: INTRODUCTION TO NUTRITION

Activity 1: Dietary Allowances, Eating Guides, and Food Selection Systems

1. A unit of energy, commonly used to indicate release of energy from food.

2. State of complete physical, mental, and social well-being, not just absence of disease.

3. A chemical substance obtained from food and needed by the body for growth, maintenance, or repair.

4. Receiving and utilizing essential nutrients to maintain health and well-being.

5. A diet that supplies sufficient energy and essential nutrients in adequate amounts for health at any stage of life.

6. Guidelines to promote healthy eating habits (*Dietary Guidelines for Americans*).

7. Levels of nutrients recommended for daily consumption for healthy individuals according to age and gender.

8. Maximum intake by an individual that is not likely to have adverse effects in a specified group.

9. A set of four reference values used for assessing and planning diets for individuals and groups.

10. An estimate of average requirements when evidence is not available to establish RDAs.

11. Food and Nutrition Board

12. National Research Council

13. American Dietetic Association or American Diabetes Association (common usage: "the associations")

14. Estimated Average Requirements

15. United States Department of Agriculture

16. American Heart Association

17. National Cholesterol Education Program

18. American Institute for Cancer Research

19. National Cancer Institute

20. Upper Limit

21. a

22. b

23. e

24. f

25. The Food Guide Pyramid is a visual representation of nutritional guidelines.

26. Coronary heart disease, strokes, hypertension, atherosclerosis, obesity, diabetes, and some cancers.

27. CHD, hypertension, obesity, and diabetes

28. The dietary guidelines designate recommended changes in lifestyle to promote good health, including weight management, physical activity, food safety, use of alcohol, and so on, whereas the pyramid concentrates on specific foods that meet the dietary recommendations and tips on how to implement the changes.

29. a) carbohydrate group, b) meat and meat substitutes, c) fat group.

30. Any three of the following: other carbohydrates, free foods list, combination food list, and fast food list.

31. RDA, Dietary Guidelines, and Food Guide Pyramid are three major sources of information.

Self-Study: Your individual answers will provide information for your personal health status.

Activity 2: Legislation and Health Promotion

1. 1 c

2. Number of servings

3. Fat, saturated fat, trans fat, cholesterol, or sodium

4. Dietary fiber, vitamin A, vitamin C, calcium, and iron

5. It is recommended that you stay below—eat "less than"—the Daily Reference Value nutrient amounts listed per day on the label.

6. If a serving of food is high or low in a nutrient

7. "Legal" conventional foods (natural or manufactured) that contain bioactive ingredients

8. Adding a bioactive ingredient especially one with nutritional value to a dietary or an OCT drug

9. According to scientists, limited evidence suggests an association between consumption of these fatty acids in fish and reduced risks of mortality from cardiovascular disease for the general population.

10. One claim, among others, is the positive effect of this vitamin on clinical disorders such as birth defects.

11. Some claims, among others, are that some chemicals in this tea can neutralize free radicals (responsible for aging) and may reduce risk of cancer.

12. One claim, among others, is that certain chemicals in this botanical or dietary supplement can improve memory and blood flow to the brain and may help cure Alzheimer's disease.

13. Primary prevention of CHD in persons with high levels of LDL.

14. Intensive management of LDL cholesterol in persons with CHD.

15. Focus on primary prevention in persons with multiple risk factors. The three approaches are more intensive LDL lowering in certain groups of people; soluble fiber as a therapeutic dietary option, with strategies for promoting adherence to the diet; and treatment beyond LDL lowering in people with high triglycerides.

16. Define these acronyms:
    a. National Institutes of Health
    b. Coronary heart disease
    c. Low-density lipoprotein
    d. High-density lipoprotein
    e. Food and Drug Administration
    f. National Cholesterol Education Program
    g. Adult treatment panel

CHAPTER 2: FOOD HABITS
Activity 1: Factors Affecting Food Consumption

1–3. Personal responses: Need to include factors that apply to your particular individual situation, such as where you live, your finances, emotions, traditions, seasonal considerations, and the like.

4. F	9. F	14. b	18. a, b, c, d
5. T	10. F	15. d	19. d
6. T	11. F	16. b	20. b
7. F	12. T	17. b	21. a, b, c, d
8. F	13. F		

Activity 2: Some Effects of Culture, Religion, and Geography on Food Behaviors

The student is responsible for submitting the answers. The instructor may wish to have the student discuss a client's diet plan, or give a grade for this assignment.

CHAPTER 3: PROTEINS AND HEALTH
Activity 1: Protein as a Nutrient

1. If you are uncertain about your answers, look at the tables provided and/or discuss with your teachers.

2. Because all essential amino acids (present in good quality protein) must be present at one time in the body or the body cannot utilize them to build body proteins.

3. No. (However, it is relatively more common among low-income groups.)

4. c	6. b	8. d	10. T
5. b	7. c	9. T	

Activity 2: Meeting Protein Needs and Vegetarianism

1. a	5. b	9. a	13. d
2. b	6. a	10. b	14. T
3. a	7. a	11. b	
4. a	8. c	12. a	

15. A diet history with as much detail as possible. List of food likes, dislikes, and allergies. Mary's present knowledge of nutritional needs and of food composition, especially protein. Her knowledge of complementary proteins and methods of food preparation. Type of vegetarianism practiced. History of pre-pregnancy eating and exercise habits.

16. Protein: 30 g extra daily; must be high quality. There is also need for 300 more kcal per day as well as extra vitamins and minerals. See RDA chart.

17. 40 g (110 lb ÷ 2.2 = 50 kg × 0.8 = 40.0).

18. Mary is underweight for her height, even if she is of small frame and very athletic. It will depend upon her physician's decision, of course, but she probably needs to gain extra weight.

19. It will be more difficult, because plant proteins have lower biological values than animal. It will also be difficult to get enough calcium and fat-soluble vitamins as well as other essential nutrients contained in animal foods. Extra soy milk, fortified with vitamin B_{12}, should be consumed with each meal. Leafy green vegetables (without oxalates), sunflower seeds, and fortified soy milk for calcium should be part of the diet.

20. To spare protein for its primary function of building new cells.

21. Positive nitrogen balance. The body retains more nitrogen than it excretes during pregnancy.

CHAPTER 4: CARBOHYDRATES AND FATS: IMPLICATIONS FOR HEALTH

Activity 1: Carbohydrates: Characteristics and Effects on Health

1. <u>4</u> 1 orange
   <u>2</u> 1 c whole kernel corn
   <u>1</u> ⅒ of a devil's food cake with icing (from a mix)
   <u>3</u> 1 slice of wheat bread
   <u>5</u> ½ c zucchini squash
   <u>3</u> ⅓ c cooked oatmeal

2. Vegetables:
   <u>3</u> ½ c green beans, cooked
   <u>3</u> ½ c cooked carrots
   <u>2</u> 1 baked potato
   <u>1</u> 1 sweet potato
   <u>4</u> 1 stalk broccoli
   <u>5</u> ½ c lettuce, chopped

3. It is converted to fat and stored in adipose tissue.

4. Any 3 of these: promotes regular elimination, helps prevent diverticulitis, helps control appetite, binds bile salts to help lower cholesterol, slows carbohydrate absorption (important in diabetes), and helps prevent cancer.

5. Good sources include raw fruits and vegetables, bran, whole grains, legumes, oats, and seeds.

6. (1) Dental caries; and (2) diets of poor nutritional quality that are high in calories can result in obesity.

7. Because they increase the risk of ketosis, dehydration, diarrhea, and loss of muscle mass.

8. c (1000 ÷ 4 = 250)

9. b	15. a	21. b	27. c
10. b	16. b	22. c	28. a
11. b and d	17. c	23. a	29. b
12. b	18. d	24. c	30. a
13. b	19. e	25. b	
14. a	20. d	26. a	

Activity 2: Fats: Characteristics and Effects on Health

1. c
2. b
3. a
4. True
5. False
6. False
7. True
8. False
9. 140/90 mmHg or higher
10. less than 40 mg/dl
11. 40%
12. low-density lipoproteins
13. A lipoprotein is made up of fats (cholesterol, triglycerides, fatty acids, etc.), protein, and a small amount of other substances.
14. Coronary heart disease
15. Eicosapentaenoic acid
16. Docosahexaenoic acid

CHAPTER 5: VITAMINS AND HEALTH

Activity 1: The Water-Soluble Vitamins

1. a	6. b	11. a and b	16. d
2. b	7. d	12. d	17. a
3. a	8. c	13. a	18. a
4. b	9. c	14. b	
5. b	10. d	15. d	

Activity 2: The Fat-Soluble Vitamins

1. b	5. d	9. c	13. d
2. c	6. a	10. a	14. c
3. d	7. d	11. b	
4. c	8. d	12. a	

Progress Check on Chapter 5

1. c	9. c	17. b	25. c
2. a	10. b	18. a	26. d
3. d	11. T	19. a	27. d
4. e	12. T	20. b	28. a
5. b	13. T	21. a	29. b
6. d	14. T	22. b	30. b
7. e	15. T	23. b	
8. a	16. T	24. a	

CHAPTER 6: MINERALS, WATER, AND BODY PROCESSES

Progress Check on Chapter 6

1. b	17. a	33. b	49. F
2. c	18. d	34. c	50. T
3. d	19. c	35. b	51. F
4. b	20. b	36. b	52. T
5. c	21. b	37. a	53. T
6. d	22. a	38. c	54. T
7. b	23. b	39. a	55. T
8. d	24. b	40. a	56. T
9. c	25. c	41. a	57. T
10. b	26. c	42. c	58. T
11. a	27. b	43. b	59. T
12. c	28. a	44. d	60. e
13. d	29. b	45. T	61. a
14. b	30. c	46. F	62. c
15. c	31. c	47. T	63. b
16. c	32. a	48. T	64. d

CHAPTER 7: MEETING ENERGY NEEDS

Activity 1: Energy Balance

1. a. The basal metabolic rate.
   b. Activity or voluntary energy expenditures.
   c. The thermic effect of food.

2. 89 kcal.
   $4 \times 4 = 16$ kcal protein
   $5 \times 9 = 45$ kcal fat
   $7 \times 4 = 28$ kcal carbohydrate
   Total $\overline{\quad 89\ \text{kcal}}$

3. Your caloric intake is in balance with your energy needs when you maintain the same weight. Excess calories are converted to fat and stored in adipose tissue (fat cells).

4. Potatoes are grouped with bread and pasta (rich in carbohydrates) and as such contain only four calories per gram.

5. a. Present intake:
      12,600 calories per week ($1,800 \times 7 = 12,600$)
      3,500 cal = 1 lb body fat $\times$ 3 (desired weight loss)
      = 10,500 cal

      $12,600$ cal
      $\underline{-10,500\ \text{cal}}$
      $2,100$ cal per week $\div$ 7 days = 300 calories per day
   b. 300 calories per day are inadequate and represent semi-starvation.

6. a. 1 c skim milk
   b. ½ c unsweetened fruit
   c. 1 slice bread
   d. ½ c. cooked vegetables
   e. 1 tsp solid fat or oil
   f. 1 oz lean meat

7. 1. c
   2. a
   3. b

Activity 2: The Effects of Energy Imbalance

1. F	11. T	21. b
2. T	12. T	22. c
3. T	13. F	23. a
4. F	14. T	24. e
5. F	15. F	25. a, b
6. F	16. F	26. b
7. T	17. T	27. c
8. T	18. T	28. a
9. F	19. a, b, c, d	29. c
10. T	20. b	

30. a. 700 calorie reduction plus 300 calories used in activity = 1,000 kcal per daily reduction;
       1,000 kcal per day $\times$ 7 days per week = 7,000 kcal deficit per week;
       7,000 $\div$ 3,500 (kcal in 1 lb body fat) = 2 lb per week.
    b. 20 lb $\div$ 2 lb per week = 10 weeks.
       October 1 to December 7 = 10 weeks.
       The answer is yes.
    c. 300 kcal burned $\times$ 7 days per week = 2,100 calories per week deficit;
       2,100 $\div$ 3,500 = .6 lb per week
    d. October 1 to December 7 = 10 weeks;
       10 weeks $\times$ 0.6 lb per week = 6.0 lb loss in 10 weeks.
       No; it would take 33⅓ weeks to lose 20 lb at 0.6 lb per week (20 lb $\div$ 0.6 = 33⅓).

Activity 3: Weight Control and Dieting

1. d	5. F
2. c	6. F
3. c	7. T
4. (a) altered metabolism;	8. T
(b) fluid and electrolyte imbalance;	
(c) nutrient deficits.	

CHAPTER 8: NUTRITIONAL ASSESSMENT AND HEALTH CARE MODEL

Activity 1: Assessment of Nutritional Status

1. Physical, anthropometric, laboratory, and historical data.

2. The health education areas needed will depend on the problems you identified with your client in the Practices.

3. *See* Table 8-1.

4. *See* Table 8-3.

5. a	7. b	9. b	
6. a	8. a	10. b	

CHAPTER 9: NUTRITION AND THE LIFE CYCLE

Activity 1: Maternal and Infant Nutrition

1. c	9. d	17. c	25. F
2. c	10. a	18. a	26. T
3. b	11. b	19. d	27. F
4. c	12. a	20. c	28. F
5. b	13. b	21. b	29. F
6. a	14. a	22. d	30. F
7. b	15. a	23. c	
8. b	16. c	24. T	

Activity 2: Childhood and Adolescent Nutrition

1. b	9. a	17. d	25. F
2. a	10. a	18. d	26. T
3. d	11. b	19. T	27. T
4. b	12. d	20. T	28. F
5. d	13. b	21. F	29. F
6. c	14. c	22. F	
7. c	15. a	23. T	
8. d	16. b	24. T	

30. Any four of these: milk, wheat, seafood, chocolate, egg white, citrus, nuts.

Activity 3: Adulthood and Nutrition

1. b	8. d	15. a	22. F
2. c	9. a	16. a	23. T
3. a	10. c	17. d	24. T
4. d	11. d	18. a	25. F
5. a	12. d	19. b	26. T
6. c	13. c	20. T	27. T
7. c	14. d	21. T	28. F

29. They may not have transportation or the stamina for lengthy shopping trips.

30. Reduced BMR; reduced activity level.

31. Remain the same.

32. a. complication of existing or developing health problems;
    b. interference with movement; and
    c. increased risk of injurious falls.

33. Decreased consumption of meat (perhaps due to high cost or difficulty in eating) and other iron-rich foods.

34. Vitamin A, ascorbic acid (vitamin C), and calcium.

35. Food is provided in group social setting; some nutrition education is provided.

Activity 4: Exercise, Fitness, and Stress Reduction Principles

1. Duration, intensity, frequency, type.

2. Predicted rate that won't cause chest pain.

3. Any three if these increased strength, flexibility, endurance. Weight control. Lower blood pressure, lower cholesterol, increase cardiovascular strength.

4. Warm up, endurance, competition, cool down.

5. Optimal nutrition, RDAs or above, adequate calories, low in fat, high in complex carbohydrates.

6. c. $365 \times 100 = 36,500 \div 3500 = 10$ lb (app.)

7. Depression, heart disease, hypertension, angina.

8. Any of these: exercise, relaxation techniques, proper diet, socialization, enough rest/sleep, counseling.

9. Scientific data only may be used to evaluate the product.

10. Those measures that enable a person to stay young and healthy in body and mind.

CHAPTER 10: DRUGS AND NUTRITION

Background Information

Answers 1–8 found in Glossary at the beginning of the chapter.

9. Any five of these:
   a. Damage intestinal walls
   b. Lower absorption
   c. Destruction of accessory organs
   d. Destroy or displace nutrients
   e. Change the nutrient
   f. Render nutrients incapable of acting
   g. Cause nutrient excretion

10. a. diarrhea/constipation
    b. nausea/vomiting
    c. altered taste/smell

11. a. drug
    b. dosage
    c. time
    d. frequency
    e. health status

12. a. Drug interference
    b. Drug-induced antagonists

13. Any five: niacin, riboflavin, pantothenic acid, ascorbic acid, folic acid, B_{12}, protein, fat, glucose, iron, copper, calcium, zinc, magnesium

14. Reabsorption/transport

15. Change in urine pH/Increase in precipitation of some

Activity 1: Food and Drug Interaction

1. a. Change absorption rate
   b. Neutralize effects
   c. Interact
   d. Influence excretion rate

2. Alcohol
   Various amines

3. Hypertensive crisis

4. a. Drug dose
   b. Amount of food
   c. Interval between drug and food ingestion
   d. Patient susceptibility
   e. Condition of the food

5. Decrease taste sensitivity

6. Causing dry mouth, constipation, and urinary retention

Fill in the blanks

7. In taking medications, the two most important precautions are:
   a. should the medication be taken on empty stomach, or 1–2 hours before or after meals.
   b. can alcohol be taken with the medication.

8. Some of the negative effects with medications when taken not according to recommendations include:
   a. irritated stomach
   b. reduced absorption
   c. nausea and/or vomiting
   d. headache
   e. irregular heartbeat and palpitation
   f. loss of potassium, calcium, and/or magnesium
   g. excessive efficiency
   h. hyperkalemia
   i. risk of bleeding
   j. flushing
   k. increased blood pressure
   l. drowsiness, impaired mental and/or motor performance

9.	c	12.	b	15.	T
10.	d	13.	a	16.	T
11.	d	14.	F	17.	T

Activity 2: Drugs and the Life Cycle

1. Renal anomalies
   CNS malformation
   Cleft palate
   Severe defects

2. a. Type of drug
   b. Concentration of drug
   c. Time lapse between drug ingestion and breast-feeding

3. Anomalies of eyes, ears, heart, CNS, mental retardation
   Male: enlargement of the mammary glands (gynecomastia)
   Female: overgrowth of vaginal lining

4. High rate of abortions
   Abruptio placenta
   Low birth weight babies

5. a. Length of time used
   b. Nutritional status
   c. Nutritional intake
   d. Susceptibility

6. a. Decreased ability to digest, absorb, and metabolize food
   b. Decreased ability to metabolize and excrete drugs
   c. Interaction of multiple drug use

7. Aspirin—bleeding (GI)
   Laxatives—inhibit vitamin absorption
   Diuretics—decreased K and Ca^+
   Alcohol—decreased folate, thiamin

8.	e	11.	F	14.	T
9.	c	12.	F	15.	F
10.	b	13.	F	16.	T

CHAPTER 11: DIETARY SUPPLEMENTS

Background Information

1.	T	3.	F	5.	h
2.	F	4.	T		

6. a. set up a new framework for FDA regulation of dietary supplements.
   b. create an office in the National Institutes of Health to coordinate research on dietary supplements.
   c. set up an independent dietary supplement commission to report on the use of claims in dietary supplement labeling.

7. a. Generally recognized as safe
   b. Good manufacturing practices
   c. Dietary Supplement Health and Education Act
   d. Food Drug and Cosmetic Act

Activity 1: DSHE Act of 1994

1. a. name and quantity of each dietary ingredient or, for proprietary blends
   b. the total quantity of all dietary ingredients (excluding inert ingredients) in the blend

c. identification of the product as a dietary supplement

d. the part of the herb or botanical ingredients used in the product

e. nutritional labeling information (U.S. regulations)

f. specification(s) in official compendium, if appropriate

2. a. nutrient-content claims
   b. disease claims
   c. nutrition support claims, which include "structure-function claims"

3. a. nutrition information
   b. ingredient information

4. d	10. F	16. T
5. b	11. T	17. T
6. F	12. T	18. T
7. F	13. T	19. T
8. T	14. T	
9. T	15. T	

Activity 2: Folate and Folate Acid

1. F	6. F	11. F
2. F	7. T	12. T
3. T	8. T	13. F
4. F	9. T	
5. F	10. F	

14. a. women of childbearing age
    b. people who abuse alcohol
    c. anyone taking anticonvulsants or other medications that interfere with the action of folate
    d. individuals diagnosed with anemia from folate deficiency
    e. individuals with malabsorption
    f. individuals with liver disease
    g. individuals receiving kidney dialysis treatment

15. a. spine (spina bifida)
    b. skull
    c. brain (anencephaly)

16. 400 micrograms of synthetic folic acid

Activity 3: Kava kava, Ginko Biloba, Golden seal, Echinacea, Comfrey, and Pulegone

1. Any five of the following: Kava Kava, *Ginkgo biloba*, Goldenseal, Echinacea, Comfrey, or Pulegone.

2. Any five of the following: ava, ava pepper, awa, intoxicating pepper, kava, kava kava, kava pepper, kava root, kava-kava, kawa, kawa kawa, kawa-kawa, kew, *Piper methysticum* Forst.f., *Piper methysticum* G. Forst, rauschpfeffer, sakau, tonga, wurzelstock, or yangona.

3. F	8. F	13. F
4. F	9. T	14. T
5. F	10. T	15. T
6. F	11. F	16. T
7. F	12. T	

Activity 4: Tips for the Savvy Supplement User: Making Informed Decision

1. F	10. F	19. F
2. F	11. T	20. T
3. F	12. T	21. T
4. F	13. F	22. T
5. F	14. T	23. T
6. T	15. T	24. F
7. F	16. T	25. T
8. F	17. F	26. F
9. T	18. F	27. T

28. a. pregnant or breastfeeding
    b. chronically ill
    c. elderly
    d. under 18
    e. taking prescription or over-the-counter medicines

29. Health status is an important clue. Overeating is a human weakness. Product description is your major weapon for self-protection. Education is invariably a part of any health program. Symptoms from taking a dietary supplement are of course valuable indications that there is something wrong with the product.

CHAPTER 12: ALTERNATIVE MEDICINE

Background Information

1. a. Taught widely in medical schools.
   b. Generally used in hospitals.
   c. Usually reimbursed by medical insurance companies.

2. a. physical
   b. mental
   c. emotional
   d. spiritual

3. Any six of the following: acupuncture, oriental massage, qi gong, herbal medicine, diet, meditation, exposure to sunlight, controlled breathing, homeopathic medicine, hydrotherapy, spine and soft-tissue spine, electric currents, ultrasound therapy, light therapy, or therapeutic counseling.

4. F	6. F	8. F
5. T	7. T	

Activity 1: Categories or Domains of Complementary Alternative Medicine

1. a. alternative medical systems
    b. mind-body interventions
    c. biologically-based treatments
    d. manipulative and body-based methods
    e. energy therapies

2. a. acupuncture
    b. herbal medicine
    c. oriental massage
    d. Qi gong

3. Any of five of the following: diet, exercise, meditation, herbs, massage, exposure to sunlight, or controlled breathing.

4. Any five of the following: diet and clinical nutrition, homeopathy, acupuncture, herbal medicine, hydrotherapy, spinal and soft-tissue manipulation, physical therapies involving electric currents, ultrasound and light therapy, therapeutic counseling, or pharmacology.

5. a. Qi gong
    b. Reiki
    c. therapeutic touch

6.	T	11.	F	16.	T
7.	T	12.	F	17.	T
8.	T	13.	F	18.	T
9.	T	14.	T		
10.	T	15.	T		

Activity 2: Products, Devices, and Services Related to Complementary Alternative Medicine

1. a. conduction electromagnetic signals
    b. activation of opioid systems
    c. changes in brain chemistry, sensations, and involuntary body functions

2. Any five of the following: nausea and vomiting, headache, dizziness, bluish discoloration of the skin due to a lack of oxygen in the blood, liver damage, abnormally low blood pressure, droopy upper eyelid, difficulty walking due to damaged nerves, fever, mental confusion, coma, or death.

3. Any three of the following: health care practitioners, medical libraries, educational organizations, research institutions, professional associations, or World Wide Web.

4. a. Who runs this site?
    b. Who pays for the site?
    c. What is the purpose of the site?
    d. Where does the information come from?
    e. What is the basis of the information?
    f. How is the information selected?
    g. How current is the information?
    h. How does the site choose links to other sites?
    i. What information about you does the site collect, and why?
    j. How does the site manage interactions with visitors?

5.	T	11.	T	17.	F
6.	T	12.	F	18.	T
7.	T	13.	T	19.	F
8.	F	14.	F	20.	T
9.	T	15.	F	21.	F
10.	F	16.	T	22.	F

CHAPTER 13: FOOD ECOLOGY

Activity 1: Food Safety

1. All of the answers below are correct:
    a. failing to wash hands after going to the bathroom
    b. not washing hands after handling meat, fish, poultry, or eggs before handling other foods
    c. failing to clean counters, cutting boards, and cooking equipment
    d. failing to wash fresh food products thoroughly before preparation
    e. failing to use clean cloths, sponges, or hand towels
    f. handling food if you have upper respiratory infections (URIs)
    g. working with sores, boils, etc., on hands, face
    h. failing to wash after touching hair, face, or other body parts before returning to food preparation
    i. talking, laughing, sneezing during food preparation
    j. poor personal hygiene: dirty clothing, body, hair, etc.

2. b

3. Bacteria—the spores themselves and/or the toxins produced from them.

4. A warm moist place is a perfect environment for bacteria to multiply. With these favorable conditions, they quickly increase by geometric progression (1-2-4-8-16-32-64, etc.).

5. All of the answers below are correct:
    a. use of pure drinking water
    b. adequate sewage disposal
    c. adequate cooking of foods
    d. proper storage of foods
    e. thorough cleaning of foods

f. sanitary handling of all foods

g. areas free of pests, rodents, vermin, etc.

6. Nausea, vomiting, diarrhea, flatulence, abdominal distention.

7. F

8. T

9. T

10. T

11. This soup may make the residents ill. It was at room temperature overnight and reheating will not destroy any microorganism, especially if contaminated by staph.

12. She should throw the cans away. Even if not bulged, there is an opening at the seam which allows for contamination.

13. Leaving ingredients such as mayonnaise and eggs out of the refrigerator to stand at room temperature for extended periods of time is a dangerous practice.

14. Handling food in this manner is dangerous because
    a. the cutting board is not washed before using and is stored near pipes
    b. the cutting board is not washed before chopping of different foodstuffs, making cross contamination possible
    c. the practice of cutting fruits and vegetables ahead of time and leaving uncovered causes excessive nutrient loss

Activity 2: Nutrient Conservation

1. a. If voluntary point-of-purchase information is provided for raw produce, meats, fish, and poultry.
    b. Eating establishments where prepared meats are provided.

2. a. It identifies the nutrients.
    b. It aids in balancing diets.
    c. It may enhance the nutritive value of food.

3. See Table 11-1.

4. See Table 11-1.

5. See Glossary for this chapter.

6. See Glossary for this chapter.

7. See Glossary for this chapter.

8. a. Enrichment: addition of iron to bread
    b. Fortification: addition of vitamin D to milk

CHAPTER 14: OVERVIEW OF THERAPEUTIC NUTRITION

Background Information

1. Therapeutic nutrition is based on modifications of the nutrients in a normal diet.

2. The purpose of diet therapy is to restore or maintain good nutritional status.

3. The diet should be altered to the specific disease (pathophysiology).

4. a. Altering basic nutrients.
    b. Altering energy value.
    c. Altering texture or consistency.
    d. Altering seasonings.

5. a. Anxiety and fear about an illness can change attitudes and personality.
    b. Immobilization compounds nutritional problems.
    c. Drug therapy may affect intake and utilization of nutrients.
    d. The disease process modifies food acceptance.

6. The nurse has a key role. He or she assists the patient at mealtimes and explains, interprets, and supports both the physician's orders and the efforts of the dietary staff. The nurse observes and charts pertinent information and coordinates the team. The nurse also involves the patient in his or her own care and provides a care plan for other staff members to follow. And, finally, the nurse plans for discharge teaching of the patient and follow-up care.

Activity 1: Principles and Objectives of Diet Therapy

1. a. Cultural aspects
    b. Socioeconomic background
    c. Psychological factors
    d. Physiological factors

2. a. The patient is often fearful and rejects hospital food.
    b. Immobilization brings about nutritional stress.
    c. The disease process alters food acceptance.
    d. Medications may interfere with nutrient utilization.

3. Diet therapy focuses on the patient's identified needs and problem.

4. Therapeutic nutrition is based upon modifications of the nutrients in a normal diet.

5. The purpose of diet therapy is to restore or maintain good nutritional status.

Activity 2: Routine Hospital Diets

1. a	5. b	9. c	13. c
2. c	6. b	10. d	
3. d	7. a	11. b	
4. c	8. b	12. c	

14. Canned fruit cup; oatmeal with milk and sugar; toast with butter (tea with sugar, if desired)

15. a. N
    b. Y
    c. Y
    d. N
    e. Y
    f. Y
    g. N
    h. Y
    i. N
    j. N

Activity 3: Diet Modifications for Therapeutic Care

1. Modify basic nutrients; modify energy value; modify texture; and modify seasoning.

2. There are numerous examples that would be correct. For instance, the diet restricted in simple carbohydrates used for the diabetic whose pancreas does not produce enough insulin. Calories are not nutrients, so a low calorie diet is not appropriate here.

3. a. When the diet imposes severe restrictions.
   b. When the patient's appetite is poor.
   c. When digestion, absorption, or metabolism is impaired.

4. Within the framework of the correctly modified diet, the individual's likes, dislikes, and tolerances should be built in. Foods of equal value should be substituted to meet the patient's ethnic and cultural desires. Participation by the patient in choosing foods within the specified diet is desirable.

Activity 4: Alterations in Feeding Methods

1. c	4. F	7. T	10. a
2. a	5. F	8. F	11. b
3. c	6. T	9. c	

12. A nutritionally adequate diet of liquified foods administered through a tube into the stomach or duodenum.

13. One advantage is that it is safer to feed enterally. Other answers may be found in the activity.

14. a. When the GI tract cannot be used.
    b. When the patient is severely depleted nutritionally.

15. a. Assist the patient's adjustment to an alternate feeding method.
    b. Monitor glucose levels.
    c. Be alert for signs of contaminated solutions and discard them.

16. a. Milk-based formula: milk and cream are primary ingredients.
    b. Blenderized formula: adds strained meats, vegetables, and fruits to the milk base.
    c. Meat-based formula: milk and cream are omitted.

CHAPTER 15: DIET THERAPY FOR SURGICAL CONDITIONS

Background Information

1. a

2. a

3. Effective wound healing

4. Increased resistance to infection

5. Lowered mortality rate

6. Shortened convalescent period (decreased probability of complications arising during and after surgery)

7. e	12. d	17. T	22. T
8. d	13. e	18. T	23. F
9. a	14. b	19. F	24. T
10. f	15. c	20. F	
11. c	16. a	21. F	

Activity 1: Pre- and Postoperative Nutrition

1. b and d	5. T
2. c	6. F
3. a	7. F
4. F	

8.

	Pro	CHO	Thia	Nia	Ribo	Fe	VitC
Oyster stew	X	X	X	_	X	X	_
Whole wheat garlic toast	X	X	X	X	X	X	_
Green pepper and cabbage slaw	X	X	_	_	_	_	X
Raisin rice pudding with orange sauce	X	X	_	_	_	X	X

Activity 2: The Postoperative Diet Regime

1. Regain normal body weight.

2. a. Correct fluid and electrolyte balance.
   b. Carefully plan dietary and nutritional support.
   c. Monitor food intake.

3. a. Prevent shock/edema.
   b. Provide for synthesis of albumin, antibodies, etc.
   c. Accelerate wound healing.

4. a. Blood.
   b. Fluids and electrolytes.
   c. 5% dextrose.
   d. Protein-sparing solutions.
   e. Vitamin supplement.
   f. Intralipids single or in any combination.

5. Clear liquid—24 hours (after bowel sounds return).
   Full liquid—1–2 days, should be supplemented with commercial formula if used longer.
   Soft to Regular—remainder of hospital stay. May need supplements.

6. $150/2.2 = 68 \times 0.45 = 30.6 \times 100 = 3060.$

7. $3060 \times 0.15 = 459$ kcal/4 = 115 g protein (rounded).

8. $3060 \times 30 = 1009.8$ kcal/9 = 112 g fat (rounded).

9. $3060 \times 0.55 = 1683$ kcal/4 = 420 g carbohydrate (rounded).

10. Your choice. Use exchange lists as needed.

CHAPTER 16: DIET THERAPY FOR CARDIOVASCULAR DISORDERS
Progress Check for Activity 1

1. a. high serum cholesterol
   b. high serum triglycerides
   c. obesity
   d. hypertension
   e. poor eating habits

2. Therapeutic lifestyle changes

3. a. reduce saturated fat and cholesterol
   b. weight reduction
   c. physical activity

4. Metabolic Syndrome

5. 25%–35% of total calories

6. abdominal obesity

7. lowering LDL cholesterol

8. nicotinic acid

9. d

10. b

11. b

12. See Nursing Implications: any 8 of 15

Practice Question

Check your answer with the sample menu in Appendix C. Your foods do not need to be the same, only within the guidelines for a TLC diet, and satisfactory to your client.

Activity 2: Heart Disease and Sodium Restriction

1. See the Low-Sodium Diet, Activity 2.

2. Example of menu for a 500 mg sodium diet.

Breakfast
Puffed wheat cereal
½ c skim milk
1 sliced banana
Sugar
2 slices low-sodium toast with unsalted soft margarine and honey
Coffee or decaffeinated

Mid morning
½ c orange juice
Unsalted crackers

Lunch
2 oz baked chicken*
½ c rice *
½ c green peas*
1 slice unsalted bread with special margarine
Sliced peaches

Lunch (continued)
½ c skim milk
1 slice unsalted bread special margarine
Canned pineapple
Coffee, tea, or decaffeinated beverage

Mid afternoon
½ c skim milk
1 cupcake*

Dinner
3 oz roast beef
Baked potato
½ c glazed carrots*
Lettuce with special dressing*

Bedtime
Fruit cup
½ c skim milk

*All food prepared without seasonings that contain sodium.

3. a. lemon juice/slices; orange juice/slices
   b. thyme, basil, marjoram, oregano, sage, bay leaf
   c. onion, garlic (fresh or powdered, not salt)
   d. chives, dill, mint, parsley, rosemary
   e. unsalted chopped nuts
   f. green pepper, pimiento
   g. cinnamon, nutmeg, brown sugar, ginger
   h. vinegar, tarragon, curry, black pepper
   i. mushrooms, cranberry sauce, dry mustard
   j. fresh tomatoes; unsalted juice

Progress Check on Nursing Implications

1. a. Reducing the workload of the heart.
   b. Improving cardiac output; promoting patient comfort.
   c. Restoring and maintaining adequate nutrition.
   d. Controlling any existing conditions such as hyperlipoproteinemia or hypertension.

2. a. Position the patient for maximal benefit; for example, allow the patient to sit up with the tray on his or her unaffected side.
   b. Place food in unaffected side of the patient's mouth.
   c. Gently stroke the patient's throat, and teach the patient to do so to relieve fear of choking (patient feels the food going down).
   d. Provide feeding devices when necessary.
   e. Protect the patient from spillage. Preserve the patient's dignity. Change linens as necessary.
   f. Take plenty of time to feed or assist self-feeding.
   g. Cut food into small bites. Open all packages and cartons.
   h. Emphasize all successes; praise attempts at self-feeding.
   i. Talk to the patient whether or not the patient can answer.
   j. Try to find out from the family what foods the patient dislikes and do not feed the patient those foods.

Activity 3: Dietary Care after Heart Attack and Stroke

1. Baking powder, baking soda, patent medicines, prescribed drugs, commercial mixes, most convenience foods, frozen and canned vegetables, softened water, cured and dried meats, and vegetables.

2. See list of acceptable alternatives to salt (Activities 2 & 3).

3. See Nursing Implications.

4. To rest the heart and reduce or prevent edema.

5. c

6. b

CHAPTER 17: DIET AND DISORDERS OF INGESTION, DIGESTION, AND ABSORPTION

Activity 1: Disorders of the Mouth, Esophagus, and Stomach

1.

Diet	Disease or Condition	Foods Allowed	Foods Limited	Foods Forbidden	Nursing Implications
Low-Residue Diet	Hiatal hernia Diverticulitis Hemorrhoidectomy Ostomics Ulcerative Colitis (U.C.)	See Table 17-2 for guidance			*See* Nursing Implications, this chapter

2a.

Diet	Disease or Condition	Foods Allowed	Foods Limited	Foods Forbidden	Nursing Implications
Regular high protein, high carbohydrate, moderate fat without interval feedings	Gastric ulcer	Any tolerated	Milk, wine*, caffeine beverage*, some seasonings*	80 proof alcohol beer, black hot chilis, caffeine	*See* Nursing Implications

2b.

Diet	Disease or Condition	Foods Allowed	Foods Limited	Foods Forbidden	Nursing Implications
Moderate low-residue, high-protein, high-carbohydrate moderate fat in 6 feedings	Dumping syndrome	*See* Table 17-4	Complex carbohydrate, milk*	Liquids with sweets, alcohol, sweetened beverages	*See* Nursing Implications

*Individual tolerance and doctors orders

3. Better understanding of the causes of gastric ulcers, and improved methods of treating them, have changed the principles of diet therapy to correspond with medical treatments.

4. Following the guidelines given in the section on gastric surgery, choose the menu from Tables 15-4 and 15-5 (antidumping diets). An example follows.

8 am	10 am	2 pm
½ rice cereal rice	½ melted cheese sandwich	2 oz white meat chicken
1 tsp margarine		½ c cooked carrots
s.c. egg		margarine

4 pm	6 pm	8 pm
2 crackers	2 oz broiled beef patty	½ sandwich:
1 tbsp smooth peanut butter	½ c mashed potatoes	1 slice white toast
		2 tsp mayonnaise
		2 oz tuna

Unsweetened beverages and water between meals.

Activity 2: Disorders of the Intestines

1. a. N   e. N   i. N
   b. Y   f. N   j. Y
   c. N   g. Y
   d. N   h. Y

2. a   6. d   10. d
3. b   7. c   11. d
4. c   8. c
5. c   9. c

12. Choose from this group:
   a. any whole grain breads/cereals
   b. any fresh fruits
   c. any fresh vegetables
   d. cooked fruits and vegetables may be used in some cases; i.e., broccoli, spinach
   e. prunes, figs, raisins
   f. nuts, legumes

13. a. correct nutrient deficits
    b. restore adequate intake
    c. prevent further losses

d. promote repair and maintenance of body tissue
e. promote healing
f. control substances that are not absorbed easily

14. *See* Nursing Implications for ileostomy, colostomy.

15. T   18. T
16. F   19. F
17. F   20. T

CHAPTER 18: DIET THERAPY FOR DIABETES MELLITUS

Activity 1: Diet Therapy and Diabetes Mellitus

1. *See* Answer Sheet for Exercise 18-1 and 18-2 following question #34.

2. b and d   9. d   16. F   23. T
3. a   10. c   17. F   24. F
4. c   11. a   18. F   25. e
5. b   12. b   19. T   26. d
6. d   13. c   20. T   27. b
7. a   14. F   21. T   28. c
8. d   15. F   22. T   29. a

30. *See* Nursing Implications.

31. *See* Patient Education: What the diabetic patient must know.

32.

	Carbo-hydrate (grams)	Protein (grams)	Fat (grams)
Milk, 2 exchanges (2%)	24	16	8
Vegetables, 3 exchanges	15	6	—
Fruit, 3 exchanges	45	—	—
Lean meat, 6 exchanges	—	42	18
Medium fat meat, 2 exchanges	—	14	10
Fat, 5 exchanges	—	—	25
Bread, 6 exchanges	90	18	—
Total	174 g	96 g	61 g

33. Your choice. Be sure to use all exchanges, but no more than the number specified.

34. c

$$174 \times 4 = 696 \text{ calories}$$
$$93 \times 4 = 372 \text{ calories}$$
$$61 \times 9 = 549 \text{ calories}$$

1617 calories (Total). Round to 1600.

35. b   7000 calories = 2 lb body fat

36. b, c   Granola bar and raisin bread each have app. 100 calories; meat, though lean, has 55 calories per oz; 8 oz whole milk has 150 calories.

37. See Answer Sheet for Exercises 18-1 and 18-2.

38. People with type 2 diabetes usually have one of the following conditions:
    a. do not always produce enough insulin.
    b. produce insulin too late to match the rise in blood sugar.
    c. do not respond correctly to the insulin that is produced.

39. The three criteria that should be considered in choosing insulin are:
    a. how soon it starts working (onset).
    b. when it works the hardest (peak time).
    c. how long it lasts in the body (duration).

40. The basic four types of insulin products are:
    a. rapid acting
    b. short acting (regular)
    c. intermediate acting (NPH)
    d. Long lasting

41. The 3 ways that diabetes pills work in the body are:
    a. stimulate the pancreas to release more insulin.
    b. increase the body's sensitivity to the insulin that is already present.
    c. slow the breakdown of foods (especially the starches) into glucose.

Answer Sheet for Exercises 18-1 and 18-2

Diet	Disease or Condition	Foods Allowed	Foods Limited	Foods Forbidden	Nursing Implications
Calculated	Diabetes mellitus	All of those listed in the food exchanges (*see* exchange list in Appendix F)	Foods are limited by amount: larger amounts for higher caloric allowances; smaller amounts for lower caloric allowances	Sugar, sweets and desserts that exceed the carbohydrate and caloric allowance of the diet plan	*See* section: Nursing Implications. Also see section on the child with diabetes mellitus.

CHAPTER 19: DIET AND DISORDERS OF THE LIVER, GALLBLADDER, AND PANCREAS
Activity 1: Diet Therapy for Diseases of the Liver

1. See Tables 16-1 and 16-2, and Nursing Implications.

2. Example: (whole day's menu)

Breakfast
Orange juice, 8 oz
Cream of Wheat, 1 c
   with sugar and
   milk
Poached egg, 1, on
   whole wheat
   buttered toast
Milk/coffee

Mid-morning
English muffin with 2
   tbsp cream cheese
Milk, 8 oz

Lunch
Tuna salad sandwich
   (3 oz tuna, 2 slices
   bread, 1 tbsp may-
   onnaise, lettuce)
Carrot/raisin salad
Assorted crackers
Fruit juice, 8 oz
Milk, 8 oz

Lunch (continued)
Sherbet with sugar
   cookies
Chicken noodle soup

Mid-afternoon
Hardboiled egg
Cottage cheese with fruit
Toast with 1 tsp butter
Juice, 8 oz

Dinner
Lean roast beef, 4 oz
Mashed potatoes, 1 c with
   butter, 1 tsp
Green beans
Fruited gelatin salad
Rolls, 1 tsp butter
Angel food cake
Milk, 8 oz

Pre-bed Snack
1 c buckwheats
1 c milk
1 banana

3. Example: (menu altered to reduce protein and sodium levels)

Breakfast
Orange juice, 4 oz
Cereal, ½ c with
   sugar and milk
Whole wheat toast, 1
   slice with butter
   and jelly
Coffee with 2 tbsp
   cream
Milk, ½ c

Mid-morning
English muffin with
   jelly
Fruit juice
Coffee with sugar

Lunch
Small baked potato
Green peas, ½ c
Carrot/raisin salad

Lunch (continued)
Bread, 1 slice with butter
Sliced peaches
Milk, ½ c
Tea with lemon and
   sugar
Fruit juice, 8 oz

Mid-afternoon
Fresh fruit
Sugar cookies
Tea

Dinner
Lean beef, 2½ oz
Potato, ½ c with
   butter
Green beans
Tossed salad with low-
   sodium dressing
Roll, 1

Dinner (continued)
Fruit cocktail, ½ c
Coffee with sugar
Juice, 4 oz

Snack
Buttered toast with jelly
Banana

Note: ½ regular amount salt in cooking; no added salt at table.

4. a. 2700 calories
   b. To cover the extra energy needs from fever, infection, and stress.
   c. For an adult, nonpregnant woman, the 1989 RDA for protein is 46 grams + 54 grams to bring the total to 100 grams as stated in the diet prescription.
   d. To repair and regenerate liver tissue.
   e. To spare protein for its primary functions and to furnish fiber, vitamins, and minerals.
   f. The vitamins are coenzymes for proper utilization of foods, especially carbohydrates. Extra vitamins replace vitamins lost through the disease process and improve overall well-being.
   g. Fatty meats, desserts high in fat content or chocolate, hard-to-digest fats, fried foods, and any foods or spices that cause discomfort or upset the patient. Alcohol is strictly forbidden.
   h. Sodium, both in products and salt at table.
   i. Isolation techniques vary somewhat from hospital to hospital, but, in general, disposable items are used. There is some problem with food getting cold unless care is taken. The nurse should visit with the patient while he or she eats, if possible, as eating in isolation usually results in decreased consumption. Consult protocol manual at institution.
   j. Cancer, severe malnutrition (marasmus), and early cirrhosis (this diet regime also is suitable for postoperative patients with no complications).

5. a. Avoid all fermented dairy products such as yogurts and cheeses.
   b. Do not eat raw vegetables, including salads and garnishes, and fruits that are not peeled.
   c. Defrost frozen foods in the refrigerator or microwave.
   d. Do not use foods kept at room temperature or kept heated for long periods of time.
   e. Serve and eat foods quickly following preparation.
   f. Cover and freeze leftovers immediately.
   g. Use refrigerated leftovers within two days.
   h. Keep the preparation and serving area very clean.
   i. Be sure that sanitary techniques are maintained throughout, and that food handlers are vigilant about personal habits and dress.

Activity 2: Diet Therapy for Diseases of the Gallbladder and Pancreas

See Table 19-1, for guidance; *also see* Nursing Implications.

1. Menu alterations for low-fat diet:

Breakfast
Orange juice
Oatmeal, skim milk, sugar
Poached egg (1)
Toast, 1 tsp butter, jelly
Coffee

Lunch
Baked chicken; no skin
Mashed potato
Green beans with pimiento

Lunch (continued)
Roll; 1 tsp butter
Skim milk
Tea/sugar

Dinner
Lean broiled hamburger patty
Parsley carrots
Tossed green salad/vinegar or lemon
French bread/1 tsp butter
Sherbet
Red wine
Coffee

2. Example only; other foods of similar type and value may be used.

Breakfast
Orange juice
Oatmeal/brown sugar/butter
Toast, butter, jelly
Skim milk

Mid-morning
Fruit
Sugar cookies
Skim milk

Lunch
Baked chicken
Mashed potato
Green beans
Roll/butter
Tapioca pudding
Skim milk

Mid-afternoon
Milkshake made with skim milk, sherbet, and fruit

Dinner
Broiled lean hamburger patty
Parsley carrots
Wild rice/mushrooms
French bread/butter
Sherbet
Fruit juice

Pre-bed Snack
Low-fat yogurt with fruit or cottage cheese and fruit
Crackers
Juice or skim milk

3. Risk of gallstone formation can be reduced with:
   a. proper food choice with small amount of fat
   b. diets with high fiber content
   c. regular physical activity

4. F   6. T   8. T
5. F   7. F

CHAPTER 20: DIET THERAPY FOR RENAL DISORDERS

Background Information and Activity 1: Kidney Function and Disease

1. c   3. d   5. d
2. a   4. c   6. c

7–12. *See* Background Information.

13–17. *See* Activity 1.

18. A proteolytic enzyme secreted by the kidney

19. Condition of soft bones with Ca+ deposited in tissues

20. High biological value protein—especially animal protein, milk, and eggs

Activity 2: Chronic Renal Failure

1. a   3. a   5. a
2. b   4. c

6–11. *See* Nursing Implications (any two from each category).

12–15. *See* section on dietary management.

Activity 3: Kidney Dialysis

1. Diffusion of solutes from one side of a semipermeable membrane to another.

2. Use of an artificial "kidney" outside the body to clear waste from blood.

3. Use of a catheter placed in the abdominal cavity to clear waste from blood.

4. Solution into which the blood waste products diffuse.

5. Continuous ambulatory peritoneal dialysis.

6. Nitrogenous wastes, sodium, potassium, and fluids.

7. Two reliable resources on renal disease information are:
   a. American dietetic Association (ADA)
   b. National Kidney Foundation (NKF)

8. Three important guideline documents for health professionals responsible for renal diseases are:
   a. A Clinical Guide to Nutrition Care in End-Stage Renal Disease (latest edition)
   b. Guidelines for Nutrition Care of Renal Patients (latest edition)
   c. National Renal Diet: Professional Guide and the National Renal Diet Client Education Guide (latest edition)

9. d   12. c   15. b   18. T
10. c   13. d   16. c   19. F
11. a   14. a   17. e   20. T

Activity 4: Diet Therapy for Renal Calculi

1. c

2. b

Check your answers to Questions 3 through 10 by referring to Table 20-3, acid-based foods.

3. c   5. a   7. a   9. c
4. b   6. c   8. b   10. c

CHAPTER 21: NUTRITION AND DIET THERAPY FOR CANCER AND HIV

Background Information

1. T   5. T   9. d
2. F   6. T   10. e
3. T   7. T   11. d
4. T   8. F   12. e

Activity 1: Nutrition Therapy in Cancer

1. a. body's response to the disease
   b. site of the cancer
   c. type of treatment
   d. specific physical response
   e. psychosocial response of patient

2. Any five of these: fatigue, asthenia, cachexia, anorexia, anemia, fluid and electrolyte balance, or many others (see text).

3. Optimum nutrition preoperatively and postoperatively, specific modifications according to surgical site and organ function.

4. a. thorough personal nutrition assessment
   b. maintenance of vigorous nutrition therapy
   c. revision of care plan as needed

5. a. hair follicle loss
   b. bone marrow dysfunction
   c. GI disturbances

6. a. personal beliefs
   b. advice of family and friends
   c. advice on Web sites and in other media

7. Three nutritional factors that will improve protein synthesis and energy metabolism are:
   a. Increase total caloric intake.
   b. Increase vitamin and mineral intake as needed.
   c. Maintain fluid and electrolyte balance.

8. See Table 21-2.

9. See Table 21-2.

10. c   17. T   24. T   31. T
11. c   18. F   25. T   32. F
12. c   19. T   26. F   33. F
13. T   20. F   27. T   34. T
14. F   21. T   28. T   35. F
15. T   22. T   29. F   36. T
16. T   23. T   30. F   37. T

Activity 2: Nutrition and HIV Infection

1. c
2. f
3. d
4. a. Delay progression of infections and improve patient's immune system.
   b. Delay wasting effects of HIV infection.
   c. Prevent opportunistic diseases.
   d. Recognize infections early and provide rapid treatment.
5. a. Phase 1. Primary stage. Manifestations: usually asymptomatic.
   b. Phase 2. Second stage. Opportunistic illnesses begin.
   c. Phase 3. Terminal stage. T lymphocyte production drops below 200/mm^3.
6. a. High-caloric, small, frequent feedings. Supplements as desired.
   b. Encourage consumption of high biological value (HBV) proteins.
   c. Use easily digested fats such as cream, butter, egg yolk, oils, and medium chain triglycerides (MCT). Keep fiber content low. Limited refined sugars.
   d. i. Serve attractive, appealing food. Cold usually better. Invite guests, friends, family to socialize.
      ii. Antiemetics administered before mealtimes. Far enough ahead to be effective, change schedule if necessary. Rearrange eating times if needed.
      iii. Use whatever method or type of feeding that is most effective. Supply HBV protein, vitamin mineral supplements as necessary. Assist with eating if patient is fatigued.
      iv. Serve cold or chilled soft bland and liquid foods in small quantities 6–8 times daily.
      v. Parenteral feedings, drug therapy as necessary, protection from others, protection of others.
7. See Nursing Implications.
8. All standard sanitation procedures that are implemented by the facility must be complied with. In addition, particular attention and compliance with stringent sanitation of food preparation areas, storage, and service must be adhered. Nursing and dietary employees should have a joint inservice session to make sure all applicable measures are being implemented.

9. T   14. T   19. T   24. F
10. T   15. F   20. T   25. T
11. T   16. T   21. F   26. F
12. F   17. F   22. T   27. T
13. T   18. T   23. F   28. F

CHAPTER 22: DIET THERAPY FOR BURNS, IMMOBILIZED PATIENTS, MENTAL PATIENTS, AND EATING DISORDERS

Activity 1: Diet and the Burn Patient

1. T	4. F	7. c
2. F	5. F	8. a
3. T	6. d	9. d

10. Anorexia, pain, inability to move head, swallow, chew

11. Body protein, fat, water

12. a. 77 lb = 35 kg
    b. 35 kg × 1 g protein/kg/bw = 35 g
    c. 40% body surface burned × 3 g/% surface burned = 120 g
    d. 35 g + 120 g = 155 g protein required

13. *See* list of 14 nursing implications.

Activity 2: Diet and Immobilized Patients

1. Four considerations in immobilized patient's nutritional and diet care are:
   a. nitrogen balance
   b. calories
   c. calcium intake
   d. urinary and bowel function

2. Actual skin breakdown can be avoided only a combination of:
   a. a high protein diet
   b. frequent position adjustment
   c. exercise if possible
   d. special bedding materials and sheets
   e. good hygiene

3. Calcium homostasis is determined by factors such as:
   a. bone integrity
   b. serum calcium
   c. intestinal function
   d. adequacy of active vitamin D
   e. kidney function
   f. parathyroid activity

4. Diseases related to excessive calcium are:
   a. hypercalcemia
   b. hypercalciuria
   c. metatastic calcification of soft tissues
   d. calcium stone formation in the bladder

5. Long-term treatment of hypercalcemia includes:
   a. mobilization as soon as possible
   b. calcium intake kept at 500–800 mg per day
   c. phosphate supplement

6. T	9. F	12. T	15. T
7. T	10. T	13. T	16. T
8. T	11. T	14. F	

Activity 3: Diet and Mental Patients

1. The health team of a mental patient includes:
   a. psychiatrist
   b. nurse
   c. social worker
   d. therapist
   e. nutritionist
   f. dietitian
   g. psychologist
   h. clinical specialist
   i. health aides

2. Criticisms on nutritional care in mental institutions include:
   a. poor food preparation facilities
   b. poor dining environment
   c. crowded and underbudget

3. Some of the basic reasons why mental patients have nutritional and dietary problems are:
   a. eating handicaps
   b. don't like the food served
   c. abnormal behavior patterns

4. General guidelines for nursing immobilized and mental patients:
   a. appropriate nutrition therapy is important
   b. use most effective method of feeding
   c. avoid interactions with medication
   d. provide nutrition education to patient, family, and caregivers

5. F	9. T	13. F
6. T	10. T	14. T
7. T	11. F	
8. T	12. F	

Activity 4: Anorexia Nervosa

1. a	3. c	5. a
2. d	4. b	

6. Any five of the nine listed under Feeding Routines.

7. Any five of the eight listed under Nursing Implications.

CHAPTER 23: PRINCIPLES OF FEEDING A SICK CHILD

Background Information

1. Any five of these: fatigue, vomiting, diarrhea, anorexia, pain, lethargy, confusion, effects of medication, fear, anxiety.

2. a. Anthropometric measures
   b. Physical assessment
   c. Laboratory tests

3. T	5. F	7. d
4. T	6. c	

Activity 1: The Child, the Parents, and the Health Team

1. Any of these: fatigue, nausea, vomiting, pain, fear, anxiety, anorexia, medications, separation from parents, treatments.

2. The nurse's primary role is that of liaison and child advocate. She coordinates and provides optimal dietary care.

3. *See* Nursing Implications.

Activity 2: Special Considerations and Diet Therapy

1. Height, weight, allergies, likes, dislikes, food and fluid intake at home, culture, and/or ethnic group.

2. Since burns cause stress to the body and require greatly increased nutrient intake, the major nutrients for wound healing as described in Chapter 12 apply. The RDAs for children are in the appendix. In general, normal requirements will double or triple, depending on the extent of the burn. Example: protein RDA for 5-year-old = 30 grams; protein requirement for Allen = 80 to 90 grams.

3. The diet should be increased in all essential nutrients. Total calories needed are high. Fats remain in the moderate range. In general, the diet prescription would read high-protein, high-carbohydrate, and moderate-fat, with supplemental vitamins and minerals as condition requires. The increases aid wound healing, restore nutrient losses, return the child to a positive nutritional status, and maintain growth and development.

4. Your choice: protein should be high quality; snacks included as part of the caloric/nutrient allowance.

5. Allow favorite foods, serve familiar food, observe likes/dislikes as diet permits, encourage group eating (if child is allowed up), establish a pleasant environment, allow food selection, provide companionship, encourage eating (take a snack with each visit to the room, unless treatment or therapy will interfere), relieve pain ahead of mealtimes, and furnish caregivers with list of acceptable foods they can bring from home.

CHAPTER 24: DIET THERAPY AND CYSTIC FIBROSIS

Background Information

1. Any five of these: frequent, large, foul-smelling stools; substandard weight gain; abdominal bloating; steatorrhea; excessive crying; sodium deficiency; circulatory collapse; frequent pneumonia.

2. b
3. b
4. c

Activity 1: Dietary Management of Cystic Fibrosis

1. No. She is undersized. The range for children seven to ten years old to the RDAs is approximately 52 inches height and 62 pounds. Susie is 8 to 10 inches shorter than average, and about 12 pounds underweight.

2. a. Diarrhea: undigested food in the stools.
   b. Lethargy: general malnutrition/fever.

3. High-calorie diet for growth and compensation for food lost in stools. High-protein diet for growth and compensation for food lost in stools. High- to moderate-carbohydrate diet to spare protein and compensate for food lost in stools (simple carbohydrates are better tolerated than starches). Low- to moderate-fat diet because fats are not tolerated well; altered types of fat such as medium-chain triglycerides may be used. High-vitamin and mineral diet: double doses of multiple vitamins in water-soluble form. Salt added generously. Pancreatic enzymes are given by mouth with meals and snacks.

4. Food from home, fast food favorites, group eating, socializing occasions, cheerful atmosphere, frequent meals, some favorite foods added, compromises.

5. Your choice. Diet should contain 90 to 100 grams protein and at least 2500 calories—3000 to 3500 calories would be better. Calories can be increased as appetite improves. Use exchange lists for figuring protein and calories, plus any caloric chart available for items not listed in exchanges.

CHAPTER 25: DIET THERAPY AND CELIAC DISEASE

Activity 1: Dietary Management of Celiac Disease

1. a

2. b

3. a

4. Gluten is the protein fraction found in wheat, rye, oats, and barley to which some people are intolerant. It may be due to an immune reaction or an inherited defect, but it has a toxic effect on the intestine. Inform Mrs. Jones of products containing gluten that must be omitted from her diet to prevent changes in the jejunum. Explain that these

changes will prevent absorption of nutrients into the cell, causing acute symptoms and malnutrition.

5. Advise Mrs. Jones to pack a lunch, as most restaurants use mixes, thickeners, and other products containing gluten. She might pack: baked chicken, potato chips, celery and carrot sticks, fruit gelatin, olives, fruit or tomato juice, vanilla tapioca pudding (homemade), crisped rice cookies (made with marshmallows), etc.

6. Pasta, breads, cereals, all breaded products, commercial mixes, thickeners, commercial candies, some salad dressings, canned cream soups, etc. (also see Table 23-1).

7. Rice and corn.

8. Any creamed, thickened and filled products, including candies, gravies, sauces, puddings, casseroles, stuffings, and meat loaf.

9. Milk in all forms: fresh, dry, evaporated, fermented or malted. All foods containing milk: cocoa, chocolate, all breads, rolls, waffles, cakes made with milk. Desserts made with milk: cookies, custard, ice cream, puddings, sherbets, cream pies. Margarine that contains milk or cream. Meats: franks, any luncheon meats containing milk powder. Candy: caramel or chocolate. Vegetables in cream sauces.

10. Yes. Medium-chain triglycerides are better tolerated than regular fats and the need for calories is high. The typical client is usually underweight.

Activity 2: Screening, occurrence, complication

1. T   3. F   5. T   7. T
2. F   4. T   6. T

8. Celiac disease could be underdiagnosed in the United States for a number of reasons:
   a. Celiac symptoms can be attributed to other problems.
   b. Many doctors are not knowledgeable about the disease.
   c. Only a handful of U.S. laboatories are experience and skilled in testing for celiac disease.

CHAPTER 25: DIET THERAPY AND CONGENITAL HEART DISEASE

Activity 1: Dietary Management of Congenital Heart Disease

1. b   4. c   7. d   10. c
2. a   5. b   8. b
3. d   6. d   9. a

11. *Breakfast*
Fruit juice, 3 oz
Salt-free cereal, 2 tbsp
Toast, ½ slice

Lunch and Dinner
Pureed or mashed vegetables, 2 tbsp
Pureed meat (prepared without salt), 1 oz

Lunch and Dinner (continued)
Pureed fruit, 2–3 tbsp
Mashed potatoes, 1 tbsp

Snacks
High-calorie, low-protein, low-sodium beverages as appropriate to age. This will assist in meeting fluid requirements.

12. *See* Managing Feeding Problems.

13. *See* Managing Feeding Problems and Nursing Implications.

14. *See* Discharge Procedures.

CHAPTER 27: DIET THERAPY AND FOOD ALLERGY

Background Information and Activity 1: Food Allergy and Children

1. Excess sensitivity to certain substances or conditions.

2. Allergens or antigens.

3. First exposure to antigen produces no overt symptoms, causes the body to form these immunoglobulins.

4. When an allergic reaction does not manifest quickly or in the usual ways, but rather over a period of time, the child shows the tension-fatigue syndrome.

5. A food allergy triggers the immunological system of the body, whereas a food intolerance is a direct result of maldigestion or malabsorption.

6. a. Amount of allergen consumed.
   b. Whether it is cooked or raw.
   c. Cumulative effects.
   d. Allergic to inhalable as well as ingestible items.
   e. Allergic at one time but not at another.
   f. Reacts to allergen when physical or emotional problems occur. Also, may be another food chemical, not protein.

7. a. Offending substances must be identified and removed.
   b. Monitors the antiallergenic diet to ensure adequate nutrient intake.

8. Breast milk does not contain beta lactoglobulins, the substance in cow's milk that may trigger reactions.

9. Skin testing and elimination diets.

Activity 2: Common Offenders

1. b
2. a
3. c
4. T

5. F
6. T
7. F
8. F

9. T
10. F

Activity 3: Inspecting Foods to Avoid Allergic Ingredients

1. T
2. F
3. T

4. FDA believes there is scientific consensus that the following foods can cause serious allergic reactions in some individuals and account for more than 90% of all food allergies:
   a. Peanuts
   b. Soybeans
   c. Milk
   d. Eggs
   e. Fish
   f. Crustaceans (e.g., shrimp)
   g. Tree nuts
   h. Wheat

CHAPTER 28: DIET THERAPY AND PHENYLKETONURIA

Background Information

1. b
2. c
3. a

4. d
5. b
6. F

7. F

Activity 1: Phenylketonuria and Dietary Management

1. a
2. c
3. b
4. b
5. b

6. a
7. c
8. d
9. d
10. T

11. T
12. T
13. F

14. a. determine age, weight, and activity level of the child;
    b. determine the client's daily requirement for phenylalanine;
    c. determine the contribution of protein from Lofenalac evaporated milk;
    d. determine calories from formula, milk, and any other food consumed; and
    e. determine total phenylalanine from formula, milk, and any other food consumed.
15. See Table 26-3. Also: the use of special, low-protein products: cookies, bread, pasta, drinks, and desserts made primarily from free foods; and the increased use of flavorings and spices as tolerated.

CHAPTER 29: THERAPY FOR CONSTIPATION, DIARRHEA, AND HIGH-RISK INFANTS

Activity 1: Constipation

1. b
2. a

3. d
4. b

5. c

6. No regular schedule for elimination (not taking time for bathroom).
7. a. Clean out the colon with enema.
   b. Continue use until a regular defecation pattern is established.
   c. Put the child on a conditioning schedule.
   d. Reduce milk to approximately 60%–80% of normal and increase other fluids and fiber until goal is attained. Keep on maintenance dosage of fiber and other fluids. Return milk to normal amount.
8. See Nursing Implications.

Activity 2: Diarrhea

1. a. Stool profile.
   b. Cause.
   c. Site of defect.

2. a. Clinical disorder.
   b. Bacteria in food/formula.
   c. Reactions to certain foods.

3. a. Restore fluid and electrolyte balance.
   b. Restore adequate nutrition.

4, 5, 6. See Table 27-2.

7. a. Add corn syrup to formula.
   b. Feed strained cereals, strained fruits.
   c. Provide extra feedings.

Activity 3: High-Risk Infants

1. c
2. d

3. a
4. a

5. b

6. a. Child can suck.
   b. Child weighs more than 2000 grams.

7. a. Manual expression.
   b. Give by tube, bottle, or dropper.
   c. Milk less than 8 hours old, unrefrigerated.

8. a. 100–130 kcal/kg/bw
   b. 3–4 g pro/kg/bw
   c. fluid = to output.
   d. Supplement calcium, iron, vitamin K, tyrosine, and cystine as needed.

9. One containing specific amounts of essential nutrients necessary for the growth of the infant.

Introduction to Nutrition

Multiple Choice

Circle the letter of the correct answer.

1. The food groups at the base of MyPyramid are:

    a. foods containing the most kilocalories.
    b. foods to be emphasized in the diet.
    c. foods that are highest in essential nutrients.
    d. foods contributing the least fiber.

2. A dietary supplement is:

    a. extra vitamins and minerals to prevent chronic diseases.
    b. a health food that alleviates illness.
    c. necessary to provide essential nutrients in the diet.
    d. a product used to increase total dietary intake.

3. Major recommendations by government health agencies for reducing chronic-disease risk include:

    a. an increase in complex carbohydrate foods.
    b. a decrease in use of foods high in fat.
    c. an increase in foods high in fiber.
    d. b and c
    e. a, b, c

4. A kilocalorie is:

    a. the release of energy from food.
    b. the amount of heat required to raise the temperature of one kilogram of water one degree centigrade.
    c. the capacity to do work.
    d. the amount of calories in a specific amount of food.

5. The recommendations to promote health and prevent or delay the onset of chronic diseases are known as:

    a. Recommended Dietary Allowances.
    b. Reference Daily Intakes.
    c. Dietary Guidelines for Americans.
    d. Daily Reference Values.

6. The levels of intake of essential nutrients considered to be adequate to meet the nutritional needs of healthy persons is known as:

    a. Dietary Guidelines for Americans.
    b. Recommended Dietary Allowances.
    c. Reference Daily Intakes.
    d. U.S. Dietary Goals.

7. Nutrition labeling information is mandatory on which of the following products?

    a. packaged foods, dairy foods
    b. raw produce, fish
    c. raw meat, poultry
    d. all of the above

8. Information on food labels may include which of these nutrients?

    a. total fat, saturated fat, cholesterol
    b. polyunsaturated fat, monounsaturated fat
    c. sodium, calcium, iron
    d. a, c
    e. a, b, c

9. The components that supply energy, promote growth, and repair and regulate body processes are termed:

    a. chemicals.
    b. nutrients.
    c. nutrition.
    d. adequate diet.

Matching

Match the foods listed on the left to the size of one serving at the right, according to MyPyramid.

_____ 10. cooked cereal   a. 1 cup
_____ 11. raw leafy vegetables   b. ¾ cup
_____ 12. fruit juice   c. ½ cup
_____ 13. milk
_____ 14. tofu

15. Define the following:

    a. AI: _____.

    b. EAR: _____.

    c. IOM: _____.

    d. USHHS: _____.

    e. %DVs: _____.

    f. Discretionary calorie allowance: _____.

    g. Functional foods: _____.

    h. Nutraceuticals: _____.

16. Which of the following is represented on MyPyramid.gov?

    a. Activity
    b. Altruism
    c. Gradual improvement
    d. Integrity
    e. Interdependency
    f. Moderation
    g. Personalization
    h. Proportionality
    i. Variety
    j. a, c, f, g, h, i
    k. a, b, c, d, e, f
    l. b, e, f, g, h, i

17. According to labeling for one serving, which of the following is recommended based on a 2000-calorie diet:

    a. 50 calories is low.
    b. 500 calories or more is high.
    c. 100 calories is moderate.
    d. 120 calories is moderate.

18. According to the sample label for macaroni and cheese, which of the following is correct?

    a. For %DV, 5% or less is low.
    b. For %DV, 20% or more is high.
    c. For trans fat, there is no %DV.
    d. For sugars, the %DV is 12%.
    e. a, b, c, d
    f. a, b, c

19. Which of the following refers to a DRI established by www.NAS.edu?

    a. Tolerable Upper Intake Levels (UL), vitamins
    b. Tolerable Upper Intake Levels (UL), elements
    c. Estimated Energy Requirements (EER) for children
    d. Acceptable Calories Distribution Ranges
    e. Recommended Intakes for Individuals, macronutrients
    f. Additional macronutrient recommendations
    g. Estimated Average Requirements for Asians
    h. a, b, c, f
    i. d, e, g, h
    j. a, b, e, f

20. Regarding omega-6-PUFA, which of the following is correct?

    a. prevalent in beef fat and corn oil
    b. may benefit persons with risk of cardiovascular disease
    c. includes EPA and DHA
    d. a, c
    e. b, c
    f. a, b

Situation

Mary is on her way to take an important examination. At a fast-food restaurant she picks up the following lunch: grilled chicken sandwich, salad with low-fat dressing, an orange juice, and a fat-free yogurt. Answer the following questions about this situation.

21. How does Mary's meal fit into MyPyramid's food selection guide?

    _____

    _____

    _____

22. List five foods that Mary should eat at dinner to round out a balanced diet.

    a. _____

    b. _____

    c. _____

    d. _____

    e. _____

23. List the objectives of the NCEP three adult treatment panels (ATP 1, 2, 3)

    a. _____

    b. _____

    c. _____

Food Habits

Multiple Choice

Circle the letter of the correct answer.

1. Which of the following mechanisms stimulates the appetite?

   a. the central nervous system
   b. the body's biological needs
   c. the sight, smell, and taste of food
   d. the time of day

2. Lack of money affects eating patterns by

   a. curtailing the kind of food bought.
   b. curtailing the amount of food bought.
   c. increasing the amount of starchy foods bought.
   d. all of the above.

3. Hunger is a mechanism controlled by

   a. the central nervous system.
   b. the body's biological needs.
   c. the sight, smell, and taste of food.
   d. the time of day.

4. The one requirement that the biological food needs of an individual must provide is

   a. adaptation to the culture and traditions of the people.
   b. essential nutrients which the body can digest, absorb, and utilize.
   c. pleasant taste, smell, and appearance of food.
   d. adequate intake.

5. Which of the following provides the best framework for changing eating behaviors?

   a. scientific knowledge
   b. relating the changes to the culture and habits
   c. teaching in a group where others have the same problem
   d. sending a home health aide out to check

6. Which of the following nutrients tend to be deficient in the diet of the Native American?

   a. calcium and riboflavin
   b. vitamins A and C
   c. protein
   d. all of these

7. The typical Chinese diet may be low in which of the following nutrients?

   a. protein, calcium, vitamin D
   b. carbohydrates, fats, fiber
   c. thiamin, niacin, riboflavin
   d. carbohydrates, iron, vitamin K

8. Which of the following meats are avoided by Muslims, Jews, and Seventh Day Adventists?

   a. beef
   b. poultry
   c. pork
   d. seafood

9. What is the condition that results when children have diets inadequate in protein?

   a. pellagra
   b. kwashiorkor
   c. PEM
   d. galactosemia

10. The diet of the Mexican-American tends to be high in

    a. fats and sodium.
    b. calcium and folacin.
    c. protein and carbohydrate.
    d. vitamins A and D.

11. Blacks, Native Americans, and Asians have a high incidence of

    a. diabetes.
    b. heart disease.
    c. lactose intolerance.
    d. marasmus.

12. Yin and yang foods refer to

    a. the soul food of Cheech and Chong.
    b. the number 1 and 2 foods used in China.
    c. hot and cold foods, not related to temperature.
    d. hot, spicy foods.

Matching

Match the statement in the left column to the type of food symbolism in the right column. (Answers can be used more than once.)

_____ 13. "I take 500 mg of   a. sociological
organic vitamin C   b. biological
three times   c. emotional
per day to keep from
getting a cold"

_____ 14. "I want the best steaks you
have; my boss is coming
to dinner"

_____ 15. "I ate a pound of chocolate
fudge after that awful day
I had at the office"

_____ 16. The food symbolism most
likely to change

True/False

Circle T for True and F for False.

17. T F Diseases of malnutrition are a problem in most countries except the United States.
18. T F A hospitalized vegetarian should not have difficulty selecting from a hospital menu.
19. T F The Jewish diet is usually high in saturated fats and cholesterol.
20. T F Hot red and green peppers, which are used liberally in the Mexican diet, contain good sources of vitamins A and C.
21. T F The practice of using lime-soaked tortillas should be discouraged.
22. T F Obesity is not a problem in United States culture.
23. T F All of the different cultures in the United States have substandard diets.
24. T F Eating behaviors develop from cultural conditioning, not from an instinct to choose adequate foods.
25. T F The economic status of an individual often changes his or her food habits.
26. T F Food has hidden meanings and may become an outlet for stress.
27. T F Poverty is a subculture in the United States.

Situation

Billy is a five-year-old who is admitted to the hospital for the first time. He will be hospitalized for approximately a week for diagnostic tests and possible surgery. When his food is not being withheld, he receives a regular diet. From this brief situation, answer the following questions by circling the letter of the best answer.

28. The breakfast tray, which has been held until 10 a.m. because of tests, has an egg, bacon, juice, and toast on it. Billy refuses it, though he has stated he was hungry. You could assume that his refusal is due to which of the following?

a. He has lost his appetite by 10 a.m.
b. The foods are unfamiliar.
c. He wants to be fed.
d. He wants his mother.

29. Billy's roommate is a one-year-old who receives a supplemental bottle feeding. When this child receives a bottle, Billy cries for one also. You could assume that this behavior is

a. a bid for attention.
b. regression to an earlier developmental stage.
c. because he still takes a bottle when he is home.
d. due to hunger.

30. You place Billy's supper tray on the bedside table and encourage him to take a few bites. He shoves the tray to the floor and starts crying loudly. The reason for this hostility is probably due to

a. being a spoiled brat.
b. anxiety and fear.
c. dislike of hospital food.
d. all of the above.

Proteins and Health

Multiple Choice

Circle the letter of the correct answer.

1. Of the twenty-two amino acids involved in total body metabolism, building and rebuilding various tissues, eight are termed essential amino acids. This means

   a. the body cannot synthesize these eight amino acids and must obtain them in the diet.
   b. these eight amino acids are essential in body processes, and the remaining fourteen are not.
   c. these eight amino acids can be made by the body because they are essential to life.
   d. after synthesizing these eight amino acids, the body uses them in key processes essential for growth.

2. A complete food protein of high biologic value would be one that contains

   a. all 22 of the amino acids in sufficient quantity to meet human requirements.
   b. the eight essential amino acids in any proportion, since the body can always fill in the difference needed.
   c. most of the 22 amino acids from which the body will make additional amounts of the eight essential amino acids needed.
   d. all eight of the essential amino acids in correct proportion to human needs.

3. Besides carbon, hydrogen, and oxygen, what other element is found in all proteins?

   a. calcium
   b. nitrogen
   c. glycogen
   d. carbon dioxide

4. The basic building blocks of proteins are

   a. fatty acids.
   b. keto acids.
   c. amino acids.
   d. nucleic acids.

5. Sufficient carbohydrate in the diet allows a major portion of protein to be used for building tissue. This is known as

   a. digestion, absorption, and metabolism.
   b. the halo effect of carbohydrate regulation.
   c. the protein-sparing action of carbohydrate.
   d. carbohydrate loading.

6. Which of the following foods contain the largest amounts of essential amino acids?

   a. soybeans and peanuts
   b. milk and eggs
   c. meat and whole wheat bread
   d. poultry and fish

7. Which two foods contain proteins that are so incomplete they will not support life if eaten alone with no other added source of protein?

   a. meat, eggs
   b. fish, cheese
   c. gelatin, corn
   d. rice, dried beans

8. Protein complementation is

   a. combining foods that taste good.
   b. combining foods with mutually supplemental amino acid patterns.
   c. combining similar protein foods.
   d. combining carbohydrates and fats with proteins.

9. Joe is a lacto-vegetarian. Which of the following would he be most likely to consume?

   a. cheese omelette
   b. strawberry yogurt
   c. tuna noodle casserole
   d. boiled egg and toast

10. The essential amino acid present in a food in the smallest amount in relation to human need is termed

    a. nonessential amino acid.
    b. limiting amino acid.
    c. target amino acid.
    d. missing amino acid.

11. Kcalories provided by excess dietary protein can be

    a. converted to muscle tissue.
    b. converted to fat.
    c. used for energy.
    d. b and c.

12. Anemia results from a deficiency of hemoglobin and/or red blood cells in the circulating blood. Can protein deficiency cause anemia?

    a. yes
    b. no
    c. only if vitamin B_{12} is also deficient
    d. only if folacin is not present

Matching

Match the protein part of the food listed in the left column to its type in the right column. (Answers can be used more than once.)

_____ 13. nuts   a. complete protein
_____ 14. fish   b. incomplete protein
_____ 15. whole wheat bread
_____ 16. cheese
_____ 17. legumes

True/False

Circle T for True and F for False.

18. T F All enzymes and hormones are protein substances.
19. T F Lipoproteins are transport forms of fat, produced mainly in the intestinal wall and in the liver.
20. T F Complete proteins of high biologic value are found in whole grains, dried beans and peas, and nuts.
21. T F Protein is best absorbed and utilized when complementary protein foods are eaten in the same meal.
22. T F 30 grams of protein yields 270 calories.
23. T F Enzymes are proteins involved in metabolic processes.
24. T F The RDA for protein for an adult is figured on 0.8 gram per kg of body weight.
25. T F Kwashiorkor is a type of malnutrition resulting from a very low-calorie diet.

Situation

Five-year-old Lisa lives in a strict vegetarian family. Lately, her mother has been concerned because Lisa has been tired, cross, and withdrawn, so she takes her to the doctor. The pediatrician who examines her tells her mother that Lisa has several nutritional deficiencies and sends her to a dietitian for a consultation. Answer the following questions regarding this situation.

26. Which of the following nutrients are likely to be low in Lisa's diet?
    a. calcium, iron, iodine
    b. vitamins B_{12}, D, riboflavin
    c. essential amino acids
    d. all of the above

Lisa eats the following foods in a 24-hour period:

Breakfast: whole wheat toast, applesauce, grape juice

Lunch: steamed rice with honey and cinnamon, carrot and raisin salad, canned pears, sweetened instant drink

Dinner: alfalfa sprouts, mushroom and tomato sandwich on whole wheat bread, vegetarian vegetable soup, apple, peach nectar

Snacks: homemade raised doughnut, applesauce

27. Based upon the foods listed above, what would you expect to happen to Lisa if the eating pattern continues?
    a. Her growth will slow or stop.
    b. She will grow up very healthy.
    c. She will become overweight.
    d. She will get scurvy.

28. List at least five foods that should be added to Lisa's diet and indicate the proper combinations.

    a. _____

    b. _____

    c. _____

    d. _____

    e. _____

Carbohydrates and Fats: Implications for Health

Multiple Choice

Circle the letter of the correct answer.

1. Which of the following is not a rich source of polysaccharides?

   a. poultry
   b. vegetables
   c. cereals
   d. potatoes

2. What organ of the body relies primarily on glucose for energy?

   a. heart
   b. lungs
   c. muscles
   d. brain

3. Which of these substances is necessary for the uptake of glucose by the cells?

   a. insulin
   b. epinephrine
   c. adrenalin
   d. thyroxin

4. Which of the following is a function of sugars?

   a. They enhance the flavor of some foods.
   b. They add kcalories to a diet.
   c. They prevent microbial growth in jams and jellies.
   d. all of the above

5. The incidence of dental caries is most influenced by

   a. the total amount of sugar consumed.
   b. the number of times a sugar food is consumed.
   c. the length of time sugar is in contact with the teeth.
   d. the type of sugar consumed.

6. A steady blood glucose level is best achieved by consuming which of the following types of diets?

   a. high-sugar foods like candy and soft drinks
   b. no fluids with meals
   c. small meals containing complex carbohydrate, protein, and fat
   d. meals high in protein, fat, and water but low in carbohydrate

7. A high-fiber diet has proven to be an effective treatment for

   a. varicose veins.
   b. coronary heart disease.
   c. appendicitis.
   d. diverticulosis.

8. A therapeutic diet frequently used in the treatment of heart disease is the low-saturated fat diet. Which of the following foods would not be allowed?

   a. whole milk
   b. corn oil
   c. special soft margarine
   d. whole grains

9. Fats provide the body with its main stored energy source. Another function of fat in the body is

   a. furnishing essential fatty acids required by the body.
   b. regulating body temperature through insulation.
   c. preventing shock to vital organs by padding.
   d. all of the above

10. The function of cholesterol in the body is to serve in the formation of

    a. hormones, bile, and vitamin D.
    b. enzymes, antibodies, and vitamin B_{12}.
    c. central nervous system tissue.
    d. vitamins, enzymes, and fats.

11. From which of these sources is cholesterol obtained?

    a. animal foods containing fat
    b. plant foods rich in polyunsaturated fats
    c. synthesis in the liver
    d. a and c

12. Which of the foods listed below contains predominantly saturated fats?

    a. fruits
    b. vegetables
    c. meats
    d. breads

13. Select the food item from the list below that does not contain cholesterol.

    a. liver
    b. cheddar cheese
    c. shrimp
    d. peanut butter

Matching

Match the phrases on the right to the terms on the left that they best describe.

_____ 14. hydrogenation
_____ 15. bile salts
_____ 16. linoleic
_____ 17. hypoglycemia
_____ 18. glycogen and lactose

a. blood sugar level below normal
b. an essential fatty acid
c. animal sources of carbohydrates
d. substance that breaks fat into small particles
e. conversion of unsaturated oil to a saturated fat

True/False

Circle T for True and F for False.

19. T F Low-density lipoproteins are thought to protect against cardiovascular disease.

20. T F Distribution of carbohydrate in the diet should range between 50 and 60 percent.

21. T F Fat should constitute approximately 40 percent of our food intake for healthful eating according to dietary guidelines.

22. T F Athletes need the same basic nutrients as all other people.

23. T F Carbohydrates are the most efficient energy source for athletes and nonathletes.

24. T F Athletes and nonathletes need some fat on their bodies.

Situation

Stacy is a sixteen-year-old high school student who is on the wrestling team. He is 5′8″ tall and weighs 150 lbs. Recently his coach told him he had to lose 10 lbs to wrestle in a lower weight division. He has 10 days before the next meet.

25. Stacy tells his mother the coach told him to eat only 1 meal a day and to increase his workouts by 1 hour. Which of the following responses is most appropriate?

a. "No son of mine is going to starve like that."
b. "You will lose weight but it will be muscle loss, not fat loss."
c. "You should lose the required amount of weight if you don't cheat on the diet."
d. "I need to lose 10 lbs. I'll go on the diet with you."

26. The foods that Stacy is allowed to eat are meats of all kinds and green salads. He gets no milk or cheese. The coach also recommends that his mother buy him a megavitamin/mineral supplement and a buddy recommends bee pollen. What is the most likely response of Stacy's body to this diet regime?

a. The extra protein and vitamins will increase his endurance and stamina.
b. The bee pollen will cause him to have an allergic reaction.
c. He will get diarrhea, dehydration, and ketosis.
d. He will improve his performance by 30 percent.

27. By decreasing his water intake the day before the match and using no salt, Stacy manages to make the 140 lb weight. Ten minutes into the match he collapses and has to be seen by a physician. The probable reason for this happening is

a. he was coming down with the flu.
b. he should have had carbohydrate loading the night before to get more energy.
c. he was dehydrated, weakened, and debilitated from the diet regime.
d. he had been to a big party and had not gotten enough rest.

28. List at least three dietary principles you would have recommended for Stacy if you had been his coach.

a. _____

b. _____

c. _____

Vitamins and Health

Multiple Choice

Circle the letter of the correct answer.

1. A dietary deficiency of vitamin A can produce

    a. xerophthalmia.
    b. a prolonged blood-clotting time.
    c. osteomalacia.
    d. all of the above.

2. Vitamin A toxicity is likely to occur from

    a. consuming too many dark green and deep orange vegetables.
    b. eating liver twice a week.
    c. consuming high dosage vitamin A supplements.
    d. drinking too much vitamin A-fortified milk.

3. The most reliable source of vitamin D in the diet is

    a. meat.
    b. fruits and vegetables.
    c. fortified milk.
    d. enriched breads and cereals.

4. Rickets is most likely to be caused by deficiencies of

    a. iron and phosphorus.
    b. calcium and vitamin D.
    c. magnesium and vitamin D.
    d. phosphorus and fluoride.

5. Major sources of vitamin E in the diet are

    a. meats.
    b. milk and dairy products.
    c. citrus fruits.
    d. vegetable oils.

6. Vitamin K deficiency is most often observed in

    a. newborns.
    b. children.
    c. teenagers.
    d. adults.

7. The vitamin that is synthesized in the intestines by bacteria is

    a. vitamin A.
    b. vitamin C.
    c. vitamin D.
    d. vitamin K.

8. Factors that may cause a deficiency of water soluble vitamins include

    a. taking no vitamin supplement.
    b. fad diets.
    c. an 1800 calorie diet from the four food groups.
    d. a regular pregnancy.

9. B complex vitamins

    a. function as coenzymes.
    b. are best supplied by supplements.
    c. include vitamin C.
    d. include laetrile.

10. A deficiency of vitamin C

    a. causes delayed wound healing.
    b. decreases iron absorption.
    c. increases capillary bleeding.
    d. all of the above

Matching

Match the statements on the left side with the letter of the corresponding vitamins listed on the right side.

_____ 11. inadequate intake causes osteomalacia and rickets

_____ 12. inadequate intake causes poor night vision and skin infection

_____ 13. promotes normal blood clotting

_____ 14. prevents destruction of unsaturated fatty acids

a. vitamin A
b. vitamin D
c. vitamin E
d. vitamin K

Match the statements on the left side with the letter of the corresponding vitamins listed on the right side.

_____ 15. deficiency causes cracked skin around the mouth, inflamed lips, and sore tongue

_____ 16. helps change one amino acid into another

_____ 17. a cobalt-containing vitamin needed for red blood cell formation

_____ 18. promotes the formation of collagen

a. ascorbic acid
b. pyridoxine
c. vitamin B_{12}
d. riboflavin

True/False

Circle T for True and F for False.

19. T F Natural and synthetic vitamins are used by the body in the same way.
20. T F Vitamin K is required for the synthesis of blood clotting factors.
21. T F B-vitamins serve as coenzymes in metabolic reactions in the body.
22. T F Natural vitamin supplements are more efficiently utilized by the body than synthetic vitamins because they are in a form the body prefers.
23. T F Vitamins are a good source of food energy.
24. T F There is no RDA for vitamin K because it is produced by the body.
25. T F A deficiency of vitamin B_{12} produces sickle cell anemia.
26. T F Niacin is found in abundance in meats, poultry, and fish.
27. T F Pyridoxine (B_6) is found in wheat, corn, meats, and liver.
28. T F Riboflavin is found abundantly in milk and cheese.

Situation

Mrs. A. is preparing dinner for visitors. She decides to do as much preparation ahead of time as she can in order to spend more time with her guests. The day before the dinner, she chops greens for a salad, puts them in a large, shallow container and refrigerates them uncovered so that they will stay crisp. The afternoon prior to the dinner she slices tomatoes and peppers and refrigerates. She peels, dices, and puts potatoes on to boil to make mashed potatoes later and reheat. She also puts green beans on about two hours prior to dinner in a large quantity of water so that they can cook slowly. She has cooked a roast which she will slice and reheat at the appropriate time. Answer the following questions.

29. Identify the practices that contribute to a loss of vitamins in the preparation and storage of this meal.

_____

_____

_____

30. Identify the vitamins that are lost.

_____

_____

_____

31. List at least three things you would teach Mrs. A. regarding conservation of nutrients.

a. _____

b. _____

c. _____

Minerals, Water, and Body Processes

Multiple Choice

Circle the letter of the correct answer.

1. Minerals most often deficient in the diet in the United States are

   a. iodine and fluorine.
   b. phosphorus and calcium.
   c. calcium and iron.
   d. potassium and sodium.

2. Iron deficiency anemia

   a. is not a major problem until age 25.
   b. is a problem for male teenagers.
   c. is a problem for young children and menstruating women.
   d. is a problem in the geriatric adult.

3. Calcium is widely involved in body processes. Among the best known functions are all except

   a. nerve transmission.
   b. muscle contraction.
   c. maintenance of heartbeat.
   d. coenzyme action.

4. The disease of later years that is primarily due to an inadequate calcium intake during younger years is

   a. osteoporosis
   b. rickets.
   c. xerophthalmia.
   d. marasmus.

5. The body survives the shortest time when _____ is lacking.

   a. protein
   b. carbohydrate
   c. fat
   d. water

6. Which of these nutrients contributes the most weight to the human body?

   a. calcium
   b. zinc
   c. water
   d. iron

7. Water functions in the body as all of these except

   a. a participant in chemical reactions.
   b. a solvent.
   c. a lubricant.
   d. a source of energy.

8. Excess consumption of meat, fish, and poultry could

   a. cause iron deficiency.
   b. increase calcium excretion.
   c. favor calcium absorption.
   d. prevent iron toxicity.

9. Fluoride deficiency is best known to cause

   a. mottling of teeth.
   b. osteoporosis.
   c. nutritional muscular dystrophy.
   d. dental decay.

10. Which of these foods provides the best source of iron?

    a. egg white
    b. oranges
    c. bananas
    d. prunes

Matching

Match the function in the left column with the letter of the mineral in the right column.

_____ 11. promotes bone calcification   a. iron

_____ 12. deficiency causes endemic goiter   b. phosphorus

_____ 13. found in some proteins   c. copper

_____ 14. part of hemoglobin molecule   d. iodine

_____ 15. necessary for hemoglobin formation combined with another mineral   e. sulphur

True/False

Circle T for True and F for False.

16. T F Most of the dietary iron ingested is absorbed.
17. T F The best food source of iron is milk.
18. T F The person constantly taking baking soda for his "acid stomach" may develop iron deficiency anemia and/or calcium deficiency.
19. T F Acidic fruits, particularly citrus and tomato, make the blood acid.
20. T F "Softened" water is usually high in sodium.
21. T F Minerals involved in maintaining the water balance of the cells are in the special form of ions.
22. T F The best source of calcium available to people who need to increase their calcium intake is calcium pills.
23. T F The major minerals are more important than the trace minerals.
24. T F The major minerals are found in larger quantities in the body than the trace minerals.
25. T F Fluoride actually forms part of the growing tooth crystal.
26. T F Manganese facilitates bone development.
27. T F Sulfur performs a structural role in the proteins of the hair, nails, and skin.

Situation

The following 24-hour intake was consumed by a 25-year-old female married graduate student.

Breakfast: coffee, cream and sugar

Lunch: green salad with blue cheese dressing
6 crackers
Jell–O with fruit cocktail
tea with lemon and sugar

Dinner: 4 oz broiled chicken
½ c rice with gravy
apple and celery salad
roll with butter
coffee, cream and sugar

Assuming that this is her typical eating pattern, answer the following questions regarding her diet:

28. Which of the following minerals would you expect to be deficient in her diet?

   a. sodium and potassium
   b. calcium and iron
   c. magnesium and zinc
   d. fluoride and iodine

29. For the minerals you identified as deficient in this diet (#28) list three good food sources and the daily amount needed according to the RDAs.

Daily Amount   *Foods*

Mineral #1

_____   a. _____

                           b. _____

                           c. _____

Mineral #2

_____   a. _____

                           b. _____

                           c. _____

30. If this person's diet remains unchanged, what nutritionally based diseases would you expect her to develop?

   a. iron deficiency anemia and osteoporosis
   b. hypertension and xerophthalmia
   c. skin lesions and dwarfism
   d. dental caries and goiter

Meeting Energy Needs

Multiple Choice

Circle the letter of the correct answer.

1. The most successful and healthful way to lose weight is to

   a. eat less but still choose a variety of foods.
   b. exercise regularly.
   c. follow an 800 kcal diet until goal weight is reached.
   d. a and b.

2. How many kcalories are in a food if it contains 10 grams of carbohydrate, 8 grams of fat, 7 grams of protein, 5 milligrams of thiamin, and 40 grams of water?

   a. 138 kcalories
   b. 140 kcalories
   c. 142 kcalories
   d. 145 kcalories

3. All of the following affect the basal metabolic rate (BMR) except

   a. muscle tone.
   b. gender.
   c. body composition.
   d. emotional state.

4. Which of the following factors is directly responsible for controlling basal metabolic energy expenditure?

   a. amount of daily physical activity
   b. thyroid hormone secretion
   c. daily caloric intake
   d. percent of body weight that is fat

5. Which of the following would influence the number of kcalories burned in a given physical activity?

   a. a person's body weight
   b. number of muscles used
   c. length of time the activity is performed
   d. all of the above

6. Which of the following are characteristics of a fad diet?

   a. It does not provide adequate carbohydrate.
   b. It severely restricts food choices.
   c. It emphasizes one or two foods.
   d. all of the above.

7. In human nutrition, the kilocalorie (calorie) is used

   a. to measure heat energy.
   b. to provide nutrients.
   c. as a measure of electrical energy.
   d. to control energy reactions.

8. Which of the following foods has the highest energy value per unit of weight?

   a. potato
   b. bread
   c. meat
   d. butter

9. The basal metabolic rate indicates the energy necessary for

   a. digestion of food.
   b. maintaining basal standard test conditions.
   c. sleep.
   d. maintaining vital life functions.

10. Growth, fever, and food intake

    a. decrease basal metabolic rate.
    b. increase basal metabolic rate.
    c. provide nitrogen equilibrium.
    d. cause basal metabolic rate to cease.

Matching

Match the statements in the left column to their equivalents in the right column. (Answers may be used more than once.)

_____ 11. calories per g of carbohydrate   a. 9
_____ 12. calories per oz of carbohydrate   b. 270
_____ 13. calories per g of protein   c. 120
_____ 14. calories per oz of protein   d. 4
_____ 15. calories per g of fat
_____ 16. calories per oz of fat

True/False

Circle T for True and F for False.

17. T F Ketosis is an abnormal metabolic condition resulting from low-carbohydrate and semi-starvation diets.
18. T F The body has an unlimited capacity to store fat.
19. T F Altering your physical activity level is usually the easiest way to change your energy expenditure.

20. T F A 20 calorie raw carrot and a 20 calorie mint candy both supply the same amount of food energy.
21. T F A hamburger probably contains more calories from fat than from protein.
22. T F A diet containing 75 g carbohydrate, 100 g protein, and 50 g fat yields 1000 calories of energy.
23. T F Mental effort requires a large output of energy.
24. T F The body is more efficient than an auto in its use of fuel.
25. T F Energy is neither created nor destroyed.
26. T F BMI is the most accurate method to estimate one's health condition.
27. T F Females with a BMI less than desirable may have a greater risk of menstrual irregularity, infertility, and osteoporosis.

Situation

Mary is a student nurse in her first semester of college. She has been very busy and usually studies late at night. Many times she and her roommate go for a snack before bedtime. She skips breakfast a lot because she gets up too late. She figures she gets enough exercise going to clinical, but she thinks wistfully of the long bicycle rides she used to take. Lately, she has been feeling sluggish and her clothes are tight. She thinks she's "holding water." Mary is 5′2″ and weighs 130 pounds. She is 21 years old. Answer the following questions.

28. Mary keeps a record of her intake for 24 hours. When she totals it, she finds she has consumed 300 grams of carbohydrate, 50 grams of protein and 150 grams of fat. What is the total caloric value of her diet?

    a. 2750 calories
    b. 500 calories
    c. 1800 calories
    d. 1250 calories

29. Based on the estimated RDA range of 1700–2300 calories per day for a female 21–25 years of age, estimate how much weight Mary is likely to gain or lose by the end of the school year (6 months).

    _____

30. Which of the following statements is true concerning Mary's present weight?

    a. She is obese.
    b. She is average weight for her height.
    c. More information is needed.
    d. She has extra muscle tissue.

31. Mary decides to go on a diet. She comes to you for advice. List five important principles for weight reduction that you would give her.

    a. _____

    b. _____

    c. _____

    d. _____

    e. _____

Nutritional Assessment

Multiple Choice

Circle the letter of the correct answer.

1. The major techniques used for assessing nutritional status are

   a. physical findings and measurements.
   b. blood tests and data collection.
   c. the problem-solving process.
   d. a and b.

2. Depletion of subcutaneous fat may be a result of

   a. dieting.
   b. undernutrition.
   c. illness.
   d. all of the above.

3. The components of the health care model consist of

   a. interviewing, testing, diagnosing, and planning health care.
   b. assessing, planning, implementing, and evaluating.
   c. testing, measuring, interviewing, and teaching.
   d. goal-setting, care plan, implementation, and follow-up care.

4. The most common biochemical tests measure

   a. creatinine clearance.
   b. hemoglobin and hematocrit.
   c. nitrogen balance.
   d. all of the above.

5. Evaluation is possible for which of the following learning objectives?

   a. Understand the rationale for a modified diet.
   b. State four foods allowed and four omitted on a modified diet.
   c. Appreciate the difference between old and new diet patterns.
   d. Tell the dietitian the diet plan will be followed.

6. Responsibilities of health personnel for community health education include all but

   a. teaching.
   b. preparing menus.
   c. acting as a liaison.
   d. providing referrals.

7. A balanced diet should contain _____ percent carbohydrate, _____ percent protein, and _____ percent fat:

   a. 50–60, 14–20, 20–30
   b. 42.5–48.9, 30.5–35.7, 30.2–35.6
   c. 60–70, 10–12, 30–35
   d. 30–35, 40–50, 10–20

8. If you decrease your food intake by 500 calories per day, you will lose

   a. 2 pounds per week.
   b. 1 pound per week.
   c. 0.5 pound per week.
   d. no weight.

9. A test useful in determining if there is a normal amount of sugar in the blood is known as a

   a. serum folate test.
   b. blood urea nitrogen test.
   c. plasma glucose test.
   d. blood transaminase test.

10. Pale nail beds, brittle nails, stomatitis, and anemia indicate a deficiency in which of the following minerals?

   a. calcium
   b. iron
   c. iodine
   d. magnesium

Matching

Match the physical indicators of nutritional status listed on the left to the type of status listed at the right. (Answers may be used more than once.)

_____ 11. thin, fine, sparse hair

_____ 12. bloodshot eyes

_____ 13. weakness and tenderness in muscles

_____ 14. dry, flaky, sandpaper skin

_____ 15. deep pink tongue, slightly rough

a. good nutritional status
b. malnutrition
c. not a positive sign of nutritional status

True/False

Circle T for True and F for False.

16. T F Approximately one-half the fat in our bodies is directly below the skin.

17. T F Assessment provides a baseline for identifying problems.

18. T F Assessment provides a baseline for later evaluation.

19. T F Nutritional needs remain the same throughout life even though people change.

20. T F All physical findings that are indicators of health are directly related to good or poor nutrition.

21. T F Subjective data are not considered helpful to the health practitioner.

22. T F Lab tests for assessing vitamins, minerals, and trace elements are routinely performed in most hospitals.

23. T F Interviewing skills affect the data obtained from a client.

24. T F Malnutrition can describe an excess of calories as well as a deficit of calories.

25. T F A health care professional's role is defined by law.

Nutrition and the Life Cycle

Multiple Choice

Circle the letter of the correct answer.

1. An expectant mother's protein intake

    a. may be related to clinical risk.
    b. affects the height of the child.
    c. may provide the child passive immunity.
    d. all of the above.

2. Pregnancy-induced hypertension (PIH)

    a. excessive sodium intake.
    b. excessive water intake.
    c. a low-protein diet.
    d. a high-protein diet.

3. Nausea and vomiting during pregnancy

    a. are uncommon.
    b. go away in the third trimester.
    c. can be counteracted to some extent by a dry, high-carbohydrate, low-fat diet.
    d. should be countered with vitamin B_{12}.

4. Advantages of breast-feeding include

    a. psychological benefits for the mother.
    b. anti-infective factors in human milk.
    c. establishing a maternal bond with the child.
    d. all of the above.

5. Advantages of bottle-feeding include

    a. greater calcium absorption by the infant.
    b. greater weight gain by the infant.
    c. a low incidence of diarrhea.
    d. all of the above.

6. The most important factor in establishing a healthy diet in children is

    a. teaching children to make adaptive food choices.
    b. withholding "junk" food so they do not acquire a taste for it.
    c. rewarding a wise choice with a special treat.
    d. requiring them to eat all food served to them.

7. Eating habits of teenagers

    a. usually demonstrate a lack of sound nutrition information.
    b. may be tied to peer acceptance.
    c. cause concern among health professionals.
    d. all of the above.

8. Nutrient needs during adulthood

    a. are the same as any other age except for different calorie needs.
    b. may require modification, dependent upon health status.
    c. affect the quality of the rest of life.
    d. all of the above.

9. The nutritional status of a female on the "Pill" may be worsened with respect to

    a. B vitamins and vitamin C.
    b. vitamin A and iron.
    c. calcium and magnesium.
    d. protein and sodium.

10. The major nutritionally related clinical conditions of old age include

    a. risk of heart disease.
    b. bone disease.
    c. weight imbalance.
    d. all of the above.

Matching

Match the description listed on the left with the infant's age listed on the right:

_____ 11. able to digest starch after this age   a. one day old
_____ 12. solids usually introduced at this age   b. 3 months old
     c. 4–6 months old
_____ 13. colostrum is the food the baby is receiving at this age   d. one year old
_____ 14. egg white usually withheld until this age

Match the items in the left-hand column with the conditions in the right-hand column.

_____ 15. body fat   a. increased in the elderly
_____ 16. periodontal disease
_____ 17. basal metabolism   b. decreased in the elderly
_____ 18. intestinal motility
_____ 19. saliva production

True/False

Circle T for True and F for False.

20. T F Aerobic exercise can increase the risk of cardiovascular disease.
21. T F Nutrition-related cancers are more prevalent during the adult years.
22. T F Elderly persons and alcoholics are at high risk for developing drug-induced nutritional deficiencies.
23. T F The nutrients most often low in the adolescent's diet are protein, iron, and vitamin D.
24. T F Iron deficiency anemia is often a problem in childhood.
25. T F Breast-fed babies may need a fluoride supplement.
26. T F Excessive use of alcohol during a pregnancy can cause the infant to be mentally retarded.

Situation

Lisa is a 2½-year-old who is brought to a well-child clinic by her grandmother, who is her guardian. Lisa says no to everything and has eaten only peanut butter sandwiches for a week. Her grandmother says her appetite has decreased since last year and she lingers over food for hours. Grandmother states that her own children were not allowed to do this. Answer the following questions in relation to this situation.

27. What developmental problem is Lisa facing and how is this affecting her eating behavior?

　_____

　_____

　_____

28. What other information do you need in order to assess Lisa's nutritional status?

　_____

　_____

　_____

29. What would you say regarding Lisa's decreased appetite?

　_____

　_____

　_____

30. How would you counsel the grandmother in regard to the peanut butter sandwiches and the difference in two generations of child-rearing practices?

　_____

　_____

　_____

Drugs and Nutrition

Multiple Choice

Circle the letter of the correct answer.

1. Drug and food interactions that compromise nutritional status include

    a. altered taste.
    b. slowed or accelerated intestinal motility.
    c. decreased or increased appetite.
    d. all of the above.

2. Foods may compromise drug actions by which of the following methods?

    a. delayed absorption
    b. altered metabolism
    c. inhibited drug response
    d. altered drug excretion
    e. all of the above

3. Drug therapy can alter which of these functions?

    a. intestinal absorption
    b. utilization of nutrients
    c. storage of nutrients
    d. synthesis of nutrients
    e. all of these

4. Absorption of drugs is accomplished by all except

    a. enzymes.
    b. gastrointestinal pH.
    c. fat solubility.
    d. particle size.

5. Persons who are malnourished are likely to respond to a drug in all except which of these ways?

    a. They respond more profoundly to the drug.
    b. They require a higher dose of the drug.
    c. They require a smaller dose of the drug.
    d. They will not exhibit toxic effects to the drug.

6. Diarrhea, steatorrhea, and weight loss are usually the result of

    a. malabsorption of drugs.
    b. poor excretory function.
    c. intolerance to foods ingested.
    d. malnutrition.

7. Foods can increase or decrease

    a. acidity.
    b. digestive juices.
    c. intestinal motility.
    d. all of the above.

8. Fatty low-fiber meals given with oral medications

    a. decrease drug absorption.
    b. slow drug action.
    c. increase drug absorption.
    d. form a neutral base for absorption.

9. High protein meals given with medications

    a. increase gastric blood flow.
    b. increase drug absorption.
    c. decrease gastric blood flow.
    d. a and b
    e. a and c

10. People who use mineral oil for a laxative should be taught that mineral oil

    a. depletes fat-soluble vitamins.
    b. depletes water-soluble vitamins.
    c. may cause rickets.
    d. a and b
    e. a and c

11. Oral contraceptives result in a deficiency of which of these vitamins?

    a. tocopherol
    b. niacin
    c. B_6
    d. B_{12}

12. Aspirin will decrease the absorption and utilization of which of these vitamins?

    a. ascorbic acid
    b. folacin
    c. B_6
    d. a and b
    e. a, b, and c

13. The drug and food components that have been identified as causing harmful effects on the course and outcome of pregnancy include

    a. alcohol.
    b. food additives.
    c. food contaminants.
    d. all of the above.

14. If a nursing mother is taking a prescribed drug that carries potential risk that passes to the infant, what should be the doctor's recommendation?

    a. Change to another drug.
    b. Warn the mother and let her decide.
    c. Stop breast-feeding.
    d. Alert her to report all signs and symptoms.

15. Administering drugs with foods is a common practice used for all except which of these reasons?

    a. reduce GI side effects
    b. disguise taste
    c. chelate the drug
    d. all of the above

16. Pregnant women who are carriers, or who have phenylketonuria, should avoid aspartame ingestion because it

    a. makes the infant hyperactive.
    b. causes birth defects.
    c. contains phenylalanine.
    d. contains caffeine.

True/False

Circle T for True and F for False.

17. T F Drug-induced malnutrition is not a problem since so many supplements are available.
18. T F Overmedicating means the person takes a larger dose than prescribed.
19. T F Prescription medications are safer than OTC medications.
20. T F OTCs and prescribed medicines usually enhance the effects of both drugs so are safer taken together.
21. T F Alcohol and OTCs are safe taken together, but prescribed medicine with alcohol is contraindicated.
22. T F Pregnant women may drink unlimited amounts of caffeine-containing beverages.
23. T F Mercury poisoning leads to permanent brain damage in the fetus.
24. T F Nicotine ingestion will cause fetal growth retardation.
25. T F Vitamin K is an essential nutrient. Foods rich in this nutrient can be taken without any precaution.
26. T F Calcium is an essential nutrient. Foods rich in this nutrient such as dairy products can be taken without any precaution.

Fill-in

27. Name the most common side effects of medication.

    _____

    _____

28. Name three drugs that increase appetite.

    a. _____
    b. _____
    c. _____

29. Name three drugs that decrease appetite.

    a. _____
    b. _____
    c. _____

30. Name three drugs that affect taste sensation.

    a. _____
    b. _____
    c. _____

31. Name two drugs that contain a large amount of glucose.

    a. _____
    b. _____

32. Name two drugs that contain large amounts of sodium.

    a. _____
    b. _____

Dietary Supplements

Multiple Choice

Circle the letter of the correct answer.

1. Labels for herbal and nutrient concoctions carry claims about

   a. relieving pain
   b. energizing the body
   c. detoxifying the body
   d. providing guaranteed results
   e. all of the above

2. Dietary supplements can be purchased through

   a. health food stores
   b. grocery
   c. drug stores
   d. discount chain stores
   e. mail-order catalogs
   f. TV programs
   g. the Internet
   h. direct sales
   i. any of the above

3. A supplement could state on its label, "Excellent source of vitamin C" when it contains, per serving, at least:

   a. 12 mg of vitamin C
   b. 15 mg of vitamin C
   c. 20 mg of vitamin C

Fill-in

4. The eight provisions of the DSHEA are:

   a. _____
   b. _____
   c. _____
   d. _____
   e. _____
   f. _____
   g. _____
   h. _____

5. A nurse must be prepared to teach clients how to:

   a. _____
   b. _____

   c. _____
   d. _____
   e. _____
   f. _____
   g. _____

6. Name the seven ways in which a dietary supplement may be harmful:

   a. _____
   b. _____
   c. _____
   d. _____
   e. _____
   f. _____
   g. _____

7. Criteria used in DSHEA to establish a formal definition of "dietary supplement" are:

   a. _____
   b. _____
   c. _____
   d. _____
   e. _____

8. Information on the statement of identity include:

   a. _____
   b. _____
   c. _____
   d. _____
   e. _____
   f. _____
   g. _____

9. The FDA authorizes disease claims showing a link between a food or substance and a disease or health-related condition based on:

   a. _____
   b. _____

10. A nutrition label must contain information in the following sequence:

a. _____

b. _____

c. _____

d. _____

e. _____

11. Name two of the questions still to be answered about Echinacea:

a. _____

b. _____

12. Gingko can cause the following side effects:

a. _____

b. _____

c. _____

d. _____

e. _____

True/False

Circle T for True and F for False.

13. T F The current definition of dietary supplement is product containing not only essential nutrients, but may be composed of herbs and other botanicals, amino acids, glandulars, metabolites, enzymes, extracts, or any combination of these.

14. T F Manufacturers must describe the supplement's effects on "structure or function" of the body or the "well-being" achieved by consuming the dietary ingredient.

15. T F Both dietary supplements and food additives have to be preapproved by the FDA before marketing.

16. T F FDA has the authority to mandate the dietary supplement supplier and retailers to withdraw a product from the market if the product is found to be adulterated.

17. T F The vitamin folic acid can be claimed to have a link with a decreased risk of neural tube defect-affected pregnancy, if the supplement contains sufficient amounts of folic acid.

18. T F Psyllium seed husk (as part of a diet low in cholesterol and saturated fat) can be claimed to lower coronary heart disease, if the supplement contains sufficient amounts of psyllium seed husk.

19. T F Nutrition support claims can describe a link between a nutrient and the deficiency disease that can result if the nutrient is lacking in the diet.

20. T F Leafy greens such as spinach and turnip greens, dry beans and peas, fortified cereals and grain products, and some fruits and vegetables are rich food sources of folate.

21. T F Women who could become pregnant are advised to eat foods fortified with folic acid or take supplements in addition to eating folate-rich foods to reduce the risk of some serious birth defects.

22. T F Lowering homocysteine with vitamins will reduce your risk of heart disease.

23. T F Supplemental folic acid should not exceed the UL to prevent folic acid from masking symptoms of vitamin B_{12} deficiency.

24. T F Use of kava-containing dietary supplements may be associated with severe liver injury.

25. T F Persons who are taking drug products that can affect the liver, should consult a physician before using kava-containing supplements.

26. T F Consumers who use a kava-containing dietary supplement do not have to consult with their physician if they are not ill.

27. T F In Europe and some Asian countries, standardized extracts from ginkgo leaves are taken to treat a wide range of symptoms, including dizziness, memory impairment, inflammation, and reduced blood flow to the brain and other areas of impaired circulation.

28. T F The extract of the ginkgo leaf contains a balance of flavone glycosides (including one suspected high-dose carcinogen, quercetin) and terpene lactones.

29. T F Ginkgo is an effective blood thinner and improves circulation. It is, therefore, effective in treating migraine headaches, depression, and a range of lung and heart problems.

30. T F Large doses of goldenseal root should not be taken internally as the side effects can be very severe.

31. T F Barberine and hydrastine are biologically effective compounds in goldenseal root.

32. T F Echinacea can be taken in large doses without serious side effects.

33. T F Comfrey is hepatotoxic and should not be used as a dietary supplement.

34. T F Allantoin is a protein that can stimulate cell proliferation.

35. T F Pennyroyal can cause hepatic, renal, and pulmonary toxicity in humans.

36. T F Herbal supplements can be taken together as they are generally safe.

37. T F Information on the functions and potential benefits of vitamins and minerals, as well as upper safe limits for nutrients are more reliable if they come from nonprofit organizations such as government agencies (e.g., FDA), university extension, American Dietetic Association, and so on.

38. T F If you are pregnant, nursing a baby, or have a chronic medical condition, such as diabetes, hypertension, or heart disease, be sure to consult your doctor or pharmacist before purchasing or taking any supplement.

39. T F Safety of dietary supplement products are reviewed by the government before they are marketed.

40. T F A nurse should counsel patients to seek expert advice from their physicians before beginning any supplement regime.

41. T F The medical profession, drug companies, and the government can suppress information about a particular treatment.

42. T F "Economic fraud" is a practice in which the manufacture substitutes part or all of a product with an ineffective, inferior, or cheaper ingredient and then passes off the fake product as the real thing but at a lower cost.

Alternative Medicine

Fill-in

1. CAM treatments and therapies are used in what three major ways?

   a. _____

   b. _____

   c. _____

2. Name five domains or categories of CAM:

   a. _____

   b. _____

   c. _____

   d. _____

   e. _____

3. Name five commonly included symptoms in depression:

   a. _____

   b. _____

   c. _____

   d. _____

   e. _____

4. Most basic questions a patient should ask the CAM practitioner are:

   a. _____

   b. _____

   c. _____

   d. _____

   e. _____

   f. _____

   g. _____

5. Ayurvedic medicine (meaning "science of life") is a comprehensive system of medicine that strives to restore the innate harmony of the individual and places equal emphasis on:

   a. _____

   b. _____

   c. _____

6. Homeopathic medicine is based on the principles that the same substance that

   a. _____

   b. _____

7. Biological-based therapies include:

   a. _____

   b. _____

   c. _____

True/False

Circle T for True and F for False.

8. T F Complementary and alternate medicine (CAM) are treatments and health care practices generally taught widely in U.S. medical schools.

9. T F Holistic treatment generally means that the health care practitioner considers the whole person's physical, mental, emotional, and spiritual aspects.

10. T F Energy therapy employs energy fields originating within the body or from electromagnetic fields outside the body.

11. T F Preventive therapy means that the practitioner educates and treats the person to prevent health problems from arising, rather than treating symptoms after problems have occurred.

12. T F The presence of qi (vital energy) and its distribution through meridians in the body have not been accepted by all conventional medical practitioners in the United States.

13. T F Acupuncture involves stimulating specific anatomic points in the body for therapeutic purposes, usually by puncturing the skin with a needle.

14. T F Meditation, certain uses of hypnosis, dance, music, and art therapy, and prayer and mental healing are categorized as complementary and alternative medicine.

15. T F Many of the biological-based therapies, including natural and biologically based practices, interventions, and products, overlap with conventional medicine's use of dietary supplements. Included are herbal, special dietary, orthomolecular, and individual biological therapies.

16. T F Treating disease with varying concentrations of chemicals, such as magnesium, melatonin, and megadoses of vitamins, is considered basically ineffective, and maybe even harmful.

17. T F Manipulative and body-based CAM methods are based on manipulation and/or movement of the body.

18. T F Massage therapists manipulate the soft tissues of the body to normalize those tissues.

19. T F Chiropractic and massage therapies are gradually being accepted as being effective in treating certain ailments.

20. T F Biofield therapies are intended to affect the energy fields, whose existence is not yet experimentally proven, that surround and penetrate the human body.

21. T F Reiki, the Japanese word representing Universal Life Energy, is based on the belief that by channeling spiritual energy through the practitioner the spirit is healed, and it in turn heals the physical body.

22. T F Therapeutic Touch is based on the premise that it is the healing force of the therapist that affects the patient's recovery and that healing is promoted when the body's energies are in balance. By passing their hands over the patient, these healers identify energy imbalances.

23. T F In Therapeutic Touch, the healer places their hands over the patient, identifies the energy imbalances, and transfers the healing force to promote patient's energy balance.

24. T F Bioelectromagnetic-based therapies involve the unconventional use of electromagnetic fields, such as pulsed fields, magnetic fields, or alternating current or direct current fields, to, for example, treat asthma or cancer, or manage pain and migraine headaches.

25. T F In traditional Chinese medicine, there are at least 2000 acupuncture points connected through 12 primary and 8 secondary meridians in the body.

26. T F Acupuncture is believed to balance yin and yang, keep the normal flow of energy unblocked, and maintain or restore health to the body and mind.

27. T F Preclinical studies have documented acupuncture's effects, but they have not been able to fully explain how acupuncture works within the framework of the Western system of medicine.

28. T F Laetrile is not approved by the Food and Drug Administration for use in the United States.

29. T F Amygdalin is found in the pits of many fruits, raw nuts, and in other plants, such as lima beans, clover, and sorghum.

30. T F Cyanide is believed to be the active cancer-killing ingredient in laetrile.

31. T F The chemical make-up of Laetrile patented in the United States is different from the laetrile/amygdalin produced in Mexico.

32. T F The patented Laetrile is a semi-synthetic form of amygdalin.

33. T F Laetrile is administered by mouth (orally) as a pill or given by injection into a vein (intravenously) or muscle.

34. T F The beneficial effects of laetrile treatment can be increased by eating raw almonds or certain types of fruits and vegetables including celery, peaches, bean sprouts, and carrots, or by taking high doses of vitamin C.

35. T F St. John's wort is an herb that is useful for treating chronic depression.

36. T F More research is required to determine whether St. John's wort has value in treating other forms of depression.

37. T F St. John's wort interacts with certain drugs, and these interactions can be dangerous.

38. T F Health care providers are becoming more familiar with complementary and alternative medical treatments, or they should be able to refer you to someone who is.

39. T F Medical regulatory and licensing agencies in your state are eligible agencies to provide information about a specific practitioner's credentials and background.

40. T F Many states license practitioners who provide alternative therapies such as acupuncture, chiropractic services, naturopathy, herbal medicine, homeopathy, and massage therapy.

41. T F Health care providers, or professional associations and organizations can provide names of local practitioners and provide information about how to determine the quality of a specific practitioner's services.

Food Ecology

Multiple Choice

Circle the letter of the correct answer.

1. Custards and cream fillings should be eaten soon after preparation and properly refrigerated when stored because

    a. bacteria such as staphylococci multiply rapidly in these foods unless they are kept at low temperatures.
    b. the fat in these foods is poisonous if it becomes rancid.
    c. all minerals and vitamins are lost if these foods are cooked at temperatures high enough to destroy the bacteria in them.
    d. cooling these foods alters their taste and destroys the vitamins.

2. If several persons become ill from food poisoning while at a picnic, which of the following foods would most likely be the cause?

    a. tuna salad
    b. Jell–O salad
    c. bean salad (kidney, wax, and green beans in oil and vinegar dressing)
    d. baked beans

3. Whenever possible, raw fruits and vegetables should be included in the menu because

    a. cooking destroys flavor.
    b. excessive heat destroys minerals.
    c. cooking removes the cellulose in plants.
    d. cooking destroys some of the minerals and vitamins.

4. The nutritive value, color, and flavor of cooked vegetables will be retained if they are prepared

    a. in an open kettle, in boiling salted water, until they are tender.
    b. in a large amount of rapidly boiling unsalted water until done.
    c. in cold water and cooked just until tender.
    d. in a covered container, in a small amount of boiling salted water just until tender.

5. The nutrients most susceptible to destruction from improper handling, processing, and cooking are

    a. niacin and iron.
    b. folacin and niacin.
    c. vitamin C and iron.
    d. vitamin C and folacin.
    e. folacin and iron.

6. Raw meats should not be stored in the refrigerator for more than _____ days, while poultry or fish can be safely stored for _____ days.

    a. 2, 2
    b. 5, 2
    c. 7, 5
    d. 9, 7

7. Which of the following temperature ranges for holding food may make it unsafe to eat?

    a. 60°–125°F
    b. 130°–140°F
    c. 160°–175°F
    d. 10°–32°F

8. The most common biological illnesses transmitted from the food supply to people are from

    a. bacteria.
    b. viruses.
    c. parasites.
    d. all of the above.

9. What is the meaning of the phrase "illness transmission by the oral-fecal route"?

    a. transmitted from beast, to human, to food
    b. transmitted from unwashed hands, to food, to mouth
    c. transmitted by improper storage methods, to food, to human
    d. transmitted by a contaminated water supply to food and liquids

10. The toxin produced by staphylococcus

    a. is seldom found in food.
    b. is anaerobic under ideal conditions.
    c. is the most common foodborne illness.
    d. will grow even in frozen foods.

Matching

Match the procedures in the left column to the statements in the right column.

_____ 11. Peel potatoes before cooking.

_____ 12. Store fresh vegetables in air-tight containers.

_____ 13. Add baking soda to cooking water of vegetables.

_____ 14. Use as little water as possible when cooking.

_____ 15. Keep freezer at constant temperature below 0°F.

a. The procedure will help to conserve nutrients.

b. The procedure will increase nutrient losses.

c. The procedure is unrelated to conservation of nutrients.

True/False

Circle T for True and F for False.

16. T F Anaerobic bacteria thrive when food is stored in open containers.

17. T F Food should be cooled before being refrigerated; otherwise the temperature in the refrigerator will get too high.

18. T F Bacteria is the major cause of foodborne illness.

19. T F Foods high in protein are the group that most commonly causes food poisoning.

20. T F Boiling a food for five minutes will make it safe to eat.

21. T F A can opener not washed after each use can cause food poisoning.

22. T F Bulging ends of a can indicate the food has spoiled.

23. T F The bacteria that thrives in low acid conditions is called perfringins.

24. T F A person who has a sore on his hand should not prepare or serve food.

25. T F Food tasting with fingers or cooking utensils during preparation is acceptable practice only at home.

Situation

Dana is a newlywed whose closest encounter with a kitchen has been to find the cook and tell her what to prepare. Her lifestyle has changed and now she is doing her own shopping and food preparation. On Wednesday afternoon she shops for fresh produce because her local market is having a sale.

26. The peaches are very pretty but she finds that the least expensive ones are not fresh. Even though they are very soft and contain some bruises, they could be used when peeled and cut up. Which of the following will happen with the peaches?

a. They will be very sweet because they are so ripe.

b. The vitamin content will be much lower because the produce is not fresh.

c. They will be fine because they will be cut and chilled ahead of time.

d. All of the above.

27. While she is shopping she buys some dry cereal and cooking oil, which she forgets and leaves in her car trunk. The result of this may be

a. she will have to buy more the next time because she forgot she had them.

b. nothing will happen; this kind of food keeps for a long time.

c. the cooking oil will get rancid and the cereal will get weevils.

d. since they are stored in a dry dark place they will probably last longer than otherwise.

28. Dana is in a hurry to fix the potatoes she bought, so she puts them on to cook without peeling them. A likely outcome of this is

a. she will get food poisoning.

b. the nutrients will be conserved.

c. she will have to change her menu as these will be unusable.

d. the caloric content will be less.

29. Dana notices that the bread she bought was labeled "enriched." This means that

a. nutrients were added that were not originally present.

b. thiamin, niacin, riboflavin, and iron were added.

c. substances were added to preserve the food from spoilage.

30. Dana should know that nutrition labeling after 1992 is mandatory

a. at all times.

b. when a nutrient is added.

c. when a claim is made.

d. b and c

Overview of Therapeutic Nutrition

Multiple Choice

Circle the letter of the correct answer.

1. The purpose of diet therapy is

    a. to modify texture and energy values.
    b. to restore and maintain good nutritional status.
    c. to interpret the diet in terms of the disease.
    d. to involve the patient in his or her care.

2. The basis of therapeutic nutrition is

    a. assisting a patient to identify his or her malnutrition.
    b. removing excess modifications.
    c. modifying the nutrients in a normal balanced diet.
    d. modifying the patient's behavior to gain appropriate acceptance.

3. Which of the following conditions is not a result of poor nutrition in the recovery to health?

    a. delayed convalescence
    b. overeating
    c. delayed wound healing
    d. anemia

4. The stress of illness may negatively affect

    a. personality.
    b. nutritional balance.
    c. developmental tasks.
    d. all of the above.

5. When planning modified diets, the major factors to be observed include altering the diet to the specific pathophysiology and

    a. considering the patient's attitude toward hospitalization.
    b. considering emotional interferences with diet.
    c. individualizing the diet to the patient's total acculturation.
    d. focusing on patient's development of a trust relationship.

6. What factor will determine a patient's nutritional requirements?

    a. nature and severity of the disease or injury
    b. functioning capacity of the hypothalamus
    c. previous nutritional state and duration of the disease
    d. a and c

7. Nutritional requirements during disease, injury, and hospitalization include

    a. increased calories and protein.
    b. increased vitamins and minerals.
    c. decreased fluids and exercise.
    d. a and b.

8. Routine hospital diets include all of these except

    a. clear- and full-liquid.
    b. low-residue.
    c. mechanical- and medical-soft.
    d. regular.

9. Blocks to nutritional adequacy that the nurse may encounter when counseling a patient on a modified diet include

    a. cultural differences.
    b. ignorance.
    c. environmental stressors.
    d. all of the above.

Matching

Match the terms listed on the left to their descriptions listed on the right.

_____ 10. ascites
_____ 11. edema
_____ 12. gastritis
_____ 13. peritoneum

  a. inflammation of the stomach
  b. membrane lining the walls of the abdominal and pelvic cavity
  c. abnormal accumulation of fluid in the peritoneal cavity
  d. abnormal accumulation of fluid in intercellular spaces

Match the diets listed on the left to their descriptions listed on the right.

_____ 14. regular
_____ 15. medical-soft
_____ 16. mechanical-soft
_____ 17. clear-liquid
_____ 18. full-liquid

  a. reduced fiber, texture and seasonings
  b. used for people who have chewing difficulty
  c. the most frequently used of all diets
  d. the most nutritionally inadequate of the standard hospital diets
  e. consists of liquids and foods that liquefy at body temperature

True/False

Circle T for True and F for False.

19. T F A modified diet is an asset rather than a stressor.
20. T F The focus of diet therapy is based upon the patient's identified needs and problems.
21. T F The regular or house diet restricts foods to the basic food groups.
22. T F A modified diet is successful only if it is accurate.
23. T F Environment and attitude affect a patient's acceptance of a modified diet.

Situation

James, age 19, is admitted to the hospital following a motorcycle accident. He has compound fractures of both legs. He is 6′ tall, weighs 130 lb, and has a past history of drug abuse.

24. Therapeutic nutrition for James would focus upon

    a. measures to restore optimal nutrition.
    b. measures to reduce liver damage.
    c. measures to increase his self-esteem.
    d. allowing him to select as he chooses.

25. Diet modification will include

    a. increasing all basic nutrients.
    b. increasing energy value.
    c. decreasing fiber content.
    d. a and b.

26. The goals of the diet therapy used for James would center upon his specific needs. These needs would include

    a. restoration of weight and nutrient reserves.
    b. promotion of bone formation.
    c. regulation of methadone dosage.
    d. a and b.

27. The nurse's role in adapting a client to a modified-diet regime includes all except

    a. diffusion of responsibility.
    b. explanation of the diet to the patient.
    c. interpretation, follow-through.
    d. discharge planning.

28. List the four most common diet modifications. Based upon your knowledge of these modifications, write the diet prescription for James.

    a. _____

    b. _____

    c. _____

    d. _____

    James's prescription:

    _____

    _____

    _____

29. State the rationale for the diet prescription you just wrote for James.

    _____

    _____

    _____

    _____

30. The greatest amount of calcium for bone healing can be provided to James through

    a. 1 egg.
    b. 2 tbsp cream cheese.
    c. 1 oz cheddar cheese.
    d. ½ c orange sherbet.

Diet Therapy for Surgical Conditions

Multiple Choice

Circle the letter of the correct answer.

1. Complete dietary protein of high biologic value is essential to tissue building and wound healing after surgery because it

   a. supplies all the essential amino acids needed for tissue synthesis.
   b. spares carbohydrate to supply the necessary energy.
   c. is easily digested and does not cause gastrointestinal upsets.
   d. provides the most concentrated source of calories.

2. Mrs. Jones is two days postoperative following a hysterectomy and tells you she wants to be on a 1000 calorie reduction diet when she is allowed to eat again. Your most appropriate response would be to

   a. ask her doctor to prescribe it.
   b. explain that a reduction diet should be at least 1200 calories.
   c. explain that tissue repair requires more nutrients.
   d. tell her a 1000 calorie high-protein diet will be okay.

3. Fluids given after surgery should

   a. be increased to replace losses.
   b. be decreased to prevent edema.
   c. be kept at maintenance levels to counteract overhydration.
   d. be withheld to prevent nausea.

4. A minimum of _____ calories per day is needed after surgery to spare protein for tissue repair.

   a. 1000
   b. 1200
   c. 1800
   d. 2800

5. Both pre- and postoperative patients need proteins of high biological value. These include

   a. milk, eggs, cheese, meats.
   b. grains, legumes, nuts, vegetables.
   c. a and b.
   d. none of the above.

6. Increased ascorbic acid is essential for wound healing. Which of these foods is highest in ascorbic acid?

   a. creamed cottage cheese.
   b. egg whites.
   c. peanut butter.
   d. coleslaw.

7. For which of the following would total parenteral nutrition be inappropriate diet therapy?

   a. a patient with 50 percent of his body surface burned
   b. a patient with a cholecystectomy
   c. a patient with advanced stomach cancer
   d. a patient admitted for surgery who has not eaten in a week

8. The most common nutrient deficiency related to surgery is that of

   a. iron.
   b. vitamin C.
   c. protein.
   d. zinc.

9. All kinds of stress related to surgery may

   a. reduce the function of the GI tract.
   b. interfere with the desire to eat.
   c. deplete liver glycogen.
   d. all of the above.

10. Good nutrition prior to surgery can

    a. shorten convalescence.
    b. increase resistance to infection.
    c. increase the mortality rate.
    d. a and b.

Matching

Match the vitamins listed on the left to their function in wound healing listed on the right.

_____ 11. vitamin C
_____ 12. folic acid
_____ 13. vitamin K
_____ 14. thiamin

a. coenzyme in carbohydrate metabolism connective tissue
b. cementing material for connective tissue
c. formation of hemoglobin
d. essential for blood clotting

True/False

Circle T for True and F for False.

15. T F Usually nothing is given by mouth for at least eight hours prior to surgery to avoid food aspiration during anesthesia.

16. T F Oral liquid feedings usually provide little nourishment regardless of the type.

17. T F Tube feedings can only be made successfully from commercial preparations.

18. T F As much as one pound of muscle tissue per day may be lost following surgery.

19. T F Vitamin D is essential to wound healing, since it provides a cementing substance to build strong connective tissue.

20. T F Most patients are at optimum nutritional status before they go to surgery.

21. T F Obese patients are high surgical risks but underweight patients are no greater risks than those of normal weight.

22. T F An inadequate protein intake will delay the healing of a fractured bone.

23. T F Inadequate diet may depress pulmonary and cardiac functions in a patient who has no history of respiratory or cardiac disease.

24. T F Malnourished patients who receive postsurgical total parenteral nutrition support have fewer noninfectious complications than controls.

25. T F Subjective global assessment (SGA) is not useful in determining the effects of malnutrition on organ function and body composition.

Situation

Mrs. H., a 40-year-old woman, was involved in an auto accident. She suffered multiple broken bones and underwent emergency surgery for a ruptured spleen. The following questions pertain to this situation.

26. The surgical team is considering placing her on total parenteral nutrition (TPN). What is the rationale for their decision?

_____

_____

_____

27. Mrs. H. finds breathing difficult because of several broken ribs. She is also 20 pounds overweight. Should she be placed on a reduction diet to ease this situation? Explain your answer.

_____

_____

_____

28. List four important nutrients necessary for Mrs. H.'s speedy recovery and two foods that are good sources for each nutrient.

a. _____

b. _____

c. _____

d. _____

29. List three nutritional nursing measures appropriate to this situation.

a. _____

b. _____

c. _____

Diet Therapy for Cardiovascular Disorders

Multiple Choice

Circle the letter of the correct answer.

1. A low-cholesterol diet would restrict all of the following foods except

   a. shellfish, cream cheese.
   b. liver.
   c. eggs, yolks.
   d. lobster.

2. Which of these seasonings may be used on a 1 gram sodium-restricted diet?

   a. lemon juice, herbs, spices
   b. soy sauce, m.s.g. (Accent)
   c. butter or margarine
   d. garlic or celery salt

3. Which of these labeling terms approved by the FDA is correct?

   a. Low calorie: contains 25% less calories than regular product
   b. Low in saturated fat: contains less than 5 g saturated fat per serving
   c. Cholesterol free: contains less than 20 mg cholesterol per serving
   d. Sodium free: contains less than 5 mg per serving
   e. All of these terms are correct

4. The amount of fiber per day recommended in the TLC diet is:

   a. 10–15 g
   b. 15–20 g
   c. 20–30 g
   d. 30–40 g

5. Which of the following meals would be most appropriate for a person on a fat-controlled diet?

   a. macaroni and cheese, avocado/grapefruit salad, Jell–O, tea
   b. roast beef, baked potato with sour cream, coconut cookie, skim milk
   c. broiled chicken breast with wild rice, tossed salad with French dressing, baked apple with walnuts and raisins, tea
   d. tuna salad on lettuce, crackers, sliced cheese, lemon pudding, skim milk

6. Poor eating habits that can increase risk of heart disease include all except

   a. consumption of large amounts of alcohol.
   b. consumption of large amounts of beef, pork, butter, ice cream.
   c. excess total daily calories.
   d. daily consumption of peanut butter, chicken, fish.

7. Which of these would be the diet therapy of choice for a patient following a myocardial infarction?

   a. clear-liquid first 24 hours
   b. regular low-residue first 24 hours
   c. limited in sodium, caffeine-restricted, soft
   d. caffeine and sodium restricted, clear-liquid

8. Following a cerebrovascular accident, the diet therapy

   a. will be an I.V. line for the first 24 hours.
   b. may be a tube feeding or oral liquids.
   c. may be semi-solid.
   d. may be any of these, or any combination.

9. The most suitable of the following food groups for a patient on TLC diet is:

   a. Lean pork, roast beef, lamb, and coconut
   b. Turkey, pasta, spinach, and graham crackers
   c. Duck, cheddar cheese, shrimp, and avocado
   d. Spareribs, bologna, ice milk, and olives

10. Total fat allowed in a LDL-lowering diet is:

    a. 10%–15% of total calories
    b. 20%–25% of total calories
    c. 25%–35% of total calories
    d. 30%–40% of total calories

Matching

Match the factors involved in heart disease listed on the left with the recommended measures to prevent or lessen the effects listed on the right.

_____ 11. hypertension
_____ 12. elevated cholesterol
_____ 13. elevated triglycerides
_____ 14. obesity
_____ 15. sedentary lifestyle

a. regular program of exercise
b. limiting sodium intake
c. limiting sugar intake
d. limiting saturated fats in diet
e. limiting total energy value of diet

True/False

Circle T for True and F for False.

16. T F About two-thirds of the total fat in the United States diet is of animal origin and therefore mainly saturated.

17. T F Coconut oil is a polyunsaturated vegetable oil, used in low-saturated-fat diets.

18. T F Optimum LDL cholesterol levels are < 100 mg/dL of blood.

19. T F Desirable total cholesterol is classified as 200–240 mg/dL of blood.

20. T F Tea, coffee, and alcohol are not used in the diet of cardiac patients.

21. T F Spices such as cinnamon, nutmeg, and garlic are high in sodium content.

22. T F HDL cholesterol levels of less than 60 mg/dL blood are considered low.

23. T F Low-potassium serum levels are not a problem for persons who are taking antihypertensive medicine.

24. T F An objective of diet therapy for a patient who has had a myocardial infarction is to reduce the workload of the heart.

25. T F Persons who must limit their intake of foods containing cholesterol should be able to eat lunchmeat and lean hamburgers.

Situation

26. Mr. J., age 45, is in the hospital recovering from a myocardial infarction. He is on a 1500 calorie diet, low in saturated fats and high in polyunsaturated fats. The chief purpose of the diet ordered for Mr. J. is to reduce weight and

    a. prevent development of edema.
    b. lower the blood cholesterol level.
    c. decrease blood clotting time.
    d. provide for ease of digestion.

27. Which of these food choices, as ordinarily prepared, would be most suitable for Mr. J.?

    a. roast turkey, baked trout, breaded veal cutlet
    b. lean roast beef, breaded veal cutlet, cheese soufflé
    c. baked trout, lean roast beef, roast turkey
    d. roast turkey, baked trout, broiled calves' liver

28. Which of these foods would be most suitable for Mr. J.'s meal?

    a. baked potato, tossed salad with French dressing, grapefruit
    b. cauliflower with cheese sauce, sliced tomato, orange sherbet
    c. hash brown potatoes, tomato salad, Jell–O with whipped cream
    d. broccoli, Waldorf salad, custard

29. In counseling Mr. J. regarding diet management, the nurse would

    a. discuss food preparation methods.
    b. need more information regarding the patient's usual habits.
    c. explain the importance of weight control.
    d. all of the above.

30. The diet for Mr. J. should be

    a. restricted only in carbohydrates.
    b. a basic pattern within the limitations imposed by the diet orders.
    c. a list of foods to be eaten at the same time each day.
    d. a weighed diet.

Diet and Disorders of Ingestion, Digestion, and Absorption

Multiple Choice

Circle the letter of the correct answer.

1. Which of these factors is most important to the healthy functioning of the gastrointestinal tract?

   a. specific food combinations
   b. physiological and psychological conditions
   c. a regular exercise program
   d. few environmental pollutants

2. Which of the following statements is true regarding the treatment of infants with cleft palate?

   a. The nutritional requirements are higher than those of unaffected infants.
   b. Surgery is performed after the age of one year.
   c. Lack of essential nutrients is the most likely cause of cleft palate.
   d. All of the above.

3. Mr. H. received a fractured mandible in an auto accident and is in the hospital. He will go home before the wires are removed. Which of the following instructions for eating will you give him?

   a. His diet, though liquid, must be high in all nutrients.
   b. He must learn to pass the tube down.
   c. He will need water and mouthwash before and after each feeding.
   d. a and c

4. Which of the following is a major cause of the high incidence of dental caries?

   a. lack of essential nutrients in the diet
   b. Vincents' disease
   c. high use of concentrated sweets
   d. pregnancy

5. The disadvantages of wearing dentures include

   a. the need for frequent realignment.
   b. lowered self-esteem.
   c. the fact that everyone knows you wear them.
   d. halitosis.

6. Which of the following are appropriate dietary measures for a person with a hiatal hernia?

   a. a low-fiber, bland diet in six feedings
   b. antacids and fluids between meals
   c. no spices, no alcohol, limited fat intake
   d. all of the above

7. The diet containing a minimum amount of residue will be deficient in which of these nutrients?

   a. calcium, iron, and vitamins
   b. carbohydrates, proteins, and fats
   c. water, sodium, and potassium
   d. cellulose, glycogen, and glucose

8. The low-residue diet would be the diet of choice for all but which of the following disorders?

   a. diverticulosis
   b. diarrhea
   c. cancer of the colon
   d. ulcerative colitis

9. Foods allowed on the very low-(minimal) residue diet include

   a. cheddar cheese, fruits, milk, creamed soup.
   b. green beans, carrots, butter, broiled steak.
   c. roast turkey, mashed potatoes, butter, tomato juice.
   d. bouillon, whole wheat toast, jelly, orange sherbet.

10. A patient had a gastrectomy and developed a "dumping syndrome." His diet must be modified. Which of these modifications would be appropriate?

    a. Lower the fat content of the diet.
    b. Avoid sugars, restrict starches.
    c. Decrease protein content of diet.
    d. All of the above.

11. Diverticulitis is best treated with a _____ diet.

    a. bland
    b. low-residue
    c. high-fiber
    d. clear-liquid

12. The dietary changes that help to reduce the incidence of constipation include

    a. using laxatives and stool softeners.
    b. increasing fiber and fluid intake.
    c. increasing protein and fat intake.
    d. all of the above.

13. The most serious consequence of functional diarrhea is

    a. weight loss.
    b. hemorrhoids.
    c. dehydration.
    d. pain and fever.

14. Research supports the high-fiber diet as a deterrent to colon cancer. Briefly describe the rationale for this conclusion:

_____

_____

_____

_____

_____

15. Mrs. Martin was on a very-low-residue diet while she was hospitalized with diverticulitis. Now that she has recovered and is going home, the doctor has told her to eat high-fiber foods. Explain the reason for this drastic change to Mrs. M.

_____

_____

_____

_____

Short answers

16. Name three serious obesity-related health problems for which GI bypass surgery would be an option.

    a. _____

    b. _____

    c. _____

17. Successful results of bypass surgery depend on what two major changes a patient must make?

    a. _____

    b. _____

18. a. A common risk of restrictive operations is vomiting. What causes vomiting to occur?

    _____

    _____

    b. Why do bypass surgeries cause the dumping syndrome to occur?

    _____

    _____

19. Briefly explain why malabsorptive operations carry a high risk for nutritional deficiencies.

_____

_____

_____

20. Name the nutritional supplements that a person will be required to take for life following a malabsorptive bypass procedure.

_____

_____

_____

True/False

Circle T for True and F for False

21. T F The state of the body system determines how food is digested and absorbed.
22. T F Cleft lip or palate is a congenital birth defect.
23. T F The G.I. tract consists of stomach, small and large intestine, and colon.
24. T F All of the teeth a person will ever have are formed before birth.
25. T F Poorly fitting dentures can lead to malnutrition.
26. T F For gastrointestinal surgery, the implication of proper enteral and parenteral nutrition revolves around the close working relationship among the doctor, the nurse, and the dietitian.
27. T F Gastrointestinal surgery for obesity does not alter the digestive process.
28. T F Restrictive surgical operation is not as successful in long-term weight loss as malabsorptive operations.

Situation

Carmen is a twenty-year-old female college student, hospitalized with ulcerative colitis. She has many food intolerances; she does not like raw fruits or vegetables, and does not drink milk. She is fond of soda pop and tacos. She will be going home soon and back to school, but is very anxious and apprehensive because she feels she will not be able to maintain her diet. The doctor has ordered a 150 gram protein, 3000 calorie diet for her. The following questions pertain to this situation.

29. Carmen has been in negative nitrogen balance. This means that she

   a. was dehydrated.
   b. was losing more tissue protein than she was replacing.
   c. was gaining tissue protein, so, therefore, excreted nitrogen.
   d. had an electrolyte imbalance.

30. Which of the following nutritional problems would the nurse not encounter in Carmen?

   a. skin lesions and inflammation
   b. anorexia and weight loss
   c. avitaminosis and anemia
   d. esophageal varices and pulmonary edema

31. If Carmen wanted tacos as part of her meals, the nurse would

   a. tell her firmly "no."
   b. tell her she will try to get them for her.
   c. explain the situation to dietary aides.
   d. compromise: if Carmen agrees to eat them with less seasoning, the nurse will ask the dietitian to include them occasionally.

32. In counseling Carmen so that she will comply with the diet, the nurse explains the rationale. List three of these reasons.

   a. _____

   b. _____

   c. _____

33. The nurse asks Carmen to keep very careful daily records. List three important records she would need in order to evaluate her progress.

   a. _____

   b. _____

   c. _____

Diet Therapy for Diabetes Mellitus

Multiple Choice

Circle the letter of the correct answer.

Mr. G., a 40-year-old man, is a newly diagnosed diabetic. He weighs 160 lb, and is 5′ 10″ tall. The diet prescribed contains 250 g carbohydrate, 100 g protein, and 70 g fat.

Answer the following questions relating to this patient.

1. Mr. G.'s daily caloric intake is

    a. 1230 calories.
    b. 1530 calories.
    c. 1830 calories.
    d. 2030 calories.

2. This caloric allowance should

    a. prevent hypoglycemia.
    b. decrease body weight.
    c. maintain body weight.
    d. promote normal potassium balance.

3. Emphasis is placed on using polyunsaturated fats and limiting foods high in cholesterol in the diet of the diabetic. This will

    a. aid in preventing cardiovascular diseases.
    b. aid in the digestive process.
    c. prevent skin breakdown.
    d. control blood sugar.

4. In counseling Mr. G. regarding diet management, the nurse should

    a. explain the importance of weight control.
    b. interpret food exchanges to him.
    c. discuss food preparation methods.
    d. all of the above.

5. Mr. G. should know that factors which can trigger hyperglycemia in a diabetic include

    a. decreased exercise.
    b. increased food intake.
    c. decreased insulin.
    d. all of the above.

6. The daily intake of foods for the diabetic is spaced at regular intervals throughout the day. This should

    a. prevent hunger pangs.
    b. avoid symptoms of hypoglycemia or hyperglycemia.
    c. modify eating habits.
    d. prevent obesity.

7. Although diabetics are taught to limit foods containing sugar, exception can be made to that rule when

    a. vigorous exercise is undertaken.
    b. there is fever.
    c. gangrene has developed.
    d. there are no exceptions.

8. The caloric value of a diabetic diet should be

    a. increased above normal requirements to meet the increased metabolic demand.
    b. decreased below normal requirements to prevent glucose formation.
    c. the same as normal energy requirements to maintain ideal weight.
    d. contributed mainly by fat to spare carbohydrate.

9. The diabetic diet is designed for long-term use and contains a balance of

    a. energy.
    b. nutrients.
    c. distribution.
    d. all of the above.

10. Sources of blood glucose include

    a. carbohydrates, proteins, and fats.
    b. amino acids, cellulose, and polysaccharides.
    c. water and vitamin and mineral compounds.
    d. by-products of metabolism.

Matching

Match the terms listed on the left to the descriptions listed on the right.

_____ 11. insulin	a.	a complete protein containing large amounts of essential amino acids
_____ 12. hypoglycemia		
_____ 13. glucagon	b.	glucose in blood exceeds the normal range
_____ 14. hyperglycemia		
_____ 15. glycogen	c.	glucose in blood below the normal range
_____ 16. ketosis		
_____ 17. high biological	d.	a hormone that raises blood sugar levels
	e.	a hormone that lowers blood sugar levels
	f.	one result of poor utilization of carbohydrate value range
	g.	emergency supply of (stored) glucose

True/False

Circle T for True and F for False.

18. T F Group teaching of diabetics is more useful than one-on-one teaching.
19. T F The exchange lists may be successfully used whenever nutrients in a diet need to be calculated.
20. T F The milk exchange list contains cheddar and cottage cheese.
21. T F Diabetic and dietetic foods are the same thing.
22. T F Large doses of vitamin C give a false urinary glucose test.
23. T F Insulin is produced by the beta cells in the islets of Langerhans in the pancreas.
24. T F People with Type 1 diabetes do not produce insulin.

Situation

Jane is a newly diagnosed ten-year-old diabetic. She weighs 70 lb and is placed on a 150 g carbohydrate, 80 g protein, 50 g fat diet with afternoon and bedtime feedings. Answer the following questions by circling the letter of the correct answer.

25. The diet prescribed for Jane furnishes

   a. 1370 calories and 1.5 g protein per kg body weight.
   b. 1370 calories and 2.5 g protein per kg body weight.
   c. 1110 calories and 1.5 g protein per kg body weight.
   d. 1110 calories and 2.5 g protein per kg body weight.

26. The night feeding, consisting of milk, crackers, and butter will provide

   a. high-carbohydrate nourishment for immediate utilization.
   b. nourishment with latent effect to counteract late insulin activity.
   c. encouragement for Jane to stay on her diet.
   d. added calories to help her gain weight.

27. In planning menus for this child, one should

   a. limit calories to encourage weight loss.
   b. allow for normal growth needs.
   c. avoid using potatoes, bread, and cereal.
   d. discourage substitutions in the menu pattern.

28. The diet should be

   a. restricted only in carbohydrates.
   b. a detailed pattern of special food and insulin.
   c. a list of foods to be eaten at some time each day.
   d. a basic pattern that can be varied by substituting foods of equal nutrient content.

29. Jane's mother should know that

   a. all of her food must be weighed.
   b. she needs a snack before she exercises.
   c. she should always carry hard candy with her.
   d. she can liberalize the diet in a few years.

Part I: Diet Therapy for Disorders of the Liver

Multiple Choice

Circle the letter of the correct answer.

1. The liver stores

    a. glycogen and vitamins.
    b. ACTH and cholecystokinin.
    c. bile and cholesterol.
    d. calcium and chlorides.

2. The symptoms of hepatitis that interfere with food intake include

    a. anorexia.
    b. confusion.
    c. constipation.
    d. internal bleeding.

3. Which of the following foods may be restricted in the diet of the hepatitis patient?

    a. milk
    b. butter
    c. noodles
    d. chocolate

4. The symptom of cirrhosis that may interfere with nutrient intake is

    a. anorexia.
    b. distention.
    c. pain.
    d. all of the above.

5. Which of the following meals would best fit the needs of a cirrhotic patient with esophageal varices who is on a 350 g carbohydrate, 80 g protein, 100 g fat diet?

    a. chicken soup, beef patty, mashed potato, stewed tomatoes, cantaloupe
    b. cranberry juice, meat loaf, hash brown potato, orange slices
    c. tuna noodle casserole, lima beans, apple juice, pineapple slice
    d. peach nectar, scrambled eggs, cooked spinach, applesauce

6. The purpose of the low-protein diet (15–20 g) is to help prevent the development of hepatic coma by

    a. decreasing ammonia production.
    b. increasing sodium excretion.
    c. decreasing serum potassium.
    d. increasing the utilization of carbohydrates.

7. Which of the following meals would be appropriate for a person on a 15 g protein diet?

    a. baked potato, green beans, fruit salad, coffee with cream
    b. sliced cheese, crackers, tossed salad, Jell–O with whipped cream
    c. meat patty, mashed potato, steamed carrots, peach half
    d. tomato stuffed with tuna fish, crackers with butter, ice cream, tea

8. Hepatic coma results from increased blood levels of

    a. glucose.
    b. fatty acids.
    c. ammonia.
    d. sodium.

9. Diet treatment for hepatic coma includes

    a. high protein tube feedings.
    b. increased fluids.
    c. N.P.O. to rest the liver.
    d. controlled I.V. fluids.

Matching

Diet therapy for hepatitis is a major part of the treatment. Match the diet modifications on the left with the rationale for their use on the right.

_____ 10. high-protein diet
_____ 11. high-carbohydrate diet
_____ 12. high-calorie diet
_____ 13. high-fluid diet
_____ 14. moderate-fat diet

a. improves total intake
b. regenerates liver cells
c. meets increased energy demands
d. restores glycogen reserves
e. compensates for losses from fever, diarrhea

Match the actions listed on the left that apply to the nutrition and elimination needs of the patient with cirrhosis with the rationale for the action listed on the right.

_____ 15. support, encouragement, small feedings, nutrition education

_____ 16. careful monitoring of patient's mental/physical status

_____ 17. individualizing the diet

_____ 18. careful measurement of all foods/fluids ingested and excreted

_____ 19. accurate charting

a. to record the patient's condition and measures taken to restore homeostasis

b. to combat anorexia, low self-esteem

c. to watch for signs of impending coma

d. to achieve adequate nutrition and changes in diet as condition indicates

e. to prevent excess accumulation of fluids in the tissues

True/False

Circle T for True and F for False.

20. T F The diet modifications for early cirrhosis are the same ones used for hepatitis.

21. T F The diet modifications for late stages of cirrhosis are the same as for hepatitis.

22. T F Optimum nutrition can help damaged liver cells regenerate.

23. T F Ascites is accumulation of fluid in the chest cavity.

24. T F The diet for a client with liver cancer is high in carbohydrates, protein, fluid, vitamins, and calories.

25. T F Diet therapy for a patient with liver disease is individualized.

Situation

Mr. L. was admitted to the hospital complaining of abdominal pain, fatigue, and anorexia. His skin showed a yellow tinge as did the sclera of his eyes. Laboratory tests and assessments revealed evidence of liver dysfunction, fluid retention, and portal hypertension. Macrocytic anemia, thiamin and zinc deficiency were also identified. The following questions pertain to this situation.

26. From the presenting symptoms, identify the probable diagnosis.

a. hepatitis
b. jaundice
c. cirrhosis
d. cancer

27. Which of the following diet modifications would be appropriate for Mr. L.?

a. 250 mg sodium
b. 60 g protein
c. fluid restriction to 1000 ml
d. all of the above

28. What daily measurements are appropriate for Mr. L.'s condition?

a. intake and output
b. weight and abdominal girth
c. skinfold thickness
d. all of the above

29. Four days after admission, Mr. L.'s condition seemed to worsen. He appeared confused, forgetful, and lethargic. His blood levels of ammonia were elevated and his skin color had deepened.

Given these symptoms, the most probable cause of his worsening condition is

a. allergic reaction.
b. impending hepatic coma.
c. esophageal varices.
d. advanced cirrhosis.

30. All except which of the following foods should be omitted from Mr. L.'s diet while he is in this stage of his illness?

a. milk and meat
b. vegetables and fruits
c. butter and honey
d. grains and legumes

Part II: Diet and Disorders of the Gallbladder and Pancreas

Multiple Choice

Circle the letter of the correct answer.

1. The gallbladder stores

   a. fats.
   b. bile.
   c. cholecystokinin.
   d. cholesterol.

2. Bile functions in the digestion of food in which of the following ways?

   a. breaks fat into fatty acids and glycerol
   b. forms lipoproteins for transport to bloodstream
   c. breaks fats into very small particles for enzyme action
   d. prevents cholesterol from entering the bloodstream

3. The function of the hormone cholecystokinin is

   a. to convert fats to cholesterol.
   b. to stimulate the gallbladder to contract.
   c. to provide the necessary enzyme for fat digestion.
   d. to prevent cholesterol from crystallizing.

4. Symptoms of cholecystitis that interfere with nutrient intake include all except

   a. distention.
   b. pain.
   c. internal bleeding.
   d. nausea and vomiting.

5. Gallstones are primarily composed of

   a. calcium.
   b. chloride.
   c. cholesterol.
   d. cholecystokinin.

6. The initial diet for acute pancreatitis is

   a. I.V. therapy.
   b. low-protein, high-carbohydrate, soft.
   c. low-fat.
   d. full-liquid.

7. The usual diet therapy for chronic pancreatitis is

   a. bland in six feedings.
   b. low-residue every hour.
   c. liquids via tube.
   d. I.V. therapy.

Matching

Match the nursing measures appropriate to diet therapy for gallbladder disease listed on the left with the rationale for the action listed on the right.

_____ 8. Evaluate diet for vitamins A, D, E, and K.

_____ 9. Provide recipes for broiling and baking foods.

_____ 10. Ask dietary personnel to remove raw apple and baked beans.

_____ 11. Ask for canned peaches and cottage cheese as a replacement for foods omitted in #10.

a. Substitute alternate sources of nutrients.
b. Fat-soluble vitamins are often inadequate.
c. Discourage use of fried foods.
d. Individual intolerance to foods requires omitting them.

True/False

Circle T for True and F for False.

12. T F Pancreatitis is a complication of cirrhosis but would not occur as a result of cholelithiasis.

13. T F Cholesterol is normally found in solution in bile.

14. T F Heredity is an important factor in gallbladder disease.

15. T F Excess polyunsaturated fats increase the risk of cholelithiasis.

16. T F Obesity is not significant in contributing to gallbladder disease.

17. T F As BMI increases, the risk for developing gallstones does not rise.

18. T F Obese people may produce high levels of cholesterol that can lead to production of bile containing more cholesterol than it can dissolve. This can lead to formation of gallstone.

19. T F Men and women who carry fat around their midsections may be at a greater risk for developing gallstones than those who carry fat around their hips and thighs.

20. T F Gallstones are common among people who undergo gastrointestinal surgery.

21. T F Weight loss should be maintained at 1 to 2 lb per week in order to avoid formation of gallstones.

Situation

Mrs. O., age 58, 5'1'' tall, 165 lb, is admitted to the hospital with a diagnosis of acute cholecystitis. Further tests confirm the presence of cholelithiasis. The doctor tells her that surgery will be necessary, but that she will be dismissed with a modified-diet plan and return for surgery at a later date. The following questions pertain to this situation.

22. From the information given, which of the following diet prescriptions would be appropriate for Mrs. O.?

    a. 500 calorie high-protein (100 g) soft diet
    b. 1000 calorie moderate-fat (100 g) diet
    c. 1200 calorie, 60 g protein, 50 g fat, regular diet
    d. low-cholesterol, regular diet

Mrs. O.'s diet history reveals the following information:

Breakfast: 2 fried eggs, sausage or bacon, 2 pieces buttered toast, 1 glass milk, coffee with cream and sugar

Mid-morning snack: 1 cup dry cereal with sugar and half-and-half cream

Lunch: sandwich (2 slices lunch meat, 1 tbsp mayonnaise, lettuce, 2 slices bread), 1 glass milk, 1 cup canned fruit in sugar syrup

Dinner: fried pork chop or hamburger steak with gravy, 1 c mashed potatoes with butter, avocado salad, pie, cake or ice cream for dessert, coffee with cream and sugar

Bedtime snack: leftover dessert or cheese and crackers or handful of peanuts, glass of cola beverage

23. This diet pattern

    a. contains adequate amounts of all the basic food groups.
    b. is short in the bread-cereal group.
    c. is short in the meat group.
    d. is short in the milk group.
    e. is short in the fruit-vegetable group.

24. In order to modify her diet to prepare for surgery,

which of the following adjustments will she need to make?

    a. change methods of preparation
    b. decrease total quantity
    c. omit all snacks
    d. change type of foods consumed
    e. a, b, and d

Alter the following items from Mrs. O.'s diet history to make them suitable for her present modified diet requirements (substitutes may be made if necessary):

25. fried eggs: _____

26. fruit in sugar syrup: _____

27. lunch meat: _____

28. pie or cake: _____

29. cheese: _____

30. avocado salad: _____

31. ice cream: _____

32. lettuce: _____

Mrs. O. returns to the hospital after a few months for a cholecystectomy and an uneventful recovery.

33. The diet she was on prior to surgery will be

    a. suitable for her convalescence.
    b. changed to meet her recovery needs.
    c. permanent to maintain her weight.
    d. discontinued and TPN used.

34. While in surgery, Mrs. O. was given an injection of vitamin K. The purpose of this was to

    a. counteract bleeding tendencies present following a cholecystectomy.
    b. prevent rapid blood clotting.
    c. prevent anemia.
    d. follow routine postoperative orders.

35. A diet very low in fat may also be low in

    a. thiamin.
    b. vitamin C.
    c. vitamin A.
    d. calcium.

Diet Therapy for Renal Disorders

Multiple Choice

Circle the letter of the correct answer.

1. Antiotensin II, which is secreted by the kidneys, is a(an)

   a. proteolytic enzyme.
   b. vasoconstrictor.
   c. precursor to erythropoietin.
   d. indicator of kidney disease.

2. Lack of erythropoietin results in

   a. anemia.
   b. albuminuria.
   c. hematuria.
   d. hypertension.

3. Lack of active vitamin D hormone will

   a. result in high blood pressure.
   b. cause an imbalance of calcium and phosphorus.
   c. cause metabolic acidosis.
   d. result in oliguria.

4. Acute glomerulonephritis is the result of

   a. hereditary defects.
   b. hypertensive crisis.
   c. acute malnutrition.
   d. streptococci infection.

5. Dietary management of renal disease requires correction of imbalances in which of these?

   a. fluids and electrolytes
   b. acidosis or alkalosis
   c. blood pressure and weight
   d. all of the above

6. Blood protein loss is _____ in hemodialysis than in peritoneal dialysis.

   a. greater
   b. lesser
   c. the same
   d. not lost in either

7. A major disruption in renal functioning affects the metabolism of which of these nutrients?

   a. carbohydrates, fats, and vitamins
   b. protein, minerals, and water
   c. blood, acids, and alkalines
   d. cellulose, chlorides, and calcium

8. Hemodialysis treatments for a person in renal failure will

   a. increase the protein requirement.
   b. decrease the protein requirement.
   c. maintain the protein synthesis.
   d. not affect the protein requirement.

9. The principles of dietary treatment for urinary calculi center around which of the following?

   a. diet therapy based on stone chemistry
   b. an attempt to change urinary pH
   c. a large fluid intake
   d. all of the above

10. The most common type of kidney stone is that composed of

    a. calcium.
    b. uric acid.
    c. cystine.
    d. magnesium.

11. The type of diet recommended for a calcium stone would be

    a. alkaline ash.
    b. acid ash.
    c. protein restricted.
    d. protein increased.

12. Which of the following foods would you expect to be prohibited on an acid-ash diet?

    a. bread, macaroni, eggs, cranberries
    b. oranges, bananas, lima beans, olives
    c. meat, cheese, eggs, plums
    d. spaghetti, prunes, eggs, meat

13. Which of the following foods would you expect to find on an alkaline-ash diet?

    a. meat, cheese, eggs, corn
    b. milk, coconut, chestnuts, oranges
    c. prunes, cranberries, plums, honey
    d. peanuts, walnuts, bacon, rice

True/False

Circle T for True and F for False

14. T F Each kidney contains over a million nephrons.
15. T F Vitamin D activity is maintained by the kidneys.
16. T F Hyperphosphaturia lowers serum calcium.
17. T F Dietary management of CRF is more moderate than the diet for acute glomerulonephritis.

18. T F Deterioration of the nephrons can cause anemia.
19. T F Diet therapy for renal disease is a standard prescription of 500 mg sodium 25 gm protein.
20. T F 500 ml of water to cover insensible loss is added to the amount of urine excreted.
21. T F Medical nutrition therapy is critical to the effective treatment of patients with renal disease, and trained dietitians are best suited to provide such nutritional intervention.
22. T F Marked improvements in the administration of dialysis have been observed by the protein and calorie therapy.

Matching

Match the terms on the left with their definitions listed on the right.

_____ 23. diaphoresis
_____ 24. glomerulus
_____ 25. nephron
_____ 26. antigen
_____ 27. antibody

a. a foreign invader of the body
b. cluster of capillaries in a capsule
c. destroyer of foreign invaders
d. profuse perspiration
e. basic unit of the kidneys

Situation

Mrs. J. has a diagnosis of uremia. After an individualized assessment of her status, she is placed on a 2000-calorie, 1000-mg sodium, 2500-mg potassium, 60-g protein diet. Her fluid intake is restricted to 500 ml plus the amount excreted the prior 24 hours.

28. This diet regime will fulfill which of the following treatment objectives?

   a. correct electrolyte imbalance
   b. minimize protein catabolism
   c. avoid dehydration/overhydration
   d. all of the above

29. If Mrs. J. is still hungry after eating all of her meal, which of the following snacks would you suggest to comply with her restrictions?

   a. banana and sugar wafers
   b. arrowroot cookies with whipped topping
   c. cottage cheese and fruit cocktail
   d. puffed wheat with milk and sugar

30. Mrs. J.'s usual eating pattern includes many protein foods with low biological value, which must be avoided. Which of the following foods would you restrict?

   a. cereal grains and vegetables
   b. milk and eggs
   c. cream, honey, and most fruits
   d. meat, fish, and poultry

31. Mrs. J.'s output for the previous 24 hours is 500 ml, so she receives 1000 ml of fluids the next 24 hours. This fluid intake

   a. should come from water and be consumed all at once.
   b. should come from foods, water, and other fluids and be divided equally throughout the day.
   c. should be given by I.V. drip.
   d. should be a saline/dextrose solution.

32. Mrs. J. develops a fever and diarrhea. Her fluid intake should

   a. remain the same.
   b. be further restricted to curtail the diarrhea.
   c. be increased to compensate for the fluid loss.
   d. be administered via tube feeding.

Nutrition and Diet Therapy for Cancer Patients and Patients with HIV Infection

Multiple Choice

Circle the letter of the correct answer.

1. The most common detection and diagnostic tools for cancer are:

   a. CT (or CAT) scans, MRI
   b. ultrasonography
   c. endoscopy
   d. biopsy
   e. any combination of the above

2. Nutritional and metabolic changes characteristic of both cancer and AIDS individuals are directly related to:

   a. the body's response to the disease
   b. treatment methods
   c. surgical procedures
   d. psychological and emotional responses
   e. any combination of the above

3. Factors that influence food intake include:

   a. Income
   b. Psychosocial factors
   c. Dependency issues
   d. Psychological factors
   e. Ethnic and cultural considerations
   f. All of the above

4. Fat intake in HIV infection and AIDS should be limited to:

   a. 0%
   b. 10%
   c. 20%
   d. 30%

5. A severely malnourished patient may require a daily intake of:

   a. 1500 to 2500 kcalories
   b. 2000 to 3000 kcalories
   c. 2500 to 3500 kcalories
   d. 3000 to 4000 kcalories

Fill-in

6. Name six characteristics of cachexia:

   a. _____
   b. _____
   c. _____
   d. _____
   e. _____
   f. _____

7. Name three metabolic changes characteristic of cancer patients:

   a. _____
   b. _____
   c. _____

8. Current cancer therapy takes four major forms:

   a. _____
   b. _____
   c. _____
   d. _____

9. The most apparent side effects in chemotherapy are changes in

   a. _____
   b. _____
   c. _____

10. The basis for planning care with patients on chemotherapy includes:

    a. _____
    b. _____
    c. _____

11. Common mouth problems with patients on chemotherapy are:

    a. _____
    b. _____
    c. _____
    d. _____

12. Name four problems associated with vitamin and mineral megadoses:

a. _____

b. _____

c. _____

d. _____

True/False

13. T F Beta cells are common lymphocytes that produce immunogloblins. They originate in the bone marrow cells and involve many cells in the body in the immune response.

14. T F Cancer occurs when cells become abnormal and keep dividing without control or order.

15. T F Anorexia, the most common symptom, is related to altered metabolism, type of treatment, or emotional distress.

16. T F Head and neck surgery or resections have no major effect on intake, and thus the diet does not require any modification.

17. T F Bone marrow effects due to radiation therapy include interference with production of both white and red blood cells, producing anemia, infection, and bleeding.

18. T F Carbohydrate should supply most of the energy intake of cancer patients with fat restricted to about 20 percent of total calories.

19. T F Vitamins A and C are components of tissue structure.

20. T F Vitamin D is not related to metabolism of blood serum.

21. T F Vitamins that are popular in megavitamin and mineral therapies are A, C, B$_{12}$, and thiamin, and the minerals iron, zinc, and selenium.

22. T F Both vitamin and mineral megadoses do not hamper immune function and are safe at high levels.

23. T F Nutrition therapy in cancer patients must be proactive but not aggressive.

24. T F Providing the patients with information regarding symptoms they are experiencing usually will discourage the patient from accepting nutrition therapy.

25. T F Enteral and/or parenteral methods of feeding patients is preferred during cancer treatment.

26. T F HIV infection has a dormant phase in the body.

27. T F Food and nutrient interactions with antiretroviral medications are common, making it difficult for a patient to adhere to the medical regime. Therefore, proactive nutrition therapy is not necessary.

28. T F The stress response of the body to the immune system's efforts to protect the body is a discrete process.

29. T F At the terminal stage of HIV infection, or AIDS, the patient is marked by declining T lymphocyte production from the normal level of $\cong 1000/mm^3$.

30. T F Death in the end stages of HIV syndrome is correlated with the degree of loss of lean body mass.

31. T F Small frequent feedings of high quality protein are better tolerated than full meals.

32. T F Planning a diet for the person with HIV infection does not have to be individualized.

33. T F Excess vitamin C often causes rebound scurvy when discontinued.

34. T F Laetrile has never been proven to be beneficial in the treatment of chronic disease.

35. T F Blue-green algae improves digestion, mental functioning, and strengthens the immune system.

36. T F Nutritional needs for children infected with HIV or with AIDS have the same RDA as their age group.

37. T F Infants with HIV or AIDS should be fed with kcal-dense formulas, supplements of MCT, or glucose polymers.

38. T F Lactaid (a commercial preparation) is added to milk products to improve their digestibility and should be fed to all HIV and AIDS patients.

39. T F The impaired immune systems of HIV and AIDS patients are unable to fight food borne infections.

40. T F Patients with HIV or AIDS should be encouraged to use self-prescribed nutrition therapy as they are complementary and alternative in nature.

Diet Therapy for Burns, Immobilized Patients, Mental Patients, and Eating Disorders

Multiple Choice

Circle the letter of the correct answer.

1. Interferences to successful feeding of burn patients include all except which of these?

   a. food brought from home
   b. difficulty swallowing or chewing
   c. psychological trauma
   d. anorexia

2. Aggressive nutritional therapy aims to keep weight loss at less than _____ percent of preburn body weight.

   a. 35
   b. 25
   c. 15
   d. 10

3. Fluid and electrolyte replacement are crucial to recovery from burns. Which of these two electrolytes are most likely to be deficient?

   a. iron and zinc
   b. glucose and calcium
   c. sodium and potassium
   d. phosphorus and magnesium

4. Immediate replacement of fluid and electrolytes is necessary to prevent

   a. edema and ascites.
   b. hypovolemic shock.
   c. hyperphosphatemia.
   d. anaphylactic shock.

5. Daily caloric need for a patient with a burn injury is calculated at _____ kcal/kg of normal body weight and _____ kcal/kg percent of body surface burned.

   a. 25, 40
   b. 10, 30
   c. 40, 40
   d. 25, 50

6. Daily protein need for a patient with a burn injury is calculated at _____ g/kg normal body weight and _____ g/kg percent of body surface burned.

   a. 2, 4
   b. 1, 3
   c. 0.8, 1.2
   d. 2, 2.5

7. The amount of vitamin C given to a burn patient is usually

   a. 2–10 times RDA.
   b. 10–20 times RDA.
   c. 20–30 times RDA.
   d. 1000 mg daily.

8. A food high in zinc includes

   a. seafood.
   b. liver.
   c. eggs.
   d. all of the above.

9. The burn patient with edema and/or ascites may also be

   a. fatigued.
   b. nervous.
   c. thirsty.
   d. confused.

10. What method(s) is/are used to combat renal calculi in an immobilized patient?

    a. provide a low-calcium diet
    b. increase fluids
    c. assist early ambulation
    d. all of the above

Fill-in

11. Untreated hypercalcemia can lead to:

    a. _____

    b. _____

    c. _____

    d. _____

12. Treatment for acute hypercalcemia may include:

    a. _____

    b. _____

    c. _____

    d. _____

13. Nutritional education programs for mental patients that have been proven successful include:

    a. _____

    b. _____

    c. _____

True/False

14. T F The likelihood of mortality from second and third degree burns decreases with age.

15. T F Immobilized patients require less protein intake than normal people.

16. T F With extended immobilization, muscle loss can be reversed with high-protein diet.

17. T F During the beginning of bed-confinement, weight loss may be avoided by a high calorie intake.

18. T F Calorie intake of all immobilized patients are generally the same.

19. T F Patients with spinal cord injury have a higher risk of genitourinary tract infection.

20. T F Intake of fluid for immobilized patients should be controlled carefully relative to their urination volume.

21. T F Immobilized patients develop either diarrhea or constipation problems easily.

22. T F In general, hospitalized mental patients have a satisfactory nutritional status.

23. T F Mental patients may be confused about food and eating.

24. T F Nutritional status of mental patients can be improved by proper care.

25. T F Malfunctioning hypothalmus can reduce the desire for food.

26. T F Anorectic patients eat better when hospitalized because they don't have to make decisions.

27. T F Most anorectics wish they didn't have a starved appearance.

28. T F A liquid diet may be more acceptable to the anorectic as it appears to contain fewer calories than solid foods.

Fill-in

29. Name eight physical symptoms of bullemia nervosa:

    a. _____

    b. _____

    c. _____

    d. _____

    e. _____

    f. _____

    g. _____

    h. _____

30. Name five manifestations of the chronic dieting syndrome

    a. _____

    b. _____

    c. _____

    d. _____

    e. _____

Principles of Feeding a Sick Child

Multiple Choice

Circle the letter of the correct answer.

1. Which of these factors decrease the probability of adequately feeding a sick child?

   a. fear, anxiety, anorexia
   b. pain, fatigue, lethargy
   c. vomiting, nausea, medications
   d. all of the above

2. Which of the following is not a factor in planning nutritional care for a hospitalized child?

   a. individual likes and dislikes
   b. personal eating patterns
   c. home feeding environment
   d. type of disease

3. Which of these considerations has little influence on the dietary care of a sick child?

   a. nutritional status of the child before hospitalization
   b. the onset and duration of symptoms
   c. rehabilitation measures needed
   d. the presence of others at mealtime

4. From which of these factors are feeding problems unlikely to develop?

   a. child's past experience with food
   b. child's nutritional status when admitted
   c. child's unreasonable demands
   d. child's fear and anxiety

5. Which of these functions would not be appropriate for the pediatric nurse to perform?

   a. Suggest changes in diet orders to the physician when deemed necessary.
   b. Request supplemental fluids/foods as needed.
   c. Ask the parents to refrain from being present at feeding time and upsetting the child.
   d. Record incidences of feeding tantrums and/or manipulation.

6. If a child must have a modified diet, which of the following guidelines will be likely to increase acceptance?

   a. Start the new regime immediately in order to teach the child to comply.
   b. Move into the new diet gradually in order to give the child time to adjust.

   c. Put the new diet in writing and let the mother start the child on the diet when they get home.
   d. Use different kinds of utensils and foods to spark interest in the new diet.

7. Which of these responses would be the most appropriate for the hospitalized child who is not eating?

   a. "If you don't eat better than this, the doctor will stick a tube down your throat."
   b. "You can't have your dessert unless you clean your plate."
   c. "Would you help me select your food for the next meal?"
   d. "Do you want to upset your mother by refusing to eat?"

8. A child's food intake may be improved by using all of the following measures except

   a. allowing self-selection.
   b. serving familiar foods.
   c. providing a cheerful environment.
   d. requiring a child to "clean the plate."

9. Instructions given to children on modified diets should be

   a. given to both parent and child.
   b. given slowly, repeated, and responses noted.
   c. based on the child's readiness to learn.
   d. all of the above.

10. The hospitalized child who is allowed freedom in choosing the foods he or she eats

    a. may become malnourished.
    b. may eat more food.
    c. may get diarrhea.
    d. may become unmanageable.

11. Sick children fail to receive adequate intake for which of the following reasons?

    a. Their gastrointestinal tract malfunctions.
    b. They have high metabolic demands.
    c. They have neurological and psychological disturbances.
    d. All of the above.

12. Diarrhea in very young children

    a. is often caused by overfeeding.
    b. causes fluid and electrolyte imbalances.
    c. requires hospitalization.
    d. causes colic.

Matching

Match the assessment data listed on the left to the type of assessment it represents at the right. (Terms may be used more than once.)

_____ 13. hemoglobin/ hematocrit

_____ 14. head circumference

_____ 15. distended abdomen

_____ 16. X-rays

_____ 17. skinfold thickness

a. anthropometric
b. physical
c. laboratory

True/False

Circle T for True and F for False

18. T F The same diet principles used for feeding a well child apply to feeding a sick child.

19. T F A diet that meets the RDAs and is based on the basic food groups satisfies the needs of all growing children.

20. T F Children of different ethnic origins should be fed the same foods in order to not discriminate.

21. T F The food choices for sick children should not be limited regardless of the disease process.

22. T F Children like to eat in groups rather than alone.

23. T F Psychosocial problems may contribute to a child's failure to eat adequately.

24. T F Children like to try new and different foods.

25. T F It is not unusual for a five-year-old to want to be fed.

Situation

Johnny, age six, was hospitalized for tests, due to weight loss, irritability, diarrhea, and a low-grade fever.

26. Which of the following statements is most accurate regarding Johnny's nutritional status?

   a. He probably has pneumonia.
   b. He has extensive nutrient and fluid loss.
   c. He has lactose intolerance.
   d. His condition may be due to neglect by his mother.

27. Johnny has food and fluids withheld for tests. When he is allowed to eat again, which of these interventions is most appropriate?

   a. Make up missed meals with supplements.
   b. Provide six small meals instead of three large ones.
   c. Ask for soft solids instead of regular food.
   d. All of the above.

28. Johnny does not seem to care for hospital food. The nurse should allow

   a. food brought in from home or a fast food outlet.
   b. him to skip meals he doesn't like.
   c. only what the diet order calls for.
   d. none of the above.

Diet Therapy and Cystic Fibrosis

Multiple Choice

Circle the letter of the correct answer.

1. Cystic fibrosis is an inherited disease that primarily affects the

   a. mucous and sweat glands.
   b. lungs and liver.
   c. pancreas and mucous and sweat glands.
   d. digestive system.

2. Malnutrition in the child with cystic fibrosis is caused primarily by

   a. lack of digestive enzymes.
   b. excessive electrolytes in sweat.
   c. lung infections.
   d. vomiting and diarrhea.

3. Failure to thrive, which is a manifestation of cystic fibrosis, describes the child who

   a. is small for gestational age.
   b. shows reduced weight gain or height appropriate for age.
   c. is malnourished.
   d. dies before reaching maturity.

4. The proper diagnosis of a child with cystic fibrosis is determined from

   a. X-rays of the chest.
   b. clinical symptoms.
   c. sodium chloride in sweat.
   d. all of the above.

5. Lack of which of the following secretions creates the malabsorption syndrome in cystic fibrosis children?

   a. lipase, trypsin, amylase
   b. sodium, potassium, iron
   c. antibodies
   d. fat-soluble vitamins

6. Early diagnosis and treatment of cystic fibrosis

   a. can restore normal body size and appearance.
   b. cannot prevent mental retardation.
   c. prevents delayed sexual development.
   d. all of the above.

7. The goals of diet therapy for cystic fibrosis include which of the following?

   a. increase body weight
   b. control or prevent rectum prolapse
   c. control or improve emotional problems associated with the disease
   d. all of the above

8. Which of these statements is correct regarding the use of pancreatic enzymes?

   a. Infants and small children are given injections of enzymes.
   b. Enzymes are given at least one hour before mealtimes.
   c. Prolonged use of enzymes can cause psychological problems.
   d. Enzymes may cause ulceration.

9. Which of the following statements is true regarding use of medium chain triglycerides?

   a. They increase energy intake.
   b. They promote fat absorption.
   c. They reduce malabsorption.
   d. All of the above.

10. Nutrient dense supplements useful in diet therapy for cystic fibrosis include all except which of these products?

    a. protein hydrolysate solutions
    b. beef serum, commercial supplements
    c. medium-chain triglycerides and glucose solutions
    d. fat polymers

Matching

Match the principles of dietary management listed on the left with the rationale listed on the right.

_____ 11. high-calorie diet	a. to compensate for pancreatic deficiency
_____ 12. high-protein diet	
_____ 13. low- to moderate-fat diet	b. to compensate for fecal losses
_____ 14. generous salt in diet	c. to meet high energy demands
_____ 15. vitamin supplements	d. to limit steatorrhea
_____ 16. pancreatic	e. to replace electrolyte losses
	f. to meet need for three times the RDA enzymes

True/False

Circle T for True and F for False.

17. T F Children with cystic fibrosis produce heavy viscid mucus.

18. T F Children with cystic fibrosis digest very little of their protein.

19. T F Up to 12 percent of cystic fibrosis patients are diagnosed at birth because of a bowel obstruction.

20. T F The child with cystic fibrosis usually is anorexic.

21. T F General feeding techniques used for all children cannot be applied to cystic fibrosis children.

22. T F Use of pancreatic enzymes definitely improves the nutritional status of the child with cystic fibrosis.

23. T F A child with cystic fibrosis may have deficient linoleic acid.

24. T F The caloric need for children with cystic fibrosis may be 80%–110% above normal requirements.

25. T F Lactose deficiency is sometimes a complication in cystic fibrosis.

26. T F When CFTR is abnormal, it blocks the movement of chloride ions and water in the lungs, pancreas, colon, and genitourinary tract with secretion of abnormal mucus.

27. T F The abnormal CFTR protein is also called deltaF508 CFTR, and accounts for all CF cases.

Situation

José is a fourteen-year-old male with cystic fibrosis admitted to the hospital with pneumonia. He is short of breath, is coughing, and has a temperature of 102°. His appetite is poor and he is approximately 20 lb underweight for his age and height. The orders are for a 3500 calorie high-protein, low-fat, soft diet. He also is prescribed pancreatic enzymes, water-miscible fat-soluble vitamin supplements, medium-chain triglyceride supplements, and extra fluid.

28. In order to increase calories, he receives a chocolate milk shake between meals, which he likes. The most probable outcome of this kind of supplement is that

    a. he will regain some lost weight.
    b. he will get diarrhea.
    c. he will receive excessive amounts of cholesterol.
    d. he will get acne.

29. Briefly explain the reason for each of the following diet orders:

    a. fat-soluble, water-miscible vitamin supplements

    _____

    _____

    b. pancreatic enzymes

    _____

    _____

    c. medium-chain triglyceride supplements

    _____

    _____

    d. extra fluids

    _____

    _____

30. List four important instructions to be given to José and his family regarding his diet when he returns home.

    a. _____

    b. _____

    c. _____

    d. _____

31. List the four major nursing implications required to adequately implement nutrition principles for a cystic fibrosis patient.

    a. _____

    b. _____

    c. _____

    d. _____

Diet Therapy and Celiac Disease

Multiple Choice

Circle the letter of the correct answer.

1. The protein to which patients are intolerant when they have celiac disease is

   a. phenylalanine.
   b. casein.
   c. gluten.
   d. glycogen.

2. Celiac patients have mucosal atrophy of the small intestine. This means that

   a. villi are lacking.
   b. the villi are flat instead of round.
   c. only small amounts of digestive enzymes are secreted.
   d. all of the above.

3. Which of the following are presenting symptoms of celiac disease?

   a. diarrhea, steatorrhea, irritability
   b. irregular heartbeat, fever, lethargy
   c. anorexia, eczema, dehydration
   d. hyperactivity, infections, weight loss

4. Which of these symptoms indicate malnutrition in the celiac patient?

   a. cheilosis, glossitis, anemia, tetany
   b. hyperosmolarity, arrhythmias, acidosis
   c. hypoglycemia, flatulence, cramps
   d. all of the above

5. The basic principle of diet therapy for celiac disease is to

   a. exclude all sources of glycogen.
   b. exclude all sources of gluten.
   c. exclude all sources of lactose.
   d. exclude all sources of casein.

6. Celiac disease in children can be cured in which of the following time frames?

   a. 1–2 weeks
   b. 1–5 years
   c. time varies with each child
   d. celiac disease is never cured

7. Which of the following foods must be excluded from the diet of the person with celiac disease?

   a. rye, wheat, barley, and oats
   b. potatoes, corn, rice, and malt
   c. arrowroot, soybean, and tapioca
   d. all of the above

8. Which of the following foods would be suitable for a celiac patient?

   a. chicken fried steak, breaded veal cutlet, fish sticks
   b. roast beef, baked chicken, broiled salmon
   c. fried chicken, meat loaf, lobster thermidor
   d. marinated herring, chili con carne, lamb chops

9. Which of the following statements is appropriate when teaching a celiac patient regarding his diet therapy?

   a. "You must read all labels carefully."
   b. "Let's talk about ways to prevent infections."
   c. "These substitutes are needed to help you balance your diet."
   d. a, b, and c are all appropriate

10. When the offending foods have been removed from the diet of the celiac patient, which of these nutrients are most likely to be deficient?

    a. vitamins A, D, E, and K
    b. thiamin, niacin, and iron
    c. sodium, protein, and carbohydrates
    d. all of the above

Matching

Match the food in the left column to its appropriate use in the right column.

_____ 11. crisped rice cereal   a. permitted
_____ 12. ice cream cone   b. prohibited
_____ 13. pancakes   c. limited
_____ 14. fruit
_____ 15. potatoes
_____ 16. chocolate candy
_____ 17. peanut butter
_____ 18. malted milk shake
_____ 19. cornbread and butter
_____ 20. catsup

True/False

Circle T for True and F for False.

21. T F Children are the major population group to have celiac disease.
22. T F A lowered prothrombin time indicates that the blood clots too quickly.
23. T F Adult patients seem to recover from celiac disease better than children.
24. T F Celiac diet therapy usually requires vitamin supplements.
25. T F The symptoms of celiac disease and cystic fibrosis are very similar.
26. T F Celiac disease is the most common genetic disease among Europeans and their descendants, about 1 in 150–200 people may have it.
27. T F Treatment is important because people with celiac disease could develop complications like cancer, osteoporosis, anemia, miscarriage, congenital malformation of the baby, short stature, convulsions, and seizures.
28. T F A person with celiac disease will show symptoms.
29. T F Diagnosis involves blood tests such as antibody tests against gluten and biopsy.

Situation

Bonnie is an 18-month-old infant brought to the clinic after her mother called the nurse there to ask what she might do to alleviate the problem of 3 or 4 foul smelling, foamy stools per day. The mother had been offering Bonnie lots of fluids but she refused them. A diagnosis of celiac disease was made.

30. What additional information would you need in order to plan diet therapy? _____

_____

_____

31. Loss of which of the following nutrients would be of greatest concern for Bonnie?

   a. water, sodium, potassium
   b. fat-soluble and water-soluble vitamins
   c. fats, calcium, carbohydrates
   d. all of the above

32. Plan a one-day menu pattern that could be used as a teaching tool for Bonnie's mother.

_____

_____

_____

33. List three commercial products useful in supplementing the diet of the child with celiac disease.

   a. _____

   b. _____

   c. _____

34. Bonnie's mother asks how long she will have to be on this diet. Your most appropriate answer would be

   a. to recommend the diet be continued indefinitely.
   b. three to six months.
   c. until she is at least six years old.
   d. until she is a teenager.

Diet Therapy and Congenital Heart Disease

Multiple Choice

Circle the letter of the correct answer.

1. Which of the following manifestations, in a child with congenital heart disease, affects nutritional status?

   a. malabsorption of nutrients
   b. elevated body temperature
   c. excessive urinary output
   d. all of the above

2. Caloric need is higher for children with congenital heart disease than for healthy children because

   a. the metabolic rate is higher.
   b. the antibody production is low.
   c. the kidneys are malfunctioning.
   d. all of the above.

3. Which of these nutrients are primarily responsible for renal overload?

   a. water, oxygen
   b. sodium, potassium
   c. calcium, iron
   d. phosphates, chlorides

4. Which of these foods are not tolerated well by children with congenital heart disease?

   a. fats and sugar in quantity
   b. proteins
   c. fluids in quantity
   d. vitamin supplements

5. Which of these factors result in vitamin/mineral deficiencies in children with congenital heart disease?

   a. amount of food consumed is too small to be adequate
   b. allergy to foods containing vitamins
   c. nonprescription vitamins do not contain all the child needs
   d. a and c

6. The introduction of solid foods to a child with congenital heart disease is delayed in order to

   a. keep the sodium content in the diet low.
   b. avoid the problem of diarrhea.
   c. reduce the workload on the heart.
   d. prevent dehydration.

7. Caretakers of children with congenital heart disease should be taught

   a. to omit sodium from the diet.
   b. principles of a balanced diet.
   c. to read labels.
   d. all of the above.

8. Which of these discharge procedures should the nurse follow when a child with congenital heart disease is going home?

   a. Provide teaching and referrals for follow up.
   b. Provide psychiatric counseling.
   c. Provide special products.
   d. All of the above.

9. Which of these guidelines provides appropriate distribution of nutrients for the child with congenital heart disease?

   a. 40% carbohydrates, 20% proteins, 30% fat
   b. 35%–65% carbohydrates, 10% proteins, 30%–50% fat
   c. 30% carbohydrates, 30% protein, 40% fat
   d. none of the above

10. Which of the following statements best describes a milliequivalent?

   a. a metric unit of volume
   b. amount of solute dissolved in a milliliter of solution
   c. concentration of an ion in solution
   d. amount of solution in a metric unit

Matching

Match the dietary alteration at the left to the correct rationale at right.

_____ 11. MCT oil	a. prevent dehydration
_____ 12. folic acid	b. prevent renal overload
_____ 13. extra juices, water	
_____ 14. extra energy supplements	c. prevent vitamin deficiency
_____ 15. limited sodium, potassium	d. provide adequate fat absorption
	e. increase caloric intake

True/False

Circle T for True and F for False.

16. T F A child with congenital heart disease may voluntarily reduce food intake.
17. T F The only cure for congenital heart disease is successful surgery.
18. T F The child should weigh at least 30 pounds before surgery is performed.
19. T F Regular foods are not used at all for children with congenital heart disease.
20. T F A congenital disease means that it is inherited.
21. T F Heart disease in children is readily identified at birth.
22. T F The cause of congenital heart disease is unknown.
23. T F The mortality rate for children with congenital heart disease is not as high for small children as for larger ones.
24. T F Children with congenital heart disease tend to be overdependent.
25. T F Children with congenital heart disease and parents may need counseling for psychological problems as well as dietary ones.

Situation

Teresa is eight months old and has a ventricular septal defect (V.S.D., a common congenital heart defect). She needs to gain a minimum of 10 pounds before she can have surgery to close the hole in the septum.

26. The major nutritional management for this child is to

   a. provide essential nutrients that are easily digested.
   b. provide high calorie food and fluids without overloading the kidneys.
   c. provide small, frequent feedings rather than three large meals.
   d. all of the above.

27. List three suitable energy supplements for Teresa that should assist in weight gain.

   a. _____

   b. _____

   c. _____

28. Provide a one-day menu pattern that Teresa's mother may use to plan her food intake.

   _____

   _____

   _____

29. Describe four feeding problems Teresa's mother may encounter and solutions to each.

   a. _____

   b. _____

   c. _____

   d. _____

30. List four important dietary principles Teresa's mother should learn.

   a. _____

   b. _____

   c. _____

   d. _____

Diet Therapy and Food Allergy

Multiple Choice

Circle the letter of the correct answer.

1. Maldigestion or malabsorption of food may be termed

   a. a food allergy.
   b. malnutrition.
   c. a food intolerance.
   d. an immunological reaction.

2. Substances that trigger allergic reactions are

   a. allergens.
   b. enzymes.
   c. antigens.
   d. a or c.

3. Less than _____ of all people in the United States have some form of food allergy.

   a. 8%
   b. 25%
   c. 50%
   d. 1%

4. Allergens are usually

   a. food additives.
   b. proteins.
   c. sugars.
   d. food preservatives.

5. Food allergies are more prevalent in

   a. adolescence.
   b. childhood.
   c. adulthood.
   d. b and c.

6. The most common food allergy in children is an allergy to

   a. nuts.
   b. wheat.
   c. soy.
   d. cow's milk.

7. The milk of choice for an infant from a family prone to allergies is

   a. cow's milk.
   b. soy formula.
   c. breast milk.
   d. evaporated milk.

Matching

Match the potential offender on the right with the food source on the left. Answers may be listed more than once.

_____ 8. mayonnaise   a. legumes
_____ 9. tartrazine   b. corn
_____ 10. chocolate   c. milk
_____ 11. tangerine   d. eggs
_____ 12. pumpkin pie   e. kola nuts
_____ 13. custard   f. citrus fruits
_____ 14. licorice   g. spices
_____ 15. corn syrup   h. artificial food colors

True/False

Circle T for True and F for False.

16. T F Most people exhibit symptoms of a food allergy, but are unaware that these symptoms are the result of a food allergy.

17. T F Skin testing is an accurate method of detecting food allergies.

18. T F An infant with a risk for developing allergies should receive solid foods as early as possible.

19. T F Depending on the number of foods eliminated, an antiallergic diet may be nutritionally inadequate.

20. T F Food allergies are relatively easy to diagnose and confirm.

21. T F Once the offending food has been determined, it should never be reintroduced into the patient's diet.

22. T F Raw foods are more likely to be allergens than the cooked form.

23. T F Occurrence of undeclared allergens usually arises from cross-contamination of allergens in ingredients or equipment used in the production of products.

24. T F Current regulations require that all added ingredients be declared on the label including allergens.

Fill-in

25. To protect the consumers, both adults and children, each FDA food inspector is asked to pay special attention to the following when inspecting an establishment that manufactures processed food products:

a. _____

b. _____

c. _____

d. _____

Situation

Bobby is exhibiting the following symptoms: skin rash, diarrhea, and nasal congestion. His mother is concerned that he may be allergic to something he is eating.

26. What would be your first course of action in determining whether a food allergy is actually the cause of the symptoms?

_____

_____

_____

_____

27. You notice that Bobby is routinely eating some of the foods listed among the top ten offenders for children. These are cow's milk, wheat, eggs, and corn. What would you suggest to Bobby's mother at this point?

_____

_____

_____

28. From close monitoring of Bobby's diet, it has been determined that Bobby is allergic to cow's milk and wheat. Besides fluid milk, name five sources of cow's milk that Bobby may also be allergic to.

a. _____

b. _____

c. _____

d. _____

e. _____

Name five sources of wheat Bobby may need to avoid.

f. _____

g. _____

h. _____

i. _____

j. _____

29. As Bobby grows older, should he try to reintroduce milk or wheat products back into his diet? Why or why not?

_____

_____

Diet Therapy and Phenylketonuria

Multiple Choice

Circle the letter of the correct answer.

1. Which of the following statements most accurately describes the etiology of PKU (phenylketonuria)?

   a. There is an inability to convert phenylalanine into tyrosine.
   b. There is a lack of synthesis of phenylalanine.
   c. There is a lack of the essential amino acids.
   d. There is a lack of leucine conversion to lysine.

2. The most serious effect of untreated PKU is

   a. behavior disturbances.
   b. convulsive seizures.
   c. mental retardation.
   d. reticulosarcoma.

3. Children with PKU usually have lighter complexions, hair, and eyes than normal children because of

   a. their genetic makeup.
   b. lack of tyrosine.
   c. failure to thrive.
   d. lack of amino acid metabolism.

4. Which of the following statements expresses the dietary management of PKU children?

   a. Rigidly restrict phenylalanine intake.
   b. Make the diet very low in tyrosine.
   c. Make the diet very low in galactose.
   d. Omit phenylalanine and tyrosine entirely.

5. If treatment is started after retardation has occurred, which of the following outcomes may be expected?

   a. Normal ability will return completely.
   b. Retardation will continue, as the process is irreversible.
   c. Growth and development will slow or stop.
   d. Normal ability will not return but the retardation will not proceed any further.

6. An infant should be provided with enough phenylalanine to maintain a serum level of

   a. 3–10 mg per 100 ml.
   b. 10–29 mg per 100 ml.
   c. 20–25 mg per 100 ml.
   d. PKU infants should not have a serum phenylalanine.

7. After the clinical condition of a one-year-old child with PKU stabilizes, what information concerning blood tests is most appropriate?

   a. The blood should be tested twice weekly.
   b. The blood should be tested daily.
   c. The blood should be tested weekly.
   d. The blood should be tested monthly.

8. The diet for PKU children must meet which of these criteria?

   a. Provide for normal growth and development.
   b. Maintain phenylalanine within safe limits.
   c. Permit liberalization to conform to culture.
   d. a and b

9. The steps necessary for planning the diet for a PKU child include which of these?

   a. Determine age, weight, and activity level.
   b. Determine daily phenylalanine required and amount of protein to be given.
   c. Determine calories received from formula, milk, and food.
   d. All of these steps are necessary.

10. Which of these techniques would promote dietary compliance in a PKU child?

    a. Remove all desserts until the child eats other food.
    b. Vary taste, texture, and variety within limits of diet.
    c. Increase the amount of milk in the diet.
    d. Omit all snacks.

Matching

Match the foods at the left with their use in the PKU diet at right.

_____ 11. meats   a. permitted
_____ 12. Lofenalac   b. prohibited
_____ 13. fruits   c. limited
_____ 14. vegetables
_____ 15. cheese

True/False

Circle T for True and F for False.

16. T F The only treatment for PKU is diet therapy.
17. T F Babies born with PKU can now be diagnosed early enough to prevent serious side effects.
18. T F Once PKU has been diagnosed, all offending substances must be omitted entirely from the diet.
19. T F Emotional support for the family is an important part of the management of PKU children.
20. T F The symptoms of PKU and cystic fibrosis are very similar.
21. T F A baby with PKU can be successfully breast-fed if the mother is willing to try.
22. T F PKU is self-limiting; the child will outgrow it.
23. T F Insufficient phenylalanine will result in mental retardation.
24. T F Excessive phenylalanine will result in mental retardation.
25. T F It is recommended that the special diet be discontinued by age four.

Situation

Terry is a three-year-old male who is seen in the pediatrician's office for a routine checkup. He has PKU but no other problems. He is 40 inches tall and weighs 36 pounds. His mother asks for a consultation with a dietitian because she believes it is time to liberalize Terry's diet. He still drinks Lofenalac and his mother monitors all the food he eats, but lately he has been crying for the hamburgers and hot dogs his father and older brothers eat. He will also start nursery school soon. His phenylalanine level is 9mg/100 ml of blood.

Circle the correct response.

26. a. Is the phenylalanine level acceptable? Yes No

    b. Is Terry's weight and height in normal range? Yes No

27. What response would be appropriate regarding liberalizing Terry's diet?

    a. "Yes, I agree it's time he got other foods."
    b. "You may ask for a second opinion, but specialists agree that three years is too early."
    c. "Why don't you stop feeding the others what Terry can't eat?"
    d. "Do you think this is just a phase he's going through?"

28. Plan a one-day menu suitable for Terry.

    _____

    _____

    _____

    _____

    _____

29. What substances must be calculated in this diet to make sure it is adequate and safe?

    a. carbohydrate, protein, fat
    b. phenylalanine, protein, calories
    c. calcium, magnesium, iron
    d. phenylalanine, vitamins, calories

Diet Therapy for Constipation, Diarrhea, and High-Risk Infants

Multiple Choice

Circle the letter of the correct answer.

1. Safe food(s) that may be used to combat constipation in infants include

   a. prune juice.
   b. 1 tsp sugar/4 oz formula.
   c. strained apricots.
   d. all of the above.

2. Recommended treatment for dry, hard stools in an infant is to

   a. increase formula feedings.
   b. increase fluids.
   c. increase laxative intake.
   d. increase activity level.

3. Two types of constipation common in children under five years old are

   a. physiological and psychological.
   b. anatomical and environmental.
   c. psychological and anatomical.
   d. environmental and physiological.

4. Parents may initiate a regular pattern of elimination by which of these methods?

   a. Put the child on a regular schedule.
   b. Increase foods with fluids and fiber.
   c. Decrease formula to 80 percent of normal.
   d. all of the above

5. If a child has diarrhea for several weeks, but continues to grow at a normal rate, the problem is classified as

   a. celiac disease.
   b. chronic diarrhea.
   c. acute diarrhea.
   d. allergy diarrhea.

6. Which of these beverages contain high amounts of both sodium and potassium?

   a. orange juice
   b. Pepsi Cola
   c. skim milk
   d. grape juice

7. The dietary management of diarrhea in children includes all except which of these steps?

   a. Restore fluid and electrolyte balance.
   b. Use an elimination diet.
   c. Restore adequate nutrition.
   d. Increase the kcal content of the diet.

8. Added foods that will increase a one year old's kcal content when the child is recovering from diarrhea include

   a. eggnog.
   b. milkshakes.
   c. strained cereal.
   d. all of the above.

9. Caloric needs of the high-risk infant are

   a. twice those of a normal infant.
   b. three to four times those of a normal infant.
   c. approximately six times those of a normal infant.
   d. the same as those of a normal infant; they have little movement.

10. High-risk infants need large amounts of fluid for all except which of these reasons?

    a. They require extra essential amino acids.
    b. They have a larger body water content than normal infants.
    c. Their kidneys can't concentrate urine.
    d. They have increased water evaporation.

11. First feedings for high-risk infants include

    a. TPN.
    b. fluid with extra calories.
    c. 10 percent glucose IVs.
    d. no feeding until stabilized.

12. A mother can breast feed her premature infant when

    a. the baby weighs more than 4 pounds.
    b. the baby has sucking reflexes.
    c. the baby gets additional supplements.
    d. all of the above.

True/False

Circle T for True and F for False.

13. T F Diarrhea is an infrequent occurrence among infants and young children.
14. T F Infants and young children with diarrhea can be managed at home unless dehydration occurs.
15. T F Milk is high in sodium.
16. T F A hypotonic solution contains excess electrolytes and glucose.
17. T F Low-residue diets are used after diarrhea has subsided.
18. T F Tyrosine and cystine are essential amino acids.
19. T F Lytren is an essential amino acid especially for children.
20. T F High-risk infants may be able to breast feed.

Matching

Match the term on the left to the definition that best defines it.

_____ 21. Meconium
_____ 22. Mucilage
_____ 23. Benign
_____ 24. Electrolyte
_____ 25. Prematurity

a. substance that dissolves in water into ions
b. interrupted before maturity
c. not recurrent
d. dark green substance in fetal intestine
e. aqueous gummy substance

Match the characteristics of normal fecal material on the right to the most likely type of feeding.

_____ 26. Commercial formula
_____ 27. Breast milk, 3 months
_____ 28. Regular foods, 10 months
_____ 29. Whole milk, 10 months
_____ 30. Mixed diet (liquid, solid), 1 year

a. similar to adult
b. intense yellow, firm
c. highly variable
d. golden, creamy texture
e. compressed, pale yellow

Answers to Posttests

Chapter 1

Multiple Choice

1. b
2. d
3. d
4. b
5. c
6. b
7. a
8. e
9. b

Matching

10. c
11. a
12. b
13. a
14. c
15. a. AI: adequate intake
    b. EAR: estimated average requirement
    c. IOM: Institute of Medicine
    d. USHHS: U.S. Department of Health and Human Services
    e. %DV: % Daily Values
    f. Discretionary Calorie Allowance: The remaining amount of calories in a food intake pattern after accounting for the calories needed for all food groups using forms of foods that are fat-free or low-fat and with no added sugars
    g. Functional foods: "legal" conventional foods (natural or manufactured) that contain bioactive ingredients
    h. Nutraceuticals: Adding a bioactive ingredient, especially one with nutritional value to a dietary or an OCT drug
16. j

17. c
18. f
19. j
20. e

21. Her lunch fits MyPyramid's recommendation.

22. a. bread
    b. fruits
    c. vegetables
    d. meat
    e. milk

23. a. ATP 1 outlined a major strategy for primary prevention of coronary heart disease (CHD) in persons with high levels of low-density lipoprotein (LDL) (>160 mg/dl) or borderline LDL of 130–159 mg/dl.
    b. ATP 2 affirmed this approach and added a new feature: the intensive management of LDL cholesterol in persons with CHD. It set a new goal of < 100 mg/dl of LDL.
    c. ATP 3 maintains the core of ATP 1 and 2, but its major new feature is a focus on primary prevention in persons with multiple risk factors. It calls for more intensive LDL lowering therapy in certain groups of people and recommends support for implementation. This approach includes a complete lipoprotein profile, high-density lipoprotein (HDL) cholesterol and triglycerides, as the preferred initial test. It encourages the use of plants containing soluble fiber as a therapeutic dietary option to enhance lowering LDL cholesterol and presents strategies for promoting adherence. It recommends treatment beyond LDL lowering in people with high triglycerides.

Chapter 2

1. c	9. b	17. F	25. T
2. d	10. a	18. T	26. T
3. a	11. c	19. T	27. T
4. b	12. c	20. T	28. b
5. b	13. b	21. F	29. b
6. d	14. a	22. F	30. b
7. a	15. c	23. F	
8. c	16. b	24. T	

Chapter 3

1. a	8. b	15. b	22. F
2. d	9. b	16. a	23. T
3. b	10. b	17. b	24. T
4. c	11. d	18. T	25. F
5. c	12. a	19. T	26. d
6. b	13. b	20. F	27. a
7. c	14. a	21. T	

28. The missing nutrients in Lisa's diet are all of those listed in question #26. Therefore, any and all of these foods need to be added to her diet:

Soy milk fortified with calcium and vitamin D, rice and bean combinations, legumes, nuts, seeds (i.e., date-nut breads), peanut butter sandwiches and peanut butter cookies, corn and beans, meat analogs, combined cereals and legumes, dark green leafy vegetables such as kale, turnip greens, mustard greens, oranges and orange juice.

Suggest: Vitamin B_{12} supplements, perhaps iron and use of iodized salt. As fiber content is high, small frequent meals may be indicated.

Chapter 4

1. a	8. a	15. d	22. T
2. d	9. d	16. b	23. T
3. a	10. a	17. a	24. T
4. d	11. d	18. c	25. b
5. c	12. c	19. F	26. c
6. c	13. d	20. T	27. c
7. d	14. e	21. F	

28. Any of these:
   1. Use the recommended distribution of nutrients.
      a. 50%–60% of total calories from carbohydrates—mainly from grains, fruits, and vegetables.
      b. Protein for a teenage athlete at 1–1.5 g/kg of body weight.
      c. Remainder of total calories from fat.

2. No reduced caloric intake at all unless percent of body fat exceeded normal range.
3. No vitamin/mineral supplements, no electrolyte solutions, no bee pollen.
4. No carbohydrate loading for a teenager.
5. High-fluid intake, especially water, at all times before, during, and after a match. If sweet drinks are used, they should be diluted.

Chapter 5

1. a	8. b	15. d	22. F
2. c	9. a	16. b	23. F
3. c	10. d	17. c	24. F
4. b	11. b	18. a	25. F
5. d	12. a	19. T	26. T
6. a	13. d	20. T	27. T
7. d	14. c	21. T	28. T

29. Storing uncovered and 24-hour advance salad preparation accelerates vitamin loss due to oxidation. Dicing potatoes and cooking ahead destroys vitamins. The smaller the cut, the greater the loss. Cooking foods in large amounts of water over long periods of time increases vitamin loss by leaching and oxidation.

30. The water-soluble vitamins, especially vitamin C which is the least stable of the vitamins, were lost.

31. Ways to conserve nutrients include:
   a. cook vegetables whole and unpared.
   b. use cooking methods that shorten cooking time.
   c. use the smallest amount of water.
   d. cook covered to use shortest cooking time possible.
   e. slice or cut fruits and vegetables just before use to prevent oxidation.

Chapter 6

1. c	8. b	15. c	22. F
2. c	9. d	16. F	23. F
3. d	10. d	17. F	24. T
4. a	11. b	18. T	25. T
5. d	12. d	19. F	26. T
6. c	13. e	20. T	27. T
7. d	14. a	21. T	28. b

29. calcium   800 mg—See calcium table for food sources.

iron   18 mg—See iron table for food sources.

30. a

Chapter 7

1. d	8. d	15. a	22. F
2. b	9. d	16. b	23. F
3. d	10. b	17. T	24. T
4. b	11. d	18. T	25. T
5. d	12. c	19. T	26. F
6. d	13. d	20. T	27. T
7. a	14. c	21. T	28. a

29. 2750 = present consumption. Using the mid-range of 2000 calories, Mary's intake is 750 kcal per day in excess of output. 750 kcal × 7 days per week = 5250 extra kcal per week. This is roughly $1\frac{1}{2}$ lb per week weight gain. Estimate 6–7 lb per month × 6 months. Mary will gain 36 to 42 lb by the end of school.

30. c

31. While there are 22 items listed under responsibilities of health personnel, 5 that are especially important in Mary's case are:
    a. Do not use any fad diets: a low-calorie diet that contains essential nutrients is to be used. (#18)
    b. Become familiar with behavior modification techniques and use them to gain control of eating patterns. (#22)
    c. Adopt a more healthful diet instead of giving up certain foods. (#20)
    d. Use a balanced diet, proper food preparation, portion control, sound food guides. (#9)
    e. Encourage regular exercise (daily), at the same time as reducing quantity of food. (#15)
    Note: #16, 19, and 21 are also important, so if you listed any of those you may count them.

Chapter 8

1. d	8. b	15. a	22. F
2. d	9. c	16. T	23. T
3. b	10. b	17. T	24. T
4. b	11. b	18. T	25. T
5. b	12. c	19. F	
6. b	13. b	20. F	
7. a	14. b	21. F	

Chapter 9

1. d	8. d	15. a	22. T
2. c	9. a	16. a	23. F
3. c	10. d	17. b	24. T
4. d	11. b	18. b	25. T
5. b	12. c	19. b	26. T
6. a	13. a	20. F	
7. d	14. d	21. T	

27. Lisa is striving for autonomy and it is reflected in the eating behavior. As she struggles for control she wants to do everything her way. It is a phase that will pass.

28. a. What and how much food does the child eat per day?
    b. Is her weight normal for her height/age?
    c. Is she gaining at a regular, slow, steady rate?
    d. Do other physical characteristics appear normal (hair, eyes, teeth, etc.)?
    e. Does she appear to be a happy child?

29. The growth rate has slowed since last year and her appetite has diminished. Accordingly, she does not need as much food as during her first year of life.

30. a. "Food jags" are common at this age. As long as the food is nutritious, the grandmother should not be concerned.
    b. Children are no longer forced to "finish everything" because obesity is a problem to be avoided at any age, but especially early childhood. After a reasonable time, remove the food from the table without comment.

Chapter 10

1. d	8. a	15. b	22. F
2. e	9. d	16. c	23. T
3. e	10. e	17. F	24. T
4. a	11. c	18. F	25. F
5. c	12. d	19. F	26. F
6. a	13. d	20. F	
7. d	14. c	21. F	

27. Anorexia, increase or decrease intestinal motility, change absorption and metabolism of nutrients, nausea, vomiting, damage intestinal walls.

28. Antidepressants, antihistamines, oral contraceptives and alcohol (small amounts only)

29. Amphetamines, Cholinergic agents, some expectorants and narcotic analgesics (Elderly: tranquilizers)

30. Penacillamine, streptomycin, KCL, vitamin B complex in liquid form and some chemotherapies

31. Cough syrup, expectorants, elixirs

32. Antibiotics and parenteral drug solutions

Chapter 11

1. e   2. i   3. a

4. a. Define dietary supplements and dietary ingredients.
   b. Establish a new framework for assuring safety.
   c. Outline guidelines for literature displayed where supplements are sold.
   d. Provide for use of claims and nutritional support statements.
   e. Require ingredient and nutrition labeling.
   f. Grant the FDA the authority to establish good manufacturing practice (GMP) regulations.
   g. Require the formation of an executive level Commission on Dietary Supplement Labels.
   h. Establish an Office of Dietary Supplements within the National Institutes of Health.

5. a. Detect fraudulent products and deceptive advertising.
   b. Purchase quality products if they intend to use supplements.
   c. Read product labels.
   d. File a report if side effects are experenced.
   e. Recognize that dietary supplements can cause harm and the reasons they can be harmful.
   f. The types of reactions that may occur.
   g. Reduce the chances of suffering adverse effects from supplement use.

6. a. Raw impurities
   b. Excess levels of ingredients used
   c. Allergic reactions to some ingredients
   d. Systemic poisoning
   e. Overdosing oneself
   f. Negative reactions in some individuals because of a specific sensitivity
   g. Safety of the product has not been carefully evaluated

7. a. A product (other than tobacco) that is intended to supplement the diet that bears or contains one or more of the following dietary ingredients: a vitamin, a mineral, an herb or other botanical, an amino acid, a dietary substance for use by humans to supplement the diet by increasing the total daily intake, or a concentrate, metabolite, constituent, extract, or combinations of these ingredients.
   b. A product intended for ingestion in pill, capsule, tablet, or liquid form.
   c. The supplement is not represented for use as a conventional food or as the sole item of a meal or diet.
   d. It is labeled as a "dietary supplement."

   e. It includes products such as an approved new drug, certified antibiotic or licensed biologic that was marketed as a dietary supplement or food before approval, certification, or license (unless specifically waived).

8. a. Net quantity of contents (e.g., "60 capsules").
   b. Structure-function claim and the statement "This statement has not been evaluated by the Food and Drug Administration."
   c. "This product is not intended to diagnose, treat, cure, or prevent any disease."
   d. Directions for use (e.g., "Take one capsule daily.").
   e. Supplement Facts panel (lists serving size, amount, and active ingredient).
   f. Other ingredients in descending order of predominance and by common name or proprietary blend.
   g. Name and place of business of manufacturer, packer, or distributor (address to write for more product information).

9. a. A review of the scientific evidence.
   b. An authoritative statement from certain scientific bodies, such as the National Academy of Sciences.

10. a. Dietary ingredients in "significant amount."
    b. Nutritional ingredients with % RDI.
    c. Nonnutritional ingredients without % RDI.
    d. Quantity per serving for each dietary ingredient (or proprietary blend).
    e. Source of dietary ingredients as appropriate.

11. a. In what form the product should be taken: orally, or is it digested to inert forms?
    b. How much of the substance is in the product and does it contain the active ingredient?

12. a. mild gastrointestinal complaints
    b. headaches
    c. dizziness
    d. palpitations
    e. allergic skin reactions

13. T	23. T	33. T
14. F	24. T	34. T
15. F	25. T	35. T
16. T	26. F	36. F
17. T	27. T	37. T
18. T	28. T	38. T
19. T	29. F	39. F
20. T	30. T	40. T
21. T	31. T	41. F
22. F	32. T	42. T

Chapter 12

1. a. alone
   b. in combination with other alternative therapies
   c. in addition to conventional therapies

2. a. alternate medicine systems
   b. mind-body interventions
   c. biologically based treatments
   d. manipulative and body-based methods
   e. energy therapy

3. Any five of the following: ongoing sad mood; loss of interest or pleasure in activities that the person once enjoyed; significant change in appetite or weight; oversleeping or difficulty sleeping; agitation or unusual slowness; loss of energy; feelings of worthlessness or guilt; difficulty "thinking," such as concentrating or making decisions; or recurrent thoughts of death or suicide.

4. a. What benefits can be expected from this therapy?
   b. What are the risks associated with this therapy?
   c. Do the known benefits outweigh the risks?
   d. What side effects can be expected?
   e. Will the therapy interfere with conventional treatment?
   f. Is this therapy part of a clinical trial, if so, who is sponsoring the trial?
   g. Will the therapy be covered by health insurance?

5. Body, mind, spirit, and strives to restore the innate harmony of the individual.

6. In large doses produces the symptoms of an illness, in very minute doses cures it.

7. a. herbal therapies
   b. orthomolecular therapies
   c. biological therapies

8. F	20. T	32. T
9. T	21. T	33. T
10. T	22. T	34. F
11. T	23. T	35. F
12. T	24. T	36. T
13. T	25. T	37. T
14. T	26. T	38. T
15. T	27. T	39. T
16. T	28. T	40. T
17. T	29. T	41. T
18. T	30. T	
19. T	31. T	

Chapter 13

1. a	9. b	17. F	25. F
2. a	10. c	18. T	26. b
3. d	11. b	19. T	27. c
4. d	12. a	20. F	28. b
5. d	13. b	21. T	29. b
6. b	14. a	22. T	30. a
7. a	15. a	23. F	
8. a	16. F	24. T	

Chapter 14

1. b	8. b	15. a	22. F
2. c	9. d	16. b	23. T
3. b	10. c	17. d	24. a
4. d	11. d	18. e	25. d
5. c	12. a	19. F	26. d
6. d	13. b	20. T	27. a
7. d	14. c	21. F	

28. The most common diet modifications are alterations in basic nutrients, energy value, texture, and seasonings. James needs an alteration in basic nutrients and energy value. Unless further assessment reveals a need for additional adjustments, the diet prescription should be a high carbohydrate, high protein, high vitamin, moderate fat, regular diet containing approximately 3500 calories.

29. Rationale: to restore and maintain nutritional status: James is underweight, apparently malnourished, and injured.

30. c

Chapter 15

1. a	8. c	15. T	22. T
2. c	9. d	16. F	23. T
3. a	10. d	17. F	24. T
4. d	11. b	18. T	25. F
5. a	12. c	19. F	
6. d	13. d	20. F	
7. b	14. a	21. F	

26. Because of extensive injuries and surgery, this patient is in a hypermetabolic state. She needs to be maintained at the high rate of TPN.

27. No. Patients are never placed on reduction diets until after healing has taken place. Other measures to relieve breathing must be considered.

28. *See* Table 13-1.

29. *See* Nursing Implications, Chapter 13.

Chapter 16

1. d	9. b	17. F	25. F
2. a	10. c	18. T	26. b
3. d	11. b	19. F	27. c
4. d	12. d	20. T	28. a
5. c	13. c	21. F	29. d
6. d	14. e	22. F	30. b
7. d	15. a	23. F	
8. d	16. T	24. T	

Chapter 17

1. b	5. a	9. c	13. b
2. a	6. d	10. b	
3. d	7. a	11. b	
4. c	8. a	12. b	

14. A high-fiber diet promotes better and faster elimination, decreasing pressure on the intestines and helping to prevent future inflammation.

15. High-fiber diets rapidly eliminate residue from the intestine, so that it is subjected to less bacterial action and harmful by-products remaining against the mucosal lining.

16. a. diabetes
    b. sleep apnea
    c. obesity-related heart problems

17. a. long-term healthy eating behaviors
    b. regular physical exercise

18. a. Vomiting occurs because the small stomach is overly stretched by food particles that have not been chewed well.
    b. Bypass surgeries cause the stomach contents to move too rapidly through the small intestines.

19. The procedure causes food to bypass the duodenum and jejunum.

20. Calcium, iron and fat-soluble vitamins (A, D, E, K). In some patients, B_{12} is also added.

21. T	25. F	29. b
22. T	26. T	30. d
23. F	27. F	31. d
24. T	28. T	

32. Any three of these: restore nutritional deficits, prevent further losses, promote healing, repair and maintain body tissue, improve chances for recovery.

33. a. fluid intake and output
    b. nutrient intake (amount of protein especially important, and vitamins)
    c. caloric intake and weight changes

Chapter 18

1. d*	8. c	15. g	22. T	29. c
2. c	9. d	16. f	23. T	
3. a	10. a	17. a	24. T	
4. d	11. e	18. F	25. b**	
5. d	12. c	19. T	26. b	
6. b	13. d	20. F	27. b	
7. a	14. b	21. F	28. d	

*$(250 \times 4) + (100 \times 4) + (70 \times 9) = 2030$
**70 lb $\div$ 2.2 = 32 kg (rounded)
  80 g protein $\div$ 32 kg = 2.5 g/kg body weight
  $(150 \times 4) + (80 \times 4) + (50 \times 9) = 1370$ calories

Chapter 19: Part I

1. a	9. d	17. d	25. T
2. a	10. b	18. e	26. c
3. d	11. d	19. a	27. d
4. d	12. c	20. T	28. d
5. d	13. e	21. F	29. b
6. a	14. a	22. T	30. c
7. a	15. b	23. F	
8. c	16. c	24. T	

Chapter 19: Part II

1. b	7. a	13. T	19. T
2. c	8. b	14. T	20. T
3. b	9. c	15. T	21. T
4. c	10. d	16. F	
5. c	11. a	17. F	
6. a	12. F	18. T	

22. boiled or poached, three times a week

23. fruit, fresh or in natural juice

24. omit, substitute chicken or tuna

25. omit, substitute fruit

26. use low-fat cottage cheese only

27. omit, use a fresh spinach or other dark green salad

28. substitute sherbet within the caloric allowance

29. no alteration necessary

30. b

31. a

32. c

Chapter 20

1. b	9. d	17. F	25. e
2. b	10. a	18. T	26. a
3. b	11. b	19. F	27. c
4. d	12. b	20. T	28. d
5. d	13. b	21. T	29. b
6. b	14. T	22. F	30. a
7. b	15. T	23. d	31. b
8. a	16. T	24. b	32. c

Chapter 21

1. e	2. e	3. f	4. c	5. d

6. Any 10 of the following: anorexia, weakness, early satiety, nonintentional weight loss, loss of muscle and fat stores, decreased mobility and physical activity, nausea, vomiting, dehydration, edema, chronic diarrhea or constipation, pain, fever, night sweats, dysphagia, candidiasis, malabsorption, or dementia.

7. Three of the following: fatigue, anemia, cachexia, hypogeusia, dysgeuisa, xerostomia, dysphagia, stomatitis, fever, altered metabolic rate, infection, nausea, vomiting, or anorexia.

8. a. surgery
   b. radiation
   c. chemotherapy
   d. combination of any of the above

9. a. bone marrow
   b. hair follicles
   c. GI tract

10. a. thorough personal nutrition assessment
    b. vigorous nutrition therapy to maintain good nutritional status and support
    c. revision of care plan as individual status changes

11. Sore mouth, dysgeusia, hypogeusia, low salivary production, candidiasis

12. Any four of the following: Toxic at high levels, increasing problems with skin, bone, central nervous system, nausea, hair loss, and depleted immune function

13. T	20. F	27. F	34. T
14. T	21. T	28. F	35. F
15. T	22. F	29. F	36. F
16. F	23. T	30. T	37. T
17. T	24. F	31. T	38. F
18. F	25. F	32. F	39. T
19. T	26. F	33. T	40. F

Chapter 22

1. a	5. a	9. c
2. d	6. b	10. d
3. c	7. a	
4. b	8. d	

11. Untreated hypercalcemia can lead to:
    a. kidney failure
    b. high blood pressure
    c. seizures
    d. hearing loss

12. Treatment for acute hypercalcemia may include:
    a. intravenous fluid therapy with saline
    b. intravenous diuretic medications and repalcement of all loss of sodium, magnesium, and postassium
    c. replacement of any excessive urine loss by fluid (intravenous saline)
    d. implement of a low-calcium diet.

13. Nutritional education programs for mental patients that have been proven successful include:
    a. teaching some basic facts and skills about food budgeting, purchasing, and preparation
    b. teaching principles of nutritional needs
    c. teaching known effects of drugs on nutritional status.

14. F	19. T	24. T
15. F	20. T	25. T
16. T	21. T	26. T
17. T	22. F	27. F
18. F	23. T	28. T

29. Any 8 of these: blood shot eyes, broken blood vessels on face, decayed teeth, bruises on hand, sore throat, swollen salivary glands, intestinal problems, fatigue, cessation of menses (women), esophageal tears, rupture of gastric mucosa

30. Any 5 of these: compulsive overeating, anxiety, emotional problems, weight cycling, loss of lean body mass, lowered BMR, altered body composition

Chapter 23

1. d	8. d	15. b	22. T
2. c	9. d	16. c	23. T
3. d	10. b	17. a	24. F
4. c	11. d	18. T	25. T
5. c	12. b	19. F	26. b
6. b	13. c	20. F	27. d
7. c	14. a	21. F	28. a

Chapter 24

1. c	8. c	15. f	22. T
2. a	9. d	16. a	23. T
3. b	10. d	17. T	24. T
4. d	11. c	18. F	25. T
5. a	12. b	19. T	26. T
6. a	13. d	20. F	27. F
7. d	14. e	21. F	28. b

29. a. He cannot absorb the fat-soluble vitamins until they are made water-miscible.
 b. These are effective in assisting the patient to utilize more of his ingested food.
 c. Medium-chain triglyceride supplements are better tolerated than regular fats and therefore increase caloric intake.
 d. He has a fever; also extra fluids help dissolve the mucus collection. Note: Extra salt may also be needed.

30. a. The essentials of the daily food guide.
 b. How to make appropriate substitutions for high-fat and poorly tolerated foods.
 c. How to keep an accurate food record for assessment and follow up care.
 d. The essentials of low-fat cookery and cooking with medium-chain triglycerides.

31. a. Maintain adequate nutrition (see Nursing Implications #1, a–e).
 b. Promote growth and development through adequate nutrition.
 c. Provide support to the family.
 d. Educate the child and its family (see Nursing Implications, #4, a–e).

Chapter 25

1. c	8. b	15. a	22. F	29. T
2. d	9. d	16. b	23. F	
3. a	10. b	17. a	24. T	
4. a	11. a	18. b	25. T	
5. b	12. b	19. a	26. F	
6. c	13. b	20. a	27. T	
7. a	14. a	21. T	28. F	

30. Weight at present. Signs of dehydration, social behavior at present. Deviations (loss) of weight. Eating behaviors (anorexia, hunger, etc.). Any physical signs of malnutrition.

31. d

32. Daily meal pattern (amounts and textures appropriate for 18-month-old child): Meat, fish, poultry or meat substitute; potato, rice, grits, sweet potatoes, vegetables (any appropriate for age); fruit (any appropriate for age); special low gluten bread or cornbread, margarine; milk.

   Between-meal snacks: Chocolate, Kool-Aid, cornstarch, rice or tapioca pudding; fruits or juices, sherbet, gelatin, cheese (no cheese foods); cookies/cakes from low gluten, rice or arrowroot flour.

33. a. low protein (gluten) flour, cookies, pastas
 b. MCT
 c. water-miscible vitamins

34. a

Chapter 26

1. d	8. a	15. b	22. T
2. a	9. b	16. T	23. T
3. b	10. b	17. T	24. T
4. a	11. d	18. T	25. T
5. d	12. c	19. F	26. d
6. c	13. a	20. F	
7. d	14. e	21. F	

27. a. Extra carbohydrate: karo syrup or polycose
 b. Extra fats: MCT and corn oil
 c. Extra low protein, low electrolyte formula in addition to solids

28. Breakfast: 3 oz juice; 2 tbsp salt-free cereal; 1 slice toast

   Lunch and dinner: 2 tbsp mashed or junior vegetables; 1 oz chopped or ground meat; 2–3 tbsp soft mashed or pureed fruit; 1 tbsp mashed potato

   Snacks: Any high calorie, low protein, low sodium beverages or formulas, such as SMA.

29. Problems: Crying; refusing to eat; using food to get their way; becoming too tired to eat; turning blue. Coping: Stay calm; avoid overconcern; do not "invalidize"; be consistent; don't feed when the child is tired; divide food into small feedings; foster independence as soon as possible.

30. All nursing implications should be reinforced for the mother to assist her in competently caring for Teresa at home. *See also* Nursing Implications, Chapter 24.

Chapter 27

1. c	7. c	13. c, d	19. T
2. d	8. b*	14. a	20. F
3. a	9. h	15. b	21. F
4. b	10. e	16. F	22. T
5. b	11. f	17. F	23. T
6. d	12. c, d, g	18. F	24. F

*(if made from corn oil, d)

25. To protect the consumers, both adults and children, each FDA food inspector is asked to pay special attention to the following when inspecting an establishment that manufactures processed food products.
    a. product development
    b. receiving
    c. equipment
    d. processing

26. Have Bobby's mother keep a detailed food record of everything Bobby eats for a certain time period.

27. Although diagnosing food allergies is difficult, the elimination diet is probably the most successful. Bobby's mother should try eliminating the four foods one at a time. When symptoms disappear, try reintroducing one food at a time until symptoms reappear, the food causing the reappearance of symptoms may be the offender. Make sure Bobby receives substitutes for the foods removed from his diet, i.e., soy milk for cow's milk, rice products for wheat products, to avoid nutritional inadequacies.

28. a. ice cream
    b. cheese
    c. custard
    d. cream and cream foods
    e. yogurt
    f–j. any of the following: most baked goods, cream sauce, macaroni, noodles, pie crust, cereals, chili, breaded foods

29. Bobby should try to reintroduce these foods into his diet occasionally because allergies may fade over time.

Chapter 28

1. a	8. d	15. b	22. F
2. c	9. d	16. T	23. T
3. b	10. b	17. T	24. T
4. a	11. b	18. F	25. F
5. d	12. a	19. T	
6. a	13. a	20. F	
7. c	14. c	21. F	

26. a. Yes   b. Yes

27. b

28. Your choice; however, the menu pattern will follow these guidelines.

    Breakfast: fruit, 1 serving; allowed cereal, ½ c; Lofenalac, 8 oz.

    Lunch: fruit, 1 serving; green vegetable, 1 serving; starchy vegetable, 1 serving; crackers (4); butter or margarine; 2 tbsp allowed dessert; Lofenalac, 4 oz.

    Snacks at 10, 2, and bedtime: fruit; arrowroot cookies (5); Lofenalac, 4 oz.

    Dinner: green vegetable, 1 serving; vegetable soup, ¼ c; potato, ½ c; butter or margarine; 2 tbsp allowed dessert; Lofenalac, 8 oz.

29. b

Chapter 29

1. d	9. b	17. T	25. b
2. b	10. a	18. T	26. e
3. c	11. c	19. F	27. d
4. d	12. d	20. T	28. a
5. b	13. F	21. d	29. b
6. c	14. T	22. e	30. c
7. b	15. T	23. c	
8. c	16. F	24. a	

Index

Photo Credits

Chapter 1
© Photodisc

Chapter 2
© Photodisc

Chapter 3
© Photodisc

Chapter 4
© Ingrid E. Stamatson/ShutterStock, Inc.

Chapter 5
© Lauren Rinder/ShutterStock, Inc.

Chapter 6
© LiquidLibrary

Chapter 7
© SW Productions/Photodisc/Getty

Chapter 8
© Losevsky Pavel/ShutterStock, Inc.

Chapter 9
© Beth Van Trees/ShutterStock, Inc.

Chapter 11
© Photodisc

Chapter 12
© Stuart Pearce/Pixtal/age footstock

Chapter 13
© Clayton Thacker/ShutterStock, Inc.

Chapter 14
© Artemis Gordon/ShutterStock, Inc.

Chapter 15
© Photos.com

Chapter 16
© Ryan Kelm/ShutterStock, Inc.

Chapter 17
© Udo Kröner/ShutterStock, Inc.

Chapter 18
Courtesy of MIEMSS

Chapter 19
© Sebastian Kaulitzki/ShutterStock, Inc.

Chapter 20
© Samual Acosta/ShutterStock, Inc.

Chapter 21
© Milan Radulovic/ShutterStock, Inc.

Chapter 22
Courtesy of Bill Branson/National Cancer Institute

Chapter 23
© Photodisc

Chapter 24
© Photodisc

Chapter 25
© Zsolt Nyulaszi/ShutterStock, Inc.

Chapter 26
© Photodisc

Chapter 27
Courtesy of James L. Horwitz, MD/Rainbow Pediatrics

Chapter 28
© LiquidLibrary

Chapter 29
© Francois Etienne du Plessis/ShutterStock, Inc.